DATE DUE

Exercise and the Heart

Exercise and the Heart

THIRD EDITION

Victor F. Froelicher, M.D.
Professor of Medicine
Director, ECG and Exercise Laboratory and
  Cardiac Rehabilitation
Division of Cardiovascular Medicine
Stanford University School of Medicine
Palo Alto Veterans Affairs Medical Center
Palo Alto, California

Jonathan Myers, Ph.D.
Assistant Clinical Professor of Medicine
Department of Cardiology
Stanford University
Palo Alto Veterans Affairs Medical Center
Palo Alto, California

William P. Follansbee, M.D.
Director, University of Pittsburgh Heart Institute
  Cardiovascular Services
Director, Nuclear Cardiology
Department of Nuclear Cardiology
University of Pittsburgh
Pittsburgh, Pennsylvania

Arthur J. Labovitz, M.D., F.A.C.C.
Professor of Medicine
Director
Echocardiography Laboratory and
  Noninvasive Hemodynamics
Department of Internal Medicine
Division of Cardiology
Saint Louis University Medical Center
St. Louis, Missouri

with 110 *illustrations*

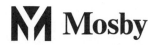 **Mosby**

St. Louis Baltimore Boston Chicago London Philadelphia Sydney Toronto

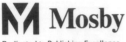

Editor: Stephanie Manning
Editorial assistant: Colleen Boyd
Project manager: Mark Spann
Production editor: Carl Masthay
Book designer: Jeanne Wolfgeher
Cover Photo: © Tony Stone Worldwide/Dennis O'Clair

THIRD EDITION

Printed in the United States of America.

Mosby–Year Book, Inc.
11830 Westline Industrial Drive
St. Louis, Missouri 63146

Library of Congress Cataloging-in-Publication Data

Froelicher, Victor F.
    Exercise and the heart / Victor F. Froelicher, coauthors,
Jonathan Myers, William P. Follansbee, Arthur J. Labovitz. —
Ed. 3.
        p.   cm.
    Includes bibliographical references and index.
    ISBN 0-8016-6819-0
    1. Exercise tests.   2. Heart function tests.   3.
Heart—Diseases—Diagnosis.   4. Radioisotope scanning.   I.
Myers, Jonathan, 1957-   .   II. Follansbee, William P.   III.
Labovitz, Arthur J.   IV. Title.
        [DNLM: 1. Exercise Test—methods.   2. Exercise
Therapy—methods.   3. Exertion.   4. Heart Diseases—
rehabilitation.   WG 141.5.F9 F926e 1993]
    RC683.5.E94F76   1993
    616.1'20754—dc20
    DNLM/DLC
    for Library of Congress   92-48415
                                                        CIP

93 94 95 96 97 CL/MY 9 8 7 6 5 4 3 2 1

Preface

Well, here's a third edition. What's new, and what's the same? New are three coauthors for this edition: Jonathan Myers, William Follansbee, and Arthur Labovitz. Jon has been with me for a decade and for about that long has been telling me that my chapter on gas analysis was just "all right." Having just finished his Ph.D. at the University of Southern California, Jon has written this section and the chapter on exercise physiology as well as improved the entire book by his careful review. Since I stopped doing nuclear cardiology after leaving the University of California, San Diego, and Professor Ashburn, it was necessary to get outside help for this area. Since we use only exercise echocardiography for physiological studies, help was needed in that area also. Bill Follansbee and Art Labovitz are excellent teachers whom I asked to join us after seeing them perform at the annual "Bernie (Chaitman) and Vic" show at the American College of Cardiology Heart House.

What else is new? Actually, I try to use current material in each edition. Thus, to have a complete picture you really have to have all three editions. Obviously the first two are out of print and therefore are now "classics" found on the shelves of scholars and libraries. Some things are repeated, but in general I've tried to present newer material. This new material is attributable to numerous people who have worked with me, and they deserve some mention. Bob Detrano seized the idea of metanalysis of diagnostic tests and took off with it (I just beat him with the first publication in 1987 in the *American Journal of Medicine*!). Previous metanalyses dealt with randomized treatment trials. His series of metanalyses summarizes the years of work in exercise testing with objectivity. Cres Miranda took my Toshiba 3300 laptop loaded with R-Base, Statgraphics, True Epistat, and the Long Beach data bases and proceeded to perform and write up one study after another. Cres helped relieve me of all the guilt that comes from not analyzing data. Charlie Morris (the poet-athlete-physician) came along the year after Cres to bring some verve to my writing and maybe even some grammar. Charlie led a team of visiting cardiologists and students to complete some studies of such basic clinical importance that they have yet to be published. Bill Herbert and Paul Ribisl are physiology professors at Virginia Polytechnic Institute and Wake Forest University, respectively, who have contributed greatly. Bill and Paul are two Southern gentlemen, best friends, who came on sabbatical at separate times. They too were excellent for transferring the guilt of unanalyzed data. I treated them like graduate students even though they are both a bit older than I, and their work is featured on these pages.

We've had some excellent visiting cardiologists who have spent time with us getting their BTA ("been-to-America") degree. From Japan came Takeo Kawaguchi, Kenji Ueshima, and Masayoshi Shimizu. Takeo worked on the influence of the right coronary artery in prognosis and hemodynamic responses to exercise testing. Kenji worked on the exercise responses of patients with atrial fibrillation. Masayoshi worked on the reproducibility of the ventilatory threshold. The Swiss connection, Paul Dubach, continues to coauthor papers wtih us, as well as perform rehabilitation studies in Chur, Switzerland.

Our students have been an exceptional group as well. Doug Walsh helped Jon with much of the gas-analysis research and wrote some lovely basic language computer programs for ramping and plotting lactate responses. Doug is currently in medical school in Irvine, California. Alisa Hideg joined us to perform the prognostic studies. Alisa is largely responsible for helping me do the follow-up study using the DHCP (decentralized computer hospital program) on our patients who underwent exercise testing. When Alisa came, my problems with hiring nearly evaporated. As her first year in medical school at Loma Linda University approached, I asked, "What are we going to do without you?" Alisa promptly found Eileen Johnson and trained her. Eileen then continued the prognostic work and worked on our Veterans Affairs cooperative trial, and when we decided to move, she trained Tiana Umann, who came with us. Kiernan Morrow became one of our group on a college elective and is our typical choice for a co-worker. He's a 30-minute 10 K runner and an excellent computer person. Kiernan helped me with the R-Base programs that we use to handle our data and also helped me use Egret for the survival analysis studies.

Jeff Froning has collaborated with me for the past 10 years. Jeff is a skilled programmer who has been responsible for our ECG analysis. Jeff keeps us current by participating in computer symposiums and cardiology conferences. Together, we continue to challenge the "silly millimeter" criteria and improve the diagnostic performance of the exercise test. Jeff shares his knowledge with much of the industry, and his influence is seen in many of the commercially available exercise systems.

Another story must be told here, since it will probably never be told anywhere else: how follow-up studies were performed at the Long Beach Veterans Affairs Medical Center. Let me give some of my background: I had considerable computer experience while at the United States Air Force School of Aerospace Medicine. Later, as part of the National Institutes of Health–sponsored specialized center of organized research (SCOR) in atherosclerosis at UCSD, I also performed data base research using minicomputers. Dr. John Ross had developed a data base for patients after myocardial infarction. When I left UCSD to go to the Long Beach VAMC, it became apparent that minicomputer support would no longer be available, and so I decided to switch to personal computers. After a little halting step with the decision that DEC Rainbows were going to be the system of the future, I narrowed down to IBM-clone personal computers. For data-base software, on the advice of friends from UCLA, I chose R-Base for data entry. We went through a series of optical scanners, supported by Bill Pewen. As a parallel effort, our computer friends at the Veterans Affairs wrote programs to follow patients. This was possible because the VA instituted a decentralized computer hospital program (DHCP) where several VA centers developed specialized programs, and then they were exchanged. This created a very large data base of patients, which is extremely valuable, since patients can be followed by their clinic visits and prescriptions. If a patient is getting prescriptions or being seen in clinic, you can assume he or she is alive. Also, death certificates are very frequently signed by VA physicians even when patients die outside the VA. Hooking a personal computer up over modem to the VA mainframes made it possible to transfer data and perform the many follow-up

studies that we have reported. These studies have led the way to the outcomes research that should be a priority. Follow-up studies have included non–Q wave myocardial infarction patients, patients with ventricular tachycardia during exercise testing, and patients after bypass surgery and have permitted development of a prognostic score similar to the Duke score. DHCP is an incredible national resource for performing outcomes research, but few researchers have taken advantage of it.

Thanks must be given to my friends in industry who generously support our work with research grants and equipment. Being a frustrated engineer and benign hacker, I have great fun working with prototypes and giving advice to the dedicated professionals making the wonderful ECG devices available to us. As in the past, though, there is one outstanding person who continues to drive the whole industry with innovation. Dave Mortara, Ph.D., made the data logger that enabled us to capture a digital data base of exercise tests and has enabled all the major manufacturers to improve their analysis software.

Jon and I moved from the Long Beach VAMC to the Palo Alto VAMC in January 1992. We are now on the faculty at Stanford University and join Eddie Atwood at our third institution together. The move marked my twentieth year practicing socialized medicine in government service. Let me add that I've never seen anything quite like that portrayed in "Article 99" during this experience. Our current major research project is Quexta, a multicenter study of quantitative exercise testing and angiography. This is a VA cooperative study program in health service research. Kenneth Lehmann and I are the principal investigators of this study. Ken is now at the Seattle VA and continues to be an outstanding collaborator. This project will fulfill my second major lifetime scientific goal. The first was to design and accomplish a randomized trial of the effects of exercise—that was PERFEXT (for perfusion, performance, and exercise trial, which was funded by the NIH at UCSD). The second goal was to design and direct a multicenter study. Completion of Quexta will leave me with little else to do but teach and see patients for the rest of my career and perhaps relieve the literature from the burden of my compulsion to write.

With Quexta needing standards for the performance of exercise testing at multiple sites, some of my ideas have coalesced on how to perform exercise testing. I believe much of the disappointment with this procedure today is attributable to the sloppiness that has crept into its performance. I hope that the rigor necessary for multicenter studies will spread into practice and we'll see a renewal of this important procedure. Exercise testing is widely available and still serves as the gatekeeper for more expensive procedures; most guidelines require it as part of the work-up for coronary artery disease. Any improvement in its use will greatly influence patient care. It is being performed more by internists and practitioners now than by cardiologists, and it is often used by them to decide who needs to see the cardiologist.

The following statement, from the guidelines Ken and I wrote for Quexta, highlights the importance of the exercise test:

The role of the exercise test as "gatekeeper" to more costly or invasive procedures places it at a critical juncture in the clinical decision-making process, with the distribution of limited health care resources often hinging on its outcome.

Frankly, I'm pleased to see exercise testing moving into the area of general medicine, but for this transfer to go well, the real challenge will be to see that the new people will be doing the test properly. The American Heart Association exercise standards published in the December 1990 issues of *Circulation* and *Journal of the American College of Cardiology* makes the best in methodology available in print inexpensively to all.

Let me outline some of my precepts regarding methodology at the outset, sort of a preview of the rest of the book: (1) hyperventilation should not be done before testing; (2) blood pressure measurements should be measured manually and not with the automated systems; (3) exercise ca-pacity should be reported in METs (metabolic equivalents) not minutes; (4) computerized ECG measurements or averages should not be relied on but used only with the raw data; (5) heart-rate targets are very misleading; (6) use the Borg scale; (7) at the end of exercise stop the treadmill abruptly and have the patient lie down; (8) follow the ECG at least 6 minutes into recovery (the recovery findings often are the most important); (9) do not be overly concerned with premature ventricular contractions, but be mindful of the "company they keep"; (10) measure the ST segment at ST0 or the J-junction, and look for horizontal or downsloping segments rather than making a measurement at ST60 or ST80; and (11) adjust the protocol to the patient utilizing ramping or versions of the Balke-Ware protocol.

Our thanks go to those who have purchased previous editions, causing the publisher to make me do this again. It is very gratifying to see students and colleagues using the book. I hope we are making a fun and interesting field more understandable. Finally, I hope no one is offended by our points of view or failure to cite his or her work. Myrv Ellestad is a good friend who is held in the highest regard and could be cited on every page, but he has his chance in the "other" book. One thing that continues to impress me is the incredible goodwill each in the "exercise group" exhibits to each other; the exercise must mellow us out.

Victor F. Froelicher, M.D.

Contents

Exercise and the Heart

1 Basic Exercise Physiology

EXERCISE PHYSIOLOGY

Exercise physiology is the study of the physiological responses and adaptations that occur as a result of acute or chronic exercise. Exercise is the body's most common physiological stress, and it places major demands on the cardiopulmonary system. For this reason, exercise can be considered the most practical test of cardiac perfusion and function. Exercise testing is a noninvasive tool to evaluate the cardiovascular system's response to exercise under carefully controlled conditions. The adaptations that occur during an exercise test allow the body to increase its resting metabolic rate up to 20 times, during which cardiac output may increase as much as six times. The magnitude of these adjustments is dependent on age, sex, size, type of exercise, fitness, and the presence or absence of heart disease. Although major adaptations are also required of the endocrine, neuromotor, and thermoregulatory systems, the major focus of this chapter is on the cardiovascular response and adaptations of the heart to acute exercise. Cardiovascular adaptations to chronic training in humans and animals are reviewed in Chapter 15.

Two basic principles of exercise physiology are important to understand in regard to exercise testing. The first is a physiological principle: total body oxygen uptake and myocardial oxygen uptake are distinct in their determinants and in the way they are measured or estimated (Table 1-1). Total body or ventilatory oxygen uptake (VO_2) is the amount of oxygen that is extracted from inspired air as the body performs work. Myocardial oxygen uptake is the amount of oxygen consumed by the heart muscle. Accurate measurement of myocardial oxygen consumption requires the placement of catheters in a coronary artery and the coronary venous sinus to measure oxygen

content. Its determinants include intramyocardial wall tension (left ventricular pressure times end-diastolic volume), contractility, and heart rate. It has been shown that myocardial oxygen uptake is best estimated by the product of heart rate and systolic blood pressure (double product). This is valuable clinically because stable exercise-induced angina often occurs at the same myocardial oxygen demand (double product) and thus is one physiological variable useful when therapy is being evaluated. When this is not the case, the influence of other factors, such as a recent meal, abnormal ambient temperature, or coronary artery spasm, should be suspected.

The second principle is one of pathophysiology: considerable interaction takes place between the exercise test manifestations of abnormalities in myocardial perfusion and function. The ECG response and angina are closely related to myocardial ischemia (coronary artery disease), whereas exercise capacity, systolic blood pressure, and heart rate responses to exercise can be determined by myocardial ischemia, by myocardial dysfunction, or by responses in the periphery. Exercise-induced ischemia can cause cardiac dysfunction, which results in exercise impairment and an abnormal systolic blood pressure response. Often it is difficult to separate the effect of ischemia from the effect of left ventricular dysfunction on exercise responses. This results in an interaction that complicates the interpretation of the exercise test findings. The variables affected by both (exercise capacity, maximal heart rate, and systolic blood pressure) have the greatest prognostic value.

The severity of ischemia or the amount of myocardium in jeopardy is known clinically to be inversely related to the heart rate, blood pressure, and exercise level achieved. However, neither resting or exercise ejection fraction, or its change

Table 1-1 Two basic principles of exercise physiology

Myocardial oxygen consumption	$\cong$ Heart rate $\times$ Systolic blood pressure (determinants include wall tension $\cong$ left ventricular pressure $\times$ volume; contractility; and heart rate)
Ventilatory oxygen consumption (VO_2)	$\cong$ External work performed, or cardiac output $\times$ a-vO_2 difference*

The arteriovenous O_2 difference is approximately 15 to 17 vol% at maximal exercise; therefore, VO_2 max is a noninvasive method for estimating cardiac output.

during exercise, correlate well with measured or estimated maximal oxygen uptake even in patients without signs or symptoms of ischemia.[1,2] Moreover, exercise-induced markers of ischemia do not correlate well with one another. Silent ischemia (that is, markers of ischemia presenting without angina) does not appear to affect exercise capacity in patients with coronary heart disease. Although not conclusive, recent radionuclide studies support this position.[3] Although maximal cardiac output is generally considered the most important determinant of exercise capacity, these studies indicate that in some patients with heart disease, the periphery may play an important role in limiting exercise capacity.

Energy and muscular contraction

Muscular contraction is a complex mechanism involving the interaction of the contractile proteins actin and myocin in the presence of calcium. The British scientist A.F. Huxley proposed that the myocin and actin filaments in the muscle slide past each another as the muscle fibers shorten during contraction. Huxley won the Nobel prize for this theory, which is still considered generally correct today. The source of energy for this contraction is supplied by adenosine triphosphate (ATP), which is produced in the mitochondria. ATP is stored as two products, adenosine diphosphate (ADP) and inorganic phosphate (P_i) at specific binding sites on the myocin heads.

The sequence of events that occurs when a muscle contracts has three other major players: calcium and two inhibitory proteins, troponin and tropomyosin. Voluntary muscle contraction begins with the arrival of electrical impulses at the myoneural junction, initiating the release of calcium ions. Calcium is released into the sarcoplasmic reticulum (which surrounds the muscle filaments) and binds to a special protein, troponin-C, which is attached to tropomyosin (another protein that inhibits the binding of actin and myocin), and actin. When calcium binds to troponin-C, the tropomyosin molecule is removed from its blocking position between actin and myocin, the myocin head attaches to actin, and muscular contraction occurs.

The main source of energy for muscular contraction, ATP, is produced by oxidative phosphorylation. The major fuels for this process are carbohydrates (glycogen and glucose), and free fatty acids. At rest, equal amounts of energy are derived from carbohydrates and fats. Free fatty acids contribute greatly during low levels of exercise, but greater amounts of energy are derived from carbohydrates as exercise progresses. Maximal work relies virtually entirely on carbohydrates. Because endurance performance is directly related to the rate at which carbohydrate stores are depleted, a major advantage exists for (1) having greater glycogen stores in the muscle and (2) deriving a relatively greater proportion of energy from fat during prolonged exercise. Both of these factors are conferred with training.

Oxidative phosphorylation initially involves a series of events that take place in the cytoplasm. Glycogen and glucose are metabolized to pyruvate through glycolysis. If oxygen is available, pyruvate enters the mitochondria from the sarcoplasm, is oxidized to a compound known as acetylcoenzyme A (acetyl CoA), which then enters a cyclical series of reactions known as the Krebs cycle, whose by-products are CO_2 and hydrogen. Electrons from hydrogen enter the electron transport chain, yielding energy for the binding of phosphate (phosphorylation) from ADP to ATP. This process, oxidative phosphorylation, is the greatest source of ATP for muscle contraction. A total of 36 ATP molecules per molecule of glucose are formed in the mitochondria during this process.

The mitochondria can produce ATP for muscle contraction only if oxygen is present. At higher levels of exercise, however, total body oxygen demand may exceed the capacity of the cardiovascular system to deliver oxygen. Historically, "anaerobic" (without oxygen) glycolysis has been the term used to describe the synthesis of ATP from glucose under these circumstances. However, several authors have recently superseded this term with the more functional description "oxygen-independent" glycolysis since "anaerobic" incorrectly implies glycolysis occurs only when there is an inadequate oxygen supply. Under such conditions, glycolysis progress in the cytoplasm much the same way as aerobic metabolism until pyruvate is formed. However, electrons released during glycolysis are taken up by pyruvate to form lactic acid. Rapid diffusion of lactate from the cell inhibits any further steps in glycolysis. Thus oxygen-independent glycolysis is quite inefficient; two ATP molecules per molecule of glucose is the total yield from this process. Although lactate can contribute to fatigue by increasing ventilation and inhibiting other enzymes of glycolysis, it can also serve as an important energy source in muscles other than those in which it was formed, and it serves as an important precursor for liver glycogen during exercise.[4,5]

Muscle fiber types

The body's muscle fiber types have been classified on the basis of the speed with which they contract, their color, and their mitochondrial content. Type I, or slow twitch fibers, are red in color and contain high concentrations of mitochondria. Type II, or fast twitch fibers, are white in color and have low concentrations of mitochondria. Fiber color is related to the degree of myoglobin, which is a protein that both stores oxygen in the muscle and carries oxygen in the blood to the mitochondria. Not surprisingly, slow-twitch fibers with their high myoglobin content are more resistant to fatigue; thus a muscle with a high percentage of slow-twitch fibers is well suited for endurance exercise. However, slow-twitch fibers tend to be smaller and produce less overall force than fast-twitch fibers. On the other hand, fast-twitch fibers are generally larger and tend to produce more force but fatigue more easily. Research indicates that the speed of contraction for each fiber type may be based largely on the activity of the enzyme myocin ATPase, which sits in the myocin head and to which ATP combines.

It is important to understand that although the two fiber types can be separated by distinct characteristics both fibers function effectively for virtually all physical activities. Recent evidence also indicates that slow-twitch and fast-twitch fibers are not as dichotomous as previously believed. Myocin ATPase activity and speed of contraction of some slow-twitch fibers approximates that of fast-twitch fibers. Moreover, type II (fast-twitch) fibers have been further divided into three subcategories: type IIA, IIB, and IIC. The type IIA fiber mimics the type I fiber in that it has a high capacity for oxidative metabolism. It has been suggested that the type IIA fiber is a type II fiber that has been adapted for endurance exercise, and endurance athletes are known to have a relatively large number of these fibers.[6] The type IIB fiber is a "true" type II fiber in that they contain few mitochondria and are better adapted for short bursts of activity. The type IIC fiber is poorly understood but may represent an "uncommitted" fiber, capable of adapting into one of the other fiber types. Historically, it has been believed that endurance athletes were obliged to be genetically endowed with larger percentages of type I fibers and the opposite was true of sprinters or jumpers. Numerous cross-sectional studies have confirmed these differences in fiber types between endurance and sprint types of athletes since the advent of the muscle biopsy technique. However, fiber types may in fact represent a continuum, some of which are capable of adapting toward the characteristics of another fiber.

ACUTE CARDIOPULMONARY RESPONSE TO EXERCISE

The cardiovascular system responds to acute exercise with a series of adjustments that assure that active muscles receive blood supply that is appropriate to their metabolic needs, that heat generated by the muscles is dissipated, and that the blood supply to the brain and heart is maintained. This response requires a major redistribution of cardiac output along with a number of local metabolic changes.

The usual measure of the capacity of the body to deliver and utilize oxygen is the maximal oxygen uptake (VO_2 max). Thus, the limits of the cardiopulmonary system are historically defined by VO_2 max, which can be expressed by the Fick equation:

$$VO_2 = \text{Cardiac output} \times \text{Arteriovenous oxygen difference}$$

Cardiac output must closely match ventilation in the lung in order to deliver oxygen to the working muscle. As outlined in detail in Chapter 3, VO_2 max is determined by the maximal amount of ventilation (VE) moving into and out of the lung and the fraction of this ventilation that is extracted by the tissues:

$$VO_2 = VE \times (FiO_2 - FeO_2)$$

where *VE* is minute ventilation, and *FiO_2* and *FeO_2* are the fractional amounts of oxygen in the inspired and expired air, respectively.

The cardiopulmonary limits (VO_2 max) are therefore defined by a central component (cardiac output), which describes the capacity of the heart to function as a pump, and peripheral factors (arteriovenous oxygen difference), which describe the capacity of the lung to oxygenate the blood delivered to it and the capacity of the working muscle to extract this oxygen from the blood. Figures 1-1 and 1-2 outline the many factors that

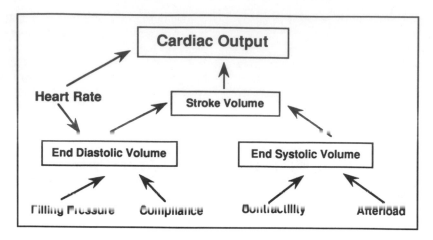

Figure 1-1 Central determinants of maximal oxygen uptake. (From Myers J, Froelicher VF: *Ann Intern Med* 115:377-386, 1991.)

affect cardiac output and arteriovenous oxygen difference. Often, an abnormality in one or more of these components dictates the presence and extent of heart disease. It may be useful at this point to review these models in the context of the cardiovascular response to exercise.

Central factors

Heart rate. Sympathetic and parasympathetic nervous system influences underlie the cardiovascular systems' first response to exercise, an increase in heart rate. Sympathetic outflow to the heart and systemic blood vessels increases, while vagal outflow decreases. Of the two major components of cardiac output, heart rate and stroke volume, heart rate is responsible for most of the increase in cardiac output during exercise, particularly at higher levels. Heart rate increases linearly with workload and oxygen uptake. Increases in heart rate occur primarily at the expense of diastolic and not systolic time. Thus, at very high heart rates (as might be observed in atrial fibrillation), diastolic time may be so short as to preclude adequate ventricular filling.

The heart rate response to exercise is influenced by several factors including age, type of activity, body position, fitness, the presence of heart disease, medications, blood volume, and environment. Of these, perhaps the most important is age; a decline in maximal heart rate occurs with increasing age.[7] This appears to be attributable to intrinsic cardiac changes rather than to neural influences. It should be noted that there is a great deal of variability around the regression line between maximal heart rate and age; thus age-related maximal heart rate is a relatively poor index

of maximal effort (see Chapter 5). Maximal heart rate is unchanged or may be slightly reduced after a program of training. Resting heart rate is frequently reduced after training because of enhanced parasympathetic tone.

Stroke volume. The product of stroke volume (the volume of blood ejected per heart beat) and heart rate determines cardiac output. Stroke volume is equal to the difference between end-diastolic and end-systolic volume. Thus a greater diastolic filling (preload) will increase stroke volume. Alternatively, factors that increase arterial blood pressure will resist ventricular outflow (afterload) and result in a reduced stroke volume. During exercise, stroke volume increases up to approximately 50% to 60% of maximal capacity, after which increases in cardiac output are attributable to further increases in heart rate. The extent to which increases in stroke volume during exercise reflect an increase in end-diastolic volume or a decrease in end-systolic volume is not entirely clear but appears to depend on ventricular function, body position, and intensity of exercise. In healthy subjects, stroke volume is higher at rest and throughout exercise after a period of exercise training. Although the mechanisms are not entirely clear, evidence indicates that this adaptation is attributable more to increases in preload, and possibly local adaptations that reduce peripheral vascular resistance, than to increases in myocardial contractility.

In addition to heart rate, end-diastolic volume is determined by two other factors: *filling pressure* and *ventricular compliance*.

Filling pressure. The most important determinant of ventricular filling is venous pressure. The

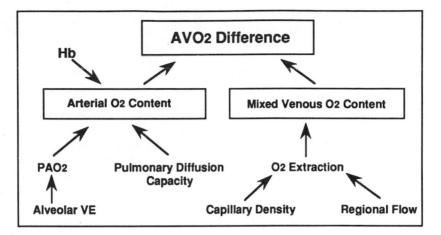

Figure 1-2   Peripheral determinants of maximal oxygen uptake. AVO$_2$ difference is the difference between arterial and venous oxygen. *Hb,* Hemoglobin; *VE,* minute ventilation; *PAO$_2$,* partial pressure of alveolar oxygen. (From Myers J, Froelicher VF: *Ann Intern Med* 115:377-386, 1991.)

degree of venous pressure is a direct consequence of the amount of venous return. The Frank-Starling mechanism dictates that, within limits, all the blood that is returned to the heart will be ejected during systole. As the tissues demand greater oxygen during exercise, venous return increases, which increases end-diastolic fiber length (preload), resulting in a more forceful contraction. Venous pressure increases as exercise intensity increases. Over the course of a few beats, cardiac output will equal venous return.

Several other factors affect venous pressure and therefore filling pressure during exercise. These include blood volume, body position, and the pumping action of the respiratory and skeletal muscles. A greater blood volume increases venous pressure and therefore end-diastolic volume by making more blood available to the heart. Because the effects of gravity are negated, filling pressure is greatest in the supine position. In fact, stroke volume generally does not increase from rest to maximal exercise in the supine position. The intermittent mechanical constriction and relaxation in the skeletal muscles during exercise also enhance venous return. Last, changes in intrathoracic pressure that occur with breathing during exercise facilitate the return of blood to the heart.

Ventricular compliance. Compliance is a measure of the capacity of the ventricle to stretch in response to a given volume of blood. Specifically, compliance is defined as the ratio of the change in volume to the change in pressure. The diastolic pressure/volume relation is curvilinear; that is, at low end-diastolic pressures large changes in volume are accompanied by small changes in pressure and vice versa. At the upper limits of end-diastolic pressure, ventricular compliance declines; that is, the chamber stiffness increases as it fills. Because of the difficulty measuring end-diastolic pressure during exercise, few data are available concerning ventricular compliance during exercise in humans.

End-systolic volume is a function of two factors: *contractility* and *afterload*.

Contractility. Contractility describes the forcefulness of the heart's contraction. Increasing contractility reduces end-systolic volume, which results in a greater stroke volume and thus cardiac output. This is precisely what occurs with exercise in the normal individual; the percentage of blood in the ventricle that is ejected with each beat increases because of an altered cross-bridge formation. Contractility is commonly quantified by the ejection fraction, the percentage of blood that is ejected from the ventricle during systole using radionuclide or angiographic techniques. Despite its wide application as an index of myocardial contractility, ejection fraction has been repeatedly shown to correlate poorly with exercise capacity.

Afterload. Afterload is a measure of the force resisting the ejection of blood by the heart. Increased afterload (or aortic pressure, as is observed with chronic hypertension) results in a reduced ejection fraction and increases in end-diastolic and end-systolic volumes. During dynamic exercise, the force resisting ejection in the periphery (total peripheral resistance) is reduced by vasodilatation because of the effect of local metabolites on the skeletal muscle vasculature.

Thus, despite even a fivefold increase in cardiac output among normal subjects during exercise, mean arterial pressure increases only moderately.

Volume response to exercise. Results of studies involving evaluation of the volume response to exercise have varied greatly. Although the advent of radionuclide techniques in the 1970s offered promise for the noninvasive assessment of ventricular volumes during exercise, the results have been disappointing. Because of technical limitations, most of these studies have been performed in the supine position. Early studies employing radionuclide or echocardiographic techniques during supine exercise among normals reported that end-diastolic volume remained constant or diminished slightly,[8-11] increased in the order of 27%,[12] or varied greatly depending on the subject.[13-15] Among patients with coronary artery disease exercised in the supine position, increases in end-diastolic volume were observed among patients with exercise-induced angina, whereas end-diastolic volume did not change in patients who were asymptomatic.[10,16] Sharma and co-workers[16] and Jones and associates[17] reported increases in both end-diastolic and end-systolic volumes in patients who developed angina during exercise. Slutsky and associates[8] reported that end-diastolic volume remained unchanged in patients with coronary artery disease whether they developed angina. Manyeri and Kostuk[18] reported large increases in both end-systolic and end-diastolic volumes during supine exercise among 20 patients with coronary artery disease, 13 of whom developed angina during exercise.

The ventricular volume response to upright exercise also varies greatly, even in similar populations. The results of some of the major studies are listed in Table 1-2. Among normals, end-diastolic volume has been reported to increase greatly,[12,18,19] increase moderately,[20,21] or decrease slightly during upright exercise.[22,23] End-diastolic volume has been reported to increase in the range of 8% to 56% among patients with coronary artery disease, whereas end-systolic volume has been shown to increase in the range of 16% to 94% in response to upright exercise.[18,20,24-28] Among normals, end-systolic volume has generally been reported to decrease in response to maximal upright exercise (range 22% to 79%).[18,20-23,29] Higginbotham and co-workers,[19] however, recently demonstrated a 48% increase in end-systolic volume among normals, whereas others have reported lesser increases.[25,26] Little is known about the ventricular response to upright exercise in patients with chronic heart failure. Sullivan and co-workers[30] observed that both end-diastolic and end-systolic volumes increased approximately 20% from upright rest to maximal exercise among 20 patients with left ventricular dysfunction.

The inconsistent results concerning the ventricular volume response to both supine and upright exercise has led investigators to raise questions concerning the validity of radionuclide techniques for assessment of ventricular function. Jensen and associates,[31] for example, studied the individual variability of radionuclide ventriculography in coronary artery disease patients over 1 year. Although differences in end-diastolic volume measurements between initial and repeat testing were small, the standard deviations of the individual differences between tests at rest and peak exercise were large, in the order of 38 and 49 ml respectively. Variability in the ejection fraction and end-systolic volume responses to exercise were of a similar magnitude.

In light of the apparent shortcomings of the radionuclide techniques, investigators have employed alternative methods for quantifying ventricular function during exercise. Crawford and associates[24] evaluated the feasibility and reproducibility of two-dimensional echocardiography for assessment of left ventricular function during exercise. A 9% test-retest difference in end-diastolic volume was demonstrated. End-diastolic volume was reported unchanged from rest to peak exercise in patients with coronary disease but increased significantly (20%) from rest to peak exercise among normals. Ginzton and associates[29] recently compared athletes with sedentary subjects during upright exercise using two-dimensional echocardiography. After a slight increase in end-diastolic volume submaximally in both groups, end-diastolic volume decreased 39% and 35% at peak exercise among athletes and sedentary subjects, respectively. Although both groups decreased end-systolic volume progressively during exercise the reduction was greater among the athletes (70% versus 52%).

Thus the ventricular volume response to exercise is not entirely clear but appears to depend on the type of disease, method of measurement (radionuclide or echocardiographic), type of exercise (supine versus upright), and exercise intensity (submaximal versus maximal). Much of the disagreement no doubt can be attributed to differences in the exercise level at which measurements were performed. With this in mind, some rough generalizations may be made concerning changes in ventricular volume in response to upright exercise.

In normal subjects, the response from upright rest to a moderate level of exercise is an increase in both end-diastolic and end-systolic volumes, in

Table 1-2 Ventricular volume response to upright exercise using radionuclide or echocardiographic techniques

Investigator	Population	Technique	Percent change EDV	Percent change ESV
Wyns 1982	Normals ($n = 10$)	RN	Decrease 7.5	Decrease 65
Rerych 1978	Normals ($n = 30$)	RN	Increase 10	Decrease 35
	CAD ($n = 20$)	RN	Increase 56	Increase 94
Iskandrian 1986	Normals ($n = 41$)	RN	Increase 6	Decrease 35
Renlund 1987	Normals ($n = 13$)	RN	Decrease 3	Decrease 79
Hakki 1985	Mixed ($n = 117$)	RN	Increased 15	—
Sullivan 1988	CHF ($n = 20$)	RN	Increase 20	Increase 20
Higgenbotham 1986	Normals ($n = 24$)	RN	Increase 45	Increase 48
Manyeri 1983	Normals ($n = 22$)	RN	Increase 31	Decrease 22
	CAD ($n = 20$)	RN	Increase 45	Increase 48
Kalischer 1984	CAD ($n = 18$)	RN	Increase 27	Increase 48
Shen 1985	CAD ($n = 14$)	RN	Increase 26	Increase 29
	Normals ($n = 17$)	RN	Increase 22	Increase 27
Freeman 1981	CAD ($n = 22$)	RN	Increase 30	Increase 38
	Normals ($n = 10$)	RN	Increase 25	Increase 10
Ginzton 1989	Normals ($n = 14$)	Echo	Decrease 26	Decrease 48
Plotnick 1986	Normals ($n = 30$)	RN	Increase 4	Decrease 50
Crawford 1985	CAD ($n = 10$)	Echo	Increase 8	Increase 22
	CAD ($n = 10$)	RN	Increase 24	Increase 38
Myers 1991	CAD ($n = 8$)	Echo	Increase 16	Increase 16

CAD, Coronary artery disease; *CHF*, congestive heart failure; *Echo*, echocardiography; *EDV*, end-diastolic volume or end-diastolic volume index; *ESV*, end-systolic volume or end-systolic volume index; *RN*, radionuclide ventriculography.

the order of 15% and 30% respectively. As exercise progresses to a higher intensity, end-diastolic volume probably does not increase further,[32] whereas end-systolic volume decreases progressively. At peak exercise, end-diastolic volume may even decline somewhat whereas stroke volume is maintained by a progressively decreasing end-systolic volume. Based on five studies that have quantified the volume response of patients with coronary artery disease to exercise in the upright position,[18,25-28] the finding is that both end-diastolic and end-systolic volume increase modestly, probably in the order of 20% to 50%. Among patients with chronic heart failure, Sullivan and co-workers[30] reported approximately 20% increases in both end-systolic and end-diastolic volumes from rest to maximal exercise during upright exercise. Few data are available in this group in the upright position.

Peripheral factors (a-vO₂ difference) (Fig. 1-2)

Oxygen extraction by the tissues during exercise reflects the difference between the oxygen content of the arteries (generally 8 to 10 ml or cc of $O_2/$ 100 ml at rest) and the oxygen content in the veins (generally 3 to 5 ml of $O_2/$100 ml at rest, yielding a typical a-vO₂ difference at rest of 4 to 5 ml of $O_2/$100 ml, approximately 23% extraction). During exercise, this difference widens as the working tissues extract greater amounts of ox-

ygen; venous oxygen content reaches very low levels, and the a-vO₂ difference may be as high as 16 to 18 ml of $O_2/$100 ml with exhaustive exercise (exceeding 85% extraction of oxygen from the blood at VO₂ max). Some oxygenated blood always returns to the heart, however, because smaller amounts of blood continue to flow through metabolically less active tissues, which do not fully extract oxygen. Generally, the a-vO₂ difference does not explain differences in the VO₂ max between subjects who are relatively homogeneous. That is, the a-vO₂ difference is generally considered to widen by a relatively "fixed" amount during exercise, and differences in the VO₂ max have been historically explained by differences in cardiac output. However, patients with cardiovascular and pulmonary disease exhibit reduced VO₂ max values that can sometimes be attributed to a combination of central and peripheral factors.

Determinants of arterial oxygen content. Arterial oxygen content is related to the partial pressure of arterial oxygen, which is determined in the lung by alveolar ventilation and pulmonary diffusion capacity and in the blood by hemoglobin content. In the absence of pulmonary disease, arterial oxygen content and saturation are usually maintained throughout exercise, even at very high levels. This is true even among patients with severe coronary disease or chronic heart failure. Patients with pulmonary disease, however, often neither ventilate the alveoli adequately nor diffuse oxygen from the lung into the bloodstream normally, and a decrease in arterial oxygen saturation during exercise is one of the hallmarks of this disorder. Arterial hemoglobin content is also usually normal throughout exercise. Naturally, a condition such as anemia would reduce the oxygen carrying capacity of the blood, along with any condition that would shift the O_2 disassociation curve leftward, such as reduced 2,3-diphosphoglycerate, PCO_2, or temperature.

Determinants of venous oxygen content. Venous oxygen content reflects the capacity to extract oxygen from the blood as it flows through the muscle. It is determined by the amount of blood directed to the muscle (regional flow) and capillary density. Muscle blood flow increases in proportion to the increase in work rate and thus the oxygen requirement. The increase in blood flow is brought about not only by the increase in cardiac output, but also by a preferential redistribution of the cardiac output to the exercising muscle. A reduction in local vascular resistance facilitates this greater skeletal muscle flow. In turn, locally produced vasodilatory mechanisms and possible neurogenic dilatation attributable to higher sympathetic activity mediate the greater skeletal muscle blood flow. A pronounced increase in the number of open capillaries reduces diffusion distances, increases capillary blood volume, and increases mean transit time, facilitating oxygen delivery to the muscle.

Cross-sectionally, fit individuals have a greater skeletal muscle capillary density than sedentary subjects. In addition, fit subjects may have a greater capacity to redistribute blood flow toward the muscle and away from nonexercising tissue. Interestingly, one of the characteristics of the patient with chronic heart failure is an "exaggeration" of the deconditioning response. These patients exhibit a reduced capacity to redistribute blood, a reduced capacity to vasodilate in response to exercise or after ischemia, and a reduced capillary-to-fiber ratio.[1]

SUMMARY

The major cardiopulmonary adaptations that are required of acute exercise make exercise testing a very practical test of cardiac perfusion and function. The rather remarkable physiologic adaptations that occur with exercise have made exercise a valuable research medium not just for the study of physical performance in athletes, but also for the study of cardiovascular disease and the normal and abnormal physiology of many other organ systems.

A major increase and redistribution of cardiac output underlies a series of adjustments that allow the body to increase its resting metabolic rate as much as 10 to 20 times with exercise. The capacity of the body to deliver and utilize oxygen is expressed as the maximal oxygen uptake. Maximal oxygen uptake is defined as the product of maximal cardiac output and maximal arteriovenous oxygen difference. Thus the cardiopulmonary limits are defined by a central component (cardiac output), which describes the capacity of the heart to function as a pump, and peripheral factors (arteriovenous oxygen difference), which describe the capacity of the lung to oxygenate the blood delivered to it and the capacity of the working muscle to extract this oxygen from the blood. Hemodynamic responses to exercise are greatly affected by the type of exercise being performed, by whether disease is present, and by the age, sex, and fitness of the individual.

Coronary artery disease is characterized by reduced myocardial oxygen supply, which, in the presence of an increased myocardial oxygen demand, can lead to myocardial ischemia and reduced cardiac performance. Despite years of study, several dilemmas remain in regard to the response to exercise clinically. Although myocardial perfusion and function are intuitively linked, it is often difficult to separate the effect of ischemia from that of left ventricular dysfunction on exercise responses. Indices of ventricular function and exercise capacity are poorly related. Cardiac output is considered the most important determinant of exercise capacity in normal subjects. However, among patients with heart disease, abnormalities in one or several of the links in the chain that define oxygen uptake contribute to the determination of exercise capacity.

The transport of oxygen from the air to the mitochondria of the working muscle cell requires the coupling of blood flow and ventilation to cellular metabolism. Energy for muscular contraction is provided by three sources: stored phosphates (ATP, creatine phosphate), oxygen-independent glycolysis, and oxidative metabolism. Oxidative metabolism provides the greatest source of ATP for muscular contraction. Muscular contraction is accomplished by three fiber types, which differ in their contraction speed, color, and mitochondrial content. The duration and intensity of activity determine the extent to which these fuel sources and fiber types are called upon.

REFERENCES

1. Myers J, Froelicher VF: Hemodynamic determinants of exercise capacity in chronic heart failure, *Am Intern Med* 115:377-386, 1991.
2. McKirnan MD, Sullivan M, Jensen D, Froelicher VF:

Treadmill performance and cardiac function in selected patients with coronary heart disease, *J Am Coll Cardiol* 3:253-261, 1984.

3. Hammond HK, Kelley TL, Froelicher VF: Noninvasive testing in the evaluation of myocardial ischemia: agreement among tests, *J Am Coll Cardiol* 5:59-69, 1985.

4. Brooks GA: Lactate: glycolytic end product and oxidative substrate during exercise in mammals—"the lactate shuttle." In Gilles R, editor: *Comparative physiology and biochemistry: current topics and trends,* vol A: *Respiration—metabolism—circulation,* New York, 1985, Springer Verlag, pp 208-218.

5. Brooks GA: The lactate shuttle during exercise and recovery, *Med Sci Sports Exerc* 18:360-368, 1986.

6. Saltin B, Henricksson J, Hugaard E, Andersen P: Fiber types and metabolic potentials of skeletal muscles in sedentary man and endurance runners, *Ann NY Acad Sci* 301:3-29, 1977.

7. Hammond K, Froelicher VF: Normal and abnormal heart rate responses to exercise, *Prog Cardiovasc Dis* 27:271-296, 1985.

8. Slutsky R, Karliner J, Ricci D, et al: Response of left ventricular volume to exercise in man assessed by radionuclide equilibrium angiography, *Circulation* 60:565, 1979.

9. Cotsamire DL, Sullivan MJ, Bashore TM, Leier CV: Position as a variable for cardiovascular responses during exercise, *Clin Cardiol* 10:137-142, 1987.

10. Stein RA, Michelli D, Fox EL, Krasnow N: Continuous ventricular dimensions in man during supine exercise and recovery, *Am J Cardiol* 41:655-660, 1978.

11. Bevegård BS, Shepherd JT: Regulation of the circulation during exercise in man, *Physiol Rev* 47:178-213, 1967.

12. Poliner LR, Dehmer GJ, Lewis SE, et al: Left ventricular performance in normal subjects: a comparison of the responses to exercise in the upright and supine positions, *Circulation* 62:528-534, 1980.

13. Bristow JD, Klosten FE, Farrahi C, et al: The effects of supine exercise on left ventricular volume in heart disease, *Am Heart J* 71:319-329, 1966.

14. Adams KF, Vincent LM, McAllister SM, et al: The influence of age and gender on left ventricular response to supine exercise in asymptomatic normal subjects, *Am Heart J* 113:732-742, 1987.

15. Granath A, Jonsson B, Strandall T: Circulation in healthy old men, studied by right heart catheterization at rest and during exercise in supine and sitting position, *Acta Med Scand* 176:425-446, 1964.

16. Sharma B, Goodwin JF, Raphael MJ, et al: Left ventricular angiography on exercise: a new method of assessing left ventricular function in ischemic heart disease, *Br Heart J* 38:59-70, 1976.

17. Jones R, McEwan P, Newman G, et al: Accuracy of diagnosis of coronary artery disease by radionuclide measurement of left ventricular function during rest and exercise, *Circulation* 64:586-601, 1981.

18. Manyeri DE, Kostuk WJ: Right and left ventricular function at rest and during bicycle exercise in the supine and sitting positions in normal subjects and patients with coronary artery disease: assessment by radionuclide ventriculography, *Am J Cardiol* 51:36-42, 1983.

19. Higginbotham MB, Morris KG, Williams RS, et al: Regulation of stroke volume during submaximal and maximal upright exercise in normal man, *Circ Res* 58:281-291, 1986.

20. Rerych SK, Scholz PM, Newman GE, et al: Cardiac function at rest and during exercise in normals and in patients with coronary heart disease: evaluation by radionuclide angiocardiography, *Ann Surg* 187:449-464, 1978.

21. Iskandrian AS, Hakki AH: Determinants of the changes in left ventricular end-diastolic volume during upright exercise in patients with coronary artery disease, *Am Heart J* 112:441-446, 1986.

22. Wyns W, Melin JA, Vanbutsele RJ, et al: Assessment of right and left ventricular volumes during upright exercise in normal men, *Eur Heart J* 3:529-536, 1982.

23. Renlund DG, Lakatta EG, Fleg JL, et al: Prolonged decrease in cardiac volumes after maximal upright bicycle exercise, *J Appl Physiol* 63:1947-1955, 1987.

24. Crawford MH, Amon KW, Vance WS: Exercise 2-dimensional echocardiography: quantitation of left ventricular performance in patients with severe angina pectoris, *Am J Cardiol* 51:1-6, 1983.

25. Freeman MR, Berman DS, Staniloff H, et al: Comparison of upright and supine bicycle exercise in the detection and evaluation of extent of coronary artery disease by equilibrium radionuclide ventriculography, *Am Heart J* 102:182-189, 1981.

26. Shen WF, Roubin GS, Choong CY-P, et al: Left ventricular response to exercise in coronary artery disease: relation to myocardial ischemia and effects of nifedipine, *Eur Heart J* 6:1025-1031, 1985.

27. Kalisher AL, Johnson LL, Johnson YE, et al: Effects of propranolol and timolol on left ventricular volumes during exercise in patients with coronary artery disease, *J Am Coll Cardiol* 3:210-218, 1984.

28. Myers J, Wallis J, Lehmann K, et al: Hemodynamic determinants of maximal ventilatory oxygen uptake in patients with coronary artery disease, *Circulation* 84:II-150, 1991.

29. Ginzton LE, Conant R, Brizendine M, Laks MM: Effect of long-term high intensity aerobic training on left ventricular volume during maximal upright exercise, *J Am Coll Cardiol* 14:364-371, 1989.

30. Sullivan MJ, Higginbotham MB, Cobb FR: Exercise training in patients with severe left ventricular dysfunction: hemodynamic and metabolic effects, *Circulation* 78:506-515, 1988.

31. Jensen DG, Genter F, Froelicher VF, et al: Individual variability of radionuclide ventriculography in stable coronary artery disease patients over one year, *Cardiology* 71:266-271, 1984.

32. Plotnick GD, Becker L, Fisher ML, et al: Use of the Frank-Starling mechanism during submaximal versus maximal upright exercise, *Am J Physiol* 251:H1101-H1105, 1986.

2 | Exercise Testing Methodology

Despite the many recent advances in technology related to the diagnosis and treatment of cardiovascular disease, the exercise test remains an important diagnostic modality. Its many applications, widespread availability, and high yield of clinical useful information continue to make it an important screening tool for more expensive and invasive procedures. The numerous approaches to the exercise test, however, have been a drawback to its proper application. Excellent guidelines have recently been updated by organizations such as the American Heart Association, American Association of Cardiovascular and Pulmonary Rehabilitation, and the American College of Sports Medicine, which are based on a multitude of research studies over the last 20 years and have led to greater uniformity in methods. Nevertheless, in many laboratories methodology remains based on tradition, convenience, equipment, or personnel available.

Recent technology, while adding convenience, has raised new questions in regard to methodology. For example, all commercially available systems today make liberal use of computers. Do computer-averaged exercise ECGs improve test sensitivity, and what should the practitioner be cautious of? What about the many computerized exercise scores? Technology has changed the exercise testing laboratory environment, and concerns such as these have arisen. Although many of these techniques are attractive, in many instances not enough data are yet available to validate them, and they should be used judiciously. In this chapter, we address basic methodology and comment on the influence these advances in technology have had.

Safety precautions and risks

The safety precautions outlined by the American Heart Association are very explicit in regard to

the requirements for exercise testing. Everything necessary for cardiopulmonary resuscitation must be available, and regular drills should be performed to ascertain that both personnel and equipment are ready for a cardiac emergency. The classic survey of clinical exercise facilities by Rochmis and Blackburn[1] showed exercise testing to be a safe procedure, with approximately one death and five nonfatal complications per 10,000 tests. Perhaps because of an expanded knowledge concerning indications, contraindications, and end points, maximal exercise testing appears safer today than 20 years ago. Gibbons and co-workers[2] recently reported the safety of exercise testing in 71,914 tests conducted over a 16-year period. The complication rate was 0.8 per 10,000 tests. They suggested that the low complication rate might be attributable to a cool-down walk, but we have observed a low complication rate despite laying patients supine immediately after the test and exercising higher risk patients.[3]

There are, of course, reports of acute infarctions and deaths associated with exercise testing. Although the test is remarkably safe, the population referred for this procedure usually is at high risk for coronary events. Irving and Bruce[4] have reported an association between exercise-induced hypotension and ventricular fibrillation. Shepard[5] has hypothesized the following risk levels for exercise: (1) three or four times normal in a cross-country foot race, (2) six to 12 times normal in a population prone to coronary artery disease performing unaccustomed exercise, and (3) as high as 60 times normal when exercise is performed by patients with coronary artery disease in a stressful environment, such as a physician's office. Cobb and Weaver[6] estimated the risk to be over 100 times in the latter situation and point out the dangers of the recovery period. The risk of exercise testing in patients with coronary artery disease cannot be disregarded even with its excellent safety record. Studies documenting the risks of exercise testing and training are presented in more detail in Chapter 16.

Indications to stop an exercise test are outlined in Table 2-1. Most problems can be avoided by having an experienced physician, nurse, or exercise physiologist standing next to the patient, measuring blood pressure, and assessing patient appearance during the test. The exercise technician should operate the recorder and treadmill, take the appropriate tracings, enter data on a form, and alert the physician to any abnormalities that may appear on the monitor scope. If the patient's appearance is worrisome, if systolic blood pressure drops or plateaus, if there are alarming electrocardiographic abnormalities, if chest pain occurs and becomes worse than the patient's usual

Table 2-1 Absolute and relative indications for termination of an exercise test

Absolute indications

1. Acute myocardial infarction, or suspicion of a myocardial infarction
2. Onset of severe angina (worse than usual)
3. Drop in systolic blood pressure with increasing work load accompanied by signs or symptoms
4. Serious dysrhythmias (second- or third-degree atrioventricular block, ventricular tachycardia, or strings of premature ventricular contractions)
5. Signs of poor perfusion, including pallor, cyanosis, or cold and clammy skin
6. CNS symptoms, including ataxia, vertigo, visual or gait problems, and confusion
7. Technical problems with monitoring any parameters (such as with the electrocardiogram)
8. Patient's request

Relative indications

1. Pronounced ECG changes from baseline including more than 0.2 mV of horizontal or downsloping ST-segment depression, or 0.2 mV of ST-segment elevation
2. Any chest pain that is increasing
3. Pronounced fatigue and shortness of breath
4. Wheezing
5. Leg cramps or intermittent claudication
6. Hypertensive response (systolic BP >260 mm Hg; diastolic BP >115 mm Hg)
7. Less serious dysrhythmias, such as supraventricular tachycardia
8. Exercise-induced bundle branch block that cannot be distinguished from ventricular tachycardia

pain, or if a patient wants to stop the test for any reason, the test should be stopped, even at a submaximal level. In most instances, a symptom-limited maximal test is preferred but is usually advisable to stop if more than 0.2 mV of flat or downsloping ST-segment depression occurs. In some patients estimated to be at high risk because of their clinical history, it may be appropriate to stop at a submaximal level, since it is not unusual for severe ST-segment depression, dysrhythmias, or both, to occur only after exercise. If the measurement of maximal exercise capacity or other information is needed, it is better to repeat the test later, once the patient has demonstrated a safe performance of a submaximal work load.

Exercise testing should be an extension of the history and physical examination. A physician obtains the most information by being present to talk with, observe, and examine the patient in conjunction with the test. A brief physical examination should always be performed to rule out significant obstructive aortic valvular disease or other contraindications. In this way, patient safety and an optimal yield of information are assured. In some instances, as when asymptomatic, apparently healthy subjects are being screened, or a repeat treadmill test is being done on a patient whose condition is stable, a physician need not be present but should be nearby and prepared to respond promptly. The physician's reaction to signs or symptoms should be moderated by the information the patient gives regarding his usual activity. If abnormal findings occur at levels of exercise that the patient usually performs, it may not be necessary to stop the test for them. Also, the patient's activity history should help determine appropriate work rates for testing.

Contraindications

Table 2-2 lists the absolute and relative contraindications to performing an exercise test. Good clinical judgment should be foremost in deciding the indications and contraindications for exercise testing. In selected cases with relative contraindications, testing can provide valuable information even if performed submaximally.

Patient preparation

Preparations for exercise testing include the following: (1) the patient should be instructed not be eat or smoke at least 2 to 3 hours before the test and to come dressed for exercise; (2) a brief history and physical examination should be performed to rule out any contraindications to testing (Table 2-2); (3) specific questioning should determine which drugs are being taken, and potential electrolyte abnormalities should be considered.

Table 2-2   Absolute and relative contraindications to exercise testing

Absolute	Relative*
Acute myocardial infarction or any recent change in the resting electrocardiogram	Any less serious noncardiac disorder
Unstable angina	Ventricular conduction defects
Serious cardiac dysrhythmias	Significant arterial or pulmonary hypertension
Acute pericarditis or myocarditis	Tachydysrhythmias or bradydysrhythmias < serious
Endocarditis	Moderate valvular or myocardial heart diseases
Severe aortic stenosis	Drug effect or electrolyte abnormalities
Severe left ventricular dysfunction	Fixed-rate artificial pacemaker
Acute pulmonary embolus or pulmonary infarction	Left main obstruction or its equivalent
Any acute or serious noncardiac disorder	Psychiatric disease or inability to cooperate
Severe physical handicap	

*Under certain circumstances, relative contraindications can be superseded.

The labeled medication bottles should be brought along so that they can be identified and recorded. Because of the life-threatening rebound phenomena associated with beta-adrenergic receptor blockers, they should not be stopped before testing is done routinely. However, if testing is performed for diagnostic purposes, they can be gradually stopped if a physician or nurse carefully supervises the tapering process, (4) if the reason for the exercise test is not apparent, the referring physician should be contacted, and (5) a 12-lead electrocardiogram should be obtained in both the supine and standing positions. The latter is an important rule, particularly in patients with known heart disease, since an abnormality may prohibit testing. On occasion, a patient referred for an exercise test will instead by admitted to the coronary care unit. There should be careful explanations of why the test is being performed, of the testing procedure including its risks and possible complications, and of how to perform the test. This should include a demonstration of getting on and off as well as walking on the treadmill. The patient should be told that he or she can hold on initially but a minute or so into the test should use the rails only for balance.

The treadmill

The treadmill should have front and side rails for patients to steady themselves, and some patients may benefit from the helping hand of the person administering the test. It should be calibrated at least monthly. Some models can be greatly affected by the weight of the patient and will not deliver the appropriate work load to heavy patients. An emergency stop button should be readily available to the staff only. A small platform or stepping area at the level of the belt is ad-

visable so that the patient can start the test by "pedaling" the belt with one foot before stepping on. Patients should not grasp the front or side rails because doing so decreases the work performed and oxygen uptake, which increases exercise time, resulting in an overestimation of exercise capacity. Gripping the handrails also increases ECG muscle artifact. When necessary, it is helpful to have patients take their hands off the rails, close their fists, and extent one finger touching the rails in order to maintain balance while walking, after they are accustomed to the treadmill. Some patients may require a few moments to feel comfortable enough to let go of the handrails, but we strongly discourage grasping the handrails after the first minute of exercise.

Consent form

In any procedure with a risk of complications, it is advisable to make certain the patient understands the situation and acknowledges the risks. Some physicians believe that informing patients of the risks involved will occasionally make them overly anxious or discourage them from performing the test. Because of this and the fact that a signed consent form does not necessarily protect a physician from legal action, there has been less insistence on consent forms. If those performing the exercise test carefully explain the possible risks and complications in detail to each patient, a consent form should be superfluous.

Legal implications of exercise testing

There are several considerations in regard to legal implications. Establishment of physician-patient communication before and after performance of the exercise test should be the first consideration. A test should not be performed without first obtainment of the patient's informed consent, orally or in writing. In the process of obtaining informed consent, the patient should be made aware of the potential risks and benefits of the procedure. A physician may be held responsible in the event of a major untoward event, even if the test is carefully performed, in the absence of informed consent. The argument can be made that the patient would not have undergone the procedure had he or she been made aware of the risks associated with the test. After the test, responsibility rests with the physician for prompt interpretation and consideration of the implications of the test. Communication of these results to the patient is necessary—with advice concerning adjustments in lifestyle—without delay. The second consideration should be adherence to proper standards of care during performance of the test. Exercise testing should be carried out only by persons thoroughly trained in its administration and in the prompt recognition of problems that may arise. A physician trained in exercise testing and resuscitation should be readily available during the test to make judgments concerning test termination. Resuscitative equipment should always be available. In 1990, a joint position statement from the American College of Physicians, American College of Cardiology, and the American Heart Association was published outlining physician competence for performing exercise testing.[7]

Blood pressure measurement

Although numerous clever devices have been developed to automate blood pressure measurement during exercise, none can be recommended. The time-proved method of the physician holding the patient's arm with a stethoscope placed over the brachial artery remains most reliable. The patient's arm should be free of the handrails so that noise is not transmitted up the arm. It is sometimes helpful to mark the brachial artery. An anesthesiologist's auscultatory piece or an electronic microphone can be fastened to the arm. A device that inflates and deflates the cuff on the push of a button can be helpful also. If systolic blood pressure appears to be increasing sluggishly or decreasing, it should be taken again immediately. If a drop in systolic blood pressure of 20 mm Hg or more occurs or if it drops below the value obtained in the standing position before testing, the test should be stopped in patients with congestive heart failure or a prior myocardial infarction or who are exhibiting signs or symptoms of ischemia. We have observed that systolic blood pressure must drop below the standing resting value to be prognostically valuable. An increase in systolic blood pressure to 260 mm Hg or an increase in diastolic blood pressure to 115 mm Hg are also indications to stop the test.

ECG recording instruments

Many technologic advances in electrocardiographic recorders have taken place. The medical instrumentation industry has promptly complied with specifications set forth by various professional groups. Machines with a high-input impedance ensure that the voltage recorded graphically is equivalent to that on the surface of the body despite the high natural impedance of the skin. There remains some concern about mismatching lead impedances, which can result in distortion. Optically isolated buffer amplifiers have ensured patient safety and machines with a frequency response from 0 to 100 Hz are commercially available. The 0 Hz lower end is possible because DC coupling is technically feasible.

Some electrocardiographic equipment has monitoring and diagnostic modes, particularly equipment used in coronary care units. The diagnostic mode follows diagnostic instrument specifications with a frequency response from 0.05 to 100 Hz. In the monitor mode, there can be distortion of the electrocardiogram. The monitor mode is available to lessen the effects of electrical interference, motion, and respiration in the ECG and should not be used for exercise testing. The type of distortion is affected by the electrocardiographic waveform that is presented. If the ECG waveform is a tall R-wave without an S-wave, the ST-segment distortion can be different from that of an R-wave followed by a large S-wave. In general, an inadequate low-frequency response can greatly decrease the Q- and R-wave amplitude and create S-waves. Alteration of the 25 to 45 Hz frequency response is the most common cause of ST-segment distortion found in tracings with abnormal ST segments. Not all ambulatory monitoring recorders or telemetry equipment meet diagnostic frequency requirements.

Waveform averaging

Analog and digital averaging techniques have made it possible to average ECG signals to remove noise. There is a need for consumer awareness in these areas, since most manufacturers do not specify how the use of such procedures modifies the ECG. Signal averaging can actually distort the ECG signal. These techniques are attractive, since they can produce a clean tracing despite poor skin preparation. However, the common expression used by computer scientists, "garbage in, garbage out," has never been more applicable than to the computerized ECG. The clean-looking ECG signal produced may not be a true representation of the actual waveform and in fact may be dangerously misleading. Also, the instruments that make computer ST-segment measurements cannot be totally reliable, since they are based on imperfect algorithms. For instance, the algorithm that measures QRS end at 70 or 80 msec after the peak of the R-wave can hardly be valid, particularly with a changing heart rate.

For some patients, it is advantageous to have a recorder with a slow paper speed option of 5 mm/sec. This speed makes it possible to record an entire exercise test and reduces the likelihood of missing any dysrhythmias when one is specifically evaluating patients with these problems. A faster paper speed of 50 mm/sec can be helpful for making accurate ST-segment slope measurements. There are many different types of electrocardiographic paper that can be used. Wax-treated paper is known to retain an electrocardiographic image for 20 years or longer. However, it is pressure sensitive and easily marked. Thermochemically treated paper is sturdy and resists marking. There are many different types of such paper, and the duration of images recorded on it is usually adequate. There has been at least one instance of ECG paper losing a recorded electrocardiographic image that resulted in legal action by a hospital against a manufacturer. Ceramic-coated paper is very sturdy and comparable in price; it has a hard finish with a high contrast, which makes it durable and easy to interpret. Untreated paper is the cheapest, but the ink jet and carbon-transfer techniques characteristically produce fuzzy images. The ink-jet and carbon-transfer recorders are available with six channels and are expensive, but they do have an excellent upper-frequency response for phonocardiography. The ceramic paper also requires an ink jet rather than a heat stylus. Ink-jet recorders are said to require more maintenance, but recent models are reliable. Copying can be a problem, since blues and reds are poorly copied by some xerographic reproduction machines.

Thermal head printers have nearly totally replaced all other types of printers. These recorders are remarkable in that they can use blank thermal paper and write out the grid as well as the ECG, vector loops, and alphanumerics. They can record graphs and figures as well as tables and typed reports. They are totally digitally driven and can produce very high resolution records. The paper price is comparable, and these devices are reasonably priced and very durable, particularly because no stylus is needed. One system uses a laser printer, but this is not suitable for the exercise environment, since recording the ECG is delayed by the 5 to 20 seconds required for the printing to occur.

Z-fold paper has the advantage over roll paper in that it is easily folded, and the study can be interpreted in a manner similar to paging through a book. Exercise electrocardiograms can be microfilmed on rolls or cartridges or in fiche cards for storage. They can also be stored in digital or analog format on magnetic media or optical discs. The latest technology involves magnetic optical discs that are erasable and have fast access and transfer times. These devices can be easily interfaced with microcomputers and can store gigabytes of digital information.

Exercise test modalities

Three types of exercise can be used to stress the cardiovascular system: isometric, dynamic, and a combination of the two. Isometric exercise, defined as constant muscular contraction without movement (such as handgrip), imposes a disproportionate pressure load on the left ventricle relative to ventricular volume. Dynamic exercise is defined as rhythmic muscular activity resulting in movement and initiates a more appropriate increase in cardiac output and oxygen exchange. Since a delivered work load can be accurately calibrated and the physiologic response easily measured, dynamic exercise is preferred for clinical testing. Using progressive work loads of dynamic exercise, patients with coronary artery disease can be protected from rapidly increasing myocardial oxygen demand. Although bicycling is a dynamic exercise, most individuals perform more work on a treadmill because a greater muscle mass is involved and most subjects are more familiar with walking than cycling.

Numerous modalities have been used to provide dynamic exercise for exercise testing, including steps, escalators, and ladder mills. Today, however, the bicycle ergometer and the treadmill are the most commonly used dynamic exercise devices. The bicycle ergometer is usually cheaper, takes up less space, and makes less noise. Upper body motion is usually reduced, but care must be taken so that isometric exercise is not performed by the arms. The work load administered by the simple bicycle ergometers is not well calibrated and is dependent on pedaling speed. It is too easy for a patient to slow pedaling speed during exercise testing and decrease the administered work load. More expensive electronically braked bicycle ergometers keep the work load at a specified level over a wide range of pedaling speeds. These are particularly needed for supine exercise testing.

Arm ergometry

Alternative methods of exercise testing are needed for patients with vascular, orthopedic, or neurologic conditions who cannot perform leg exercise. To determine the sensitivity of arm exercise in detecting coronary artery disease, Balady and co-workers[8,9] tested 30 patients with angina pectoris using both arm ergometry and a treadmill before coronary angiography. All patients had at least 70% diameter reduction in one or more major coronary arteries. Ischemic ST-segment depression (≥ 0.1 mV) or angina occurred more frequently with leg exercise (86%, 26 patients) than with arm exercise (40%, 12 patients). There was no significant difference in peak rate-pressure product achieved with either test, though the peak oxygen consumption was greater during leg exercise than during arm exercise (18 versus 13 ml/kg/min). For concordantly positive tests, the oxygen uptake at the onset of ischemia was significantly lower during arm testing than during leg testing (12 versus 17 ml/kg/min). There was no significant difference in heart rate during either test at the onset of ischemia. Thus arm exercise testing is a reasonable but not equivalent alternative to leg exercise testing in patients who cannot perform leg exercise.

Supine versus upright exercise testing

A great deal of the information available on hemodynamic responses to exercise has come from supine exercise, mostly because cardiac catheterization is required to obtain much of this information. However, there are considerable differences between the body's response to acute exercise in the supine versus upright positions. During supine bicycle exercise, stroke volume and end-diastolic volume do not change much from values obtained at rest, whereas in the upright position these values increase during mild work and then plateau. Naturally, exercise capacity is considerably lower in the supine position compared to upright cycling. In patients with heart disease, left ventricular filling pressure is more likely to increase during exercise in the supine position than in the upright position. When patients with angina perform identical submaximal bicycle work loads in supine and upright positions, for the supine position the heart rate is higher, the maximal work load is lower, and angina will develop at a lower double product. ST-segment depression is often greater in the supine position because of the greater left ventricular volume.

As with upright exercise, a linear relationship between cardiac output and oxygen uptake during supine bicycle exercise has been observed and has been used to separate patients with heart disease

from normals. Exercise factor, or the increase in cardiac output for a given increase in oxygen uptake, is based on studies of normal persons. For every 100 ml increase in oxygen consumption, cardiac output should increase by 500 ml. Left ventricular filling pressure does not increase in proportion to work in normal persons but often increases in patients with heart disease. Radionuclide imaging has shown that the ejection fraction usually increases in normal subjects but can decrease during exercise in patients with ischemia or left ventricular dysfunction. However, many patients with heart disease demonstrate discordance between their disease and ventricular function and can respond normally to exercise.

Bicycle ergometer versus treadmill

In most studies comparing upright cycle ergometer with treadmill exercise, maximal heart rate values have been demonstrated to be roughly similar, whereas maximal oxygen uptake has been shown to be 6% to 25% greater during treadmill exercise.[10-13] Early hemodynamic studies by Bruce, Niederberger and co-workers[14] concluded that bicycle exercise constitutes a greater stress on the cardiovascular system for any given oxygen uptake than treadmill exercise does. The clinical importance of these findings in relation to patients with cardiovascular disease undergoing exercise testing is that slightly higher maximal oxygen uptakes are achieved with slightly less hemodynamic stress when treadmill exercise is used. Wickes and co-workers[15] reported similar ECG changes with treadmill testing as compared with bicycle testing in patients with coronary artery disease. Rather than for any clinical reason, however, the treadmill is the most commonly used dynamic testing modality in the United States because patients are more familiar with walking than they are with bicycling. Patients are more likely to give the muscular effort necessary to increase myocardial oxygen demand adequately by walking than by bicycling.

Exercise with intracardiac catheters

Exercise testing with intracardiac catheters has significant advantages over alternative diagnostic methods for (1) separation of cardiac from pulmonary dyspnea, (2) separation of left ventricular systolic from diastolic dysfunction, and (3) quantitative evaluation of the clinical significance of valvular disease.

Cardiac versus pulmonary dyspnea. Patients with severe chronic obstructive pulmonary disease (COPD) have clinical findings that make the assessment of left ventricular function extremely difficult. Many patients with COPD have left-sided heart disease secondary to coronary artery disease, hypertension, or left-sided valvular disease. In left-sided heart disease, there is a common denominator for cardiac dyspnea: elevation of the left atrial pressure. This leads to elevation of the pulmonary wedge pressure, which leads to increased pulmonary interstitial fluid, decreased pulmonary compliance, and dyspnea. In contrast, significant elevation of left atrial or pulmonary wedge pressure is unusual in uncomplicated COPD. Therefore measurement of the rest and exercise wedge pressure allows one to distinguish the pathophysiology of COPD from left-sided heart disease. In the former case, pulmonary artery pressure may rise considerably, but pulmonary wedge pressure will remain below 20 mm Hg even with maximal supine exercise. In left-sided heart disease, a pulmonary wedge pressure greater than 25 mm Hg often occurs at maximal exercise.

Left ventricular systolic versus diastolic dysfunction. Left ventricular systolic dysfunction with a resultant increase in left ventricular volume leads to an increase in diastolic filling pressure. The patient with heart failure after a myocardial infarction is the classic example of systolic dysfunction. In hypertrophic cardiomyopathy, systolic or contractile function can be normal or even better than normal, but a thick noncompliant ventricle that cannot readily fill leads to an increased pulmonary wedge pressure. Diastolic dysfunction is characterized by a normal cardiac output for a given work load, but this output comes at the expense of an elevated filling pressure. The distinction between systolic and diastolic function requires the measurement of cardiac output.

Quantitation of valvular disease. Patients whose symptoms seem out of proportion to their valvular disease can be assessed by use of these invasive techniques. In the case of significant valvular lesions, exercise leads to an increase in pulmonary wedge pressure. Forward output may be maintained until late in their course. Elevation of exercise pulmonary wedge pressure at symptom-limited exercise indicates that valve disease rather than concomitant pulmonary disease may be the cause of clinical symptoms.

Exercise protocols

The many different exercise protocols in use has led to some confusion regarding how physicians compare tests between patients and serial tests in the same patient. The most common protocols, their stages, and the predicted oxygen cost of each stage are illustrated in Figure 2-1. When treadmill and cycle ergometer testing were first introduced into clinical practice, practitioners adopted protocols used by major researchers, that is, Balke,[16] Åstrand,[17] Bruce,[18] and Ellestad[19] and their co-workers. In 1980, Stuart and Ellestad[20] surveyed 1375 exercise laboratories in North America and reported that of those performing treadmill testing, 65.5% use the Bruce protocol for routine clinical testing. This protocol uses relatively large and unequal 2 to 3 MET increments in work every 3 minutes. Large and uneven work increments such as these have been shown to result in a tendency to overestimate exercise capacity.[21] Investigators have since recommended protocols with smaller and more equal increments.[10,22,23]

Redwood and associates[24] performed serial testing in patients with angina and reported that work-rate increments that were too rapid resulted in a reduced exercise capacity and could not be reliably used for studying the effects of therapy. When excessive work rates were used, the reduction in myocardial oxygen demand after administration of nitroglycerin was minor, an indication that protocols placing heavy and abrupt demands on the patient may mask a potential salutatory effect of an intervention. These investigators recommended that the protocol be individualized for each patient to elicit angina within 3 to 6 minutes. Smokler and associates[25] reported that, among 40 pairs of treadmill tests conducted within a 6-month period, tests that were less than 10 minutes in duration showed a much greater percentage of variation than those that were greater than 10 minutes in duration. Buchfuhrer and co-workers[12] performed repeated maximal exercise testing in five normal subjects while varying the work-rate increment. Maximal oxygen uptake varied with the increment in work; the highest values were observed when intermediate increments were used. These investigators suggested that an exercise test with work increments individualized to yield a duration of approximately 10 minutes was optimal for assessment of cardiopulmonary function. Lipkin and co-workers,[26] on the other hand, observed that, among patients with chronic heart failure, small work increments yielding a long test duration (31 ± 15 minutes) resulted in reduced values for maximal oxygen uptake, minute ventilation, and arterial lactate compared with tests using more standard increments. These observations have led several investigators to suggest that protocols should be individualized for each patient such that test duration is approximately 8 to 12 minutes.

Ramp testing

An approach to exercise testing that has gained interest in recent years is the ramp protocol, in

Figure 2-1 Estimated ventilatory oxygen cost per stage for most of the commonly used treadmill protocols

FUNCTIONAL CLASS	CLINICAL STATUS	O₂ COST ML/KG/MIN	METS	BICYCLE ERGOMETER (1 WATT = 6 KPDS) FOR 70 KG BODY WEIGHT — KFDS	BRUCE (3 MIN STAGES) MPH	BRUCE %GR	KATTUS MPH	KATTUS %GR	BALKE WARE % GRAD AT 3.3 MPH (1-MIN STAGES)	ELLESTAD (3/2–3 MIN STAGES) MPH	ELLESTAD %GR	USAFSAM (2 OR 3 MIN STAGES) MPH	USAFSAM %GR	"SLOW" USAFSAM MPH	"SLOW" USAFSAM %GR	McHENRY MPH	McHENRY %GR	STANFORD % GRADE AT 3 MPH	STANFORD % GRADE AT 2 MPH	METS
NORMAL AND I	HEALTHY, DEPENDENT ON AGE, ACTIVITY	56.0	16		5.5	20			26											16
		52.5	15		5.0	18	4	22	25	6	15									15
		49.0	14	1500					24											14
		45.5	13		4.2	16	4	18	22	5	15	3.3	25			3.3	21	22.5		13
		42.0	12	1350	—				20			3.3	20			3.3	18	20.0		12
		38.5	11	1200					18					2	25			17.5		11
		35.0	10	1050	3.4	14	4	14	15	5	10	3.3	15			3.3	15	15.0		10
		31.5	9	900					13					2	20			12.5		9
	SEDENTARY HEALTHY	28.0	8	750	2.5	12	4	10	11	4	10	3.3	10	2	15	3.3	12	10.0		8
		24.5	7						9					2	10	3.3	9	7.5	17.5	7
II		21.0	6	600	1.7	10	3	10	7	3	10	3.3	5	2	5	3.3	6	5.0	14	6
	LIMITED	17.5	5	450	1.7	5	2	10	5	1.7	10	3.3	0	2	0			2.5	10.5	5
III		14.0	4	300	1.7	0			4							2.0	3		7	4
		10.5	3	150					3			2.0	0					0.0	3.5	3
	SYMPTOMATIC	7.0	2						2											2
IV		3.5	1																	1

which work increases constantly and continuously (Figure 2-2). The recent call for "optimizing" exercise testing would appear to be facilitated by the ramp approach, since work increments are small and because it allows for increases in work to be individualized, a given test duration can be targeted.

To investigate this, our laboratory recently compared ramp treadmill and bicycle tests to protocols more commonly used clinically. Ten patients with chronic heart failure, 10 with coronary artery disease who were limited by angina during exercise, 10 with coronary artery disease who were asymptomatic during exercise, and 10 age-matched normal subjects performed three bicycle tests (25 watts/2 min stage, 50 watts/2 min stage, and ramp) and three treadmill tests (Bruce, Balke, and ramp) in randomized order on different days. For the ramp tests, ramp rates on the bicycle and treadmill were individualized to yield a test duration of approximately 10 minutes for each subject. Maximal oxygen uptake was significantly higher (18%) on the treadmill protocols versus the bicycle protocols collectively, findings that confirm previous observations. Only minor differences in maximal oxygen uptake, however, were observed between the treadmill protocols themselves or between the cycle ergometer protocols themselves.

The relationships between oxygen uptake and work rate (predicted oxygen uptake), defined as a slope for each protocol, are illustrated in Table 2-3. These relationships, which reflect the degree of change in oxygen uptake for a given increase in work (a slope of unity would indicate that the cardiopulmonary system is adapting in direct accordance with the demands of the work), were highest for the ramp tests and lowest for the protocols containing the greatest increments in work. Further, the variance about the slope (standard error of the estimate, in oxygen uptake, ml or cc kg/min) was largest for the tests with the largest increments between stages (Bruce treadmill and 50 watts/stage bicycle) and smallest for the ramp tests. These observations indicate that (1) oxygen uptake is overestimated from tests that contain large increments in work and (2) the variability in estimating oxygen uptake from the work rate is much greater on these tests than for an individualized ramp treadmill test.

It is also interesting how oxygen uptake kinetics were influenced by the presence of disease. The oxygen uptake slopes were generally steeper (closer to unity) among normal subjects regardless of the protocol used (Table 2-4). Patients with heart disease had reduced slopes compared with normal subjects, confirming previous investigations. However, we observed a pronounced improvement in the slope of oxygen uptake in these patients when using an individualized protocol. In fact, the response of patients with heart failure was similar to that of normal subjects when both groups performed ramp treadmill tests (Figure 2-3).

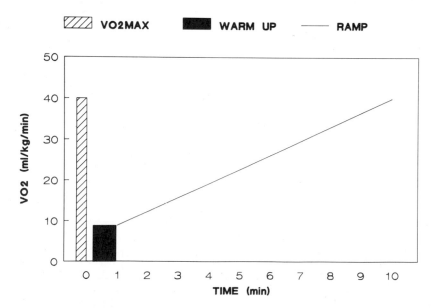

Figure 2-2 Ramp treadmill test. After a 1-minute warm-up at 2.0 mph/0% grade, the rate of change in speed and grade is individualized to yield a work rate (x axis) corresponding to an estimated exercise capacity (y axis) in approximately 10 minutes.

Table 2-3 Slopes in oxygen uptake versus work rate for 40 subjects performing six exercise protocols

	Treadmills			Bicycles		
	Bruce	Balke	Ramp	25 W	50 W	Ramp
Slope	0.62	0.79	0.80	0.69	0.59	0.78
SEE	4.0	3.4	2.5	2.3	2.8	1.7

Each slope ≥ 0.78 was significantly different from each slope ≤ 0.69 ($p < 0.05$ except Balke versus 25 watts, $p = 0.07$). If the change in ventilatory oxygen uptake was equal to the change in work rate, the slope would be equal to 1.0. *SEE*, Standard error of the estimate (ml or cc of O_2/kg/min); 25 W = 25 W/stage; 50 W = W/stage.

Table 2-4 Slopes in oxygen uptake versus work rate for each patient subgroup performing each of the six exercise protocols

	CAD	Angina	CHF	Normal
Slope	0.51	0.53	0.53	0.71*
SEE	2.6	3.1	2.8	4.2

*$p < 0.001$ versus other groups. *CAD*, Coronary artery disease; *CHF*, chronic heart failure; *SEE*, standard error of the estimate (ml or cc of O_2/kg/min). If the change in ventilatory oxygen uptake was equal to the change in work rate, the slope would be equal to 1.0.

Because this approach appears to offer several advantages, we presently perform all our clinical and research testing using the ramp. This approach is empirical, however, and more data from other laboratories are necessary to confirm its utility. Moreover, recent recommendations for individualizing the exercise test depending on the patient tested and the purpose of the test are, of course, taken to an extreme by the individualized ramp approach. To our knowledge, only three equipment manufacturers have developed or are

in the process of developing treadmills that can perform such a test. Nevertheless, recent studies from different laboratories indicate that there may be better ways of testing patients than the traditional, single-protocol approaches.

Walking tests

Guyatt and co-workers[27] point out that bike and treadmill exercise tests can be difficult for many patients with heart failure and may not reflect the capacity to undertake day-to-day activities. Also, walking tests have proved useful as measures of outcome for patients with chronic lung disease. To investigate the potential value of the 6-minute walk as an objective measure of exercise capacity in patients with chronic heart failure, the test was administered six times over 12 weeks to 18 patients with chronic heart failure and 25 with chronic lung disease. The subjects also underwent bike testing, and their functional status was evaluated by means of conventional measures. The walking test proved highly acceptable to the patients, and reproducible results were achieved after the first two walks. The results correlated with the conventional measures of functional status and exercise capacity. The "6-minute" or other walking tests are now frequently incorporated into pharmaceutical trials among patients with heart disease as an additional measure of efficacy.

Submaximal versus maximal exercise testing

Submaximal exercise testing is useful clinically for predischarge postmyocardial infarction evaluations (see Chapter 9) and is a method commonly used for fitness screening evaluations, as in health clubs. Such tests are rather limited for the latter purpose because most of them use an extrapolation of the heart rate response to estimate fitness. A common submaximal cycle ergometer test is outlined by the YMCA, in which work is incre-

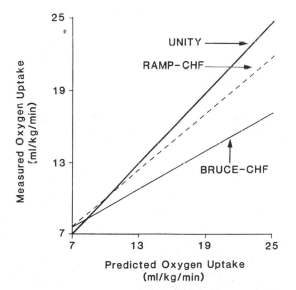

Figure 2-3 Relation between the change in measured and predicted oxygen uptake for the ramp and Bruce treadmill protocols among patients with chronic heart failure (CHF). The unity line is achieved when predicted oxygen uptake is equal to measured oxygen uptake. The regression equation was $y = 0.80x + 2.0$ for the ramp test and $y = 0.54x + 3.8$ ($p < 0.01$ for slope) for the Bruce test.

mented based on the heart rate response up to a submaximal level.[28] Many exercise testing laboratories terminate the test when the patient reaches 85% or 90% of predicted maximal heart rate for age. Unfortunately, there is a wide spread of maximal heart rate around the regression line for age (standard deviation of 12 beats/min). Thus the target heart rate is maximal for some subjects, beyond the limits of some, and submaximal for others. This testing procedure has the advantage that patients can be tested in street shoes and clothes and are not usually uncomfortable, since most patients are not stressed to a maximal effort. When using submaximal tests, there exists a paradox that the most vulnerable patients are stressed to a relatively greater extent whereas the less impaired are limited by submaximal target heart rates. A submaximal test is clinically indicated in patients in the immediate period after myocardial infarction and in patients with dangerous dysrhythmias. In the latter group, even if dysrhythmias are overridden during exercise, they can occur in the postexercise period.

Borg scale. Rather than using heart rate to determine the intensity of exercise, it is preferable to use either the 6-to-20 Borg scale (Table 2-5) or his later, nonlinear 1-to-10 scale of perceived exertion[29,30] (Table 2-6). The 6-to-20 scale was developed by noting that young men could approximate their exercise heart rate if a scale ranging from 60 to 200 was aligned with labels of very, very light for 60 to very, very hard for 200. One zero was dropped and the scale was used for all ages. Because sensory perception of pain or exertion is nonlinear, Borg developed the 1-to-10 scale (Table 2-6).

Skin preparation

Proper skin preparation is essential for the performance of an exercise test. During exercise, because noise increases with the square of resistance, it is extremely important to lower the resistance at the skin-electrode interface and thereby improve the signal-to-noise ratio. It is often difficult to make technicians consistently prepare the skin properly because doing so may cause the patient discomfort and minor skin irritation. The performance of an exercise test with an electrocardiographic signal that cannot be continuously monitored and accurately interpreted because of artifact is worthless and can even be dangerous.

The general areas for electrode placement are cleansed with an alcohol-saturated gauze pad, and then the exact areas for electrode application are marked with a felt-tipped pen. The mark serves as a guide for adequate removal of the superficial layer of skin. The electrodes are placed using anatomic landmarks that are found with the patient supine. Some persons with loose skin can have a considerable shift of electrode positions when they assume an upright position. The next step is to remove the superficial layer of skin either with a hand-held drill or by light abrasion with fine-grained emery paper. Skin resistance should be reduced to 5000 ohms or less, which can be verified before the exercise test with an inexpensive AC impedance meter driven at 10 Hz. A DC meter should not be used, since these can polarize the electrodes. Each electrode is tested against a common electrode with an ohmmeter, and when 5000 ohms or less is not achieved, the electrode must be removed and skin preparation repeated. This maneuver saves time by obviating the need to interrupt a test because of noisy tracings.

Electrodes and cables. The only suitable electrodes are constructed with a metal interface that is sunken to create a column that can be filled

Table 2-5 The linear 6-to-20 Borg scale of perceived exertion or pain

6	
7	Very, very light
8	
9	Very light
10	
11	Fairly light
12	
13	Somewhat hard
14	
15	Hard
16	
17	Very hard
18	
19	Very, very hard
20	

Table 2-6 The nonlinear 0-to-10 Borg scale of perceived exertion or pain

0	Nothing at all	
0.5	Extremely light	(Just noticeable)
1	Very light	
2	Light	(Weak)
3	Moderate	
4	Somewhat heavy	
5	Heavy	(Strong)
6		
7	Very heavy	
8		
9		
10	Extremely heavy	(Almost maximal)
●	Maximal	

with either an electrolyte solution or a saturated sponge. These fluid column electrodes greatly decrease motion artifact as compared with those with direct metal-to-skin contact. There are many disposable electrodes that perform excellently. Silver plate or silver–silver chloride crystal pellets are the best electrode materials. Platinum is too expensive, and the frequently used German silver is actually an alloy. If electrodes of different types of metals are used together, there can be generated an offset voltage that makes it impossible to record an electrocardiogram. The disposable electrodes have the advantages of quick application and no need for cleansing for reuse. They are more expensive to use than nondisposable electrodes, since the better nondisposable electrodes can be used for over 100 tests. A disposable electrode that has an abrasive center that is spun by an applicator after the electrode is attached to the skin called Quickprep is available from Quinton Instrument Company, Seattle. This approach does not require skin preparation. A clever feature of the applicator is a built-in impedance meter that stops it from spinning when the skin impedance has been appropriately lowered.

Developing suitable connecting cables between the electrodes and the recorder has been a problem in gathering exercise ECG data. The earliest versions of these cables were subject to wire continuity problems, frequent failures, and motion artifact; they were improperly shielded and utilized inadequate connectors. Shielding of the electrode wires and cables is especially important in metropolitan areas or near high-voltage x-ray equipment. Several commercial companies have concentrated on solving these problems, and now there are exercise cables available that are constructed to avoid these problems. Buffer amplifiers carried by the patient are no longer advantageous. Cables develop continuity problems over time with use and require replacement rather than repair. We often find replacement to be necessary after 500 tests. Some systems have utilized analog-to-digital converters carried by the patient in the electrode junction box. Digital signals are relatively impervious to noise, and so the patient cable can be unshielded and is very light.

Lead systems. Electrodes have been placed in a variety of ways using many different lead systems. This situation has complicated making comparisons of the ST-segment response to exercise. The four major exercise electrocardiographic lead systems are the bipolar, the Mason-Likar 12-lead, a simulation of Wilson's central terminal, and the three-dimensional (orthogonal or nonorthogonal systems).

Bipolar lead systems have been used because of the relatively short time required for placement, the relative freedom from motion artifact, and the ease with which noise problems can be located. Figure 2-4 illustrates the electrode placements for most of the bipolar lead systems. The usual positive reference is an electrode placed the same as the positive reference for V_5. The negative reference for V_5 is Wilson's central terminal, which consists in connecting the limb electrodes—right arm (RA), left arm (LA), and left leg (LL). The only other notable bipolar lead system is the roving bipolar lead, which was introduced by McHenry. In this system, beginning with a CC_5 placement, the electrodes are moved around to obtain the maximal R-wave with a small S-wave.

The problem with comparing the results of ST-segment analysis if different leads are used has been demonstrated by a computer analysis study.[31] ST-segment depression and slope measurements were made on signals gathered simultaneously from CC_5, CM_5, and V_5. A common positive reference electrode was used. CM_5 consistently had a more negative J-junction and a more positive slope than V_5 and CC_5 did, whereas V_5 and CC_5 were essentially identical on the basis of standard analysis but differed statistically when computer measurements were compared. This difference in the leads most likely explains why investigators using CM_5 have reported an inadequate ST slope to be as serious as horizontal depression. Specific ST-segment responses relative to test sensitivity and different lead systems is presented in more detail in Chapter 6.

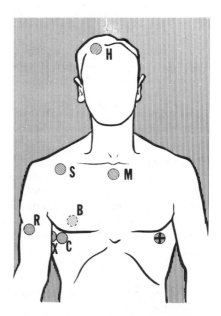

Figure 2-4   The common bipolar ECG leads used during exercise testing.

Vector leads. There are several three-dimensional or vectorcardiographic lead systems that can be used during exercise. The corrected Frank lead system has the advantage that the electrical activity of the heart is orthogonally represented in the three derived signals. The relative ease of placement of only seven electrodes required for the Frank system has made it the most popular orthogonal lead system. Care should be taken so that the X and Z electrodes are placed as described by Frank in his original paper, at the fifth intercostal space level and the sternum. The vectorcardiographic (VCG) approach makes it possible to evaluate the spatial changes of the ST segment vector. The Frank X is a left precordial lead but is about 25% smaller in amplitude in V_5 because of the Frank network resistance, which is an attempt to electrically move the heart to the center of the chest. However, ST-segment criteria have not been adjusted for this. When using both the 12-lead and Frank systems, several electrodes can be shared. V_4 and V_6 are I and A, LF can also be F, and in this way 14 electrodes can be used to obtain both systems.

The Dalhousie square is a simple way to assist with the proper and reproducible placement of the Frank electrodes and of the Wilson precordial electrodes.[32] It is a simple right-angled device that is held to the chest. Proper placement is necessary for the application of ECG/VCG interpretive criteria. Reproducible placement is essential for assessment of serial changes.

Mason-Likar electrode placement. Since a 12-lead ECG could not be obtained accurately during exercise with electrodes placed on the wrists and ankles, Mason and Likar suggested that adhesive electrodes be placed at the base of the limbs for exercise testing. In addition to providing a noise-free exercise tracing, their modified placement apparently showed no differences in electrocardiographic configuration when compared to the standard limb-lead placement. However, this has been disputed by others who have found that the Mason-Likar placement causes amplitude changes and axis shifts when compared to standard placement. Since this could lead to diagnostic changes, it has been recommended that the modified exercise electrode placement not be used for recording a resting ECG. The preexercise test ECG has been further complicated by the recommendation that it should be obtained standing, since that is the same position maintained during exercise. This is worsened by the common practice of moving the limb electrodes onto the chest in order to minimize motion artifact.

It is clinically important to obtain an accurate preexercise ECG, because it should be compared to previous tracings in order to see if any changes have occurred, and to use it as a baseline ECG for testing. We hypothesized that much of the confusion regarding distortion of the preexercise ECG has been attributable to misplacement of limb electrodes medially on the torso and by obtaining the ECG in the standing position. Therefore we compared 12-lead ECGs utilizing the standard limb placement (electrodes on wrists and ankles) to two modified exercise placements in the supine and standing positions in the same patients.[33]

Figure 2-5 illustrates the Mason-Likar torso-mounted limb lead system. The conventional ankle and wrist electrodes are replaced by electrodes mounted on the torso at the base of the limbs. In this way, the artifact introduced by movement of the limbs is avoided. The standard precordial leads use Wilson's central terminal as their negative reference, which is formed by connecting the right arm, left arm, and left leg. This triangular configuration around the heart results in a zero voltage reference through the cardiac cycle. The use of Wilson's central terminal for the precordial leads (V leads) requires the negative reference to be a combination of three additional electrodes rather than the single electrode used as the negative reference for bipolar leads. Simulation of Wilson's central terminal by other combinations of electrodes has not been validated, and therefore such alternative configurations should be avoided.

The UCSD electrode placement. Before exercise testing, 104 male patients with stable coronary heart disease were studied.[33] Included were 30

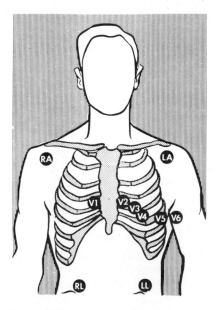

Figure 2-5   Mason-Likar simulated standard 12-lead ECG electrode placement for exercise testing.

men with ECG criteria for an inferior myocardial infarction, 13 with anterior myocardial infarction, five with diagnostic Q-waves in multiple locations, six with right bundle branch block (three with diagnostic Q-waves), 33 with other abnormalities, and 17 with normal ECGs. Just before a treadmill test, each patient had 12-lead ECGs recorded with lead placements as illustrated in Figure 2-6. The four electrode placements included placement 1—the standard limb lead electrode placement on the wrist and ankles, supine ("standard"); placement 2—arm electrodes placed medially on the torso, 2 cm below the midpoint of the clavicle and leg electrodes below the umbilicus ("misplaced"); placement 3—the "correct" Mason-Likar placement with the arm electrodes placed at the base of the shoulders against the deltoid border 2 cm below the clavicle and with the leg electrodes the same as placement 2 with the patient supine ("exercise-supine"); and placement 4—the same as placement 3 except with the patient standing ("exercise-standing"). In addition, the Frank X, Y, Z leads were recorded at the same time as the exercise-supine and exercise-standing ECGs.

The tracings were read by two blinded observers looking for definite diagnostic changes that might be clinically important (including "new" Q-waves in aV_L or III), and other obvious changes. Q-waves were considered diagnostic if they were 25% or greater of the following R-wave amplitude and 40 msec or longer in duration. Visual analysis of each of the 104 patients' four ECGs were performed independently and by consensus of two observers. The tracings were interpreted separately and then compared to the standard limb lead ECG to search for "serial" changes in the other three tracings.

Differences between the standard limb lead ECG and the other ECGs were grouped into three categories: (1) diagnostic changes, (2) important changes, and (3) other obvious changes (Table 2-7). The category "diagnostic changes" contained tracings whose waveforms had changed by alteration of the lead placement or by standing such that the diagnosis was different from that of the supine limb lead ECG. In all cases except one, the change in diagnosis was either the loss or appearance of an inferior infarct. The one exception was a standing tracing that the change in position had caused an anterior infarct pattern to disappear. The "exercise standing" placement had a total of 12 diagnostic changes: seven where a new diagnosis of inferior infarct was made; four where an inferior infarct diagnosis was lost; and the aforementioned exception of losing an anterior infarct diagnosis. The "misplaced" electrode placement had six diagnostic changes: one where the criteria for an inferior infarct was reached and five where it was lost. The "supine exercise" placement had three diagnostic changes, all showing a loss of the criteria for an inferior infarct compared to the standard ECG.

The category "important changes" comprised changes that may be clinically important but do not of themselves alter the electrocardiographic diagnosis. Such changes included significant Q-waves in III or aV_L alone, ST-segment and T-wave changes such as flipped or flattened T-waves or ST-segment depression, and one instance of a Q-wave appearing in V_6. The "misplaced exercise" placement had 19 important changes: eight where a new Q-wave appeared in aV_L, seven where a Q-wave in only III disappeared, three where a Q in III appeared, two ST-

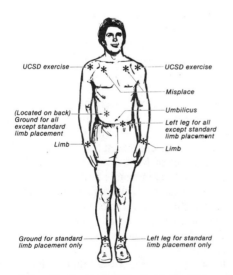

Figure 2-6 Electrode placement of the University of California, San Diego (UCSD) study of the effects of limb lead placement and standing on the routine ECG.

Table 2-7 Differences noted by standard visual interpretation between exercise-test electrode placements and standard supine electrocardiogram*

	Misplaced	Exercise-standing	Exercise-supine
Diagnostic changes	6	12	3
Important changes	19	12	7
Other obvious changes	3	6	0
Total changes	28	30	10

*See the text for an explanation of the changes.

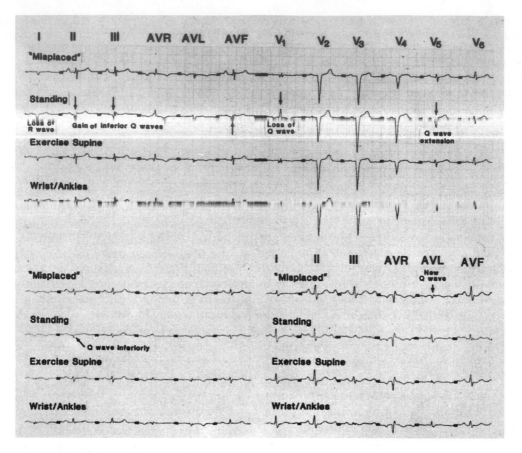

Figure 2-7 Examples of the artifact seen in the preexercise test 12-lead ECG study.

segment or T-wave changes, and one where a Q appeared in aV_L. The "exercise-supine" placement had seven important changes: four where a Q in III disappeared, one where it appeared, and two where a Q in aV_L appeared. Figure 2-7 illustrates the changes seen in three patients; in the bottom two tracings changes occurred only in the limb leads.

QRS frontal axis means, standard deviations, and differences analyzed by computer for the four electrode placements are given in Table 2-8. When compared to the standard electrode placement, "misplaced" showed an average of 26 degrees of deviation to the right ($p < 0.01$), "supine-exercise" showed an average of 9 degrees of rightward deviation (not significant), and "standing-exercise" showed an average of 3 degrees of deviation to the left (not significant). "Standing-exercise" showed the greatest amount of variability, with a standard deviation of +53 degrees.

Other electrode-placement studies. Kleiner and co-workers compared ECGs gathered on 75 patients using the standard wrist and ankle place-

ment to the Mason-Likar placement.[34] Fifty of the 75 patients had a rightward axis shift of 30 degrees or more on the modified ECG compared to the standard. In addition, 11 of these patients had a rightward shift in axis on their modified ECG that resulted in Q-wave and T-wave inversion in lead aV_L without prior history of myocardial infarction by ECG. Seventeen patients had diagnostic criteria for an old inferior myocardial infarction, and seven (41%) of them had these criteria erased by the rightward axis shift on the modified placement. They cautioned that the modified exercise placement of Mason and Likar should not be considered interchangeable with the standard electrodes placement. However, it was not stated where the shoulder electrodes were placed or if the modified ECG was recorded supine or standing. Rautaharju and co-workers[35] came to a similar conclusion.

The preexercise ECG is further complicated by positional differences when it is recorded. Shapiro and colleagues studied the differences between supine and sitting Frank lead vectorcardiograms

Table 2-8 Computer analysis of QRS axis measured in frontal plane presented as mean values, standard deviation, mean of the differences, and standard deviation of the difference*

	Standard	Supine-exercise	Misplaced	Standing-exercise
Mean	18	27	44	18
Standard deviation	43	48	48	53
Mean difference		9	26	−3
Standard deviation of the differences		36	41	48
Significant difference		NS	$p < 0.01$	NS

*The differences are presented as modified ECG measurements minus standrd limb electrode placement measurements. Only the "misplaced" electrode placement measurements were significantly different from standard electrode placement measurements.

in 59 adult male patients with suspected coronary artery disease.[36] They observed that QRS spatial and R-wave amplitudes in lead Z were significantly higher and R amplitudes in lead Y lower for sitting than for supine positions. They concluded that the preexercise ECG should be obtained before the test with the patient in the same position as that maintained during exercise. Other studies have also shown differences between ECGs taken supine versus sitting or standing. Sigler studied 100 patients and found a tendency for the QRS axis to shift to the left for abnormal tracings and to the right for normal tracings when changing from supine to standing.[37] Dougherty correlated changes in the frontal-plane QRS axis with changes in heart position measured with a chest x-ray film brought about by moving from supine to standing.[38] He found that every degree of positional heart change caused a 3-degree shift in QRS frontal axis throughout the normal range in the same direction. A higher prevalence of false-positive polar cardiographic criteria for myocardial infarction was found standing than supine by Bruce and co-workers in 72 normal men and women.[39]

Another complicating factor is the effect of respiration on inferior Q-waves. Because it was suggested that inspiration caused a Q in III to diminish or disappear in normal subjects and to persist among patients with inferior myocardial infarction, Mimbs and colleagues studied the effect of respiration on the Q in III in normals and patients with documented inferior myocardial infarction.[40] They found that the Q in III decreased on inspiration in 82% of the patients with a recent myocardial infarction and in 44% of patients with an old infarction. In eight normals with a Q in III, only one showed a decrease in amplitude and others showed no change. They concluded that the effect of inspiration on the ECG was variable though they did not report specific amplitude changes.

As part of a thorough study of 194 patients,

Riekkinen and Rautaharju analyzed the effects of respiration and sitting on the vectorcardiogram.[41] Because of the great variability of the changes, rarely with any significant differences in the means, they reported the percentage of patients who increased or decreased specific values beyond an arbitrary threshold. The changes with deep inspiration were much more prominent than deep expiration. With inspiration, 35% of the patients had a posterior shift in the horizontal plane, and 8% had an anterior shift; 45% had a rightward shift in the frontal plane, and 3% had a leftward shift. R-wave amplitude in lead Z decreased a mean of 0.5 mV, Q-wave amplitude decreased, and the QRS-T angle increased. During sitting, R-wave amplitude increased in Z, Q-wave amplitude decreased in Y, and the mean QRS maximal spatial magnitude increased. Sitting also caused 26% of patients to have posterior shift in the horizontal plane and 10% to have anterior shifts, 15% had rightward and 10% had leftward shifts in the frontal plane, and 36% had an increase in the QRS-T angle.

The results of the UCSD lead study clarify much of the confusion regarding the preexercise test electrocardiogram. Misplacement of the Mason-Likar arm leads is common and has even been published as the correct exercise modification. When the leads are placed medially, near the midclavicular line, it has been shown that the frontal plane axis shifts rightward on the average of 26 degrees. This shift caused decreased amplitudes in the Q in III and in the R in I and aV_L and caused increased amplitudes in the Q in aV_L and in the R-waves in II, III, and aV_F. Of clinical importance is what these shifts did to the visual interpretation of the ECG. In five patients the ECG diagnosis of old inferior infarct was lost. In addition, seven patients lost significant Q-waves in III alone. There were instances of Q-waves gained. Eight patients had no Q-waves in aV_L; one had a new Q in III, one with a new Q in II, one with a new Q in V_6; and one patient gained an inferior infarct diagnosis. Although these "serial" changes are merely artifacts produced by electrode misplacement, they could be very misleading. The changes caused by misplaced electrode arrangement were very similar to those reported by Kleiner.

Standing can cause many changes in the visual interpretation of the electrocardiogram including those that would be most alarming, that is, appearance of new Q-waves (particularly inferiorly). The misplacement of the arm electrodes in the midclavicular area also cause many clinical changes including the appearance of Q-waves in aV_L as well as large axis shifts and amplitude changes. The correct Mason and Likar modification can also cause amplitude and duration changes, but they are less clinically important than the aforementioned ones. The modified exercise electrode placement should not be used for routine electrocardiography. However, the changes caused by the exercise electrode placement can be kept to a minimum if one keeps the arm electrodes off the chest and puts them on the shoulders while having the patient supine. In this situation, the modified exercise limb lead placement of Mason and Likar can serve well as the reference resting ECG before an exercise test.

Relative sensitivity of leads. Numerous studies comparing the relative sensitivity of different ECG leads were reported in the 1970s. Robertson and associates reported their results using 12-lead exercise tests in 39 patients with both abnormal exercise tests and abnormal coronary angiograms.[42] Eighteen percent had an abnormal response in leads other than V_5. Patients with right coronary artery lesions usually showed ST-segment depression in inferior leads, and patients with left coronary system lesions usually showed ST-segment depression in leads I and aV_L and in the chest leads. However, almost a third of the patients showed ST-segment depression in leads other than those anticipated from their angiographic anatomy. Tucker and colleagues reported 12-lead exercise test results in 100 consecutive patients who were also studied with coronary angiography.[43] Forty-eight had abnormal tests, with 30% of the abnormal responses occurring in leads other than V_5 (17% in aV_F and 13% in other leads). Two false-positive results occurred in V_5 and two in aV_F, whereas 16 true-positive results occurred in leads other than V_5 or aV_F. Of those abnormal in aV_F alone, five had lesions in the right coronary or left circumflex artery and two had disease in the left anterior descending artery.

Chaitman and colleagues reported the role of multiple-lead electrocardiographic systems and clinical subsets in interpreting treadmill test results.[44] Two hundred men with normal ECGs at rest had a maximal treadmill test using 14 ECG leads and then underwent coronary angiography. This study included standard leads plus three bipolar leads. The prevalence of significant *coronary stenosis* was 86% in 87 men with typical angina, 65% in 64 men with probable angina, and 28% in 49 men with nonspecific chest pain. The predictive value of *ST-segment deviation* in any one of 14 leads was 45% in men with nonspecific chest pain versus 70% in men with probable angina, and 55% in men with typical angina. In the latter, recording a single lead such as CM_5 was adequate. In men with typical or probable angina, a normal response in 14 leads associated with treadmill work time longer than 9 minutes reduced the chance of three-vessel disease to less than 10%. The likelihood of multivessel disease in a patient with an abnormal ST response and a treadmill time equal to or less than 3 minutes was approximately 90%. In patients with angina, the use of 14 leads increased sensitivity over that of V_5 alone from 52% and 65% to 75%. This value was increased even further to 86% by the additional consideration of bipolar leads.

Miranda and associates[45] recently studied 178 males who had undergone both exercise testing and coronary angiography to evaluate the diagnostic value of ST-segment depression occurring in the inferior leads. Lead V_5 had a better sensitivity (65%) and specificity (84%) than that of lead II (sensitivity and specificity 71% and 44% respectively) at a single cut point. Receiver operating characteristic curve analysis demonstrated that lead V_5 (area = 0.759) was greatly superior to lead II (area = 0.582) over multiple cut points. Moreover, the area under the curve in lead II was not significantly greater than 0.50, an indication that, for the identification of coronary artery disease, isolated ST-segment depression in lead II is unreliable.

It remains to be demonstrated what the specificity of leads other than V_5 eventually will be, but one has the impression that inferior leads have more false-positive results and may require different criteria. This apparent lack of specificity may be attributable to the effect of atrial repolarization in inferior leads, which causes depression of the ST-segment. With adequate experience, atrial repolarization can be recognized as causing ST segment depression. The end of the PR segment can be seen to be depressed in a curved fashion to the same level that the ST segment begins. Such findings also support the concept of intercoronary artery steal during exercise; that is, ischemic areas obtain blood flow through collaterals. This phenomenon makes it impossible for ST-segment depression with multi-lead exercise testing to allow prediction of the location of coronary artery occlusions.

Body-surface mapping studies in normal subjects

The normal repolarization response to exercise using large electrode arrays has been described by Mirvis and co-workers[46] and by Miller and co-workers.[47] Mirvis and co-workers used a 42-electrode left precordial lead system in 15 normal volunteers during supine exercise. Analyses of the exercise isopotential maps revealed a minimum during the early portions of the ST segment located below the standard V_3 and V_4 chest positions with negative potentials involving most of the precordial region. Isopotential "difference" maps were constructed by subtraction of potentials at the beginning of the ST from potentials later in the ST. These maps characterized the direction and magnitude of ST-segment slopes and revealed upsloping ST segments over regions of negative ST potentials.

Miller and co-workers obtained total thoracic surface exercise maps in 20 normal subjects, recording from 24 electrode sites and deriving the remaining potentials at 150 locations using previously developed mathematical transformations. Isopotential maps during the early ST segment were less negative than those described by Mirvis and co-workers primarily because of Miller's "zero" reference potential. The end of the PR segment was chosen in contrast to that of Mirvis, who used the ST segment (which shortens when heart rate increases). Exercise isopotential maps in normals were characterized by a left anterior maximum during ST-T.

Studies of patients with coronary artery disease

Fox and colleagues from London have used very simple exercise ECG mapping techniques to detect myocardial ischemia.[48] Using a 16-lead precordial map and visual interpretation of the scaler ECG data, contour maps were drawn for each patient illustrating regions on the precordial surface where significant ST-segment depression was observed. The first study involved 100 patients undergoing coronary angiography for evaluation of chest pain. In that study the sensitivity of the precordial mapping technique (96%) for diagnosing coronary disease was better than the modified 12 leads (80%), using 0.1 mV horizontal ST-segment depression as being abnormal. This improved sensitivity was attributed to the improved recognition of patients with single vessel disease.

Also of interest was the regional localization of the ischemic ST contours in single vessel disease. ST-segment depression involving the uppermost horizontal row of electrodes was highly specific for proximal left anterior descending or left-main coronary artery disease. This was done without a loss in specificity (90%).

In a second exercise study involving 200 patients undergoing coronary angiography Fox and others again compared the 12-lead ECG to a 16-lead map and found that the standard precordial leads sampled only 41% of the ST-segment depression projected to the front of the chest.[49] In only 7% of patients, however, was the ST-segment depression not apparent in the standard precordial leads. The rightmost column of electrodes never recorded ST-segment depression that was not seen in one or more of the remaining 12 electrodes on the precordial surface. The authors concluded that these 12 precordial leads along with the standard limb leads would optimize the detection of ST-segment changes.

Yanowitz and co-workers at the University of Utah has reported using a 32-lead electrode array to derive torso potential distributions at 192 locations by means of a mathematical transformation.[50] He evaluated this system during exercise testing in 25 patients with documented coronary artery disease. In this study the distribution of 80 msec ST-segment isochoric (equal-area) contours (ST80 isochoric maps) was plotted and compared to the standard precordial leads. He found that in 25% of patients with ischemic ECG changes the maximal ST change was located at sites distant to the standard leads. In addition, there was some evidence of localization in patients with single vessel disease.

Simoons and Block recorded exercise body surface maps in 25 normal subjects and 25 patients with coronary disease using a system of 120 thoracic surface electrodes.[51] Evaluation of normal subjects revealed a low-level (less than 90 μV) precordial minimum during early ST followed by the development of a prominent maximum later in the ST-T wave, similar to the observations of Miller and co-workers. In the coronary patients, exercise maps frequently showed a prolonged negative area in the precordium with varying locations of the minimum. There was no relation between the specific ST isopotential distributions and either the coronary anatomy or the location of thallium scan defects. The maps, however, were more sensitive (84%) in detecting abnormal repolarization patterns in coronary patients as compared to the 12-lead exercise ECG (60%), using a ST-segment minimum of >90 μV at 60 msec after the J-point as the criterion for an abnormal map. None of the normal subjects had negative ST potentials of this magnitude (specificity of 100%).

It is oversimplistic to consider ST-segment mapping data as having the ability to directly quantitate ischemic myocardium. The physiological mechanisms responsible for ST-segment (and TQ segment) shifts in ischemic injury are complex and depend on the shape and location of the ischemic region in relation to the electrode sites on the body surface. Since currents of injury primarily occur at the boundaries between normal and abnormal tissue, cancellation of forces will likely distort the relationships between body-surface ST-segment changes and the degree of ischemia. The subendocardial and nontransmural locations of most exercise-induced ischemia make it unreasonable to expect that body-surface ECG recordings would reflect the extent, magnitude, and location of the ischemic tissues.

Experimental confirmation of these concerns has been provided by Mirvis and co-workers.[52] Body-surface maps were obtained in dogs with previously placed amaroid constrictors around one of the three major coronary arteries. Reversible myocardial ischemia was induced by atrial pacing. Although the location of the ischemic repolarization abnormalities on the maps varied with the particular artery involved, significant spatial overlap was observed so as to preclude any identification of discrete ischemic zones unique to a given arterial lesion. These findings as well as the added cost of specialized recorders and more electrodes leave mapping as a research tool without much clinical applicability.

Number of leads to record

In patients with normal resting ECGs, a V_5 or similar bipolar lead along the long axis of the heart usually is adequate. In patients with ECG evidence of myocardial damage or with a history suggestive of coronary spasm, additional leads are needed. As a minimal approach, it is advisable to record three leads: a V_5 type of lead, an anterior V_2 type of lead, and an inferior lead such as aV_F; or Frank X, Y, and Z leads may be used. This approach is also helpful for the detection and identification of dysrhythmias. It is advisable also to record a second three-lead grouping consisting of V_4, V_5, and V_6. Occasionally, abnormalities may be seen as borderline in V_5, whereas they will be clearly abnormal in V_4 or V_6. The medical electronics industry has made 12 leads the standard available in all machines.

Postexercise period

If maximal sensitivity is to be achieved with an exercise test, patients should be supine during the postexercise period. It is advisable to record about 10 seconds of electrocardiographic data while the patient is standing motionless but still experiencing near maximal heart rate and then to have the patient lie down. Some patients must be allowed to lie down immediately to avoid hypotension. Having the patient perform a cool-down walk after the test can delay or eliminate the appearance of ST-segment depression.[53] According to the law of Laplace, the increase in venous return and thus ventricular volume in the supine position increases myocardial oxygen demand. Recent data from our laboratory[54] indicates that having patients lie down may enhance ST-segment abnormalities in recovery. However, a cool-down walk has been suggested to minimize the postexercise chances for dysrhythmic events in this high-risk time when catecholamines are high. The supine position after exercise is not so important when the test is not being performed for diagnostic purposes. When testing is not performed for diagnostic purposes, it may be preferable to walk slowly (1.0 to 1.5 mph) or continue cycling against zero or minimal resistance (0 to 25 watts when one is testing with a cycle ergometer) for several minutes after the test.

Monitoring should continue for at least 6 to 8 minutes after exercise or until changes stabilize. In the supine position 4 to 5 minutes into recovery, approximately 85% of patients with abnormal responses in a large series were abnormal at this time only or in addition to other times. An abnormal response occurring only in the recovery period is not unusual. All such responses are not false-positive results, as has been suggested. Experiments confirm mechanical dysfunction and electrophysiologic abnormalities in the ischemic ventricle after exercise. A cool-down walk can be helpful when one is performing tests on patients with an established diagnosis undergoing testing for other than diagnostic reasons, when testing athletes, or when patients have dangerous dysrhythmias.

Indications for treadmill test termination

The absolute and relative indications for termination of an exercise test listed in Table 2-1 have been derived from clinical experience. Absolute indications are clearcut, whereas relative indications can sometimes be disregarded if good clinical judgment is used. Absolute indications include a drop in systolic blood pressure despite an increase in work load, anginal chest pain becoming worse than usual, central nervous system symptoms, signs of poor perfusion (such as pallor, cyanosis, and cold skin), serious dysrhythmias, technical problems with monitoring the patient, patient's request to stop, and pronounced electrocardiographic changes, such as more than 0.3 mV of horizontal or downsloping ST-segment depression, and 0.2 mV of ST-segment elevation. Relative indications for termination include other worrisome ST or QRS changes such as excessive junctional depression; increasing chest pain; fatigue, shortness of breath, wheezing, leg cramps, or intermittent claudication; worrisome appearance, hypertensive response (systolic pressure greater than 260 mm Hg, diastolic pressure greater than 115 mm Hg), and less serious dysrhythmias including supraventricular tachycardias. In some patients estimated to be at high risk by their clinical history, it may be appropriate to stop at a submaximal level, since the most severe ST-segment depression or dysrhythmias may occur only after exercise. If more information is required, the test can be repeated later.

SUMMARY

Utilization of proper methodology is critical to patient safety and for obtainment of accurate results. Preparing the patient physically and emotionally for testing is necessary. Good skin preparation must cause some discomfort but is necessary for good conductance and to avoid artifacts. The use of specific criteria for exclusion and termination, physician interaction with the patient, and appropriate emergency equipment are essential. A brief physical exam is always necessary to rule out significant aortic valve disease. Pretest standard 12-lead ECGs are needed in both the supine and standing positions. The changes caused by exercise electrode placement can be kept to a minimum if one keeps the arm electrodes off the chest, places them on the shoulders, and records the pretest reference ECG with the patient supine. In this situation, the modified exercise limb lead placement of Mason and Likar can serve well as the reference resting ECG before an exercise test.

Few studies have correctly evaluated the relative yield or sensitivity and specificity of different electrode placements for exercise-induced ST-segment shifts. Studies show that using other leads in addition to V_5 will increase the sensitivity; however, the specificity is decreased. ST-segment changes isolated to the inferior leads are often false-positive responses. Vectorcardiographic and body-surface mapping lead systems do not appear to offer any advantage over simpler approaches for clinical purposes.

The exercise protocol should be progressive with equal increments in speed and grade whenever possible. Smaller, even, and more frequent work increments are preferable to larger, uneven, and less frequent increases because the former yield a more accurate estimation of exercise ca-

pacity. The value of individualizing the exercise protocol, rather than using the same protocol for every patient, has recently been emphasized by many investigators. The optimal test duration is from 8 to 12 minutes, and so the protocol work loads should be adjusted to permit this duration. Because ramp testing uses small increments, it permits a more accurate estimation of exercise capacity and can be individualized for every patient to yield a targeted test duration. As yet, however, only a few equipment companies manufacture a controller that performs such tests using a treadmill.

Target heart rates based on age should not be used because the relationship between maximal heart rate and age is poor, and there is wide scatter around many different recommended regression lines. Such heart rate targets result in a submaximal test for some individuals, a maximal test for some, and an unrealistic goal for others. The Borg scales are an excellent means of quantifying an individual's effort. Exercise capacity should not be reported in total time but rather as the VO_2 or MET equivalent of the work load achieved. This permits the comparison of the results of many different exercise testing protocols. Hyperventilation should be avoided before testing. Subjects both with and without disease may or may not exhibit ST-segment changes with hyperventilation; the value of this procedure in lessening the number of false-positive responders is no longer considered useful by most researchers. The postexercise period is critical diagnostically, and the patient should be placed in the supine position immediately after testing for this reason.

REFERENCES

1. Rochmis P, Blackburn H: Exercise tests: a survey of procedures, safety, and litigation experience in approximately 170,000 tests, *JAMA* 217:1061-1066, 1971.
2. Gibbons L, Blair SN, Kohl HW, Cooper K: The safety of maximal exercise testing, *Circulation* 80:846-852, 1989.
3. Yang JC, Wesley RC, Froelicher VF: Ventricular tachycardia during routine treadmill testing, *Arch Intern Med* 151:349-353, 1991.
4. Irving JB, Bruce RA: Exertional hypotension and post exertional ventricular fibrillation in stress testing, *Am J Cardiol* 39:849-851, 1977.
5. Shepard RJ: Do risks of exercise justify costly caution? *Physician and Sports Med* 5:58, 1977.
6. Cobb LA, Weaver WD: Exercise: a risk for sudden death in patients with coronary heart disease, *J Am Coll Cardiol* 7:215-219, 1986.
7. Schlant R, Friesinger GC, Leonard JJ, et al: Clinical competence in exercise testing: a statement for physicians from the ACP/ACC/AHA task force on clinical privileges in cardiology, *Ann Intern Med* 107:588-589, 1987.
8. Balady GJ, Schick EC, Weiner DA, et al: Comparison of determinants of myocardial oxygen consumption during arm and leg exercise in normal persons, *Am J Cardiol* 57:1385-1387, 1986.
9. Balady GJ, Weiner DA, McCabe CH, et al: Value of arm

exercise testing in detecting coronary artery disease, *Am J Cardiol* 55:37-39, 1985.

10. Myers J, Froelicher VF: Optimizing the exercise test for pharmacological investigations, *Circulation* 82:1839-1846, 1990.

11. Hermansen L, Saltin B: Oxygen uptake during maximal treadmill and bicycle exercise, *J Appl Physiol* 26:31-37, 1969.

12. Buchfuhrer MJ, Hansen JE, Robinson TE, et al: Optimizing the exercise protocol for cardiopulmonary assessment, *J Appl Physiol* 55:1558-1564, 1983.

13. Myers J, Buchanan N, Walsh D, et al: Comparison of the ramp versus standard exercise protocols, *J Am Coll Cardiol* 17:1334-1342, 1991.

14. Niederberger M, Bruce RA, Kusumi F, Whitkanack S: Disparities in ventilatory and circulatory responses to bicycle and treadmill exercise, *Br Heart J* 36:377, 1974.

15. Wicks JR, Sutton JR, Oldridge NB, Jones NL: Comparison of the electrocardiographic changes induced by maximum exercise testing with treadmill and cycle ergometer, *Circulation* 57:1066-1069, 1978.

16. Balke B, Ware R: An experimental study of physical fitness of air force personnel, *US Armed Forces Med J* 10:675-688, 1959.

17. Åstrand PO, Rodahl K: *Textbook of work physiology,* New York, 1986, McGraw-Hill, pp 331-365.

18. Bruce RA: Exercise testing of patients with coronary heart disease, *Ann Clin Res* 3:323-330, 1971.

19. Ellestad MH, Allen W, Wan MCK, Kemp G: Maximal treadmill stress testing for cardiovascular evaluation, *Circulation* 39:517-522, 1969.

20. Stuart RJ, Ellestad MH: National survey of exercise stress testing facilities, *Chest* 77:94-97, 1980.

21. Sullivan M, McKirnan MD: Errors in predicting functional capacity for postmyocardial infarction patients using a modified Bruce protocol, *Am Heart J* 107:486-491, 1984.

22. Webster MWI, Sharpe DN: Exercise testing in angina pectoris: the importance of protocol design in clinical trials, *Am Heart J* 117:505-508, 1989.

23. Panza JA, Quyyumi AA, Diodati JG, et al: Prediction of the frequency and duration of ambulatory myocardial ischemia in patients with stable coronary artery disease by determination of the ischemic threshold from exercise testing: importance of the exercise protocol, *J Am Coll Cardiol* 17:657-663, 1991.

24. Redwood DR, Rosing DR, Goldstein RE, et al: Importance of the design of an exercise protocol in the evaluation of patients with angina pectoris, *Circulation* 43:618-628, 1971.

25. Smokler PE, MacAlpin RN, Alvaro A, Kattus AA: Reproducibility of a multi-stage near maximal treadmill test for exercise tolerance in angina pectoris, *Circulation* 48:346-351, 1973.

26. Lipkin DP, Canepa-Anson R, Stephens MR, Poole-Wilson PA: Factors determining symptoms in heart failure: comparison of fast and slow exercise tests, *Br Heart J* 55:439-445, 1986.

27. Guyatt GH, Sullivan MJ, Thompson PJ, et al: The six-minute walk: a new measure of exercise capacity in patients with chronic heart failure, *Can Med Assoc J* 132:919-923, 1985.

28. Golding LA, Myers CR, Sinning WE, editors: *The Y's way to physical fitness,* ed 3, Champaign, Ill, 1989, Human Kinetics.

29. Borg G: Perceived exertion as an indicator of somatic stress, *Scand J Rehabil Med* 23:92-93, 1970.

30. Borg G, Holmgren A, Lindblad I: Quantitative evalution of chest pain, *Acta Med Scand* 644:43-45, 1981.

31. Froelicher VF, Wolthuis R, Keiser N, et al: A comparison of two bipolar electrocardiographic leads to lead V$_5$, *Chest* 70:611, 1976.

32. Rautaharju PM, Wolf HK, Eifler WJ, Blackburn H: A simple procedure of positioning precordial ECG and VCG electrodes using an electrode locator, *J Electrocardiol* 9:35-40, 1976.

33. Gamble P, McManus H, Jensen D, Froelicher VF: A comparison of the standard 12-lead electrocardiogram to exercise electrode placements, *Chest* 85:616-622, 1984.

34. Kleiner JP, Nelson WP, Boland MJ: The 12-lead electrocardiogram in exercise testing, *Arch Intern Med* 138:1572-1573, 1978.

35. Rautaharju PM, Prineas RJ, Crow RS, et al: The effect of modified limb positions on electrocardiographic wave amplitudes, *J Electrocardiol* 13:109-114, 1980.

36. Shapiro W, Berson AS, Pipberger HV: Differences between supine and sitting Frank-lead electrocardiograms, *J Electrocardiol* 9:303-308, 1976.

37. Sigler LH: Electrocardiographic changes occurring with alterations of posture from recumbent to standing positions, *Am Heart J* 15:146-152, 1938.

38. Dougherty JD: Change in the frontal QRS axis with changes in the anatomic positions of the heart, *J Electrocardiol* 8:299-311, 1970.

39. Bruce RA, Detry JM, Early K, et al: Polarcardiographic responses to maximal exercise in healthy young adults, *Am Heart J* 83:206-212, 1972.

40. Mimbs JW, deMello V, Roberts R: The effect of respiration on normal and abnormal Q-waves, *Am Heart J* 94:579-584, 1977.

41. Reikkinen H, Rautaharju P: Body position, electrode level, and respiration effects on the Frank lead electrocardiogram, *Circulation* 53(1):40-45, 1976.

42. Robertson D, Kostuk WJ, Ahuja SP: The localization of coronary artery stenoses by 12-lead ECG response to graded exercise test: support for intercoronary steal, *Am Heart J* 91:437, 1976.

43. Tucker SC, Kemp VE, Holland WE, et al: Multiple lead ECG submaximal treadmill exercise tests in angiographically documented coronary heart disease, *Angiology* 27:149, 1976.

44. Chaitman BR, Bourassa MG, Wagniart P, et al: Improved efficiency of treadmill exercise testing using a multiple lead ECG system and basic hemodynamic exercise response, *Circulation* 57:71-78, 1978.

45. Miranda CP, Liu J, Kadar A, et al: Usefulness of exercise-induced ST-segment depression in the inferior leads during exercise testing as a marker for coronary artery disease, *Am J Cardiol* 69:303-307, 1992.

46. Mirvis DM, Keller FW, Cox JW, et al: Left precordial isopotential mapping during supine exercise, *Circulation* 56:245, 1977.

47. Miller WT, Spach MS, Warren RB: Total body surface potential mapping during supine exercise, *Circulation* 56:245, 1977.

48. Fox KM, Selwyn AP, Shillingford JP: A method for precordial surface mapping of the exercise electrocardiogram, *Br Heart J* 40:1339-1343, 1978.

49. Fox KM, England D, Jonathan A, et al: Precordial surface mapping of the exercise ECG, *Br J Hosp Med* 29:291-299, 1982.

50. Yanowitz FG, Vincent GM, Lux RL, et al: Application of body surface mapping to exercise testing: S-T80 isoarea maps in patients with coronary artery disease, *Am J Cardiol* 50:1109, 1982.

51. Simoons M, Block P, Ascoop C, et al: Computer processing of exercise ECGs—a cooperative study. In van Bemmel JH, Willems JL, editors: Trends in computer-pro-

cessed electrocardiograms, Amsterdam, 1977, North-Holland Publishing, p 383.

52. Mirvis DM, Ramanathan KB: Alterations in transmural blood flow and body surface ST segment abnormalities produced by ischemia in the circumflex and left anterior descending coronary arterial beds of the dog, *Circulation* 76(3):697-704, 1987.

53. Gutman RA, Alexander ER, Li YB, et al: Delay of ST depression after maximal exercise by walking for two minutes, *Circulation* 42:229-233, 1970.

54. Lachterman B, Lehmann KG, Abrahamson D, Froelicher VF: "Recovery only" ST segment depression and the predictive accuracy of the exercise test, *Ann Intern Med* 112:11-16, 1990.

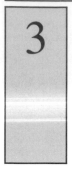

3 Special Methods: Ventilatory Gas Exchange

Ventilatory gas exchange techniques have generally been used in human performance laboratories, and applications in clinical settings have been minimal. However, recent technological advances have lessened the difficulty with which gas-exchange analysis can be performed during exercise, and an increase in the application of this technology has occurred. Such measurements permit a more accurate and reproducible assessment of cardiopulmonary function as compared to estimating work from treadmill speed and grade.[1] This makes them essential when the need exists for accurate quantification of the effect of interventions.[2] For this reason, many research protocols are now conducted using gas-exchange techniques.

It is frequently argued whether the additional and more accurate information gained from exercise testing using gas-exchange techniques justifies the added expense, time, and discomfort to the patient. Unfortunately, there is not a yes or no answer to this question. The answer depends on the purpose of the test and who is conducting the test. In regard to the first consideration, if the purpose of the test is to evaluate an intervention, for example, for research purposes, the limitations in predicting exercise capacity (outlined at right) dictate, in our view, the use of gas-exchange techniques. Alternatively, if the purpose of the test is to increase myocardial oxygen demand to an optimal level while obtaining a general estimation of METs, gas-exchange techniques would generally not be as useful. In regard to the second consideration, the absence of a good understanding of gas exchange and basic exercise physiology by physicians will likely always be a limitation to the widespread application of gas-exchange technology. Gas-exchange analysis requires a degree of expertise by the technician because proper attention to data collection and calibration are essential. At the same time, clinical application of the data requires that the physician possess a basic understanding of ventilatory gas-exchange analysis. This chapter presents some basic methodology and illustrates the clinical utility of gas-exchange techniques for testing patients with heart disease.

PREDICTING OXYGEN UPTAKE

Because the measurement of oxygen uptake requires added cost, time, equipment, and potential discomfort to the patient, the question is frequently raised whether these techniques are necessary in clinical practice. As mentioned, the answer to this question probably depends on the purpose of the test and how important the added precision is to the user. In regard to measuring work with precision, it may be useful to review some of the major research studies to put this question into perspective.

Predicting oxygen uptake from treadmill or cycle ergometer work load is common clinically, but it can be very misleading. Although the two are directly related, with correlation coefficients ranging between 0.8 and 0.9, there is a wide scatter around the regression line. Figure 3-1 illustrates that the 95% confidence limits for predicting oxygen uptake based on treadmill time range roughly 20 ml or cc kg/min (nearly 6 METs). This inaccuracy has been attributed to such factors as subject habituation (less variation occurs with treadmill experience), fitness (less variation occurs with increased fitness), the presence of heart disease (oxygen uptake is overpredicted for diseased individuals), handrail holding (the oxygen cost of the work is greatly reduced if the subject is allowed to hold on to the handrails), and the exercise protocol (less variation occurs when using more gradual, individualized protocols)

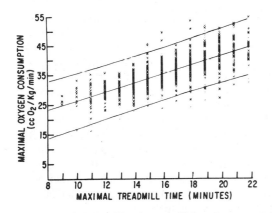

Figure 3-1 Relationship of treadmill time to measured ventilatory oxygen consumption (VO₂) using a progressive treadmill protocol in healthy pilots.

(Table 3-1). Thus, if quantifying work with precision is an important objective, as in research studies, a direct measurement is essential.

Studies describing the factors that affect the relationship between measured and predicted oxygen uptake are numerous; it may be useful to review some of them here. The wide scatter around the regression line between oxygen uptake and exercise time or work load is well documented yet poorly appreciated, and most pharmaceutical trials continue to report work in terms of the relatively unreliable measure—exercise time. This is particularly a concern, since many studies have shown that the presence of heart disease can greatly increase the error associated with predicting oxygen uptake. Sullivan and McKirnan[3] reported that, among patients with coronary disease, measured oxygen uptake was 13% lower than normal subjects for the same treadmill work at higher levels of exercise. Roberts and associates[4] plotted the relationship between measured and predicted oxygen uptake in a heterogeneous

group of patients with heart disease and a group of normals (Figure 3-2). Measured oxygen uptake was lower at matched work rates throughout exercise among the patients. Moreover, the discrepancy between the two groups became progressively greater as exercise progressed; at higher levels of exercise, differences as large as 1 MET were observed.

We recently compared the slope of the relationship between patients with heart disease and age-matched normals on a variety of treadmill and cycle ergometer protocols.[5] The slope represents a change in an independent variable (in this case, an increment in treadmill or cycle ergometer work) for a given change in a dependent variable (in this case measured oxygen uptake). Thus a slope equal to 1 would be observed if the variables changed in direct proportion to one another. This is never the case, however, even among normals. Table 3-2 illustrates that patients with chronic heart failure, coronary disease, and those limited by angina on the treadmill have significantly reduced slopes (ranging from 0.51 to 0.53) compared to normals (slope = 0.71). The explanation suggested by many investigators to account for the reduced oxygen uptake values at matched work rates (sometimes called oxygen uptake lag, or "drift") is an inability of the cardiopulmonary system to adapt to the demands of the work. Not surprisingly, patients with chronic heart failure are particularly known to exhibit this response, and the effects of beta-blockade on this response must also be considered when one is using work load to predict oxygen uptake.[6,7]

The choice of exercise protocol is also known to influence the relationship between measured and predicted work. Haskell and co-workers,[8] for example, reported that estimating oxygen uptake among patients with heart disease was valid only if a gradual protocol was used. Using an accelerated protocol, peak VO₂ was significantly overes-

Table 3-1 Factors affecting the relationship between measured and predicted oxygen uptake

Factor	Effect
Habituation	Oxygen uptake and variability decrease; reproducibility improves with treadmill experience.
Fitness	Oxygen uptake and variability in oxygen uptake for a given work load decrease with increased fitness.
Heart disease	Oxygen uptake is overpredicted in patients with heart disease.
Handrail holding	Oxygen uptake is reduced by holding handrails.
Exercise protocol	Oxygen uptake is overpredicted; variability is greater with rapidly incremented, more demanding protocols.
Mechanical efficiency	Oxygen cost of work is increased by obesity (on treadmill) but reduced by stride length, training specificity, habituation, and coordination.

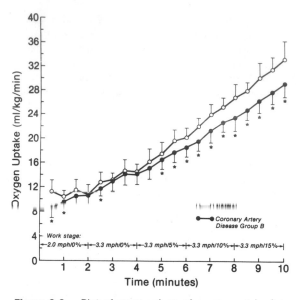

Figure 3-2 Plot of mean values of oxygen uptake for matched treadmill work loads in normals and patients with coronary heart disease. At higher levels of work, oxygen uptake is significantly reduced among patients with heart disease.

timated. Our laboratory recently evaluated differences between six protocols in terms of the relationship between measured and predicted oxygen uptake.[5] Three treadmill and three bicycle ergometer protocols were compared. The three treadmill protocols used were a gradual (modified Balke), a rapid (standard Bruce), and a moderately incremented test (individualized ramp). The three bicycle ergometer protocols were a rapid (50 watts/stage), gradual (25 watts/stage), and a moderately incremented test (individualized ramp). Among 31 patients with heart disease and 10 normals, the slope of the relationship between measured and predicted oxygen uptake was quantified throughout exercise.

Table 3-3 presents the slopes of these relation-

ships for each protocol. The protocols with the largest increments in work (that is, Bruce treadmill and 50 watts/stage cycle ergometer) have slopes that were significantly lower that those with smaller increments in work. This indicates that protocols that increase rapidly or have large increments in work overpredict exercise capacity. In addition, the standard error of the estimate (oxygen uptake, ml/kg/min) was largest for the Bruce test and smallest for the individualized ramp tests, an indication that the variability in estimating oxygen uptake from the work load is greater on rapidly incremented tests versus tests that are more gradual and individualized.

Reproducibility

An important consideration, particularly when one is serially testing patients for research protocols such as pharmaceutical trials, is the reliability and reproducibility of the data. This has been one of the most important arguments in favor of the use of gas-exchange techniques. The tendency to increase treadmill time with serial testing without an increase in maximal oxygen uptake is well documented. Many major multicenter drug trials in cardiology have shown significant increases in exercise time on placebo treatment, which could be attributed only to repeated testing, in some cases causing a "masking" of the effects of therapy.

Changes in treadmill time with serial testing have even been observed without changes in maximal heart rate or double product.[9] Elborn and co-workers[10] performed three consecutive treadmill tests on separate days in patients with heart failure and reported that the first test underestimated exercise time by approximately 20%. Pinsky and co-workers[11] performed repeated treadmill tests among patients with heart failure until test duration on three consecutive tests varied by less than

Table 3-2 Slopes in oxygen uptake versus work rate for each patient subgroup performing each of the six exercise protocols

	CAD	Angina	CHF	Normal
Slope	0.51	0.53	0.53	0.71*
SEE, ml of O₂/kg/min	2.6	3.1	2.8	4.2

*p < 0.001 versus other groups. *CAD,* Coronary artery disease; *CHF,* chronic heart failure; *SEE,* standard error of the estimate. If the change in ventilatory oxygen uptake was equal to the change in work rate, the slope would be equal to 1.0

Table 3-3 Slopes in oxygen uptake versus work rate for 41 subjects performing six exercise protocols

	Treadmills			Bicycles		
	Bruce	Balke	Ramp	25 W	50 W	Ramp
Slope	0.62	0.79	0.80	0.69	0.59	0.78
SEE	4.0	3.4	2.5	2.3	2.8	1.7

Each slope ≥0.78 was significantly different from each slope ≤0.69 (p <0.05 except Balke versus 25 W, p = 0.07). If the change in ventilatory oxygen uptake were equal to the change in work rate, the slope would be equal to 1.0. *SEE,* Standard error of the estimate (ml of O₂/kg/min); 25 W = 25 W/stage; 50 W = 50 W/stage.

60 seconds. This stability criteria was achieved within three tests on only nine of 30 patients, whereas 13 patients required four or five tests and eight patients required more than six tests.

Sullivan and associates[1] compared intraclass correlation coefficients for treadmill time and oxygen uptake among patients with angina tested on three different days within a week. Measured oxygen uptake had a higher intraclass correlation coefficient ($r = 0.88$) than treadmill time ($r = 0.70$) across the three exercise tests on different days (Table 3-4). The 90% confidence intervals for the intraclass correlation coefficients were higher for measured oxygen uptake ($r = 0.76$ to 0.95) than for treadmill time ($r = 0.48$ to 0.86). Thus, gas-exchange techniques yield a more reliable, reproducible, and accurate assessment of exercise capacity and cardiopulmonary function than treadmill time or work load achieved. In our view, this technology is essential when one is using exercise as an efficacy parameter when studying interventions.

INSTRUMENTATION

The measurement of oxygen uptake can be roughly described as simply the product of ventilation (VE) in a given interval and the fraction of oxygen in that ventilation that has been consumed by the working muscle:

$$VO_2 \text{ ml/min (STPD)} = VE \times (FiO_2 - FeO_2)$$

where FiO_2 is the fraction of inspired oxygen and FeO_2 is the fraction of expired oxygen. FiO_2 is equal to 20.93% at sea level and 0% humidity, and ventilation is converted to standard temperature and pressure, dry (STPD). Thus $FiO_2 - FeO_2$ represents the amount of oxygen consumed by the working muscle for a given sample, sometimes called "true O_2."

For the sake of explanation, the above equation is oversimplified because it assumes that expired air is dry and that inspired and expired volumes are not different. Because this is generally not the case (unless respiratory exchange ratio equals one), several additional calculations are necessary for accurate determination of oxygen uptake. First, the sample of air that is analyzed for O_2 and

CO_2 content must be dried, or the humidity in the room must be measured and FiO_2 adjusted accordingly. Second, because oxygen uptake is the difference between the fraction of oxygen in the inspired and expired ventilation, both inspired and expired ventilation must be known precisely. Ventilatory volume is frequently measured only from the expired air. Inspired volume, however, can be determined from the expired volume and the fractions of oxygen and carbon dioxide. This is possible because nitrogen (N_2) and other inert gases do not affect the body's gas-exchange processes. Thus, given that the concentrations of N_2, CO_2, and O_2 of the inspired air are known to be 0.7904, 0, and 0.2093 respectively, the fraction of inert gases (N_2) in the expired air (Fe_{N2}) becomes:

$$Fe_{N2} = 1 - FeO_2 - FeCO_2$$

Thus inspiratory volume (V_I) can be expressed as the difference between the fraction of inert gases in the expired air and the fraction of inert gases in the atmosphere:

$$V_I = \frac{VE \times (1 - FeO_2 - FeCO_2)}{0.7904}$$

And the equation for oxygen uptake becomes:

$$VO_2 \text{ L/min STPD} = \frac{(1 - FeO_2 - FeCO_2)}{0.7904} \times (FiO_2 - FeO_2) \times VE \text{ STPD}$$

Collection of expired ventilation

The measurement of gas exchange variables during exercise requires that the patient have a mouthpiece in place that seals tightly and the nose sealed with a clip. Although face masks are available that cover the nose and mouth (making speaking possible), these sometimes leak during exercise at high ventilation rates. According to the above equation, expired gas analysis requires that the gases be analyzed for total volume as well as oxygen and carbon dioxide content. Accurate measurement requires water content to be accounted for by adjustment for standard pressure and temperature (thus the correction for STPD). As originally performed, expired gases were collected in a Tissot spirometer. This device is an in-

Table 3-4 Mean ± standard deviation of treadmill time and oxygen uptake at maximal angina-limited exercise

	Day 1	Day 2	Day 3	Intraclass correlation coefficient (ICC)	ICC, 90% confidence interval
Time (seconds)	503 ± 72	516 ± 85	526 ± 66	0.70	0.48-0.86
Oxygen uptake (L/min)	1.559 ± 0.289	1.553 ± 0.334	1.557 ± 0.294	0.88	0.76-0.95

verted open metal cylinder suspended in a large container filled with water. Filling the inner cylinder with expired air caused it to rise in the water, and ventilation was measured as the degree of displacement of the cylinder. Other methods of measuring air volume required Douglas bags or weather balloons, using a turret that rotated from one bag to the next at each time interval. These methods required a great deal of technician time and limited precision because sampling was dictated by the size of the collection bags and slowly responding analyzers. Because of the many advances recently in gas analysis systems, these methods are virtually obsolete.

Today, gas analysis is being performed on-line; various types of flowmeters including mass transducers, Fleisch pneumotachometers, hot-wire devices, small propellers or turbines, or dry gas meters, are used. A mixing chamber from which expired gases are sampled is frequently required. The Fleisch device measures the pressure drop because of the Venturi effect caused by airflow through a tube; the "hot wires" drop in temperature when cooled by air, and the propellers are spun by airflow. One of the problems with these devices is the difficulty in measurement of ventilatory gas volume directly from a rapidly breathing individual. The phasic nature of breathing affects these devices. It is often suggested that most commercial devices that measure flow directly from a patient are not as accurate as "off-line" methods. However, many technological advances have occurred in this area in recent years, these systems are now the norm commercially, and studies on their validation are available.

Gas-exchange data sampling

The recent availability of these rapidly responding gas analyzers, though facilitating precision and convenience, has lead to confusion regarding data sampling. For example, differences in sampling (that is, breath by breath, 30 seconds, 60 seconds, or "running" breath averaging) can greatly affect precision and variability in measuring oxygen uptake. Figure 3-3 illustrates the standard deviation of various oxygen-uptake samples during steady-state exercise in 10 subjects.[49] The variability in oxygen uptake is greater as the sampling interval shortens (that is, 4.5 ml/kg/min for breath by breath versus 0.8 ml/kg/min for 60-second samples). Thus a given value for oxygen uptake carries an inherent variability, and this variability depends on the sampling interval. Shorter sampling intervals increase precision but also increase the variability.

Data derived from small sampling intervals should be interpreted with caution, and one should resist the tendency to use breath-by-breath

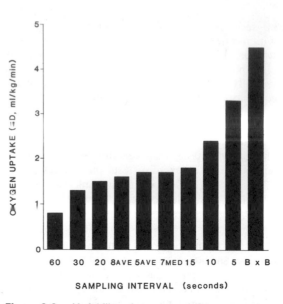

Figure 3-3   Variability of oxygen uptake expressed as standard deviation of oxygen uptake for each sampling interval during 5 minutes of steady-state exercise. *AVE*, Average; *MED*, median.

data simply because the technology is available. Breath-by-breath sampling can be invaluable for certain research applications, such as oxygen kinetics, but it is inappropriate for general clinical applications. Breath averaging would appear to represent a reasonable balance between precision and variability. Regardless of the sample chosen, investigators should report the sampling interval used, and the intervals should be consistent throughout a given trial when one is studying interventions.

INFORMATION FROM VENTILATORY GAS-EXCHANGE DATA DURING EXERCISE

Maximal oxygen uptake is the most common and most important measurement derived from gas-exchange data during exercise. Unfortunately, it is frequently the only variable used in many laboratories. Gas-exchange techniques can, however, provide a great deal of additional information regarding the capacity of the heart and lungs to deliver oxygen to the working muscle during exercise. In the following, variables other than oxygen uptake are outlined with particular emphasis on their applications to testing patients with heart disease. For reference, formulas for calculating these variables are outlined in Table 3-5.

Minute ventilation (VE)

Minute ventilation is the volume of air moving into and out of the lungs expressed as liters per

Table 3-5   Calculations for basic gas-exchange data

1. Oxygen uptake (VO_2 L/min, STPD) $= \left[\dfrac{(1 - FeO_2 - FeCO_2)}{0.7904} \times (FiO_2 - FeO_2)\right] \times$ VE STPD

2. Minute ventilation (VE, L/min, BTPS) = Respiratory rate × Tidal volume. For calculations of VO_2 and VCO_2, VE in BTPS is converted to STPD by the following:

   VE (STPD): VE (BTPS) $\times \dfrac{(273)}{273 + 37} \times \dfrac{(Pb - 47)}{760}$

3. Carbon dioxide production (VCO_2 L/min, STPD) = VE (L/min, STPD) × $FeCO_2$

4. Respiratory exchange ratio (RER) $= \dfrac{VCO_2}{VO_2}$

5. Oxygen pulse (O_2 pulse, cc of O_2/beat) $= \dfrac{VO_2 \text{ cc, STPD}}{\text{heart rate, beats/min}}$

6. Ventilatory equivalents for O_2 and CO_2 $= \dfrac{\text{VE L/min, BTPS}}{VO_2 \text{ L/min, STPD}}$ and $\dfrac{\text{VE L/min, BTPS}}{VCO_2 \text{ L/min, STPD}}$

7. End-tidal PCO_2 ($PETCO_2$, mm Hg) = $FeTCO_2$ × (Pb − 47)

8. Ventilatory dead space (Vd) = Vt $\times \dfrac{PaCO_2 - PeCO_2}{PaCO_2}$ − Valve dead space, ml

   Where $PeCO_2$ = $FeCO_2$ × (Pb − 47).
   $PaCO_2$ is estimated by use of $PaCO_2$ = 5.5 + 0.90 $PETCO_2$ − 0.0021 × Vt.
   One calculates the ventilatory dead space–to–tidal volume ratio (Vd/Vt) by dividing by Vt.

9. Breathing reserve $= \dfrac{\text{Maximal VE, L/min}}{\text{MVV, L/min}}$

   Where VE is equation 2 and MVV is the maximal voluntary ventilation at rest.

Some abbreviations in table: *BTPS,* Body temperature and pressure, saturated—gas volume at body temperature and pressure saturated with water vapor (37° C and 47 mm Hg); *FeCO₂,* fraction (%) of carbon dioxide in the expired air; *FeO₂,* fraction (%) of oxygen in the expired air; *FeTCO₂,* fraction (%) of end-tidal carbon dioxide in the expired air; *FiO₂,* fraction (%) of oxygen in the inspired air; *PaCO₂,* partial pressure of carbon dioxide in arterial blood; *Pb,* barometric pressure, mm Hg; *PeCO₂,* mixed expired CO_2 pressure, mm Hg; *PETCO₂,* end-tidal carbon dioxide pressure, mm Hg; *PETO₂,* end tidal oxygen pressure, mm Hg; *STPD,* standard temperature and pressure, dry—gas volume at standard temperature (0° C) and barometric pressure (760 mm Hg), dry; *VE,* minute ventilation; *Vt,* tidal volume, ml.

minute (BTPS). Because true O_2 (the difference between inspired and expired oxygen content) does not differ that much between individuals, even with widely varying fitness levels, ventilation is the major component of oxygen uptake during exercise. Fit individuals with high maximal ventilations and thus high maximal oxygen uptakes, however, must also have cardiac outputs that roughly match ventilation in the lung. On the other hand, abnormal hyperventilation is an important characteristic of both patients with chronic heart failure and pulmonary disease, attributable in part to a mismatching of ventilation and perfusion. The ventilatory response of patients with chronic heart failure to exercise has been of particular interest in recent years, and gas-exchange data can be important both in identifying this disorder and gauging their response to therapy.

Carbon dioxide production (VCO_2)

Carbon dioxide produced by the body during exercise is usually expressed in liters per minute, STPD. VCO_2 is a byproduct of oxidative metabolism. An elevation in carbon dioxide in the blood can quickly result in respiratory acidosis. Fortu-

nately, the major determinants of ventilation during exercise are metabolic CO_2 and the CO_2 resulting from the buffering of lactate, which are reflected in the expired air as VCO_2. Thus VCO_2 closely matches VE during exercise, and the body maintains a relatively normal pH during most exercise.

Respiratory exchange ratio (RER)

The respiratory exchange ratio represents the amount of carbon dioxide produced divided by the amount of oxygen consumed. Normally, roughly 75% of the oxygen consumed is converted to carbon dioxide. Thus RER at rest generally ranges from 0.70 to 0.85. Because RER depends on the type of fuel used by the cells, it can provide an index of carbohydrate or fat metabolism. If carbohydrates were the predominant fuel, RER would equal one given the formula:

$C_6 H_{12} O_6$ (glucose) + $6O_2 \rightarrow 6CO_2$ + $6H_2O$
RER = VCO_2 divided by VO_2 = $6CO_2$ divided by $6O_2$ = 1.0

Because relatively more oxygen is required to burn fat, the respiratory exchange ratio for fat metabolism is lower, roughly 0.70. At high levels of exercise, CO_2 production exceeds oxygen uptake; thus an RER exceeding 1.0 to 1.2 is often used to indicate that the subject is giving a maximal effort. However, peak RER values vary greatly and generally are not a precise cut point for "maximal" exercise.

Oxygen pulse (O_2 pulse)

Oxygen pulse is an indirect index of combined cardiopulmonary oxygen transport. It is calculated by dividing oxygen uptake (ml/min) by heart rate. In effect, O_2 pulse is equal to the product of stroke volume and arteriovenous O_2 difference. Thus circulatory adjustments that occur during exercise, that is, widening arteriovenous O_2 difference, increased cardiac output, and redistribution of blood flow to the working muscle, will increase the O_2 pulse. Maximal O_2 pulse is higher in fitter subjects, lower in the presence of heart disease, and, more importantly, higher at any given work load in the fitter or healthier individual. On the other hand, O_2 pulse will be reduced in any condition that reduces stroke volume (left ventricular dysfunction secondary to ischemia or infarction) or reduces arterial O_2 content (anemia, hypoxemia).

Ventilatory equivalents for oxygen and carbon dioxide (VE/VO_2 and VE/VCO_2)

The ventilatory equivalents are calculated by dividing ventilation (L/min) by VO_2 or VCO_2 in liters per minute. A great deal of ventilation (25 to 40 liters) is required to consume a single liter of oxygen; thus VE/VO_2 is often in the 30s at rest. A decrease in VE/VO_2 is frequently observed from rest to submaximal exercise, followed by a rapid increase at higher levels of exercise when VE increases in response to the need to buffer lactate. VE/VO_2 reflects the ventilatory requirement for any given oxygen uptake; thus it is an index of ventilatory efficiency. Patients with a high fraction of physiologic dead space or uneven matching of ventilation to perfusion in the lung ventilate inefficiently and have high values for VE/VO_2. High VE/VO_2 values characterize the response to exercise among patients with lung disease or chronic heart failure[11a] (Figure 3-4).

VE/VCO_2 represents the ventilatory requirement to eliminate a given amount of CO_2 produced by the metabolizing tissues. Since metabolic CO_2 is a strong stimulus for ventilation during exercise, VE and VCO_2 closely mirror one another, and after a drop in early exercise, VE/VCO_2 normally does not increase significantly throughout submaximal exercise. However, in the presence of chronic heart failure, VE/VCO_2 is shifted upward compared to normals, and high

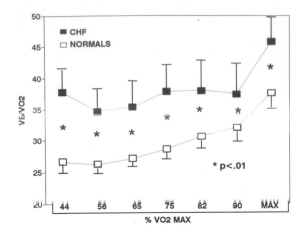

Figure 3-4 Changes in VE/VO_2 expressed as a percentage of maximal oxygen uptake for patients with heart failure and normal subjects (Mean ± 2 SEM).

VE/VCO_2 values are one of the characteristics of the abnormal ventilatory response to exercise in this condition.

Caiozzo and co-workers[12] compared gas-exchange indices used to detect the ventilatory threshold and found that the use of the ventilatory equivalents for O_2 and CO_2 most closely reflected a lactate inflection point and thus were the best indices to detect the ventilatory threshold. Many laboratories define the ventilatory threshold as the beginning of a systematic increase in VE/VCO_2 without an increase in VE/VO_2.

Ventilatory dead space–to–tidal volume ratio (Vd/Vt)

Vd/Vt measured by gas exchange is an estimate of the fraction of tidal volume that represents physiologic dead space. Physiologic dead space ventilation is the difference between minute ventilation and alveolar ventilation. Thus Vd/Vt is an estimate of the degree to which ventilation matches perfusion in the lung. When significant ventilation/perfusion mismatching is present, Vd/Vt is high.

In normal subjects, Vd/Vt falls from roughly one third to between one tenth to one fifth at peak exercise. However, in the presence of pulmonary disease or heart failure, in which there is significant ventilation/perfusion mismatching, Vd/Vt is elevated and often remains relatively unchanged throughout exercise. Ventilation/perfusion mismatching and thus a high Vd/Vt accounts in large part for the abnormally high ventilation observed in patients with pulmonary disease and heart failure. Figure 3-5 illustrates the relationship between maximal Vd/Vt and VO_2 max in a group of patients with chronic heart failure and a group of aged-matched normals.[11a] Not only do patients

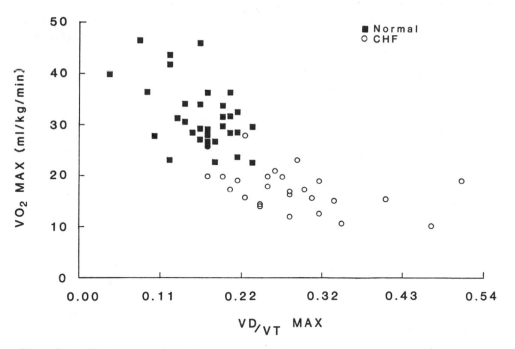

Figure 3-5   The relationship between maximal estimated ventilatory dead space–to–tidal volume ratio (Vd/Vt max) and maximal oxygen uptake (VO₂ max) for normal subjects *(darkened squares)* and patients with chronic heart failure *(open circles)*. The correlation coefficient between the two variables was −0.73 (SEE = 6.2, $p < 0.001$).

with heart failure have poorer exercise capacity, but considerably higher Vd/Vt values are also observed; for some patients, nearly half of the tidal volume is dead space. With such a large fraction of dead space and thus "wasted" ventilation, it is not surprising that a significantly higher ventilation is required for the same relative work among patients with heart disease (Figure 3-4).

Breathing reserve

The breathing reserve is calculated as the ratio of maximal voluntary ventilation at rest (MVV) to maximal exercise ventilation. Most healthy subjects achieve a maximal ventilation of only 60% to 80% of MVV at peak exercise. One characteristic of chronic pulmonary obstruction is a maximal ventilation that approximates or equals the individual's MVV. These patients reach a "ventilatory" limit during exercise, whereas normal subjects generally have a substantial ventilatory reserve (20% to 40%) at peak exercise and are limited by other factors.

Ventilatory threshold

A physiological link between exercise capacity, lactate accumulation in the blood, and respiratory gas exchange was made by Hill and Lupton[13] more than 60 years ago. A sudden rise in the blood lactate level during exercise has long been

associated with muscle anaerobiosis and has therefore been termed the "anaerobic threshold."[14] Historically the anaerobic threshold has been defined as the highest oxygen uptake during exercise above which a sustained lactic acidosis occurs. When this level of exercise is reached, excess H⁺ ions of lactate must be buffered to maintain physiological pH. Because bicarbonate buffering yields an additional source of CO_2, ventilation is further stimulated. This point of nonlinear increase in ventilation has been used to detect the anaerobic threshold noninvasively and is often termed the "gas-exchange anaerobic threshold" or the "ventilatory threshold" (VT) (Figure 3-6). A great deal of confusion presently exists concerning the mechanism underlying this point and how it might be determined and applied clinically.[15,16]

Changes in oxygen uptake at the VT have been used clinically during pharmacological and other investigations to imply that a change in oxygen supply to the working muscle has occurred. The anaerobic threshold has recently come under scrutiny, however, on the basis of both theoretical[16] and pragmatic[17-19] grounds. Connet and colleagues[20] studied dog gracilis muscle, which is a pure red fiber containing only type I and type IIA fibers, and observed lactate accumulation during fully aerobic, mild (10% VO₂ max) conditions. These investigators also observed that lactate ac-

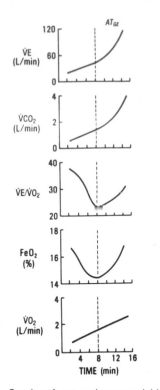

Figure 3-6   Graphs of gas exchange variables that can be measured during exercise to determine the ventilatory threshold.

cumulation was not altered by changes in blood flow and that lactate accumulation occurred even though no anoxic areas were present in the muscle. This indicates that lactate production and muscle hypoxia may be unrelated. Additionally, the advent of tracer technology has raised strong questions about the cause-and-effect relation between oxygen availability to the muscle and the anaerobic threshold. Many studies now indicate that lactate production occurs at all times, even in resting conditions.[16] Further, the turnover rate of lactate (the ratio of appearance and disappearance) is linearly related to oxygen uptake during exercise.[16,21,22] Recent arguments have also addressed whether lactate during exercise in fact increases in a pattern that is mathematically "continuous" rather than as a threshold.[23-25] The cumulative effect of these studies has led to the conclusion that the "anaerobic" threshold is not related to muscle anaerobiosis but instead reflects simply an imbalance between lactate appearance and disappearance.[16] The term "ventilatory threshold" has been suggested as preferable to "anaerobic threshold" because it does not imply the onset of anaerobiosis.

The precise mechanism underlying the VT remains to be delineated. Irrespective of whether the VT is directly related to anaerobiosis, lactate does accumulate in the blood during exercise, ventilation must respond to maintain physiological pH, a breakpoint in ventilation appears to occur reproducibly,[1] and this point is related to various measures of cardiopulmonary performance in normals[26-28] and patients with heart disease.[14,29-33] A common argument clinically in favor of the use of the VT is that, as a submaximal parameter, it is better associated with a patient's everyday activities than maximal exercise is, and using the VT avoids the increased risk and discomfort of maximal exercise. On the basis of recent studies, the following suggestions might be made concerning the use of the VT during exercise testing: (1) regardless of the mechanism, ventilatory changes appear strongly correlated with the accumulation of lactate, and (2) an alteration in the VT reflects a change in the balance between lactate production and removal, and references to muscle anaerobiosis should be avoided. Because lactate is strongly associated with muscle fatigue, a change in this relation that can be attributed to an intervention may add important information concerning the intervention. In this context, the VT during exercise testing remains an interesting and applicable index for use during exercise studies.

An additional consideration concerns the method of choosing the VT. Our laboratory,[19] in agreement with others,[17,18] has observed that the VT can vary greatly depending on both the observer and the method of determination. Although a number of methods of determination have been proposed, Caiozzo and co-workers[12] reported that the use of the ventilatory equivalents for oxygen uptake (VE/VO_2) and carbon dioxide (VE/VCO_2) most closely reflected a lactate inflection point. Many laboratories have therefore defined the VT as the beginning of a systemic increase in VE/VO_2 without a concomitant increase in VE/VCO_2. We have successfully used a method outlined by Sullivan and colleagues[1] in which two experienced, blinded (to patient name and test purpose, that is, whether the test represents a drug or placebo phase) observers independently choose the VT for each exercise test. When a discrepancy exists, a third observer is also blinded and chooses the VT independently. The VT is determined as the minute sample in which two of the three observers agree. The VT is not included in the analysis for that particular patient when all observers differ. We have found that two observers agree 72% of the time, and two of the three observers agree on 100% of the tests.[1] In a more recent study, this method resulted in 7% of tests being excluded.[19] This technique avoids interobserver bias and provides a means by which the

VT can be determined objectively. Methods, problems, and advantages and disadvantages of various methods of choosing the VT or lactate inflection points have been the subjects of numerous reports.[12,15-19,23-25,34-37]

Oxygen kinetics

Although the measurement of oxygen kinetics often requires a specialized exercise test, is defined differently by various laboratories, and requires mathematical computations not familiar to most clinicians, this measurement is probably underutilized as an index of cardiopulmonary function clinically. Put simply, oxygen kinetics quantify the ability of the cardiopulmonary system to respond to the demands of a given amount of work; it is usually defined as the rate at which oxygen uptake reaches a steady-state value. However, measures such as the oxygen uptake–to–work rate relation, oxygen debt, the steepness of the slope of the relationship between work rate and oxygen uptake (see Table 3-2), and various other measures of the difference between predicted and measured oxygen uptake generally describe oxygen kinetics. Although mainly limited thus far to applications in human performance laboratories among healthy subjects, this is an untapped area for quantifying interventions in patients with heart disease.

Models of oxygen kinetics have been used to study cardiovascular function before and after beta-blockade in which oxygen kinetics are slowed by propranolol and metoprolol.[38-40] Hypoxia slows oxygen kinetics and causes a greater deficit and intramuscular lactate,[41,42] whereas hyperoxia appears to enhance oxygen kinetics.[41,42] Oxygen kinetics are greater below versus above the ventilatory threshold,[43] and greater after a program of physical conditioning.[44] The implications of these findings for the study of pharmacologic interventions, exercise training, or other therapies in patients with heart disease are intriguing, but few such studies have been performed in the clinical setting.

Plateau in oxygen uptake

Maximal oxygen uptake is considered the best index of aerobic capacity and maximal cardiorespiratory function. By defining the limits of the cardiopulmonary system, it has been an invaluable measurement clinically for assessment of the efficacy of drugs, exercise training, or invasive procedures. No other measure of work is as accurate, reliable, or reproducible as ventilatory maximal oxygen uptake. The collection and analysis of an expired gas sample taken during the last minute of an exercise test has generally been used to determine maximal oxygen uptake. From early studies using interrupted protocols a test was considered "maximal" only when there was no further increase in oxygen uptake despite further increases in work load. On the other hand, oxygen uptake has been considered "peak" when the subject reaches a point of fatigue while no plateau in oxygen uptake was observed. Unfortunately, the many problems associated with the determination and criteria for the "plateau" in oxygen uptake makes these definitions more semantic that physiological. A brief history of this concept and its inherent problems are outlined below.

In 1955, Taylor and associates[45] established the criteria of plateauing as a failure to increase oxygen uptake more than 150 ml/min, or 2.1 ml/kg/min, with an increase in work load. His original research was done using interrupted progressive treadmill protocols. With interrupted protocols, stages of exercise could be separated by rest periods ranging from minutes to days. Taylor and co-workers found that 75% of the subjects fulfilled these criteria. Using continuous treadmill protocols, Pollock and co-workers[46] found that 69%, 69%, 59%, and 80% of subjects plateaued when tested using the Balke, Bruce, Ellestad, and Åstrand protocols respectively. Froelicher and co-workers[47] found that only 33%, 17%, and 7% of healthy subjects met these criteria during testing with the Taylor, Balke, and Bruce protocols respectively, despite the fact that there were no significant differences between the protocols in maximal heart rate, VO₂ max, or blood pressure. Taylor and co-workers later reported that plateauing did not occur when using continuous treadmill protocols. More recent studies, using a variety of empirical criteria, report the occurrence of a plateau ranging from 7% to 90% of tests.

The plateau concept has been subjected to many interpretations and criteria. The newer, automated gas-exchange systems that allow breath-by-breath or any specified sampling interval have raised new questions in regard to interpreting a plateau. Although the definitions of plateauing vary greatly, all focus on the concept that oxygen uptake at some point will fail to continue to rise as work increases. Using ramp treadmill testing in which work increases constantly at an individualized rate, we measured the slope of the change in work versus the change in oxygen uptake using different sampling intervals.[48,49] In this way, if oxygen uptake were no longer increasing (while work increases continuously), the slope of the relationship between the two variables would be equal to, or not differ from, zero. To increase the possibility of observing a plateau, a large sampling interval of 30 consecutive eight-breath averages was used. Figure 3-7 illustrates the slope of each sample during the last several minutes of exercise in a healthy subject limited by fatigue. The open squares represent samples that were significantly greater than zero (that is, both work and oxygen uptake were increasing), and the closed squares represent samples that were not different from, or were less than, zero (that is, work was increasing while oxygen uptake was not). This subject appeared to "plateau" at peak exercise. However, there was also a "plateau" submaximally. Figure 3-8 illustrates the same subject using the same ramp protocol several days later. In this case, there were several "plateaus" submaximally, and no plateau was observed at peak exercise. Figure 3-9 illustrates the effect of reducing the sampling interval to 10 consecutive eight-breath averages, in which the variability is much greater. Thus the slope of the change in oxygen uptake throughout progressive exercise varies greatly, despite a constant, consistent change in external work and the use of large, averaged samples. This degree of variability would appear to preclude the determination of a plateau by common definitions.

The plateau concept is long ingrained in exercise physiology. Intuitively, the body's respiratory and metabolic systems must reach some finite limit beyond which oxygen uptake can no longer increase, and some subjects who are highly motivated may exhibit a plateau. However, the occurrence of a plateau depends as much on the criteria applied, the sampling interval, and methodology as the subject's health, fitness, and motivation. Recent data from our laboratory[48,49] and of others[50,51] indicate that the plateau concept has limitations for general application during standard exercise testing.

NORMAL VALUES FOR EXERCISE CAPACITY

Maximal oxygen uptake declines with increasing age, and higher values are observed among men compared with women. Thus, when measuring or estimating maximal oxygen uptake, it is useful to have reference values for comparison. Numerous investigators have developed reference values for measured maximal oxygen uptake that are adjusted for age and sex, and one is referred to these sources for more detail.[52-59] The following are commonly used generalized equations based on data published in North America and Europe in the 1950s to 1970s:[56-59]

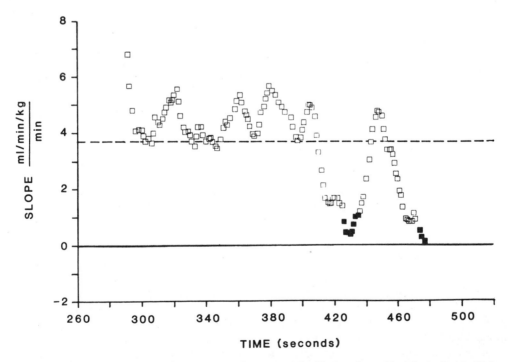

Figure 3-7   Individual slopes in oxygen uptake regressed with time for subject 1 on day 1. Each *darkened square* represents a 30 eight-breath average sample in which the slope was not significantly greater than zero. Each *open square* denotes those that were greater than zero. *Dashed line* represents the mean of the observed change in oxygen uptake (3.73 $\frac{ml/kg/min}{min}$). (From Myers J et al: *Chest* 96:1312-1316, 1989.)

Men

$$VO_2 \text{ max (L/min)} = 4.2 - 0.032 \text{ (age) (SD} \pm 0.4)$$
$$VO_2 \text{ max (ml/kg/min)} = 60 - 0.55 \text{ (age) (SD} \pm 7.5)$$

Women

$$VO_2 \text{ max (L/min)} = 2.6 - 0.014 \text{ (age) (SD} \pm 0.4)$$
$$VO_2 \text{ max (ml/kg/min)} = 48 - 0.37 \text{ (age) (SD} \pm 7.0)$$

Hansen and associates[54] and Wasserman and associates[53] have published predicted values for measured oxygen uptake that consider sex, age, height, and weight and whether testing was performed on a treadmill or a cycle ergometer:

Men	Over-weight	VO_2 max (ml/min)
Cycle*	No	$W \times (50.72 - 0.372 \times A)$
	Yes	$(0.79 \times H - 60.7) \times$ $(50.72 - 0.372 \times A)$
Treadmill†	No	$W \times (56.36 - 0.413 \times A)$
	Yes	$(0.79 \times H - 60.7) \times$ $(56.36 - 0.413 \times A)$
Women		
Cycle*	No	$(42.8 \times W) \times (22.78 -$ $0.17 \times A)$
	Yes	$H \times (14.81 - 0.11 \times A)$
Treadmill‡	No	$W \times (44.37 - 0.413 \times A)$
	Yes	$(0.79 \times H - 68.2) \times$ $(44.37 - 0.413 \times A)$

W, weight in kg; *H*, height in cm; *A*, age in years
*Overweight is W $>(0.79 \times H - 60.7)$
†Overweight is W $>(0.65 \times H - 42.8)$
‡Overweight is W $>(0.79 \times H - 68.2)$

Unfortunately, relatively few clinical exercise laboratories measure oxygen uptake directly, and a variety of methods have been developed using estimated values from exercise times or work loads. One of the early techniques was developed by Bruce and co-workers[55] who suggested the use of a nomogram for estimating functional aerobic impairment (FAI). In this nomogram, one side shows treadmill time using his protocol, and the other shows age. Between these two lines are percent increments of FAI for sedentary and active individuals. By drawing a straight line through age (from which the maximal oxygen uptake can be predicted) and the treadmill time, an estimate of aerobic impairment can be read from the sloped lines. Normally FAI would be zero, since observed maximal oxygen uptake should be the same as that predicted. One problem with this approach is that studies have demonstrated relatively poor correlations between age and maximal oxygen uptake in healthy males even when activity levels were considered (Figure 3-10). This is attributable to the many factors that affect an indi-

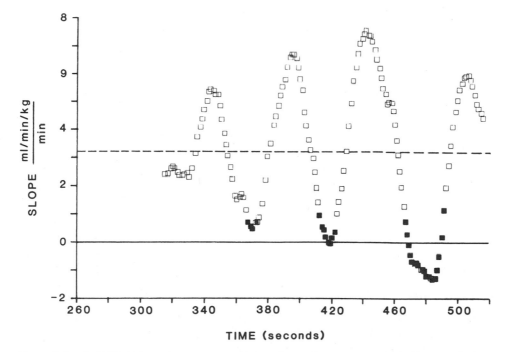

Figure 3-8   Individual slopes in oxygen uptake regressed with time for subject 1 on day 2. Each *darkened square* represents a 30 eight-breath average sample in which the slope was not significantly greater than zero. Each *open square* denotes those that were greater than zero. *Dashed line* represents the mean of the observed change in oxygen uptake (3.26 $\frac{\text{ml/kg/min}}{\text{min}}$). (From Myers J et al: *Chest* 96:1312-1316, 1989.)

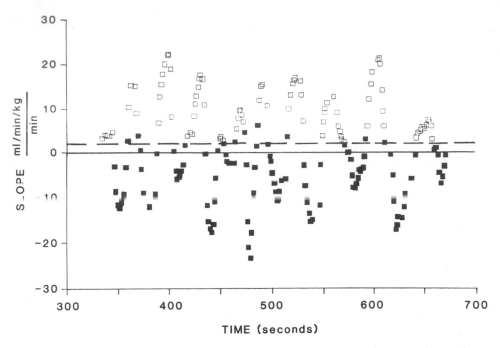

Figure 3-9 Slope of the change in oxygen uptake regressed with time for one subject using a smaller (10 eight-breath average) sampling interval. *Darkened squares* represent slopes that were not significantly greater than zero; *open squares* are those that were significantly greater than zero.

vidual's aerobic capacity beside current activity level, including past activity level, genetic endowment, mechanical efficiency, previous testing experience, and the specificity of training. Thus this nomogram was based on two relatively poor relationships, which thereby limit its ability to predict functional capacity.

Morris and associates[60] recently developed a similar nomogram from 1388 veteran patients. These data are presented in more detail in Chapter 5 and are mentioned only briefly here. This nomogram may be more applicable clinically because (1) it is based on METs achieved from treadmill speed and grade and does not restrict one to using the Bruce protocol and (2) it was derived from a group of males who were referred for exercise testing for clinical reasons. The regression equations derived from the group were as follows:

All subjects: METs = 18.0 − 0.15 (age); SEE = 3.3; $r = -0.46$; $p < 0.001$
Active subjects: METs = 18.7 − 0.15 (age); SEE = 3.0; $r = -0.49$; $p < 0.001$
Sedentary subjects: METs = 16.6 − 0.16 (age); SEE = 3.2; $r = -0.43$; $p < 0.001$

When one is using regression equations or nomograms for reference purposes, it is important to consider several points. First, as mentioned, the relationship between exercise capacity and age is

rather poor ($r = -0.30$ to -0.60). Second, nearly all equations are derived from different populations using different protocols; thus, to some extent, they are both population and protocol specific. Moreover, since treadmill time or work load tends to overpredict maximal METs, it is important to consider whether gas-exchange techniques were used in developing the equations. For example, the equations developed by Morris and co-workers[60] were derived from a large group of veterans referred for testing for clinical reasons. Thus they had a greater prevalence of heart disease than the other studies, and it is not surprising that a greater slope was present with a faster decline in VO_2 max with age.

To account for the differences in measured versus predicted oxygen uptake, Morris and co-workers[60] also developed a nomogram using measured oxygen uptake among 244 active or sedentary apparently healthy males (Figures 5-8 and 5-9). The MET values are shifted downward roughly 1.0 to 1.5 METs for any given age, reflecting the lower but more precise measures of exercise capacity.

All subjects: METs = 14.7 − 0.11 (age)
Active subjects: METs = 16.4 − 0.13 (age)
Sedentary subjects: METs = 11.9 − 0.07 (age)

Thus such scales are specific both to the population tested and to whether oxygen uptake was

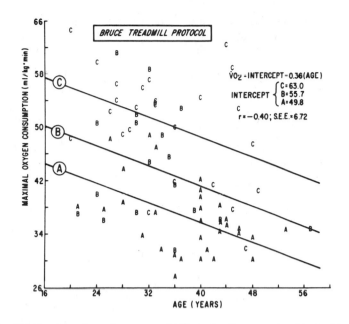

Figure 3-10   Relationship of age to measured VO₂ in the Bruce protocol in healthy subjects with activity status considered.

measured directly or predicted. Within these limitations, these equations and the nomograms derived from them can provide reasonable references for normal values and can facilitate communication with patients and between physicians regarding their level of exercise capacity in relation to their peers. The figures corresponding to each of these equations, along with equations developed by other investigators, are presented in Chapter 5.

SUMMARY

The use of gas-exchange techniques can greatly supplement exercise testing by adding precision and reproducibility and increasing the yield of information concerning cardiopulmonary function. Quantifying work from treadmill or cycle ergometer work load introduces a great deal of error and variability. In addition to some inherent variability in predicting oxygen uptake from external work, factors such as treadmill experience, the exercise protocol, and the presence of heart disease contribute to these errors. The limitations of quantifying work in terms of exercise time or work load make gas-exchange techniques essential when one is using exercise as an efficacy parameter in research protocols.

Maximal oxygen uptake is considered the best index of aerobic capacity and maximal cardiorespiratory function. By defining the limits of the cardiopulmonary system, it has been an invaluable measurement clinically for assessment of the efficacy of drugs, exercise training, or invasive procedures. No other measurement of work is as accurate, reliable, or reproducible as ventilatory maximal oxygen uptake. Oxygen uptake is quantified by measurement of the volume of expired ventilation and determination of the difference in the oxygen content of inspired and expired air. Hemodynamically, oxygen uptake is equal to the product of cardiac output and arteriovenous oxygen difference. Historically, the maximal cardiopulmonary limits have been considered to be achieved when oxygen uptake does not increase further with an increase in work (plateau). However, many criteria and definitions used to describe this point and differences in data sampling limit its utility.

In addition to the measurement of oxygen uptake, the use of gas exchange techniques can provide additional information concerning cardiopulmonary function during exercise. Various methods of expressing efficiency of ventilation, breathing patterns, physiological dead space, and oxygen kinetics can be useful in characterizing the presence of certain heart and lung diseases and in gauging their responses to therapy. The additional accuracy and information provided by this technology must be balanced against potential increases in cost, time, and inconvenience to the patient. In addition, the quality of the test is dependent on some basic skills required of the technician, who must properly calibrate the system and perform the test, and the physician, who must interpret the test. Thus the decision to employ gas-exchange techniques should be based on the purpose of the test and the personnel available to perform the test.

REFERENCES

1. Sullivan M, Genter F, Savvides M, et al: The reproducibility of hemodynamic, electrocardiographic, and gas exchange data during treadmill exercise in patients with stable angina pectoris, *Chest* 86:375-381, 1984.
2. Myers J, Froelicher VF: Optimizing the exercise test for pharmacologic investigations, *Circulation* 82:1839-1846, 1990.
3. Sullivan M, McKirnan MD: Errors in predicting functional capacity for postmyocardial infarction patients using a modified Bruce protocol, *Am Heart J* 107:486-491, 1984.
4. Roberts JM, Sullivan M, Froelicher VF, et al: Predicting oxygen uptake from treadmill testing in normal subjects and coronary artery disease patients, *Am Heart J* 108:1454-1460, 1984.
5. Myers J, Buchanan N, Walsh D, et al: Comparison of the ramp versus standard exercise protocols, *J Am Coll Cardiol* 17:1334-1342, 1991.
6. Brown H, Wasserman K, Whipp BJ: Effect of beta-adrenergic blockade during exercise on ventilation and gas exchange, *J Appl Physiol* 41:886-892, 1976.
7. Reybrouck T, Amery A, Billiet L: Hemodynamic response to graded exercise after chronic beta-adrenergic blockade, *J Appl Physiol* 42:133-138, 1977.
8. Haskell W, Savin W, Oldridge N, DeBusk R: Factors influencing estimated oxygen uptake during exercise testing soon after myocardial infarction, *Am J Cardiol* 50:299-304, 1982.
9. Starling MR, Moody M, Crawford MH, et al: Repeat treadmill exercise testing: variability of results in patients with angina pectoris, *Am Heart J* 107:298-303, 1984.
10. Elborn JS, Stanford CF, Nichols DP: Reproducibility of cardiopulmonary parameters during exercise in patients with chronic cardiac failure: the need for a preliminary test, *Eur Heart J* 11:75-81, 1990.
11. Pinsky DJ, Ahern D, Wilson PB, et al: How many exercise tests are needed to minimize the placebo effect of serial exercise testing in patients with chronic heart failure? *Circulation* 80(suppl II):II-426, 1989.
11a. Myers J, Salleh A, Buchanan N, et al: Ventilatory mechanisms of exercise intolerance in chronic heart failure, *Am Heart J* 124:710-719, 1992.
12. Caiozzo VJ, Davis JA, Ellis JF, et al: A comparison of gas exchange indices used to detect the anaerobic threshold, *J Appl Physiol* 53:1184-1189, 1982.
13. Hill AV, Lupton H: Muscular exercise, lactic acid, and the supply and utilization of oxygen, *Q J Med* 16:135-171, 1923.
14. Wasserman K, McElroy MB: Detecting the threshold of anaerobic metabolism in cardiac patients during exercise, *Am J Cardiol* 14:844-852, 1964.
15. Davis JA: Anaerobic threshold: review of the concept and directions for future research, *Med Sci Sports Exerc* 17:6-18, 1985.
16. Brooks GA: Anaerobic threshold: review of the concept and directions for future research, *Med Sci Sports Exerc* 17:22-31, 1985.
17. Gladden LB, Yates JW, Stremel RW, Stamford BA: Gas exchange and lactate anaerobic thresholds: inter- and intra-evaluator agreement, *J Appl Physiol* 58:2082-2089, 1985.

18. Yeh MP, Gardner RM, Adams TD, et al: "Anaerobic threshold": problems of determination and validation, *J Appl Physiol* 55:1178-1186, 1983.
19. Shimizu M, Myers J, Buchanan N, et al: The ventilatory threshold: method, protocol, and evaluator agreement, *Am Heart J* 122:509-516, 1991.
20. Connett RJ, Gayeski TEJ, Honig GR: Lactate accumulation in fully aerobic working dog gracilis muscle, *Am J Physiol* 246:H120-H128, 1984.
21. Issekutz B, Shaw WAS, Issekutz AC: Lactate metabolism in resting and exercising dogs, *J Appl Physiol* 40:312-319, 1976.
22. Stanley WC, Neese RA, Wisneski JA, Gertz EW: Lactate kinetics during submaximal exercise in humans: studies with isotopic tracers, *J Cardiopulmonary Rehabil* 9:331-340, 1988.
23. Beaver WL, Wasserman K, Whipp BJ: Improved detection of lactate threshold during exercise using a log-log transformation, *J Appl Physiol* 59:1936-1940, 1985.
24. Hughson RL, Weisiger KH, Swanson GD: Blood lactate concentration increases as a continuous function during progressive exercise, *J Appl Physiol* 62:1975-1981, 1987.
25. Myers J, Walsh D, Buchanan N, et al: The lactate response revisited: continuous versus "threshold" increase. (Submitted, 1992.)
26. Davis JA, Frank MH, Whipp BJ, Wasserman K: Anaerobic threshold alterations caused by endurance training in middle-aged men, *J Appl Physiol* 46:1039-1046, 1979.
27. Ready AE, Quinney HA: Alterations in anaerobic threshold as the result of endurance training and detraining, *Med Sci Sports Exerc* 14:292-296, 1982.
28. Tanaka K, Matsuura Y, Matsuyaka A, et al: A longitudinal assessment of anaerobic threshold and distance running performance, *Med Sci Sports Exerc* 16:278-282, 1986.
29. Sullivan MJ, Cobb FR: The anaerobic threshold in chronic heart failure: relationship to blood lactate, ventilatory basis, reproducibility, and response to exercise training, *Circulation* 81:1147-1158, 1990.
30. Matsumura N, Nishijima H, Kojima S, et al: Determination of anaerobic threshold for assessment of functional state in patients with chronic heart failure, *Circulation* 68:360-367, 1983.
31. Weber KT, Kinasewitz GT, Janicki JS, Fishman AP: Oxygen utilization and ventilation during exercise in patients with chronic cardiac failure, *Circulation* 65:1213-1223, 1982.
32. Myers J, Atwood JE, Sullivan M, et al: Perceived exertion and gas exchange after calcium and β-blockade in atrial fibrillation, *J Appl Physiol* 63:97-104, 1987.
33. Sullivan M, Atwood AE, Myers J, et al: Increased exercise capacity after digoxin administration in patients with heart failure, *J Am Coll Cardiol* 13:1138-1143, 1989.
34. Dickstein K, Barvik S, Aarsland T, et al: A comparison of methodologies in detection of the anaerobic threshold, *Circulation* 81(suppl II):II-38–II-46, 1990.
35. Hughes EF, Turner SC, Brooks GA: Effects of glycogen depletion and pedaling speed on "anaerobic threshold," *J Appl Physiol* 52:1598-1607, 1982.
36. Whipp BJ, Wand SA, Wasserman K: Respiratory markers of the anaerobic threshold, *Adv Cardiol* 35:47-64, 1986.
37. Gaesser GA, Poole DC: Lactate and ventilatory threshold: disparity in time course of adaptations to training, *J Appl Physiol* 61:999-1004, 1986.
38. Hughson RL: Alterations in the oxygen deficit-oxygen debt relationships with beta-adrenergic receptor blockade in man, *J Physiol* (Lond.) 349:375-387, 1984.
39. Petersen ES, Whipp BJ, David JA, et al: Effects of β-adrenergic blockade on ventilation and gas exchange during exercise in humans, *J Appl Physiol* 54:1306-1313, 1983.

40. Twentyman OP, Disley A, Gribbin HR, et al: Effect of β-adrenergic blockade on respiratory and metabolic responses to exercise, *J Appl Physiol* 51:788-792, 1981.
41. Linnarsson D: Dynamics of pulmonary gas exchange and heart rate changes at start and end of exercise, *Acta Physiol Scand* 415:1-68, 1974.
42. Linnarsson D, Karlsson J, Fagraeus L, Saltin B: Muscle metabolites and oxygen deficit with exercise in hypoxia, *J Appl Physiol* 36:399-402, 1974.
43. Sietsema KE, Daly JA, Wasserman K: Early dynamics of O_2 uptake and heart rate as affected exercise work rate, *J Appl Physiol* 67:2535-2541, 1989.
44. Hickson RC, Bomze HA, Holloszy JO: Faster adjustment of O_2 uptake to the energy requirement of exercise in the trained state, *J Appl Physiol* 44:877-881, 1978.
45. Taylor HL, Buskirk E, Heuschel A: Maximal oxygen intake as an objective measurement of cardiorespiratory performance, *J Appl Physiol* 8:73-80, 1955.
46. Pollock ML, Bohannon RL, Cooper KH, et al: A comparative analysis of four protocols for maximal treadmill stress testing, *Am Heart J* 92:39-46, 1976.
47. Froelicher VF, Brammell H, Davis G, et al: A comparison of the reproducibility and physiologic response to three maximal treadmill exercise protocols, *Chest* 65:512-517, 1974.
48. Myers J, Walsh D, Buchanan N, Froelicher VF: Can maximal cardiopulmonary capacity be recognized by a plateau in oxygen uptake? *Chest* 96:1312-1316, 1989.
49. Myers J, Walsh D, Sullivan M, Froelicher VF: Effect of sampling on variability and plateau in oxygen uptake, *J Appl Physiol* 68:404-410, 1990.
50. Katch VL, Sady SS, Freedson P: Biological variability in maximum aerobic power, *Med Sci Sports Exerc* 14:21-25, 1982.
51. Noakes TD: Implications of exercise testing for prediction of athletic performance: a contemporary perspective, *Med Sci Sports Exerc* 20:319-330, 1988.
52. Jones NL: Clinical exercise testing, Philadelphia, 1988, WB Saunders, pp 306-311.
53. Wasserman K, Hansen JE, Sue DY, Whipp BJ: Principles of exercise testing and interpretation, Philadelphia, 1987, Lea & Febiger, pp 72-86.
54. Hansen JE, Sue DY, Wasserman K: Predicted values for clinical exercise testing, *Am Rev Respir Dis,* Suppl 549-555, 1984.
55. Bruce RA, Kusumi F, Hosmer D: Maximal oxygen uptake and nomographic assessment of functional aerobic impairment in cardiovascular disease, *Am Heart J* 85:546-562, 1973.
56. Shephard RJ: Endurance fitness, Toronto, 1969, University of Toronto Press.
57. Åstrand P: Human physical fitness, with special reference to sex and age, *Physiol Rev* 36(suppl 2):307-335, 1956.
58. Åstrand I: Aerobic work capacity in men and women with special reference to age, *Acta Physiol Scand* 49(suppl 196):1-92, 1960.
59. Lange-Anderson K, Shephard RJ, Denolin H, et al: Fundamentals of exercise testing, Geneva, 1971, World Health Organization.
60. Moris CK, Myers J, Kawaguchi T, et al: Nomogram for exercise capacity using METs and age, *J Am Coll Cardiol,* 1993. (In press.)

Special Methods

Computerized Exercise ECG Analysis

A digital computer was first used for electrocardiographic analysis by Taback and colleagues in 1959.[1] They pointed out the advantages of digital versus analog data processing including more precise and more accurate measurements, less distortion in recording, and direct accessibility to digital computer analysis and storage techniques. Other advantages include rapid mathematical manipulation (averaging), avoidance of the drift inherent in analog components, digital algorithm control permitting changing analysis schema with ease (software rather than hardware changes), and no degradation with repetitive playback. Advantages of digital processing apparent when outputting data include higher plotting resolution and facile repetitive manipulation.

The two critical problems posed by exercise ECG testing are (1) reduction of the amount of electrocardiographic data collected during the testing and (2) the elimination of electrical noise and movement artifact associated with exercise. Since the total period of an exercise test can exceed 30 minutes, and many physicians want to analyze all 12 leads during and after testing, the resulting quantity of ECG data and measurements can quickly become excessive. The three-lead vectorcardiographic (or "3-D," that is, aV_F, V_2, V_5) approach would reduce the amount of data; however, clinicians favor the 12-lead electrocardiogram (ECG). The exercise electrocardiogram often includes both random and periodic noise of both high and low frequency that can be attributable to respiration, muscle artifact, electrical interference, wire continuity, and electrode-skin contact problems. In addition to reducing noise and facilitating data reduction, computer processing techniques have also demonstrated the potential to make precise and accurate measurements, to separate and capture dysrhythmic beats, to per-

form spatial analysis, and to apply optimal diagnostic criteria for ischemia.

With the advent of large-scale integrated electronics, microcomputers have been developed to process the exercise ECG, thus eliminating the need for the larger, more expensive digital computers required in the past. Microcomputers can be used to digitize electrocardiographic signals and immediately apply digital techniques while the data are being gathered; that is, on-line and in real time. Earlier approaches to computer processing required that analog data be initially recorded during the test, digitized later, and then subsequently analyzed off line.

CAUSES OF NOISE

There are many reasons noise appears in the exercise ECG signal that cannot be corrected, even by meticulous skin preparation. Noise is defined here as any electrical signal that is foreign to or distorts the true electrocardiographic waveform. With this definition of noise, the types of noise that may be present can be attributable to any combination of line frequency (60 Hz), muscle, respiration, contact, or continuity artifact. Line-frequency noise is generated by the interference of the 60 Hz electrical energy with the electrocardiogram. This noise can be reduced by use of shielded patient cables. If despite these precautions this noise is still present, the simplest way to remove it is to design a 60 Hz notch filter and apply it in series with the ECG amplifier. A notch filter removes only the line frequency; that is, it attenuates all frequencies in a narrow band around 60 Hz. This noise can also be removed by attenuation of all frequencies above 59 Hz; however, this method of removing line-frequency noise is not recommended, since it causes waveform distortion and results in a system that does not meet American Heart Association specifications. The most obvious manifestation of distortion caused by such filters is a decrease in R-wave amplitude; therefore a true notch filter is advisable. An example of 60 Hz noise and its removal by a notch filter is given in Figure 4-1.

Muscle noise is generated by the activation of muscle groups and is usually of high frequency. This noise, along with other types of high-frequency noise, can be reduced by signal averaging. Motion noise, another form of high-frequency noise, is caused by the movement of skin and the electrodes, which in turn causes a change in the contact resistance. Respiration causes an undulation of the waveform amplitude and the baseline value varies with the respiratory cycle. Baseline wander can be reduced by low-frequency filtering; however, low-frequency filtering results in distortion of the ST segment and can cause artifactual ST-segment depression and slope changes. Other baseline removal approaches have been used, including linear interpolation between isoelectric regions, high-order polynomial estimates,

and cubic-spline techniques, which can each smooth the baseline value to various degrees (Figure 4-2). The new class of digital filters has just been implemented by most manufacturers and results in only several seconds of delay before on-line processing. Changes in waveform amplitude with respiration are physiological in nature and may have clinical significance; however, these changes can be modified by signal averaging. This method can result in some problems when one is comparing the average beats between rest and exercise because the ratio of inspiratory to expiratory beats is greater during exercise than at rest.

Contact noise appears as low-frequency noise or sometimes as step discontinuity baseline drift. It can be caused by either poor skin preparation resulting in high skin impedance, or by air-bubble entrapment in the electrode gel. It is reduced by meticulous skin preparation and by rejection of beats that show large baseline drift. Also, by using the median rather than the mean for signal averaging, this type of drift can be reduced. Continuity noise caused by intermittent breaks in the

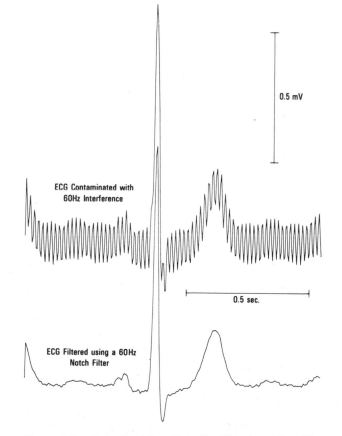

0.5 mV

ECG Contaminated with
60Hz Interference

0.5 sec.

ECG Filtered using a 60Hz
Notch Filter

Figure 4-1   Example of the effect of a 60-hertz notched filter.

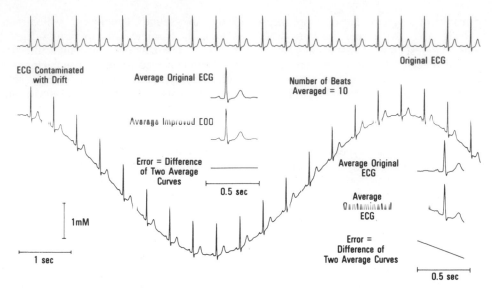

Figure 4-2 Example of the effect of a cubic spline filter on baseline wander.

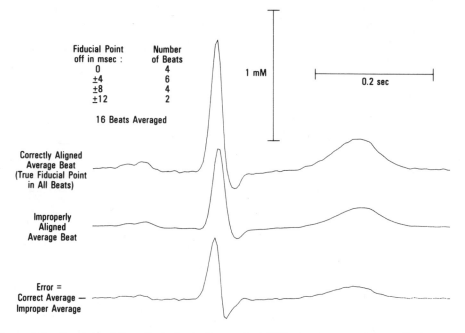

Figure 4-3 Example of the effect of misalignment of QRS complexes on the resultant averaged waveform.

cables is rarely a problem because of technologic advances in cable construction, except, of course, when cables are abused or overutilized.

Most of the sources of noise can be effectively reduced by beat averaging. However, two types of artifact that can actually be caused by the signal-averaging process are attributable to (1) the introduction of beats that are morphologically differ- ent from others in the average and (2) the misalign- ment of beats during averaging (exemplified in Fig- ure 4-3). As the number of beats included in the average increases, the level of noise reduction is greater. Electrocardiographic waveforms change in morphology over time, however, and consequently averaging time and the number of beats to be in- cluded in the average has to be compromised.

OUTLINE OF COMPUTER FUNCTIONS

The computer converts the original continuous analog electrocardiographic signal into a discrete, digital representation of voltages sampled at regular fixed intervals that can be easily handled during subsequent computer processing. Provided that the frequency of signal sampling is appropriate, the duration of the sampling window is long enough, and the computer word size is adequate, the resultant digital signal will faithfully describe and reproduce the shape of the original electrocardiographic waveform. The following functions are found in all computerized exercise systems:

Recognition of electrocardiographic complexes

The ECG complex is detected either on the basis of the largest amplitude, specific frequency components, or the rate of voltage change.

Finding a fiducial point or landmark

Serial beats can be accurately time aligned with reference to a recognizable feature or point in each complex; this alignment point can be the downslope of the R-wave using rate of voltage change, frequency components, or a maximum correlation.

Choosing the beats to be averaged

This process excludes all premature ventricular contractions, all aberrant beats, and regions of excessive noise by choosing beats that are as similar as possible; this is accomplished by use of one or more methods such as recognition of R R interval duration and polarity differences, classification by multivariate cluster analysis, calculation of the area differences, template comparison, and maximal cross-correlation of complexes.

Averaging the selected beats

Averaging is accomplished by use of either the mean or the median approach and results in a single representative ECG cycle with reduced noise; the median has the advantage of being relatively insensitive to the inclusion of premature ventricular complexes or abrupt baseline shifts (Figure 4-4).

Waveform recognition

Once the representative ECG cycle is formed, the algorithms for recognizing the beginning and end of the P-wave, QRS complex, and T-wave are implemented. These algorithms can recognize the waveform complexes and intervals by one of three ways: (1) the peak of the R-wave or the nadir of the S-wave is located and measurements of the ST-segment amplitude at a fixed interval beyond this landmark are taken; (2) the onset or off-set of a complex can be identified by use of time derivatives from a single lead such as V_5; and (3) the beginning and end of the QRS complex can be demarcated by use of a variety of mathematical constructs, such as change in spatial velocity. The third approach is the most accurate, but surprisingly little validation has been done of the various algorithms that have been empirically derived to accomplish this recognition process.

Once the boundaries of the P, QRS, and T-wave components are demarcated, measurements can then be made of the ST segment. These measurements are made with reference to an isoelectric baseline located within the PR segment. This can be found by use of a fixed interval before the Q- or R-wave or by various other algorithms that search for a flat region.

COMPUTER PRINCIPLES

The following is an explanation of the principles of computerized exercise ECG signal processing. Figure 4-5 illustrates analog-to-digital conversion. An analog signal can be represented by a continuous signal that varies in amplitude with time. Converting the analog signal into a digital signal requires sampling it periodically at fixed time intervals and converting the amplitudes at any point in time into binary numbers that have a time index or sequence. The digital signal is recorded as a binary number with each bit corresponding to a fixed voltage level determined by the analog-to-digital converter.

The basic computer storage unit is the byte, or word, that has a certain number of bits for a given computer and reflects how large or small an integer can be represented within the computer. Analog-to-digital conversion resolution is determined in part by the word size. Storage-unit size affects the resolution by controlling the range of measurements that are possible, according to the formula 2^n minus 1 where n equals the number of bits in the word or byte size being used. An eight-bit digitizer divides the analog input range into 2^8 minus 1, or 255 fixed voltage units in the range -127 to $+127$. In general, the more bits per word, the greater the resolution. Resolution is also dependent on the sampling rate. The greater the sampling rate, the greater the detail of the analog signal that is retained. The more points sampled, however, the more digital data that must be analyzed and stored. The usual sampling rates used for electrocardiography are 250/sec (4 msec increments) or 500/sec (2 msec increments). In addition to sampling rate and word size, signal resolution is also determined by the positive-to-negative analog input voltage window. The ana-

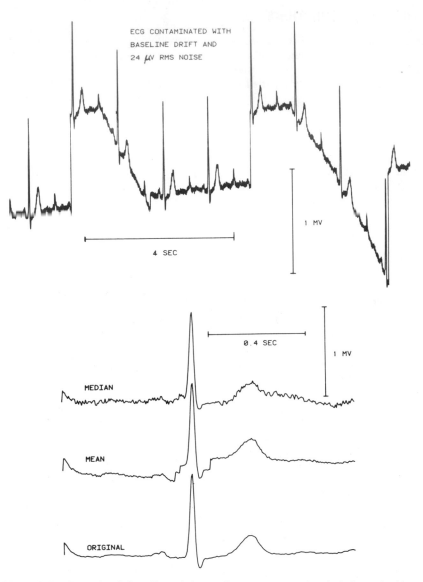

Figure 4-4 Example of the effect of the median process on electrical discontinuities.

log window must be large enough to accept the largest possible ECG signal-amplitude excursions; however, a large window will decrease the resolution for small ECG signals dependent on the number of analog-to-digital bits.

Figure 4-6 illustrates the effects of analog-to-digital converter resolution and input signal range, or window, on the details of the electrocardiogram. The top line is the actual electrocardiogram. The second line shows this ECG signal after being digitized and then being reconstructed as an analog signal. Five-bit resolution of the analog-digital converter loses details but roughly follows the S-, R-, and T-waves. The three-bit analog-digi-

tal converter distorts the P-, S-, and T-waves. When only half of the input range of the three-bit converter is used, the P- and T-waves are completely lost and the S-wave is considerably distorted, roughly equivalent to a two-bit analog-digital converter. The bottom figure shows the effects of sampling rate on the original ECG when reconstructed back as an analog signal. Sampling at 100 samples/sec accurately represents the P-, R-, S-, and T-wave amplitudes but loses some detail. Sampling at 10 samples/sec loses either the P- or R-wave and distorts the T-wave. A slight shift of the point in time when digitization begins (a phase shift) greatly affects resolution.

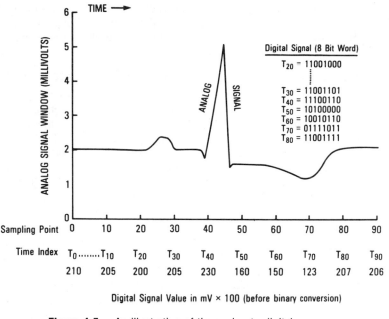

Figure 4-5 An illustration of the analog-to-digital process.

The American Heart Association and others have recommended that 16-bit resolution and 500 samples/sec are minimal digitizing specifications for computer processing of an electrocardiogram. High-frequency information can be lost, but now the industry can deliver instruments with higher resolution. Research indicates the value of higher-frequency components of the ECG, and so these rigorous digitizing specifications are necessary.

Mathematical constructs

Mathematical constructs applied by computers to digital electrocardiographic data are used for three purposes: (1) to locate and characterize QRS complexes, (2) to obtain a reference, or fiducial point, in the QRS complex, and (3) to determine the beginning and the end of the P-wave, QRS, and T-wave. The crucial purpose for these constructs, however, is the definition of a reference point to align beats and thus permit averaging. Peak R-wave was first used, but because of the rapid amplitude changes at each peak, different peak regions could be sampled during digitizing and result in misalignment of complexes. The point of most rapid change in electrocardiographic amplitude (dx/dt), which usually occurs in the downslope of the R-wave or in upslope of QS, can be consistently found and has been used.

Particularly for one-lead analysis, the mathematical construct of maximal dx/dt can be a reliable and efficient fiducial point. More recently, investigators have used spatial constructs from three time-coherent leads to achieve alignment. Figure 4-7 illustrates the major spatial mathematical constructs.

Thresholds set in these mathematical constructs also permit the localization of a waveform's beginning and end. Intuitively, the spatial recognition of the QRS, ST segment, and T-waves that requires multiple leads would be more accurate than algorithms applied to only one lead. Electrical activity may appear to end in a single lead but continue in a perpendicular direction with later activity seen in another lead.

Averaging is performed after beats are aligned by a fiducial point specified in a mathematical construct derived from the electrocardiogram. After alignment, each time indexed sample referenced to the fiducial point has an aligned series of values from each beat included in the averaging. These values can then be averaged in two ways. The easiest way is to sum the values of the samples at each aligned point and divide them by the number of beats included in the alignment array yielding the mean. The second approach is to determine the median. The median requires calculation of the 50th percentile, or midpoint value, at each time-index point. Because of its mathematical characteristics, the median has a greater central tendency and thus is less affected by discrepant values. When the median is used, however, the amount of random noise is not reduced as much as when the mean is used, since the mean has a higher signal-to-noise ratio. If a few prema-

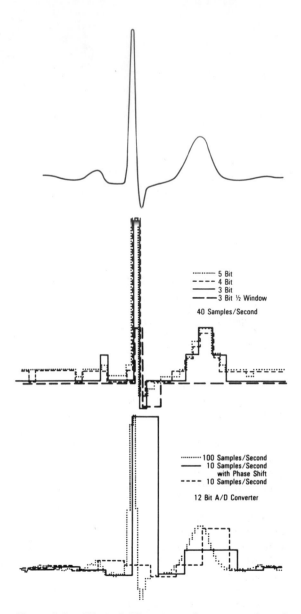

.... 5 Bit
---- 4 Bit
——— 3 Bit
——— 3 Bit ½ Window

40 Samples/Second

.... 100 Samples/Second
——— 10 Samples/Second
with Phase Shift
---- 10 Samples/Second

12 Bit A/D Converter

Figure 4-6   Effect of different sampling rates and word size on signal resolution.

ture ventricular contractions or aberrancies are included in beats used to generate an average, the median beat will not be affected; however the mean beat will be distorted. Thus the median beat appears to be a better estimate of the so-called true complex, though it is slightly higher in random noise content. Calculation of median requires larger computer memory and more processing time. A practical compromise frequently used is the trimmed mean.

Many researchers have utilized approximately 10 seconds of sampling time rather than a specific number of beats. This sample usually includes

sufficient beats for averaging techniques and lessens the chances of physiologic changes occurring and disturbing the average, particularly during exercise.

Computer-derived criteria for ischemia

Several investigators have proposed various computer criteria for detecting ischemia during exercise testing. Some of these are shown in Figure 4-8 and described in Table 4-1 (on page 57). In 1965, Blomqvist reported a computerized quantitative study of the Frank vector leads.[2] He divided the PR, QRS, and ST-T segments into eight subsegments of equal duration (that is, time normalized). He found that the maximal information for differentiation of patients with angina pectoris from normals was obtained by measurement of the ST amplitude at the time-normalized midpoint (ST_4) of the ST-T segment.

In 1969, Hornstein and Bruce reported using a computer of average transients to analyze exercise electrocardiographic data gathered from bipolar lead CB_5.[3] They reported that in apparently healthy middle-aged men, ST-segment depression with exercise was found to be more prevalent and of greater magnitude than anticipated. They concluded that a single bipolar precordial lead appeared to be as reliable as the three-dimensional Frank lead system.

McHenry (at the U.S. Air Force School of Aerospace Medicine) and colleagues reported results with a computerized exercise electrocardiographic system developed at USAFSAM and later applied at the University of Indiana.[4] ST-segment amplitude was measured over the 10 msec interval of the ST segment, starting at 60 msec after the peak of the R-wave. The slope of the ST-segment was measured from 70 to 110 msec beyond the R-wave peak. The PQ, or isoelectric, interval was found by scanning before the R-wave for the 10 msec interval with the least slope (rate of change). If the ST-segment depression was 1.0 mm or greater and if the sum of ST-segment depression in millimeters and ST slope in millivolts per second equaled or was less than 1.0 during or immediately after exercise, the response was defined as abnormal. This measurement, called the "ST index," was developed by comparison of two groups of subjects, one with angina pectoris and the other consisting of age-matched clinically normal people. When applied in clinical practice, it did not outperform standard criteria.

The magnitude of the ST-segment deviation from the baseline value has been expressed by some investigators in terms of the ST-area or integral (μV-sec). Sheffield and colleagues measured the area from the end of the QRS to either

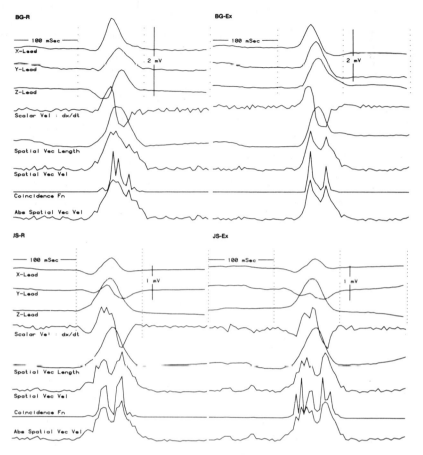

Figure 4-7   Major mathematical constructs utilized in digital signal processing.

the beginning of the T-wave or to where the ST-segment first crossed the isoelectric baseline.[5] In this study, normals demonstrated a modest increase in ST-integral with increasing heart rate, with the mean integral at maximal heart rate being −4.3 microvolts (for a reference comparison, 25 mm/sec paper speed and gain of 1 cm equals 1 mV, a 1 mm block thus equals 4 μV-sec. Patients with angina pectoris had a mean integral of −15.3 μV-sec, and this occurred at significantly lower heart rates. They computed the time-voltage integral of the ST-segment beginning at QRS end and continuing until crossing the isoelectric line or until reaching 80 msec after QRS end. This integral expresses the area of ST-segment deviation from the baseline. An ST-integral greater than −10 μV-sec was found to be an abnormal exercise electrocardiographic response, and the normal range was from 0 to −7.5 μV-sec. By arbitrarily taking −7.5 μV-sec as the cutoff range for normals, Sheffield obtained a sensitivity of 81% and a specificity of 95% on 41 normal subjects and 31 patients with angina. This measure-

ment has the advantage of "combining" slope and depression in one measurement. Using a cutoff point of −16 μV-sec, the MRFIT group found a sensitivity of 34% and a specificity of 96%.[6]

Simoons and colleagues reported using a PDP-8E computer on-line to process the Frank orthogonal leads.[7] The interactive computer system also controlled the exercise test so that the physician and technician could interact with the patient. In trying to decide the optimal criteria for the detection of ischemic heart disease, Simoons compared the computerized criteria of other investigators.[8] These criteria included ST-area, ST-index, polar coordinates, time-normalized ST-T amplitudes, and Chebyshev polynomials. These criteria were applied to a population of 95 coronary artery disease patients and 129 healthy males. He obtained the best results with ST-segment amplitude at 60 msec after the end of the QRS complex. A range of amplitudes for exercise heart rates was established by consideration of the response of the normal group. This approach is a logical one, since ST-segment depression in-

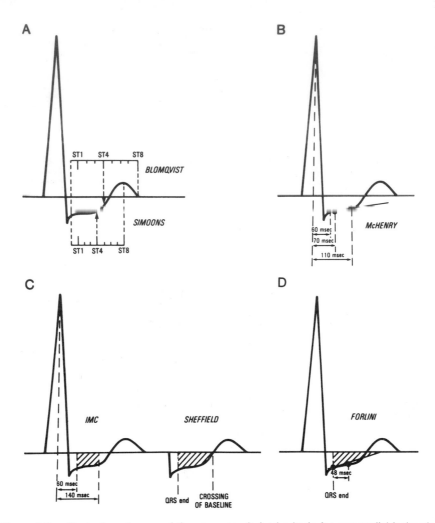

Figure 4-8   Illustration of some of the computer-derived criteria for myocardial ischemia.

creases in proportion to heart rate. He obtained a sensitivity of 81% and a specificity of 93% using this new criterion. In comparison, previous computer criteria were not superior to this ST-amplitude measurement adjusted for heart rate.

Sketch and colleagues conducted a study to evaluate the validity and usefulness of the Viagraph, a system made by International Medical Corp, for automated exercise ECG analysis.[9] Here, 107 patients who were referred for evaluation for chest pain underwent a Bruce test and coronary angiography. Patients who had a previous myocardial infarction and those on digitalis were excluded. Twenty-nine patients were considered to have performed submaximal testing because of not reaching 85% of maximal heart rate predicted for age. Lead V_5 was continuously sampled at 500 samples/sec, and 16 complexes were averaged sequentially. They measured the ST-integral over an interval from 60 to 140 msec after the peak of the R-wave and chose -6 μV-sec as the cutoff point for normals. This area measurement began at 60 msec after the peak of the R-wave and extended for 80 msec. Postexercise areas were more specific, whereas areas measured during exercise were more sensitive. Also, as the criteria for ischemia were lessened, sensitivity increased while specificity decreased, and these values varied over the range of ST-area criteria presented. It appeared that automated analysis of the ST-area was valid and comparable to visual analysis. They concluded that it should not negate the need for visual confirmation or for the physician's consideration of hemodynamic responses.

In an attempt to test the diagnostic value of an isolated ST-integral, Forlini and colleagues exercise-tested 133 subjects.[10] In this study, there were 62 normals (group 1), 29 patients with cor-

Table 4-1 Some of the computer-derived criteria for diagnosing coronary artery disease

Method	Criteria for abnormal (ischemia)
Classic ST-segment depression	With junctional depression of 0.1 mV (1 mm) or more: exercise-induced ST-segment depression must be flat or downsloping to be abnormal.
Upsloping ST 80	For upsloping ST segment with junctional depression of >2 mm from the isoelectric baseline: abnormal if ST segment is depressed 2 mm or more at 0.08 sec (80 msec) after J point (QRS end); normal if less depressed at that point.
ST midpoint (ST_4)	Blomqvist divided the ST segment from QRS end until the end of the T-wave into eight equal time periods. He found ST_4, or the midpoint, to provide the most discrimination between normal and abnormal. Simoons used a midpoint from QRS end until peak of the T-wave, since peak is easier to identify than T-end.
ST index	Abnormal when ST-segment depression is 1.0 mm or greater and the sum of ST-segment depression in mm plus ST slope in mV/sec is equal to or greater than 1.0. (Mean ST depression measured at 60 to 70 msec after R-wave peak, slope in 40 msec window afterward.)
ST integral	ST integral below isoelectric line greater than 10 μV-sec (1 square mm on electrocardiographic paper at standard speed and calibration = 4 μV-sec) is considered abnormal. Sheffield originally described measuring the ST integral from the end of the QRS complex to the beginning of the T-wave or where the ST segment crossed the isoelectric line. Others have implemented this by using the peak of the R-wave and measuring the area from 60 to 140 msec after the R-wave.
Spatial ST-T magnitudes	Dower and Bruce analyzed magnitudes and slopes at time-normalized areas of $\sqrt{X^2 + Y^2 + Z^2}$.
ST 60 for heart rate	A range of amplitudes at 60 msec after QRS end for exercise heart rate with measurements outside of a normal band and considered abnormal.

onary disease and an abnormal visual exercise test (group II), and 42 patients with congenital heart disease but with normal visual exercise tests (group III). Using the isolated ST-integral measurement, Forlini found an overall sensitivity of 85% and a specificity of 90%. In group III, 79% of the patients were diagnosed as abnormal despite having normal or nondiagnostic exercise tests as determined by visual criteria. In addition, more than 50% of the patients in group II manifested abnormal isolated ST-integrals before development of typical "ischemic" ST changes as detected visually. Also, in more than half of these patients the isolated ST-integral continued to be abnormal long after the disappearance of classic visual criteria for ischemia.

In 1977, Ascoop and colleagues reported on the diagnostic performance of automatic analysis of the exercise ECG studied in 147 patients with coronary angiography.[11] The computer-determined results were compared with visual analyses of the same recordings. Using bicycle ergometry and recording two bipolar thoracic leads, computer processing was performed on the electrocardiograms

gathered only during the stage of maximal exercise. A single, averaged beat was obtained, and onset and the offset of the QRS complex were determined using a template method. The ST depressions at 10 and 50 msec after QRS end, ST slope, and ST integral were measured. A group of patients with a mean age of 48 were divided into a learning and testing set. Many of the patients were referred from other hospitals where they had negative exercise tests. Of the 87 patients in the learning set, 57 had abnormal coronary angiograms, and 30 essentially had no coronary lesions. In the test population of 60 patients, 39 had significant coronary disease, whereas 21 had no angiographic disease. The integral value of 8 μV-sec was similar to a previous value used by Sheffield. Ascoop concluded that the bipolar leads he used were superior to vector leads and that the computer criteria yielded higher sensitivities and specificities than visual analysis.

In 1979, Turner and colleagues reported their findings in 125 consecutive patients who had undergone exercise treadmill tests and coronary angiography.[12] The Quinton model 740 ECG data

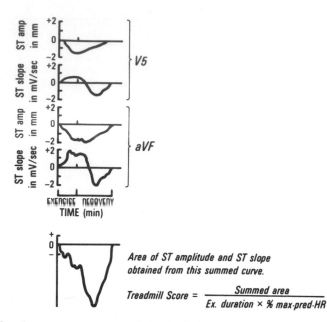

Figure 4-9   Area measurements made by the CASE-I for the Hollenberg scoring system.

computer analyzed V_5 and calculated the ST-index. Of the 125 patients studied, 38 had normal coronary arteries, and the rest had significant disease. Unfortunately, their results were confounded by consideration of angina in the determination of abnormal results and a vague classification of "inadequate test."

The Hollenberg Treadmill Exercise Score (TES). Hollenberg and associates have developed a treadmill score that grades the ST-segment response to exercise by combining the total of all changes in ST amplitude and slope measured during the entire exercise test and throughout recovery.[13] This treadmill score is derived by summation of the areas of the time curves that describe the ST-segment amplitude and slope changes in two leads (aV_F and V_5) and division of this summed area by the duration of exercise (in minutes) and the percent maximal predicted heart rate achieved during the exercise test (Figure 4-9). These area measurements were obtained using a Marquette CASE-I computerized exercise system. They reported that the treadmill exercise score could distinguish patients with three-vessel or left main disease from those with no significant disease.

In their first study, 70 patients who had coronary angiography and 46 healthy volunteers were included. Using the treadmill exercise score shown below, sensitivity and specificity were 85% and 98% respectively:

Treadmill exercise score =

$$\frac{\text{J-point amplitude and ST-slope curve areas score}}{\text{Duration of exercise} \times \text{Percent predicted max heart rate achieved}}$$

This score includes the following measures of severity: depth of J-point depression, slope, occurrence of depression in relation to heart rate, decreased heart rate response to exercise, and functional capacity. The area under the curves were considered during hyperventilation and when ST-segment abnormalities were present at rest. Subsequent refinements by this group included validation of adjusting the amplitude of ST depression by R-wave amplitude using a thallium ischemia score.[14] They then applied the modified TES to asymptomatic army officers.[15] Detrano at Cleveland clinic, in a large series of patients without prior myocardial infarction, found visual analysis to outperform the original, uncorrected Hollenberg treadmill exercise score. Vergari and colleages[16] also reported poor results with the Hollenberg score.

ST/HR slope

Although accomplished originally manually, the measurement of the ST-segment/heart rate slope is included here because it is more practical when performed by computer. In 1980, Elamin, Linden, and colleagues reported results with a new exer-

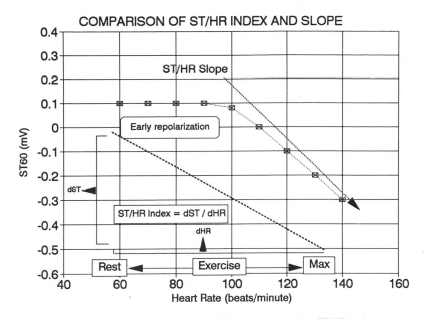

COMPARISON OF ST/HR INDEX AND SLOPE

Figure 4-10   Comparison of the ST/HR slope and the ST/HR index.

cise test criteria proposed to detect the presence and severity of coronary artery disease.[17] In 206 patients with anginal pain and using recordings from 13 electrocardiographic leads (including CM_5), the maximal rate of progression of ST-segment depression relative to increases in heart rate (maximal ST/HR ratio) was measured. Displacement of the ST segment was measured at 80 msec after QRS end. Curves were constructed, relating the values of the ST segment to heart rate during rest and exercise in each of the 13 leads. Rate of development of ST-segment depression with respect to increments in heart rate observed in any one lead was represented as the slope of a computed regression line. The ranges of maximal ST/HR slopes in the 38 patients with no disease, 49 with single-vessel, 75 with double-vessel, and 44 with triple-vessel disease were different from each other, and there was no overlap in the data between the adjacent groups. They claimed they had no false-positive, false-negative, or indeterminate results. This procedure required 3 hours of analysis time per test by a knowledgable person and a special protocol that resulted in a linear heart rate increase of 10 bpm per stage.

Thwaites and co-workers performed a study to determine whether the maximal ST/HR slope using a bicycle ergometer is better than the standard 12-lead analysis using a Bruce treadmill protocol.[18] The maximal ST-segment/HR slope was calculated in 81 patients and compared with the results of a standard 12-lead exercise test. In 21 patients (26%), the ST/HR slope could not be cal-

culated. In 60 patients with ST/HR slope values, the extent of the coronary artery disease was predicted in 24 patients (40%). The sensitivity and specificity of the ST/HR slope in allowing prediction of the presence of coronary artery disease in the 60 patients with slope values were 91% and 27% respectively. The sensitivity and specificity of the usual treadmill test in the 81 patients were 81% and 64% respectively.

Kligfield and co-workers compared the exercise ECG with radionuclide ventriculography and coronary angiography in 35 patients with stable angina to assess the value of the ST/HR slope.[19] An ST/HR slope of 6.0 or more allowed identification of three-vessel coronary disease with a sensitivity of 89% and specificity of 88%. The exercise ST/HR slope was directly related to the exercise ejection fraction, but there was considerable scatter. Somewhat poorer results were obtained when they enlarged their series, and such results have demonstrated considerable variability in the maximal slope measurement particularly as effected by the rate of heart rate changes and the frequency with which the ST measurements are made. Quyyumi and colleagues assessed these criteria in 78 patients presenting with chest pain and found that the maximum ST-segment/heart rate slope had a sensitivity of 90% but a specificity of only 40% and was not useful in predicting the extent of coronary disease.[20]

ST/heart rate index. Fortunately, Kligfield and co-workers[21] subsequently obtained similar results by simply dividing the change in the ST segment from baseline value to maximum exercise by the change in heart rate over the same time period. This measurement has been called the ST/HR index, and in Figure 4-10 it is compared to the ST/HR slope. Kligfield and co-workers excluded tests with upsloping ST segments from standard visual analysis; such results occurred in 17% of their patients. As is advisable and done in clinical practice, such tests should be considered borderline or normal. By excluding them, Kligfield and co-workers found the standard criteria of 1 mm to have a significantly poorer performance than the ST/HR index or slope.

ST amplitude at ST60 or ST0 for ST/HR index?

The most recent paper in *Circulation* by Okin and co-workers[22] is a rebuttal to our paper,[23] wherein we published results dissimilar to those in their first paper in *Circulation*,[21] in which they found the ST/HR index to have improved sensitivity and specificity compared to standard ST measurements. Our results showed equal efficacy of the standard measurements and the index. Whereas they used the ST amplitude at ST60 without considering slope, we made ST measurements at ST0 and then only when the ST segment was horizontal or downsloping. At the time, we utilized visual measurements. Subsequently we have employed a personal computer to obtain computerized measurements[24] similar to what Okin and co-workers report using a Quinton work station. This permitted us to analyze optical discs containing exercise ECG data that we have been gathering since 1987.[25]

They hypothesize that the ST measurement point affects the ST/heart rate index but not standard measurements. We performed a similar analysis to theirs to test this hypothesis. We selected 202 patients with cardiac catheterization and exercise tests referred initially for evaluation of possible coronary artery disease but without a history or ECG evidence of a prior myocardial infarction. All tests were performed using a modified Balke-Ware or ramp protocol resulting in nearly linear increases in heart rate. All were males, with a mean age of 60 years. Using 70% or greater diameter narrowing as a criterion for coronary artery disease, we found that 71 (35%) had no significant coronary disease and 60 (30%) had three-vessel or left main disease. There were no significant differences in these measurements as to their discriminating performance. We have since been able to implement several other twists on the ST/heart rate measurement. We have implemented the actual ST/heart rate slope, have summed depression in all leads, and have chosen the lead

with the greatest depression for division by change in heart rate.

We could not duplicate the findings of Okin and colleagues in our population or support their hypothesis. The measurement point does not appear to affect the ST-measurement characteristics when made without slope considered. Once again, we explain our divergent results by population differences between ours and Cornell's and not methodology. Our population is more typical of that seen by a clinician, and all patients underwent cardiac catheterization, unlike those in the study by Okin and colleagues. We utilized a purely male population, which should, if anything, give improved test performance.

The effect of limited challenge

Concern must be directed to the unusual populations the Cornell group has used to validate the ST/HR slope or index. Separating the most sick from the most well is not a fair evaluation. The challenge in clinical practice is to separate those in the middle group. They included patients with prior myocardial infarctions, normals who did not present a diagnostic problem, angina patients without cardiac catheterization, and a few patients with confirmed angiographic disease. This mixture of patients explains why their receiver operating characteristic (ROC) curves have such large areas and do not exhibit 0% sensitivity at 100% specificity. It is inappropriate to use specificity from a group of normals and sensitivity from a group of abnormals to assess test performance. Another problem is the difference of mean maximal heart rate between their three groups, that is, 165 bpm for the normals versus 134 bpm for the patients with angina versus 115 bpm for the catheterization-confirmed coronary disease patients. ROC curves based on heart rate alone would yield results comparable to their ST-segment analysis.

The obvious differences between our study and that of Kligfield and co-workers include the following: (1) they considered upsloping ST segments to be equivocal for standard analysis, whereas we did not; (2) only 100 of their patients had cardiac catheterization, all with angina pectoris, whereas we had 298 patients who underwent catheterization for clinical reasons without further selection for angina; (3) they considered ST amplitudes at 70 msec after J-junction, whereas we used J-junction; (4) they included post–myocardial infarction patients without distinguished test performance in those with and without MI; and (5) they used 50% luminal reduction, whereas we used 75%. We chose 75% versus 50% luminal reduction as the criterion for angiographic disease because the former has a higher short-term prognostic value, but we found, as Kligfield did, that there was little difference in patient classification and no difference between the criteria in test performance. We chose J-junction instead of 60 msec later to avoid the T-wave at high heart rates but have demonstrated little difference in test classification between these two points. We included all patients who underwent both procedures because this is the group clinicians would like to be better able to classify. Typical angina patients, as studied only by Kligfield, have a high probability of coronary disease regardless of the test results, and clinicians usually do not test such patients for diagnostic purposes. Patients with myocardial infarction are presumed to have coronary artery disease, and so, unlike Kligfield and co-workers, we distinguished them for diagnostic evaluation but included them for identifying severe coronary disease. In addition, Kligfield and co-workers did not consider pretest probability of disease or the performance of the criteria for identifying severe disease. Since the ROC analysis showed no difference in the criteria compared, we emphasized the portion of the curve that would be used by clinicians and considered the dependence of test performance on clinical subsets. Herbert and co-workers did not find beta-block administration to influence the diagnostic performance of the ST analysis method (Figure 4-11).[26]

The question arises as to a fair comparison of these criteria. Certainly excluding tests with depressed but upsloping ST segments from analysis, as done by Kligfield and co-workers, is not a practical approach in clinical practice. They excluded 17% of patients tested from analysis in a group already selected by baseline ECGs and medication status that would not invalidate ST analysis. Considering ST depression with an inadequate upward slope (that is, ST depression 1 mm at 60 or 80 msec after J-junction) to be abnormal increases sensitivity and decreases specificity. Our approach was to consider them negative as is done in most clinical laboratories and as recommended by the American Heart Association guidelines. Adding recovery measurements to the ST/HR index may improve its performance. In our data set, consideration of recovery increased the sensitivity of standard analysis from 50% to 59% without a decline in predictive value.

Sato and colleagues[27] have reported applying the Leeds methods but using a Bruce protocol and computerized ECG analysis. They selected 142 patients out of 1026 who had undergone coronary angiography and exercise testing and 402 low-risk asymptomatics. For any disease, they used stan-

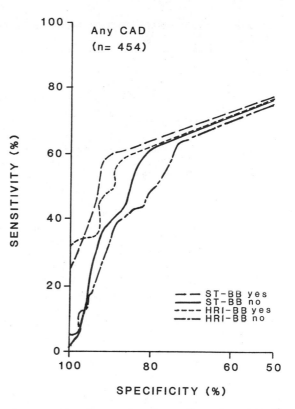

Figure 4-11 Comparative diagnostic performance of the most ST depression in exercise or recovery (ST) and the ST/HR index (HRI) in patients receiving or not receiving beta-blocker therapy (BB). *CAD*, Coronary artery disease.

dard criteria of 1 mm if horizontal or downsloping and 1.5 mm at 80 msec after J-junction if upsloping; for left main/three-vessel disease they used the considerably positive criteria of Weiner and co-workers. For the ST/HR slope, aV_F and V_5 changes appeared to be combined resulting in slope values twice as high as those reported by other investigators. ST/HR slope could not be calculated for technical reasons in nearly 20% of their patients. They chose slope values of 7.5 and 16 μV/bpm as partition criteria for any and left main/three-vessel disease respectively.

Metanalysis

Table 4-2 compares the results of the major studies evaluating the ability of the exercise test to identify coronary artery disease using standard as well as heart rate–adjusted criteria. Differences in test performance between studies can be explained by population selection, particularly "limited challenge," and by methodological differences. Although it is always difficult to compare

Table 4-2 Major studies that have evaluated the computer criteria for diagnosing coronary artery disease

First author	Number in study	Age (average or range)	Computer criteria for ischemia	Standard visual analysis		Computer analysis	
				Sensitivity (%)	Specificity (%)	Sensitivity (%)	Specificity (%)
McHenry	86 patients	50	ST index	68	—	82	95
Sheffield	31 patients	48	ST integral	—	—	81	95
	41 normals	56	(using QRS end)				
Sketch	107 patients	48	ST integral (using R-wave on Viagraph)	59	92	58	88
Turner	123 patients	48	ST index (Quinton analog system	—	—	82	83
Forlini	71 patients	53	Isolated ST	—	—	85	90
	62 normals	44	integral				
Hollenberg	70 patients	53	Treadmill score	71	82	85	91
	46 normals	23	(Marquette CASE I)				
Simoons	Initial:						
	52 patients	21-65	ST 60 with heart rate	50	94	85	91
	86 normals		considered				
	Test:						
	43 patients	21-65		51	95	84	88
	53 normals						
Ascoop	39 patients	52	0.035 mV 50 msec after J-junction in CC_5	28	100	67	95
	21 normals						
Detrano	122 patients	54	0.1 mV 80 msec after J-junction in V_5 and Hollenberg Score	51	86	50	85
	149 normals						
AVERAGES				44	91	77	90

studies with different populations and protocols, some conclusions seem appropriate. The ST/HR index or slope have yet to be reliably verified by other investigators as superior to standard interpretation. As Bobbio and Detrano pointed out in a metanalysis of this subject, only half of the published studies have supported heart rate adjustment and most of these positive studies came from Leeds and Cornell.[28] Morise and Duvall found no difference in test performance when comparing standard criteria and the heart rate index in an appropriate clinical population.[29] Further investigation into proving ST interpretation of ischemia can only be applauded despite the fits and starts that are inherent in such a pursuit.

To the clinician, what does our dispute mean? Our findings support the surprising power of the standard one-millimeter criteria. We find that visual analysis at the J-junction with the ST slope horizontal or downward in exercise or recovery has considerable power for diagnosing coronary artery disease. Computer simulation of this visual criteria in our hands matches or outperforms all the proposed computer criteria including the ST/heart rate index or ST/heart rate slope, even when they are measured at ST60. The clinician must consider the wisdom of switching to a new technique when it has not consistently been shown to improve upon established methods.

ST60 OR ST0 WITH OR WITHOUT SLOPE CONSIDERED

Uniform criteria for an abnormal exercise-induced ST-segment response that maximizes its diagnostic accuracy is essential, not only for obvious reasons, but also for internal consistency in direct comparisons of the exercise response in different populations. Unfortunately, a single method of interpretation has never been uniformly accepted.[30] There have been proponents of patterns of ST-segment depression that include upsloping as an abnormal response,[31] whereas others believe that the consideration of horizontal or downsloping

ST-segment depression significantly affects the accuracy of exercise testing beneficially. Points of contention regarding the interpretation of the exercise ECG still arise. Should the ST-segment depression be measured at the J-point or ≥60 msec after the J-point? Does the consideration of the slope of the ST-segment depression, using only horizontal or downsloping, improve diagnostic accuracy? Savvides and co-workers demonstrated little difference in the classification of patients between measurements made at the J-point and 70 msec later.[32] A metanalysis performed by Gianrossi and associates revealed that the consideration of slope had a significant influence on the accuracy of exercise testing,[33] but a study by Stuart and Ellestad suggests that upsloping ST-segment depression should still be considered an abnormal response.[31] Kurita and colleagues evaluated 230 patients referred for coronary arteriography, with standard exercise testing, and found that 60% (46/77) of patients with ≥1.5 mm junctional and upsloping ST-segment depression had at least one ≥75% coronary stenosis.[34] Stuart and Ellestad found that of 70 patients with upsloping ST-segment depression 40 (57%) had multivessel coronary disease.

The issue of whether the consideration of slope, in other words, excluding upsloping as an abnormal response, significantly improves diagnostic accuracy is another question. Rijneke and colleagues studied 623 patients with bicycle exercise testing and coronary angiography.[35] The criterion for an abnormal response was ST-segment depression of ≥0.1 mV measured 80 msec after the J-junction. There was no significant difference between measurements that included upsloping ST-segment depression as an abnormal response (sensitivity 66%/specificity 89%) and measurements that involved consideration of only horizontal or downsloping ST-segment depression as being abnormal (sensitivity 58%/specificity 92%). The positive (93% versus 94% respectively) and negative (56% versus 52%) predictive values were also virtually identical.

To clarify these issues a retrospective study of 173 males without prior myocardial infarction was performed (108 patients in a training population and 65 patients in a validation population).[36] By chi-square, the following order was demonstrated: measurements made at the J-junction with slope considered (ST0 + slope) ($\chi^2 = 24$; $p < 0.001$), measurements made 60 msec after the J-junction with slope considered (ST60 + slope) ($\chi^2 = 20$; $p < 0.001$), measurements made 60 msec after the J-junction (ST60) ($\chi^2 = 13$; $p < 0.001$), and measurements made at the J-junction (ST0) ($\chi^2 = 6$; $p = 0.01$). When one considers

only horizontal or downsloping slope as an abnormal response, measurements of ST-segment depression at either the J-junction (ST0 + slope) or 60 msec after the J-junction (ST60 + slope) were not significantly different as markers for the presence of any coronary disease. Receiver operating characteristic (ROC) curve analysis confirmed this in that no significant difference in the area under the ST0 + slope curve (0.76) and the ST60 + slope curve (0.76) was found ($z = 0.2$; two-tailed $p = 0.80$). ROC curve analysis did reveal that the additional consideration of slope added significant diagnostic discrimination to measurements made at the J-junction: area of curve with slope considered (0.76), without slope considered (0.6) ($z = 2.4$; two-tailed $p = 0.02$). However, slope did not significantly improve the discriminatory ability of exercise testing when measurements were made 60 msec after the J-junction: with slope considered (0.76), without slope considered (0.73) ($z = 1$; two-tailed $p = 0.33$). Similar results were obtained in the validation population of 65 patients.

When quantitating the depth of horizontal or downsloping exercise-induced ST-segment depression, there was no significant difference between measurements made at the J-junction or 60 msec after the J-junction as markers for coronary artery disease. Slope considerations were a significant improvement in the identification of coronary disease when measurements are made at the J-junction but not when they are made 60 msec after the J-junction. When using the computer-generated analysis of ST-segment depression measured at ST0 + slope the cut point of ≥0.7 mm of ST-segment depression had the best combination of sensitivity and specificity, not ≥1.0 mm of ST-segment depression, which was the best cutoff point for visual interpretation of the exercise electrocardiogram. The computer can measure the ST-segments more accurately than the human eye, and when evaluating ST-segments visually there is a "rounding off" of values; for example, 0.7 mm of ST-segment depression is often rounded up to 1.0 mm visually. For ST60 + slope the cutoff point of ≥0.6 mm, for ST0 without slope considered the cutoff point ≥1.4 mm, and for ST60 without slope considered the cutoff point ≥0.9 mm of exercise-induced ST-segment depression gave the best combinations of sensitivity and specificity.

Why slope improves measurements made at the J-junction and not at a point 60 msec later in the ST-segment is unclear. Let us assume that the cutoff point of ≥0.1 mV measured 60 msec after the J-junction is the optimal marker for coronary disease during exercise testing. To fulfill this criterion, a patient would need to have more ST-segment depression at the J-junction if it were upsloping so that at 60 msec after the J-junction it would still be measured ≥0.1 mV, but it would not have to be a greater amount of ST-segment depression at the J-junction if the slope were horizontal or downsloping because it would be the same measurement or even greater measured 60 msec later. Therefore the simplest measurement may be one taken at 60 msec after the J-junction with slope being disregarded.

Measurements of exercise-induced ST-segment depression at either the J-junction or 60 msec after the J-junction, regardless of slope, are reliable markers for coronary disease. When one is considering only horizontal or downsloping ST-segment depression as an abnormal response, there is no significant difference between measurements made at the J-junction or 60 msec later. Slope considerations significantly improve diagnostic accuracy when measurements are made at the J-junction but not for measurements made 60 msec after J-junction.

Multivariate approaches

Pruvost and co-workers in 1987 used the Marquette CASE II to process the exercise ECG on 558 men without prior myocardial infarction.[37] They considered computer-measured ST depression and slope, change in ST depression, and ST index. Using multivariate analysis, they found exercise duration, angina, age, and maximal heart rate to have a greater predictive accuracy for coronary artery disease than ST-segment measurements.

Detry and co-workers evaluated 387 men without prior myocardial infarction and not receiving beta-blockers who underwent computer-assisted exercise testing; 284 symptomatic patients had angiography and 103 healthy men were assumed to be free of coronary artery disease.[38] The computer-averaged ECG signal (x, y, and z) recorded only at maximal exercise, and maximal heart rate, systolic blood pressure, work load, and angina pectoris during the test were submitted to multivariate stepwise discriminant analysis. Pretest probability of coronary artery disease was calculated from age and chest pain history, and the above-mentioned variables were then used to calculate post-test probability. Of the ST measurements investigated, only ST60 amplitude and slope in lead X provided independent information. A compartmental rather than a categoric model provided the best performances (that is, 82% sensitivity, 92% specificity, and 83% predictive accuracy).

Direct comparison of computer criteria

Three studies have systematically compared several of the computer criteria described by other investigators. Simoons obtained the best separation of normals from patients with coronary disease with a single computer measurement, ST60 (ST-segment amplitude 60 ms after the QRS end) in Frank lead X when adjusted for heart rate.[39] This amplitude was considered relative to heart rate to adjust for the normal ST-segment depression that occurs with increasing heart rate. Subsequently, Decker and Simoons evaluated the ST/HR index, ST60 adjusted for heart rate, the Hollenberg score, and Detry's multivariate technique.[40] They studied 345 men with a computerized exercise ECG bicycle test. None had prior myocardial infarction or were taking digoxin, but half were receiving beta-blockers. Two hundred twenty-two of the subjects had undergone catheterization for chest pain, whereas the other 123 healthy men were considered to be free of coronary artery disease. The following ST measurements were made: (1) ST60 adjusted for instantaneous heart rate; (2) the Hollenberg score as well as just the time-area portion of the score including ST60 and slope in x and $y;$ (3) the discriminant function described by Detry and co-workers; and (4) the ST/HR index in lead X.

They found the diagnostic value of the TES to be low, but it was improved when the ST amplitude and slope time-areas were considered without adjustment for heart rate or time. The Detry discriminant function model and the ST/HR index functioned the best (that is, sensitivity 70% to 80%, specificity 90%) and were least affected by beta-blocker therapy. They found the Hollenberg score to function the poorest but the ST area components to perform reasonably well. Since the 12-lead ECG was not used, these studies must be confirmed. Also, Decker's study did not consider visual analysis. Our group has accomplished a similar comparison. We performed a retrospective analysis on 442 men, 200 without prior myocardial infarction, all with cardiac catheterization correlates. Surprisingly, slope in V_5 during recovery and the Hollenberg area-time plot of this measurement exhibited the greatest discriminating power for any or severe coronary artery disease.

Table 4-2 lists the results of most of the studies described above. For comparison, Table 4-3 lists the results of these studies, 33 studies relating angiographic findings with standard visual interpretation of the exercise test, 16 studies using thallium scintigraphy, and 12 studies using radionuclide ventriculography. It is apparent from these studies that computerized ECG analysis has outperformed the more expensive modalities.

Table 4-3   Comparison of the diagnostic performance of four exercise testing methods.

	Visual ECG $n = 33$	Computer ECG $n - 10$	Thallium scintigraphy $n = 16$	Radionuclide ventriculography $n = 12$
Sensitivity	66%	80%	76%	93%
Specificity	84%	91%	89%	79%

n, Number of reported studies.

REFINEMENTS BY THE MEDICAL INSTRUMENTATION INDUSTRY

Computers are being widely utilized as part of commercial exercise testing systems for processing exercise electrocardiograms gathered during clinical testing for three reasons: (1) inexpensive microprocessors can use software for filtering, averaging, and measuring ECG signals that previously could be performed only on larger, more expensive computers; (2) these microprocessors can present and summarize the exercise ECG responses in an attractive series of waveforms along with tables or graphs and can make a variety of measurements not previously possible or accurate when using standard visual techniques; and, (3) prior research has demonstrated that computerized measurements, particularly of the ST segment, significantly improve both the sensitivity and specificity of exercise testing.

In 1977, Marquette Electronics introduced a commercial on-line exercise system using a LSI-11 computer (CASE I). The computer performed test-control functions, signal conditioning, beat averaging, and on-line ST-segment measurements. Instead of simple mean beat averages, a new technique of averaging was introduced in this system. Called "incremental averaging" by the developers, it is a method well suited to a continuous input with slow changes. In this method of averaging, each digital sample of a new, time-aligned QRS complex is compared with its corresponding member in the currrent average. Alignment is accomplished using frequency components of the QRS complex. Wherever the average is low (or high) it is incremented (or decremented) by a small, fixed amount (3.5 µV) independent of the size of the difference. ST-level and ST-slope measurements were displayed and recorded. These measurements were made from the average cycle by use of the onset and offset of QRS determined during initialization. ST-slope measurements were made to correlate with visual impressions by dynamic adjustment of the ST-slope interval with heart rate. The ST-interval for slope measurement was one eighth of the average RR-interval. After sales exceeding 1000 units worldwide this unit was replaced by the CASE II. Also designed by David Mortara, Ph.D., it added 12-lead analysis, analog-to-digital signal conversion at the patient junction box, and a remote infrared hand-held controller. Two subsequent models developed by other engineers have been the CASE 12 and the Maxiply. They continue a tradition of mechanical and technical excellence that have made them popular around the world. The incremental average was a major breakthrough, almost simulating how the human reader learns from previous complexes what to look for even with noise present. Also, it was implemented when practical computer chips available to manufacturers did not have the power to average on line the waveforms as was previously done off line. Although there is some concern that the average may not follow changes quickly enough, this does not seem to be a problem in the clinical setting.

In 1983, a microprocessor-based commercial system called the Status 1000 was introduced by Quinton Instrument. The strong point of this system is that the exercise testing protocols and methodology can be easily programmed into the system by the operator. Since then, four subsequent models have been released (Q2000 to Q5000) that have improved on their concept. The Q5000 uses a touch screen, and its software can be updated by floppy disc. Time histograms of all parameters are recorded on a summary report at the end of the test. Quinton recently became the first company to offer a work station where exercise ECG data can be reviewed and measurements edited.

Siemens and Burdick have joined forces to develop a wide assortment of ECG devices. The Mega-Cart has the best new signal-processing software to come on the market in some time. Their ABC baseline filter will be patented. The liquid-crystal diode screen is very sharp, but many physicians find them difficult to use, and so a standard video monitor can be slaved. Schiller from Switzerland have presented a series of technically elegant devices for exercise testing. They have integrated gas analysis and use robotics to keep their prices low.

In 1985 Mortara Instruments released the ELIXIR exercise testing device. This system used a liquid-crystal diode screen similar to those used in lap-top computers. Particularily revolutionary though was the ability to connect this to a personal computer and collect continuous exercise ECG data by use of specialized software developed by Mortara for a planned Veterans Affairs cooperative study. Twelve-lead ECG data were sampled at 500 samples per second and stored on optical discs. With only minor compression (differences stored of 8 leads), 20 minutes of total exercise per recovery time required 5 megabytes per patient. With up to 640 megabytes per side available per $100 disc, it was now practical to create a digital exercise data base that could be used to validate scores and software. This device was followed in 1990 by the X-Scribe: a special board enabled a DOS personal computer to collect and process ECG data from patients and play them out on a thermal head printer. Color graphics, pop-down windowing menus, and a track ball make this a unique system.

The Mortara Data Logger

We have gathered a digital library of exercise ECG signals on patients who also have cardiac catheterization data using the Mortara Data Logger. The digital unprocessed ECG signals are stored on inexpensive optical discs similar to compact discs. These can be analyzed by use of various software or devices enabling comparisons of waveform processing as well as diagnostic performance of various algorithms or scores. Since the modern application of exercise testing utilizes computerized techniques, validations and comparisons will have a great influence on practice. Clinicians are not certain as to how and what measurements should be made or if published scores offer an advantage over visual methods. Since the exercise ECG is the most widely used procedure for deciding who should have further testing or interventions, clarification of its utility will greatly affect the practice of medicine. One outcome could be validation of a score or algorithm that will perform as well as more expensive modalities such as echocardiography or radionuclides. The digital data library will be available to resolve many secondary practical clinical as well as highly complicated software problems. The potential scientific information eminating from this library is enormous.

There are at least two reasons for utilizing commercial computerized exercise testing sys-

tems. First, a computerized system can decrease the time the referring physician must wait for the results of a test. The tests are facilitated by automation of the procedure and by the rapid generation of a final report. Systems using thermal head printers can mix graphics with alphanumerics producing a printed report that does not need typing. Secondly, if they meet their promise of improved diagnostic and prognostic information, this could result in more cost-effective and higher quality health care. Unfortunately, despite sales in the thousands, none of the commercial units have had independent validation of their signal-processing or signal-measurement algorithms, and their diagnostic capacities have not been adequately compared to standard visual techniques. However, most manufacturers use digital data bases to improve their software and should soon be presenting the performance of their machines on validated patient data.

Although cardiologists agree that computerized analysis simplifies the evaluation of exercise ECG, there has been less agreement as to whether accuracy is enhanced.[41] A recent comparison of computerized resting ECG analysis programs led to the conclusion that physician overreading is necessary.[42]

THE SUNNYSIDE BIOMEDICAL EXERCISE ECG PROGRAM

The advancement of digital integrated circuit technology has made it possible to use increasingly sophisticated methods to process exercise ECGs in real time. This section describes a combination of techniques developed by Olson, Froning, and Froelicher for beat classification and temporal alignment, baseline removal, and representative beat extraction, which can be incorporated into a microprocessor system. The introduction of ever-faster single-chip general purpose microprocessors makes possible the implementation of increasingly sophisticated algorithms at reasonable cost. As more powerful ECG signal-processing techniques become affordable, previously acceptable standards of performance must be reevaluated.

Our signal-processing techniques used for processing of exercise ECG were refined over a period of several years in several of off-line minicomputer testbed systems. These techniques can be applied in a real-time microprocessor-based exercise system. Four areas of signal processing for the exercise ECG are described: (1) absolute spatial vector velocity generation, (2) baseline removal, (3) beat classification and temporal alignment, and (4) representative beat extraction.

Absolute spatial vector velocity (ASVV)

In any approach to the processing of ECG data, a central issue is the choice of the methods to be used for identification and comparison of the various waves and intervals in the ECG signal. Determination of onset and offset of waves should be based on the earliest onset and latest offset seen in any lead. This necessitates the use of a mathematical construct or combination waveform derived from three orthogonal (that is, statistically independent) leads where electrical activity in all orientations will be represented. The approach taken is to use a filtered ASVV curve as the basis for all similarity measures and temporal alignments.

Submitting a low- and high-pass filtered signal derived from one or more ECG leads to a threshold detection algorithm is a standard technique for R-wave detection. The low-pass filter tends to minimize effects of power-line interference and high-frequency muscle noise while the high-pass filter reduces low-frequency baseline drift and wander.

It was discovered empirically that a greater immunity to noise is preserved when the slope calculations from each of the orthogonal leads is separately filtered before the nonlinear operation of taking the absolute value of this sum. This is apparent when this approach is contrasted to the results of performing the computationally faster method of first summing the absolute slopes and then filtering only the sums (that is, the ASVV curve itself). To reduce the computational requirements of this multiple-lead filtering operation, the filter was redesigned into a prefilter/equalizer form. The prefilter is a simple moving average (recursive running sum), which does much of the stop-band attenuation at an insignificant cost in processing time. The equalizer is a standard filter designed to act in concert with the prefilter to improve the passband and stopband performance where needed. This optimization resulted in the same filter performance characteristics while only 60% of the coefficients required for the more conventional approach are being used.

It is important to note that these filtering operations do not disturb the ECG data set itself; they are used to generate a derived waveform (the ASVV) that is convenient for internal processing. The ASVV curve is subsequently used to detect R-waves, align beats for fiducial marking, and determine onsets and offsets of the major ECG waveform components. Later measurements on the unfiltered ECG signals from individual, simultaneously recorded leads are made in relation to these detected fiducial points and markers along the ASVV curve.

Baseline removal

The baseline value for the ECG often wanders or drifts in an unpredictable and undesirable manner during exercise. This wander can take several forms such as sharp discontinuities, ramps, or cyclical swings. Such baseline wander can be induced by electrode impedance changes resulting from perspiration, motion, respiration, or other sources.

A commonly used technique for removing unwanted baseline fluctuations is to pass the ECG signal through a high-pass filter. The low end of the passband of this type of filter is designed to remove much of the baseline wander. Since the clinically relevant portion of the ECG power spectrum often has most of its energy at frequencies above those of the baseline drift, this simple technique can work fairly well and is still popular. However, it is not without dangers. If this type of filter design attenuates frequencies that are clinically relevant, the diagnostic accuracy of many measurements can be affected.

Another method of dealing with baseline wander takes advantage of an *a priori* knowledge of the underlying morphology of the ECG signal. The degree of baseline wander present in an individual QRS complex is estimated by measurement of the relative levels of the TP segments both before and after the QRS complex. If the amplitude difference between these levels exceeds some threshold, the beat is discarded from further processing. This technique has the advantage of not introducing any distortion into the waveform and works best for detecting and avoiding QRS complexes that have sharp discontinuities or ramps in their baseline.

Removing an estimate of the baseline wander from the signal is not the same as removing the true baseline wander. All baseline compensation methods have theoretical and practical limits, and all are capable of introducing a certain amount of distortion. In the case of the cubic spline, the fundamental limit is the lack of sufficient baseline estimation points to unambiguously specify the form of the baseline wander. In other words, it is likely that the set of PR-segment values and their locations does not contain enough points to satisfy the Nyquist sampling criterion, given the power spectrum of the baseline wander.

Beat classification and alignment

The major increase in the signal-to-noise ratio is achieved by coherent processing of the ECG signal by QRS fiducial alignment and averaging point by point. Thus a representative ECG complex is extracted from many beats that have been temporally aligned. It is imperative that only similar beats be used in this extraction process. Distorted complexes, arrhythmic or aberrant complexes, and noise must be excluded. Cross-correlation of segments of the ASVV is used both to determine which template a QRS complex will be assigned to and to adjust the final temporal alignment point for each classified QRS complex.

A threshold-detection algorithm applied earlier to the ASVV curve generates several candidate R-waves. Templates are then formed by computation of the cross-correlation of 200 msec regions of the ASVV curves containing the candidate QRS complexes. The cross-correlations are computed for alignments at every point from 20 to +20 msec of each initial point considered. The point at which the maximum correlation is achieved is then considered to be the final alignment that is fiducial for the complexes being correlated. Also, a minimum correlation coefficient of +0.90 is needed to classify a beat into a template. Choosing the alignment corresponding to the maximum correlation is more accurate than using the threshold-selected alignment and gives increased immunity for the template-selection process to noise. A short burst of noise in a critical spot (such as one near the temporary alignment point selected earlier) may cause the alignment point to be missed, since thresholds use properties of the signal that are local to only a few points. Cross-correlation, on the other hand, uses properties of the signal that are distributed over the entire range being correlated and thus is more immune to the effects of short bursts of noise, which may be present.

Representative beat extraction

It is desired to produce, from the set of aligned and similar beats, one ECG complex that is representative of the set. This composite ECG complex should emphasize those characteristics that are characteristic of the set and should minimize those characteristics that appear only in a few ECG complexes in the set. Thus, such a composite, representative ECG complex would have an increased signal-to-noise ratio largely because most of the noise in the signal should not be aligned consistently between all the ECG complexes and is effectively "averaged" out.

An arithmetic mean is the linear process that produces the greatest increase in signal-to-noise ratio when the noise satisfies several constraints including that it be gaussian distributed. However, in the case of exercise ECG data, the noise is not distributed in a gaussian manner particularly because of the presence of skeletal muscle artifact. In addition, the noise often contains significant transient components that are attributable to either sharp discontinuities in the baseline or the "hump" effect of cyclical baseline swing. Taking a point-by-point mean from a set QRS complexes with this type of noise would pass $1/N$ of the noise level to the representative complex (where N is the number of QRS complexes in the original set).

A process that gives less of an increase in the signal-to-noise ratio for gaussian noise but that is relatively immune to the effects of sharp discontinuities or "humps" is the median. Also, the attenuation of muscle noise by use of the median seems adequate for consistent measurements. However, the median is a computationally expensive operation requiring a sorting procedure on each of the representative beat epochs on a point-by-point basis. An algorithm that uses an estimate based on the previous median point index can speed up the sorting for the next point. In most cases, this implementation of the median operation is five times faster than a standard median computation implementation, thus allowing use of this attractive extraction method.

A hybrid method sometimes referred to as a trimmed mean combines some advantages of both of the two methods described above. It computes an arithmetic mean based only on the "center" points surrounding the median point, throwing out several extreme points on both the high and low side. This gives an added increase in the signal-to-noise ratio compared to the median while retaining some of the immunity to discontinuities and humps. However, one would like to adjust the number of trimmed points based on some estimate of the types of noise in the set of aligned, similar beats. Estimators of discontinuities exist but are computationally expensive; estimators of humps would have to gauge qualitatively the nature of the removed baseline wander and might also tend to be expensive. For these reasons, the median was chosen as our preferred method because it possesses both superior immunity to discontinuities and humps and because it has adequate attenuation of muscle artifact.

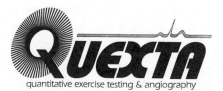

(Veterans Affairs cooperative study of *Q*uantitative *Ex*ercise *T*esting and *A*ngiography)

These Quexta techniques have been the basis for a multicenter Veterans Affairs prospective study of quantitative exercise ECG and coronary angiography. The key to this study is that work-up bias will be reduced when patients with angina agree to undergo both procedures before being tested. All ECG data will be gathered on optical disc and sent to us for analysis. This study will include 12 sites and evaluate 4000 patients in 2 years. In addition to calipered angiograms, cardiac end points will also be considered during a 5-year follow-up period.

SUMMARY

Although computers can record very clean representative ECG complexes and neatly print a wide variety of measurements, the algorithms they use are far from perfect and can result in serious differences from the raw signal. The physician who uses commercially available computer-aided systems to analyze the results of exercise tests should be aware of the problems and always review the raw analog recordings to see if they are consistent with the processed output. However, our colleagues in industry are working hard to improve their techniques. They must be congratulated for their admirable efforts, which have done much to improve the quality of the exercise test our patients now receive. Even if computerization of the original raw analog ECG data could be accomplished without distortion, the problem of interpretation still remains. Numerous algorithms have been recommended for obtaining the optimal diagnostic value from the exercise electrocardiogram. These algorithms have been shown to give improved sensitivity and specificity compared to standard visual interpretation. All too often, this improvement has been documented and substantiated only by the investigator who proposed the new measurement. Thus none of them can be recommended for widespread use. We hope that the ability to store the entire exercise ECG in digital format will enable extraction of information that will improve diagnosis. It is amazing to consider how well the simple one-millimeter criterion functions—surely something else lies hidden in the ECG to improve interpretation! Perhaps neural networks and other discriminant function techniques will uncover new criteria. Our preliminary efforts in applying these techniques have indicated that the ST-segment slope during recovery in the lateral leads may provide a breakthrough for interpretation.

REFERENCES

1. Taback L, Marden E, Mason HL, et al: Digital recording of electrocardiographic data for analysis by digital computer, *Med Electronics* 6:167, 1959.
2. Blomqvist G: The Frank lead exercise electrocardiogram, *Acta Med Scand* 178:1-98, 1965.
3. Hornsten TR, Bruce RA: Computer ST forces of Frank and bipolar exercise electrocardiograms, *Am Heart J* 78:346-350, 1969.
4. McHenry PL, Stowe DE, Lancaster MC: Computer quantitation of the ST segment response during maximal treadmill exercise, *Circulation* 38:691-702, 1968.
5. Sheffield LT, Holt TH, Lester FM, et al: On-line analysis of the exercise ECG, *Circulation* 40:935-944, 1969.
6. Rautaharju PM, Prineas RJ, Eifler WJ, et al: Prognostic value of exercise electrocardiogram in men at high risk of future coronary heart disease: multiple risk factor intervention trial experience, *J Am Coll Cardiol* 8:1010, 1986.
7. Simoons ML, Boom HD, Smallenberg E: On-line processing of orthogonal exercise electrocardiograms, *Comput Biomed Res* 8:105-117, 1975.
8. Simoons ML: Optimal measurements for detection of coronary artery disease by exercise electrocardiography, *Comput Biomed Res* 10:483-499, 1977.
9. Sketch MH, Mohiuddin MS, Nair CK, et al: Automated and nomographic analysis of exercise tests, *JAMA* 243:1052-1055, 1980.
10. Forlini FJ, Cohn K, Langston ME: ST segment isolation and quantification as a means of improving diagnostic accuracy in treadmill stress testing, *Am Heart J* 90:431-438, 1975.
11. Ascoop CA, Distelbrink CA, DeLang PA: Clinical value of quantitative analysis of ST slope during exercise, *Br Heart J* 39:212-217, 1977.
12. Turner AS, Nathan MC, Watson OF, et al: The correlation of the computer quantitated treadmill exercise electrocardiogram with cinearteriographic assessment of coronary artery disease, *NZ Med J* 89:115-118, 1979.
13. Hollenberg M, Budge WR, Wisneski JA, Gertz EW: Treadmill score quantifies electrocardiographic response to exercise and improves test accuracy and reproducibility, *Circulation* 61:276-285, 1980.
14. Hollenberg M, Wisneski JA, Gertz EW, Ellis RJ: Computer-derived treadmill exercise score quantifies the degree of revascularization and improved exercise performance after coronary artery bypass surgery, *Am Heart J* 106:1096-1104, 1983.
15. Hollenberg M, Zoltick JM, Go M, et al: Comparison of a quantitative treadmill exercise score with standard electrocardiographic criteria in screening asymptomatic young men for coronary artery disease, *N Engl J Med* 313:600-606, 1985.
16. Vergari J, Hakki H, Heo J, Iskandrian AS: Merits and limitations of quantitative treadmill exercise score, *Am Heart J* 114:819-826, 1987.
17. Elamin MS, Mary DASG, Smith DR, Linden RJ: Prediction of severity of coronary artery disease using slope of submaximal ST segment/heart rate relationship, *Cardiovasc Res* 14:681-691, 1980.
18. Thwaites BC, Quyyumi AA, Raphael MJ, et al: Comparison of the ST/heart rate slope with the modified Bruce exercise test in the detection of coronary artery disease, *Am J Cardiol* 57:554-556, 1986.
19. Kligfield P, Okin PM, Ameisen O, Borer JS: Evaluation of coronary artery disease by an improved method of exercise electrocardiography: the ST segment/heart rate slope, *Am Heart J* 112:589-598, 1986.
20. Quyyumi AA, Raphael MJ, Wright C, et al: Inability of the ST segment/heart rate slope to predict accurately the severity of coronary artery disease, *Br Heart J* 51:395-398, 1984.
21. Kligfield P, Ameisen O, Okin PM: Heart rate adjustment of ST segment depression for improved detection of coronary artery disease, *Circulation* 79:245-255, 1989.
22. Okin PM, Bergman G, Kligfield P: Effect of ST segment measurement point on performance of standard and heart

rate–adjusted ST segment criteria for the identification of coronary artery disease, *Circulation* 84:57-66, 1991.

23. Lachterman B, Lehmann KG, Detrano R, et al: Comparison of ST segment/heart rate index to standard ST criteria for analysis of exercise electrocardiogram, *Circulation* 83:44-50, 1990.

24. Froning JN, Froelicher VF: Detection and measurement of the P-wave and T-wave during exercise testing using combined heuristic and statistical methods, *J Electrocardiology* October: 145-156, 1987.

25. Froning JN, Froelicher VF, Olson MD: A real-time datalogger system using an optical disk WORM for archiving continuous 12-lead ECG data during exercise testing, *J Electrocardiology* S141-S148, 1988.

26. Herbert WG, Dubach P, Lehman KG, Froelicher VF: Effect of β-blockade on the interpretation of the exercise ECG: ST level versus ST/HR index, *Am Heart J* 122(4):993-1000, 1991.

27. Sato I, Keta K, Aihara N, et al: Improved accuracy of the exercise electrocardiogram in detection of coronary artery and three vessel coronary disease, *Chest* 94:737-744, 1989.

28. Bobbio M, Detrano R: A lesson from the controversy about heart rate adjustment of ST segment depression, *Circulation* 84:1410-1413, 1991.

29. Morise AP, Duvall RD: Accuracy of ST/heart rate index in the diagnosis of coronary artery disease, *Am J Cardiol* 69:603-606, 1992.

30. Miranda CP, Lehmann KG, Froelicher VF: Indications, criteria for interpretation, and utilization of exercise testing in patients with coronary artery disease: results of a survey, *J Cardiopulmonary Rehabil* 9:479-484, 1989.

31. Stuart RJ Jr, Ellestad MH: Upsloping S-T segments in exercise stress testing: six year follow-up study of 438 patients and correlation with 248 angiograms, *Am J Cardiol* 37:19-22, 1976.

32. Savvides M, Ahnve S, Bhargava V, Froelicher VF: Computer analysis of exercise-induced changes in electrocar-

diographic variables: comparison of methods and criteria, *Chest* 84:699-706, 1983.

33. Gianrossi R, Detrano R, Mulvihill D, et al: Exercise-induced ST depression in the diagnosis of coronary artery disease: a meta-analysis, *Circulation* 80:87-98, 1989.

34. Kurita A, Chaitman BR, Bourassa MG: Significance of exercise-induced junctional S-T depression in evaluation of coronary artery disease, *Am J Cardiol* 40:492-497, 1977.

35. Rijneke RD, Ascoop CA, Talmon JL: Clinical significance of upsloping ST segments in exercise electrocardiography, *Circulation* 61:671-678, 1980.

36. Miranda C, Froelicher, V, Froning J: Should ST amplitude be measured at ST0 or ST60? *J Am Coll Cardiol* 17:192A, 1991 (Abstract).

37. Pruvost P, Lablanche JM, Beuscart R, et al: Enhanced efficacy of computerized exercise test by multivariate analysis for the diagnosis of coronary artery disease: a study of 558 men without previous myocardial infarction, *Eur Heart J* 8:1287-1294, 1987.

38. Detry JM, Robert A, Luwaert RJ, et al: Diagnostic value of computerized exercise testing in men without previous myocardial infarction: a multivariate, compartmental and probabilistic approach, *Eur Heart J* 6:227-238, 1985.

39. Simoons ML, Hugenholtz PG, Ascoop CA, et al: Quantitation of exercise electrocardiography, *Circulation* 63: 471-475, 1981.

40. Deckers JW, Rensing BJ, Tijssen JG, et al: A comparison of methods of analysing exercise tests for diagnosis of coronary artery disease, *B Heart J* 62:438-444, 1989.

41. Milliken JA, Abdollah H, Burggraf GW: False-positive treadmill exercise tests due to computer signal averaging, *Am J Cardiol* 65:946-948, 1990.

42. Willems J, Abreu-Lima C, Arnaud P, et al: The diagnostic performance of computer programs for the interpretation of electrocardiograms [see comments], *N Engl J Med* 325:1767-1773, 1991.

5 | Interpretation of Hemodynamic Responses to Exercise Testing:

Exercise Capacity, Heart Rate, and Blood Pressure

When the exercise test is being interpreted, it is important to consider each of its responses separately. Each type of response has a different effect on making a diagnostic or a clinical decision and must be considered along with clinical information. A test should not be called abnormal (or positive) or normal (or negative), but rather the interpretation should specify which responses were abnormal or normal. And the results should not be called subjectively or objectively positive or negative, but the particular responses should be recorded. The objective responses to exercise testing (exercise capacity, heart rate, blood pressure, electrocardiographic changes, and dysrhythmias) and subjective responses (patient appearance, the results of physical examination and symptoms, particularly angina) require interpretation and are discussed below. The final report should be directed to the physician who ordered the test and who will receive the report. It should contain information that helps in patient management and not vague medical language. Interpretation is actually very dependent on the application for which the test is used and on the population tested, and so this chapter must be considered a preparation for information available in later chapters.

EXERCISE CAPACITY OR FUNCTIONAL CAPACITY

The functional status of patients with heart disease is frequently classified by symptoms during daily activities (New York Heart Association, Canadian, or Weber classifications are common examples). However, the standard is directly measured maximal oxygen uptake. Maximal ventilatory oxygen uptake (VO_2 max) is the greatest amount of oxygen that a person can extract from inspired air while performing dynamic exercise involving a large part of the total body muscle mass. Since maximal ventilatory oxygen uptake is equal to the product of cardiac output and arteriovenous oxygen ($a\text{-}vO_2$) difference, it is a measure of the functional limits of the cardiovascular system. The maximal $a\text{-}vO_2$ difference is physiologically limited to roughly 15 to 17 vol%. Thus the maximal $a\text{-}vO_2$ difference behaves more or less as a constant, making maximal oxygen uptake an indirect estimate of maximal cardiac output.

Maximal oxygen uptake is dependent on many factors, including natural physical endowment, activity status, age, and sex, but it is the best index of exercise capacity and maximal cardiovascular function. As a rough reference, the maximal oxygen uptake of the normal sedentary adult is often considered approximately 30 cc or ml of O_2/kg/min, and the minimal level for physical fitness is often considered roughly 40 ml of O_2/kg/min. Aerobic training can increase maximal oxygen uptake by up to 25%. This increase is dependent on the initial level of fitness and age as well as the intensity, frequency, and length of training sessions. Individuals performing aerobic training such as distance running can have maximal oxygen uptakes as high as 60 to 90 ml of O_2/kg/min. For convenience, oxygen consumption is often expressed in multiples of basal resting requirements (metabolic equivalents, METS). The MET is a unit of basal oxygen consumption equal to approximately 3.5 ml of O_2/kg/min. This value is the oxygen requirement to maintain life in the resting state.

Figure 5-1 illustrates the relationship between maximal oxygen uptake to exercise habits and age.[1] Although the three activity levels have regression lines that fit the data as one would expect, there is much scatter around the lines, and the correlation coefficients are poor. This finding demonstrates the inaccuracy involved with trying

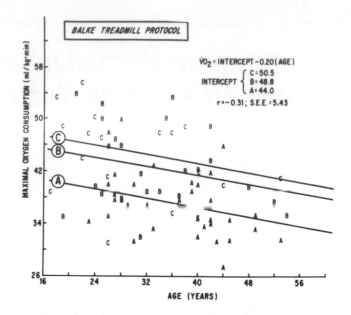

Figure 5-1   Relationship of maximal oxygen uptake (VO₂ max) to current exercise status and age.

to predict maximal oxygen uptake from age and habitual physical activity. It is preferable to estimate an individual's maximal oxygen uptake from the work load reached while performing an exercise test. Maximal oxygen uptake is of course, most precisely determined by direct measurement using ventilatory gas exchange-techniques (Chapter 3).

Patterson and colleagues studied 43 patients with cardiac disease and compared their functional classification by maximal oxygen uptake and clinical assessment.[2] When a discrepancy occurred, the hemodynamic data from cardiac catheterization usually indicated that maximal oxygen uptake more accurately reflected the degree of impairment. Patients began to experience limiting symptoms when maximal oxygen uptake was less than 22 ml of O_2/kg/min (6 METS) and considered themselves severely limited when maximal oxygen uptake was 16 ml of O_2/kg/min (4 METS) or less. When a patient's exercise capacity is estimated from testing at less than 4 METS, many studies have shown that prognosis is not so good as those with normal exercise capacity.

Questionnaire assessment

Functional classifications have been found to be too limited and poorly reproducible. One problem is that "usual activities" can decrease, and so an individual can become greatly limited without having a change in functional class. A better approach is to use the specific activity scale (SAS) of Goldman[3] shown in Table 5-1, or the Duke ac-

tivity scale in Table 5-2, or to question a patient regarding usual activities that have a known MET cost. Hlatky and co-workers at Duke developed a brief, self-administered questionnaire to estimate accurately functional capacity and allow assessment of aspects of quality of life.[4] Fifty subjects undergoing exercise testing with measurement of peak oxygen uptake were studied. All subjects were questioned about their ability to perform a variety of common activities by an interviewer blinded to exercise test findings. A 12-item scale (the Duke Activity Status Index) that correlated well with peak oxygen uptake was then developed.

Exercise capacity and cardiac function

Exercise capacity determined by exercise testing has been proposed as a means to estimate ventricular function. A direct relationship would appear to be supported by the fact that both resting ejection fraction (EF) and exercise capacity have prognostic value in patients with coronary heart disease. However, a noticeable discrepancy between resting ventricular function and exercise performance is frequently seen clinically. Additionally, exercise capacity is poorly related to ventricular function in patients with cardiomyopathies. Exercise-induced ischemia could limit exercise despite normal resting ventricular function, and so patients with angina must be excluded, and silent ischemia must be considered when one is evaluating an interaction.

We investigated the relationship between rest-

Table 5-1   Specific activity scale (SAS) of Goldman

Class I (≥7 METs)	A patient can perform any of the following activities: Carrying 24 pounds up eight steps Carrying an 80-pound object Shoveling snow Skiing Playing basketball, touch football, squash, or handball Jogging/walking 5 mph
Class II (≥5 METs)	A patient does not meet class I criteria but can perform any of the following activities to completion without stopping: Carrying anything up eight steps Having sexual intercourse Gardening, raking, weeding Walking 4 mph
Class II (≥2 METs)	A patient does not meet class I or class II criteria but can perform any of the following activities to completion without stopping: Walking down eight steps Taking a shower Changing bed sheets Mopping floors, cleaning windows Walking 2.5 mph Pushing a power lawn mower Bowling Dressing without stopping
Class IV (≤2 METs)	None of the above

Table 5-2   The Duke activity scale index

Activity	Weight
Can You?	
1. Take care of yourself, that is, eating, dressing, bathing or using the toilet?	2.75
2. Walk indoors, such as around your house?	1.75
3. Walk a block or two on level ground?	2.75
4. Climb a flight of stairs or walk up a hill?	5.50
5. Run a short distance?	8.00
6. Do light work around the house like dusting or washing dishes?	2.70
7. Do moderate work around the house like vacuuming, sweeping floors, or carrying in groceries?	3.50
8. Do heavy work around the house like scrubbing floors, or lifting or moving heavy furniture?	8.00
9. Do yard work like raking leaves, weeding, or pushing a power mower?	4.50
10. Have sexual relations?	5.25
11. Participation in moderate recreational activities like golf, bowling, dancing, doubles tennis, or throwing a basketball or football?	6.00
12. Participate in strenuous sports like swimming, singles tennis, football, basketball or skiing?	7.50

DASI = Sum of weights for "yes" replies
$VO_2 = 0.43 \times DASI + 9.6$

ing ventricular function and exercise performance in patients with a wide range of resting EFs able to exercise to volitional fatigue.[5] Radionuclide measurements of left vetricular perfusion and EF were compared with treadmill responses in 88 patients with coronary heart disease free of angina pectoris. The exercise tests included supine bicycle radionuclide ventriculography, thallium scintigraphy, and treadmill testing with expired gas analysis. The number of abnormal Q-wave locations, EF, end-diastolic volume, cardiac output, exercise-induced ST-segment depression, and thallium scar and ischemia scores were considered. Resting and exercise ejection fraction was highly correlated with thallium scar score but not with maximal oxygen uptake. Fifty-five percent of the variability in predicting treadmill time was explained by the change in heart rate (39%), thallium ischemia score (12%), and resting cardiac output (4%). The change in heart rate induced by the treadmill test explained only 27% of the variability in measured maximal oxygen uptake. Myocardial damage predicted resting ejection fraction, but the ability to increase heart rate with treadmill exercise was the most important determinant of exercise capacity. Exercise capacity and VO$_2$ max were only minimally affected by asymptomatic ischemia and were relatively independent of ventricular function.

A plot of resting ejection fraction versus measured maximal oxygen consumption is shown in Figure 5-2. This poor relationship ($r = 0.25$) confirms other studies among patients with chronic heart failure and coronary heart disease. The relationship was not improved by exclusion of patients with a respiratory quotient less than 1.1 or with a perceived exertion less than 17. However, maximal ejection fraction, maximal end-diastolic volume, and thallium ischemia were significantly correlated with exercise capacity. Resting ejection fraction correlated negatively with the sum of Q-wave areas on the resting electrocardiogram ($r = -0.40$), and the thallium scar score explained most of the variability in resting ejection fraction (44%) with ST-segment depression adding only 6%. The change in ejection fraction poorly correlated with the amount of ST-segment depression and thallium ischemia score. When

routine treadmill parameters were considered alone, a change in the rate-pressure product was selected first but could explain only 6% of the variability in resting ejection fraction.

When one is using cardiac parameters to predict treadmill time or VO$_2$ max, thallium ischemia, resting cardiac output, and maximal end-diastolic volume were chosen sequentially and combined to explain 19% of the variability. When these patients were separated into those with normal and those with abnormal resting ejection fraction (0.50 being the discriminant value), predictive variables changed, but no real improvement in explaining the variability in estimated VO$_2$ max was achieved. When treadmill parameters were added, the change in heart rate during treadmill exercise entered first, explaining 39% of the variability, followed by the thallium ischemia score (51%) and resting cardiac output (4%) to account for 55% of the variability in estimated VO$_2$ max or treadmill time. Again, separating patients by normal and abnormal resting ejection fraction did not improve the prediction. When treadmill parameters alone were considered, the change in heart rate with exercise alone explained 38% of the variability in the relationship with treadmill time or estimated VO$_2$ max.

Ehsani and colleagues published a study similar to ours.[6] Extensive measurements of systolic ventricular function were considered, but none of these were found to be good predictors of maximal oxygen uptake. Resting ejection fraction did not correlate with maximal oxygen uptake, and there was a weak correlation with peak exercise ejection fraction and maximal oxygen uptake. In contrast to our study, however, they did find that the change in ejection fraction from rest to maximal exercise ($r = 0.77$) and maximal heart rate ($r = 0.61$) correlated significantly with maximal oxygen uptake. It is not quite clear why different findings are made with regard to the change in ejection fraction. Both studies indicated that chronotropic incompetence is a significant factor in determining maximal oxygen uptake, but considerable variance in maximal oxygen uptake remains unexplained.

Weber and colleagues classified 62 patients with chronic stable congestive heart failure into functional classes based on VO$_2$ max.[7] Pulmonary capillary wedge pressure and direct Fick measurements of cardiac output were made at rest and during upright exercise. The most limited patients increased cardiac output by heart rate alone and had lower maximal heart rates, oxygen pulses, and changes in oxygen pulse from rest to maximal exercise. Patients were symptom-limited by exercise cardiac output rather than high filling

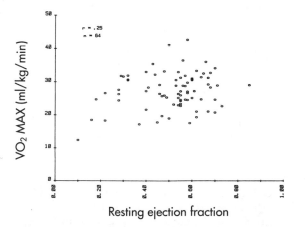

Figure 5-2 A plot of resting ejection fraction versus measured maximal oxygen consumption illustrating the poor relationship even in patients not limited by angina.

pressures. Patients achieved a normal exercise capacity by increasing both heart rate and stroke volume and tolerating a very high filling pressure during upright exercise. These findings are supported by those of Litchfield and colleagues in six patients with severe ventricular dysfunction.[8] Other compensatory mechanisms included an increase in end-diastolic volume and elevated circulating catecholamines. Higginbotham and colleagues also examined determinants of upright exercise performance in 12 patients with severe left ventricular dysfunction using radionuclide angiography and invasive measurements.[9] Multivariate analysis identified changes in heart rate, cardiac output, and a-vO_2 difference with exercise as important predictors of VO_2 max. The resting ejection fraction did not correlate with VO_2 max, nor did changes in ejection fraction, stroke counts, or end-diastolic counts during exercise. These results are similar to our findings, but our study included patients with coronary artery disease having a wide range of ejection fractions.

The discrepancy between ventricular function and exercise capacity is now well known. Studies have employed radionuclide, angiographic, and echocardiographic measures of ventricular size and function to document this finding in patients with heart disease. Correlations between exercise capacity and various indices of ventricular function have ranged from -0.10 to 0.24.[10] Increasing heart rate and cardiac index appear to be the most important determinants of exercise capacity, but they often leave more than 50% of the variance in exercise capacity unexplained. Radionuclide techniques add little to the explanation of variance in exercise capacity. The change in ejection fraction from rest to maximal supine exercise has a poor association probably because of the complex nature of this response. The established clinical impression today is that good ventricular function does not guarantee normal exercise capacity and vice versa. Thus, even in patients free of angina, exercise limitations or expectations should not be determined by ventricular function but rather by the their symptomatic response to exercise.

Adaptations in anaerobic metabolism may contribute to the poor ability of cardiac and treadmill parameters to allow prediction of measured and estimated VO_2 max. However, differences in a-vO_2 difference may more simply explain these findings. The fact that patients with severely limited ventricular function can improve their exercise capacity after training without altering resting ventricular function[11] provides further evidence for the poor relationship between resting ventricular function and exercise capacity. One could even hypothesize that exercise training could be used to increase exercise capacity and improve the poor prognosis associated with cardiac dysfunction.

Myocardial damage and exercise capacity

The relationship between myocardial damage, ventricular function, and exercise capacity are poorly understood. Pfeiffer and colleagues reported that ventricular performance was directly related to the amount of myocardium remaining after inducing myocardial infarctions in rats.[12] However, rats with smaller infarctions (4% to 30% of the left ventricle) had no discernible impairment in either baseline hemodynamics or peak indices of pumping and pressure-generating ability when compared to sham operated controls. This indicates that considerable damage to the left ventricle can occur before pump performance or oxygen transport are affected.

Carter and Amundsen reported a significant inverse correlation ($r = -0.68$) between infarct size estimated from serum creatinine phosphokinase and exercise capacity at approximately 3 months after myocardial infarction.[13] This relationship improved ($r = -0.84$) after exercise training, an implication that infarct size affects the response to training. In contrast, Grande and Pedersen reported an insignificant correlation between the enzyme estimate of infarct size and duration of work ($r = -0.15$) performed in a progressive steady-state protocol within 2 months after infarction.[14] They observed significant correlations between infarct size and maximal heart rate ($r = 0.39$), maximal systolic blood pressure (SBP) ($r = -0.32$), and the increases in both SBP ($r = -0.46$) and heart rate ($r = 0.39$) from rest to 100 watts. In our study, the thallium scar score, an estimate of myocardial damage, was not significantly correlated with VO_2 max or change in heart rate. However, there was a significant negative correlation with maximal SBP, rate pressure product, and change in rate pressure product from rest to maximal exercise.

DePace and colleagues studied resting left ventricular function, thallium-201 scintigraphy, and a QRS scoring scheme in patients remote from a myocardial infarction.[15] They reported significant correlations between resting EF and QRS score ($r = -0.51$) and between resting EF and thallium score ($r = 0.61$) similar to the values for Q-wave areas ($r = -0.40$) and thallium scar score ($r = -0.72$) we obtained. The thallium score correlated poorly with the QRS score in their study but the Q-wave sum was significantly correlated to the thallium scar score in our study ($r = 0.48$). The thallium scar score was highly correlated to and predictive of resting ejection fraction. However, both parameters had very poor correlations with exercise capacity. Thus data reported from both animal and human studies confirm that cardiac function has only a minor influence on determining VO_2 max.

Use of nomograms for exercise capacity

As experience with exercise testing has progressed, many protocols have been developed for best assessment of certain patient populations. Rapidly paced protocols may be suited to screening of younger or active individuals (that is, Bruce, Ellestad), whereas more moderate ones are adapted to older or deconditioned patients (that is, Naughton, Balke-Ware, USAFSAM). The main disadvantage to having so many techniques has been determining equivalent work loads between them (that is, What does 5 minutes on a modified Bruce protocol mean in terms of a Balke-Ware protocol or real-life activities such as hiking or grocery shopping?). An estimation of maximal ventilatory oxygen uptake from treadmill or ergometer work load during dynamic exercise has been proposed and validated as an excellent common language with which investigators and clinicians can communicate to assess these widely different exercise protocols and everyday physical activities of their patients.

It has been well established that maximal oxygen uptake (VO_2) can be reasonably estimated from the work load achieved in accord with a given protocol (see discussion in Chapter 2). The term "metabolic equivalent" (MET) was coined to describe the quantity of oxygen consumed by the body from inspired air under basal conditions and is equal on the average to 3.5 ml of O_2/kg/min.[16] One may translate VO_2 into METs by dividing by 3.5, thus providing a unitless, convenient, and accurate manner for referring to a patient's exercise capacity. Despite its practicality and acceptance by exercise physiologists, common usage of the MET has not been adopted in clinical practice. Because VO_2 is dependent on age, gender, activity status, and disease states, tables that take these factors into account must be referred to so that one can accurately categorize a certain MET value as either normal or abnormal. Morris from our group therefore developed a nomogram that would make it convenient for physicians to translate a MET level into a percentage of normal exercise capacity for males based on age and activity status, similar to that published by Bruce,[17] except that we utilized METs instead of time in the Bruce protocol.[18] We retrospectively reviewed the exercise test results of 3583 male patients referred to our laboratory during the period of April 1984 to January 1990 for the evaluation of possible or probable coronary artery disease. Excluded were those who had a submaximal test, a prior myocardial infarction by history or Q wave, history of congestive heart failure, beta blocker or digitalis use, prior coronary artery bypass surgery or coronary angioplasty, valvular heart disease, chronic obstructive pulmonary disease, or claudication. Since less than 2% of our population were women, they were excluded as well. This left us with a male "referral" population of 1388 with a mean age of 57 years (range 21 to 89). For those who could be so classified, a further subgrouping was done into sedentary ($n = 253$) and physically active ($n = 346$). We classified activity status by asking, "Do you perform 20 minutes or more of brisk walking three times a week or do you regularly participate in an aerobic sport?" An additional grouping was made of those under 54 years of age with similar subgroupings. As exercise capacity has been shown to be a significant independent predictor of cardiovascular mortality,[19] use of such nomograms can facilitate discussions between physicians and their patients regarding prognosis as well as disability.

A separate nomogram was developed from 244 "normal" males who volunteered for maximal exercise testing with ventilatory gas exchange analysis. These subjects differed from the former in that they were not referred for any clinical reason and were a healthy, younger (mean age 45 ± 14 years, range 18 to 72), free-living population. Exercise testing was performed for research purposes in these subjects and not for clinical reasons. They were also classified into sedentary ($n = 74$) and active ($n = 122$) groups.

All referred patients underwent exercise testing using the USAFSAM treadmill protocol with 2-minute stages, starting at 2.0 mph/0% grade and increasing to 3.3 mph followed thereafter by grade increases of 5% per stage.[20] The completion of each subsequent stage was associated with an estimated additional 2 MET expenditure. If a patient completed less than 1 minute of exercise in his highest stage, he was assigned the MET level corresponding to the previous completed stage. The MET values were calculated using commonly used equations based on speed and grade.[21] Blood pressure, heart rate, Borg scale, and electrocardiographic measurements were recorded for each stage and with the onset of symptoms. Standard criteria for terminating the test were followed,[22] but no heart rate or time limits were imposed and a maximal effort was encouraged.

Among volunteers who performed exercise testing with ventilatory gas exchange, an individualized ramp treadmill protocol was employed.[23] Oxygen uptake, obtained from the 1-minute sample at peak exercise divided by 3.5, was used to represent maximal METs. Only subjects who were limited by fatigue, leg fatigue, or shortness of breath were included. Simple univariate linear regression was performed, with age as the independent variable, and the various hemodynamic responses including METs, maximum heart rate, maximum systolic blood pressure, and maximum double product were the dependent variables. These relationships were studied for all patients together and for the subgroups classified as sedentary and active. Age limits were chosen for selected relationships for comparison with other populations. Analysis of variance (ANOVA) was also used to create boxplots of METs for selected age categories and to test for differences between age categories.

The predicted METs for age were calculated by the formulas obtained from the regression analysis using age as the independent variable. This was done for the entire group as well as for the "sedentary" and "active" groups separately. All equations are numbered in sequence for convenience. A percent exercise capacity was obtained from the following equation:

1. $\text{Exercise capacity} = \dfrac{\text{Observed MET level}}{\text{Predicted METS}} \times 100$

Exercise capacity represents the actual percentage capacity for a given age based on METs performed, with 100% being the average for age.

Values for percent exercise capacity were calculated for various ages using the above equation. A nomogram was fashioned by plotting specific ages and observed MET levels for differing values of exercise capacity. A "best fit" line was then drawn through the various intercepts to complete the nomogram (see Figures 5-3 to 5-5).

Among patients tested for clinical reasons ("referrals"), regression analyses of METs against age for the entire group and for each of the two subgroups yielded the following equations:

2. All "referrals": Predicted METs = 18.0 − 0.15(Age); $n = 1388$; SEE = 3.3; $r = -0.46$; $p < 0.001$
3. Active: Predicted METs = 18.7 − 0.15(Age); $n = 346$; SEE = 3.0; $r = -0.49$; $p < 0.001$
4. Sedentary: Predicted METs = 16.6 − 0.16(Age); $n = 253$; SEE = 3.2; $r = -0.43$; $p < 0.001$

The nomogram for equation 2 is illustrated in Figure 5-3; the nomogram for equations 3 and 4 is illustrated in Figure 5-4; and a plot of the rela-

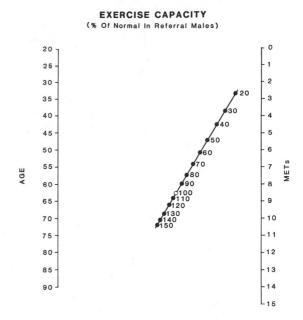

Figure 5-3   Nomogram of percent normal exercise capacity for age in total population of "referral" males.

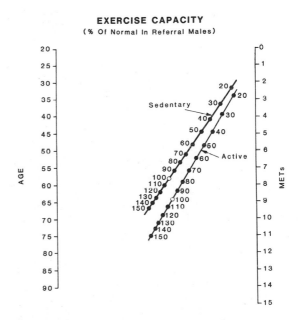

Figure 5-4   Nomogram of percent normal exercise capacity in sedentary and active "referral" males.

tionship reflecting equation 2 is presented in Figure 5-5.

For the entire group of 1388 "referrals" the mean maximal Borg score and mean maximal heart rate were 18 and 144 respectively, which are consistent with a maximal effort. Maximal

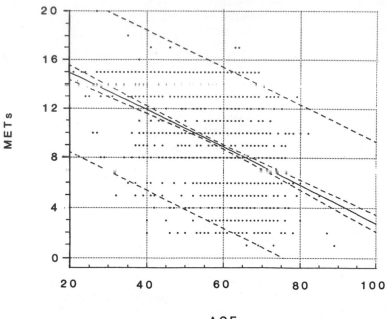

Figure 5-5   Graph of regression equation of METs (1 metabolic equivalent = 3.5 cc of O_2/kg/min) on age for all "referral" patients. *Inner lines* represent 95% confidence limits, and *outer lines* represent 95% prediction limits ($r = -0.49$; $p < 0.001$).

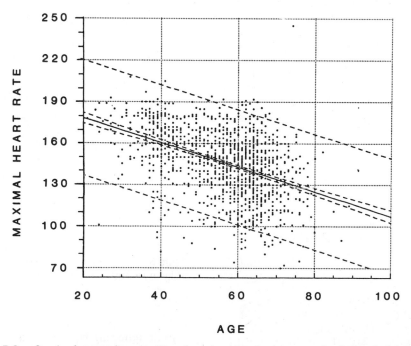

Figure 5-6   Graph of regression equation of maximal heart rate on age for "referrals." *Inner lines* represent 95% confidence limits, and *outer lines* represent 95% prediction limits ($r = -0.43$; $p < 0.001$).

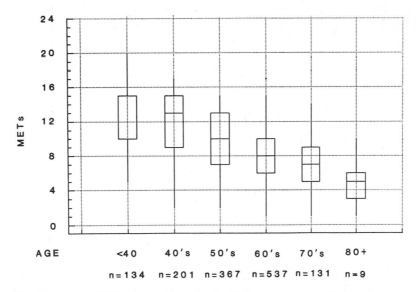

Figure 5-7   Box plots of METs by age decades for "referrals." Each *horizontal line* represents a quartile, and the extremes of the age decade are represented by the *ends of the vertical line*.

heart rate regressed with age (shown in Figure 5-6) led to the following equation:

5. Maximal heart rate = 196 − 0.9(Age); SEE = 21.2; $r = -0.43$; $p < 0.001$

When maximum systolic blood pressure was regressed with age, the slope of the regression line was not significantly different from zero ($p = 0.32$), an indication that no significant relationship existed between the two variables.

ANOVA was performed for METs by the age grouping <40, 40-49, 50-59, 60-69, 70-79, and 80-89 years ($p < 0.001$), and respective box plots are illustrated in Figure 5-7.

The relationships were then reanalyzed, with exclusion of referrals 54 years of age or older in order to match a prior study population. Examination of this new grouping (mean age 43, $n = 442$) led to regression equations not appreciably different from those shown above for all ages.

Healthy volunteers tested with ventilatory gas exchange analysis ("normals"). Regression analysis of METs (measured maximal oxygen uptake, ml/kg/min, divided by 3.5) against age for the normals and for active and sedentary subgroups yielded the following equations:

6. All ("normals"): Predicted METs = 14.7 − 0.11(Age); $n = 244$; SEE = 2.5; $r = -0.53$; $p < 0.001$
7. Active: Predicted METs = 16.4 − 0.13(Age); $n = 122$; SEE = 2.5; $r = -0.58$; $p < 0.001$
8. Sedentary: Predicted METs = 11.9 − 0.07(Age); $n = 74$; SEE = 1.8; $r = -0.47$; $p < 0.001$

The nomogram for equation 6 is illustrated in Figure 5-8, and the nomogram for equations 7 and 8 is illustrated in Figure 5-9.

For these subjects, the values observed for maximal heart rate and maximal perceived exertion were 167 ± 19 and 19.0 ± 1.2 respectively, consistent with a maximal effort.

Maximal heart rate regressed with age yielding the following equation:

9. Maximal heart rate = 200 − 0.72(Age); SEE = 15.3; $r = -0.55$; $p < 0.001$

The term "METs" is a more meaningful and useful expression of exercise capacity than the various conglomerations of protocol times and stages often used. Use of the term facilitates comparisons of data using different protocols and tailoring of protocols for particular patients. MET levels can be used for exercise prescription and for estimation of levels of disability by use of tables listing the MET demands of most common activities (Table 5-3).

Many physicians find exercise capacity relative to the peers in an age group to be a useful means of assessing a patient's cardiovascular status. In addition, the patients themselves seem to have a better understanding of this concept. Thus it seems clear that "METs" is a term that can improve communication between physicians, whereas "percent normal exercise capacity" can do the same for dialog between physicians and their patients.

Comparison with other populations. The regression analysis of this group of 1388 referred males

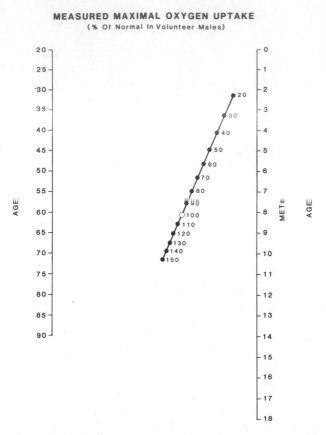

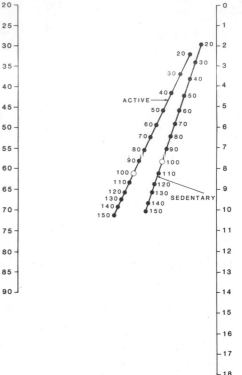

Figure 5-8 Nomogram of percent normal exercise capacity among healthy "normals" tested using ventilatory oxygen uptake.

Figure 5-9 Nomogram of percent normal exercise capacity among active and sedentary healthy "normals" tested using ventilatory oxygen uptake.

from the Long Beach Veterans Affairs Medical Center differs from those developed by Froelicher and co-workers in 1975 using U.S. Air Force military personnel.[24] They regressed measured VO_2 against age and obtained the following equations for 710 asymptomatic men of all activity levels (age range 20 to 53 years):

10. Predicted METs = $13.1 - 0.08$(Age); $n = 710$); SEE = 1.7, $r = -0.32$

Compare this to that obtained from our population of patients less than 54 years old:

11. Predicted METs = $18.8 - 0.17$(Age); $n = 442$; SEE = 3.3; $p < 0.001$; $r = -0.33$

The slope and intercept show an apparent difference, which reflects the different populations (see below). Bruce derived his nomogram for functional capacity from 138 healthy men (mean age 49) and calculated the observed exercise capacity from the following equation:

12. Observed MET level = $1.11 + 0.016$ (duration in seconds)

They then obtained the predicted exercise capacity for age by regressing treadmill duration on age in order to obtain the following equation:

13. Predicted METs = $13.7 - 0.08$(Age); $n = 138$; SEE = 1.37

From the values for observed MET levels and predicted METs, they were able to calculate the relative impairment. Their group consisted of healthy volunteers, like those in the USAF study and the healthy volunteers from Long Beach, and all three populations were roughly the same age (equation 6, 10, and 13). Thus these equations yield approximately the same results for any given age. These contrast the population of patients who were referred to our hospital-based laboratory for evaluation of possible coronary artery disease (equation 2).

When Dehn and Bruce conducted a review of the literature[25] regarding VO_2 max and its variation with age and activity, they derived a regression equation from a compilation of 17 previous studies encompassing 700 observations in healthy males of all ages:

14. Predicted METs = 16.2 − 0.11(Age)

All these equations are listed in Table 5-4 for comparison.

Several factors account for the differences between the regression equations obtained from the referred group in Long Beach and those of Froelicher and colleagues' study and Bruce and associates. Our greater slope is consistent with a faster decline in VO$_2$ max with age than that found in these previous studies. Regression analyses can vary because of population differences, including age, activity status, state of health, definition of normal or healthy individuals, and gender. The last is not a question in this context because all studies dealt with males. There are significant differences in the mean ages and age ranges of the studies quoted, with the VAMC population being the oldest. For this reason, we included a separate analysis of patients under 54 years of age, but a steeper slope was still obtained. The decline in maximal heart rate with age is also steeper in our "referrals", paralleling the VO$_2$ slope. Thus maximal heart rate decreased with age at a greater rate than in prior studies,[26] which could be attributed to a submaximal effort or complicating illnesses in older patients or may simply be attributable to the wide scatter that has been observed for this measurement in past studies.

The classification of the study population was done by a "cardiac screening exam" in Bruce's study, by exclusion criteria in our study, and, most stringently, by a requirement to fulfill criteria to achieve "flying status" in the USAF study. Cardiac patients have lower VO$_2$ max values than "normals" and thus failure to adequately exclude such patients could cause variations in the results. Activity status was not classified in the study by Bruce, whereas activity status was classified by a similar method in the VAMC and USAF studies. However, varying levels of conditioning could be a factor in the divergence of the regression equations.

One must also consider differences in methodology when examining divergent results. Only the healthy volunteers at the VAMC and the USAF study used measured VO$_2$ values. Additionally, the treadmill protocols were quite different, and controversy exists as to whether some are more accurate than others when METs are estimated. For instance, longer more gradual protocols may favor the elderly and thus alter the regression line. Nevertheless, the mean MET levels for age in our study agree quite well with those of prior investigations (Table 5-5).

It would be difficult to sort out which study has produced the most "universal" regression equations because all have weaknesses in either population selection or methodology. Ours applies to a typical population referred to a hospital or clinic for evaluation of possible heart disease, excluding those with obvious medical problems, which might compromise their exercise capacity. The earlier studies by Bruce and Froelicher were primarily

Table 5-3 MET demands for most common activities

Activity	METs
Mild	
Baking	2.0
Billiards	2.4
Bookbinding	2.2
Canoeing (leisurely)	2.5
Conducting an orchestra	2.2
Dancing, Ballroom (slow)	2.9
Golf (with cart)	2.5
Horseback riding (walking)	2.3
Playing a musical instrument	2.0
Volleyball (noncompetitive)	2.9
Walking (2 mph)	2.5
Writing	1.7
Moderate	
Calisthenics (no weights)	4.0
Croquet	3.0
Cycling (leuisurely)	3.5
Gardening (no lifting)	4.4
Golf (without cart)	4.9
Mowing lawn (power mower)	3.0
Playing drums	3.8
Sailing	3.0
Swimming (slowly)	4.5
Walking (3 mph)	3.3
Walking (4 mph)	4.5
Vigorous	
Badminton	5.5
Chopping wood	4.9
Climbing hills	7.0
Cycling (moderate)	5.7
Dancing	6.0
Field hockey	7.7
Ice skating	5.5
Jogging (10-minute mile)	10
Karate or judo	6.5
Roller skating	6.5
Rope skipping	12
Skiing (water or downhill)	6.8
Squash	12
Surfing	6.0
Swimming (fast)	7.0
Tennis (doubles)	6.0

These activities can often be done at variable intensities if one assumes that the intensity is not excessive and that the courses are flat (no hills) unless so specified.

From the American Heart Association Exercise Standards.

Table 5-4 Equations for predicting maximal METs from age

Study	Equation	Number of patients	Mean age (range)	Assessment of activity	Definition of normal	Ventilator oxygen (VO$_2$)	Protocol
Morris	Pred METs = 18.1 − 0.16 (age)	1388	57 (21-89)	Simple questionnaire	No history of CABS, CHF, BB or digoxin, COPD, claudication, angina, prior MI, arrhythmias, or greater than 1 Q-wave on ECG	Est	USAFSAM
Morris (<54 years of age)	Pred METs = 18.8 − 0.17 (Age)	479	45 (21-53)	Simple questionnaire	No history of CABS, CHF, BB or digoxin, COPD, claudication, angina, prior MI, arrhythmias, or greater than 1 Q-wave on ECG	Est	USAFSAM
Morris	Pred METs = 14.7 − 0.11 (Age)	244	45 (20-72)	Simple questionnaire	Apparently healthy	Meas	Ramp
Froelicher[9]	Pred METs = 13.1 − 0.08 (Age)	710	N/A (20-53)	None	Normal exam, normal resting and exercise ECG, no HTN	Meas	3.3 mph 1% grade increment/min
Bruce[18]	Pred METs = 13.7 − 0.08 (Age)	2092	44.4 (N/A)	None	Cardiac screening exam	Est	Bruce
Wolthius[19]	Pred METs = 13 − 0.05 (Age)	704	37 (25-54)	Questionnaire interview	Normal history and physical exam, CXR, resting and exercise ECG, and Holter. No arrhythmias, HTN, or medications	Meas	Balke (long) 3.3 mph 1% grade increment/min
Dehn[10]	Pred METs = 16.2 − 0.11 (Age)	700	52.2 (40-72)	—	—	Mixed	Mixed

BB, Beta-adrenergic receptor blockade; *CABS*, coronary artery bypass surgery; *CHF*, congestive heart failure; *COPD*, chronic obstructive pulmonary disease, *CXR*, chest x-ray film; *ECG*, electrocardiogram; *Est*, estimated; *HTN*, hypertension; *Meas*, measured; *MI*, myocardial infarction; *N/A*, not applicable; *Pred METs*, predicted metabolic equivalents; *USAFSAM*, U.S. Air Force School of Aerospace Medicine.

with apparently healthy "normals" and volunteers, which is not so applicable to the patients seen by practicing physicians. The regression lines from our "referred" group may differ from those done on "free living populations" because of varying levels of disease prevalence and activity. This seems a more likely explanation than a difference attributable to protocol selection because the regression lines were almost identical when obtained by Froelicher using the Balke and Bruce protocol.

The aforementioned factors likely combine to explain the upward shift in the slope of the nomogram scale among volunteers whom oxygen uptake was determined directly from ventilatory gas exchange analysis. It is well established that estimating MET levels from treadmill work results in an overestimation of exercise capacity.[27] The approximate 1.0 to 1.5 higher predicted MET values for any given age among referred patients whom exercise capacity was estimated from treadmill work load is not surprising given that differences of this magnitude between measured and estimated maximal oxygen uptake have been reported previously.[28] Moreover, the fact that the larger group was referred for testing for clinical reasons naturally makes it a group more inclined to have disease, even though "obvious" disease was excluded. Not only does the presence of cardiovascular disease exacerbate the overprediction of oxygen uptake, but also the slope of the maximal heart rate versus age relationship was steeper in the group of patients. The resultant lower maximal heart rate contributes to the lower measured oxygen uptake at a given work rate for any given age. These data underscore two important points: (1) the scales are population specific; and (2) although measured oxygen uptake is the more precise measure of work, the scales are also specific to whether oxygen uptake was measured or predicted.

Although one solution would be for each center to develop its own "normals," doing so is neither economical nor likely. Instead, given the imprecision that is inherent in estimating METs and activity status, investigators and clinicians alike can use the nomograms developed from populations of clinically referred patients (equation 2 to 4) or healthy volunteers (equation 6 to 8) and apply them to the population they are likely to be testing. Despite the wide scatter of METs for age even in normals, physicians should consider norms for age. This can be done by age decade as presented in Figure 5-7, or by use of nomograms as previously presented. The latter concept is popular because it adjusts for age.

An advantage to these nomograms is that they are relatively simple to use, requiring only values for age and observed MET levels in order to draw a line between them to obtain the percent normal exercise capacity. For instance, if a patient were to complete 6 minutes of a Bruce protocol (stage 2), he would have achieved an exercise capacity of 7 METs. If he were 55 years of age, this would calculate to be an exercise capacity of 70% using the nomogram. Similarly, if the same patient completed 8 minutes of a Balke protocol, he would also have achieved 7 METs and have an exercise capacity of 70%. Values obtained below 100% indicate exercise impairment relative to one's age group, whereas values above 100% indicate supernormal performance.

Also, equations based on time in a protocol, that is, METs = 1.11 + 0.016 (duration in seconds), for the Bruce protocol; or on treadmill speed and grade, that is, METs = (mph × 26.8) × [0.1 + (Grade × 0.018) + 3.5]/3.5; or as ergometer work load, that is, METs = [(2 × kilogrammeter/min + 300)/body weight in kilograms]/3.5, can be used to obtain particular MET levels.

The total population nomograms are appropriate if activity status is unknown. The "referral" nomograms may be used for patients referred for testing for clinical reasons, and the "normal" nomograms may be more appropriate for individuals tested for screening or pre-exercise program evaluations.

Maximal cardiac output. Maximal cardiac output

Table 5-5 MET levels for age decades from previous studies

	Froelicher[24]	Hossack[30]	Pollock (Cooper's Clinic)[22]	Morris (referrals)
20-29	11 ± 2	13 ± 1	12 ± 2	—
30-39	10 ± 2	12 ± 2	12 ± 2	—
40-49	10 ± 2	11 ± 2	11 ± 2	11 ± 4
50-59	—	10 ± 2	10 ± 2	9 ± 4
60-69	—	8 ± 2	8 ± 2	8 ± 3
70-79	—	5 ± 1	8 ± 2	7 ± 3
80-89	—	—	—	5 ± 3

is believed by most physiologists to be the major factor limiting maximal oxygen uptake; numerous studies have demonstrated a linear relation between the two. The rate of increase in cardiac output is commonly considered to be roughly 6 liters per 1 liter increase in oxygen uptake. However, there is a wide biologic scatter of maximal cardiac output and VO_2 max in healthy persons even when age, sex, and activity status are considered. Because both maximal cardiac output and maximal oxygen uptake decline with age, the effects of age and disease are usually difficult to separate. McDonough and colleagues measured maximal cardiac output in cardiac patients and found a decline in maximal cardiac output to be the major hemodynamic consequence of symptomatic coronary artery disease and one that resulted in exercise impairment.[29] Reductions in left ventricular performance at high levels of exercise, manifested by decreasing stroke volume and increasing pulmonary artery pressure, appeared to be the mechanism limiting cardiac output. Hossack and co-workers studied 100 patients (89 men, 11 women) to determine their aerobic and hemodynamic profiles at rest and during upright treadmill exercise.[39] The mean maximal cardiac output (CO), measured by use of the direct Fick equation, was 57% ± 14% of average normal values. The reduction in maximal heart rate (63% ± 13% of normal) was a greater factor in the reduction in cardiac output than stroke volume (88% ± 16% of normal). Maximal oxygen consumption (VO_2 max) was 48% ± 15% of normal and the greater reduction in VO_2 max compared with CO was attributable to lower peripheral extraction in the coronary patients. Variables that correlated with maximal CO in a univariate analysis included angina severity ($r = -0.45$), VO_2 max ($r = 0.67$), maximal heart rate ($r = -0.31$), left ventricular dysfunction ($r = -0.45$), maximal systolic blood pressure ($r = -0.31$), and number of vessels with greater than or equal to 50% diameter reduction ($r = -0.3$). Resting ejection fraction did not correlate with maximal CO using a multivariate analysis, four variables correlated significantly ($r = 0.77$) with maximal CO in the following order: VO_2 max, number of vessels with greater than or equal to 50% stenosis, magnitude of ST-segment depression, and sex. These data were used to estimate limits of maximal cardiac output and stroke volume in normal subjects, and these normal standards were then used to evaluate the results in the patients. Patients with an ejection fraction of less than 50% had significantly impaired age-adjusted cardiac output and stroke volume.

MAXIMAL HEART RATE
Methods of recording

Although measuring a patient's maximal heart rate (HR max) should be a simple matter, the different ways of recording rate and differences in the type of exercise used may affect its measurement. The best way is to use a standard ECG recorder and use the R-R intervals to calculate instantaneous heart rate. Methods using the arterial pulse or capillary blush technique are much more affected by artifact than electrocardiographic techniques are. Some investigators have used averaging over the last minute of exercise or in immediate recovery; both of these methods are inaccurate. Heart rate drops quickly in recovery and can climb steeply even in the last seconds of exercise. Premature beats can affect averaging and must be eliminated so that one can obtain the actual heart rate. Cardiotachometers are available but may fail to trigger or may trigger inappropriately on T-waves, artifact, or aberrant beats thus yielding inaccurate results. Not all cardiotachometers have the accuracy of the ECG paper technique.

Atwood and associates compared nine different sampling intervals (1, 2, 3, 6, 10, 15, 20, 30, and 60 seconds) using calipers at rest and during exercise to determine the "ideal" method of measurement in subjects with normal sinus rhythm and patients with atrial fibrillation.[31] This is particularly a problem in atrial fibrillation because of the irregularity of the ventricular response. The heart rate obtained from each interval was compared with the true heart rate (determined by a 4-minute sample at rest and by the last 30 seconds of each minute during exercise). Among patients with atrial fibrillation, large differences were observed between the heart rate obtained and the true heart rate, both at rest and during exercise, with small sampling intervals being used. The mean of these differences ranged between 16 ± 11 beats/min (range 14 to 22) with use of 1-second sampling intervals and 2.2 ± 2.0 beats/min (range 1.6 to 4.4) using 20-second sampling intervals during progressive exercise. Variability of the heart rate obtained from random heart rate samples was also high when short sampling intervals were used among patients with atrial fibrillation. These observations were contrasted by subjects in normal sinus rhythm, among whom neither variability nor measurement error were influenced remarkably when the sampling interval was changed or the heart rate increased. It was concluded that the number of R-R intervals from a 6-second rhythm strip at the end of each minute multiplied by 10 represented a reasonable balance between convenience and precision for measuring heart rate in both atrial fibrillation and normal sinus rhythm.

Factors limiting maximal heart rate

Several factors may affect the HR max during dynamic exercise (Table 5-6). Maximal heart rate declines with advancing years and is affected by gender. Height, weight, and even lean body weight apparently are not independent factors affecting maximal heart rate. Sheffield and colleagues treadmill tested 100 asymptomatic females 19 to 69 years of age, and concluded that the regression of maximal heart rate on age in women was different from that in men, being about 5 beats/min lower.[32] Some investigators report a substantial decrease in maximal heart rates in well trained athletes. Perhaps blood volume changes and cardiac hypertrophy can explain this. However, this has not been a consistent finding. A group of elite marathon runners underwent maximal exercise testing and were found to have similar maximal heart rates to age-matched sedentary controls. Although this point remains unsettled, it is possible that training in early life may result in cardiac hypertrophy or dilatation, or both. Perhaps cardiac dimensions determine the maximal heart rate in individuals with a healthy sinus node.

Age, fitness, cardiovascular disease. Many studies have reported the HR max during treadmill testing in a variety of patients. Regressions with age have varied depending on the population studied and other factors. Table 5-7 and Figure 5-10 summarize these studies of maximal heart rate and are self-explanatory. Some of the major studies are discussed below.

Bruce and colleagues attempted to separate the effects of aging from the effects of cardiovascular disease on HR max by analyzing data on over 2000 healthy middle-aged men and subgroups of over 2000 ambulatory male patients with hypertension, coronary heart disease, or both.[33] All men were given maximal treadmill tests, and the data from each subgroup were regressed on age and compared. Any substantial difference in slope would imply that disease, independently from age, influenced maximal heart rates. Bruce found

an age-related decline in all groups, with correlation coefficients ranging from −0.3 to −0.5. Applying the derived equations for a 50-year-old man would yield an estimated maximal heart rate of 177 for healthy men, 168 for hypertensives, and 151 beats/min for those with coronary heart disease.

Cooper and associates examined the maximal heart rate response to treadmill testing in over 2500 men ranging in age from 10 to 80 years with a mean of 43.[34] Patients with abnormal resting electrocardiograms and those unable to give a maximal effort were eliminated from the study. Levels of cardiovascular fitness were determined by age-adjusted treadmill times using the Balke-Ware protocol; subjects were grouped into below average, above average, or average based on their results. Although their population as a whole showed a regression line and a slope similar to other studies, the data based on cardiovascular fitness showed significantly different slopes. These data suggested that those with lower fitness achieved lower maximal heart rates and that these differences were more divergent at older ages. Those who were cardiovascularly fit tended to show less rapid declines in their maximal heart rates with age.

In an effort to clarify the relationship between maximal heart rate and age, Londeree and Moeschberger performed a comprehensive review of the literature compiling over 23,000 subjects 5 to 81 years of age.[35] A stepwise multiple regression revealed that age alone accounted for 75% of the variability; other factors added only about 5% and included mode of exercise, level of fitness, and continent of origin but not sex. The 95% confi-

Table 5-6 Several factors affecting the maximal heart rate in response to dynamic exercise

Age	Bed rest
Gender	Altitude
Level of fitness	Type of exercise
Cardiovascular disease	True maximal exertion

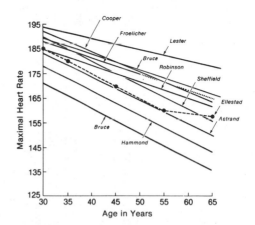

Figure 5-10 Plots of regression lines from the studies of maximal heart rate during dynamic exercise. See Table 5-7 for additional details.

Table 5-7   Summary of studies of maximal heart rate

Study	Number	Population studied	Mean age (SD or RANGE)	Mean HR max (SD)	Regression line	Correlation coefficient	Standard error of the estimate (beats/min)
Åstrand*	100	Asymptomatic men	50 (20-69)	166 ± 22	y = 211 − 0.922 (age)	NA	NA
Bruce	2091	Asymptomatic men	44 ± 8	181 ± 12	y = 210 − 0.662 (age)	−.44	14
Cooper	2535	Asymptomatic men	43 (11-79)	181 ± 16	y = 217 − 0.845 (age)	NA	NA
Ellestad†	2583	Asymptomatic men	42 ± 7 (10-60)	173 ± 11	y = 197 − 0.556 (age)	NA	NA
Froelicher	1317	Asymptomatic men	38 ± 8 (28-54)	183	y = 207 − 0.64 (age)	−0.43	10
Lester	148	Asymptomatic men	43 (15-75)	187	y = 205 − 0.411 (age)	−0.58	NA
Robinson	92	Asymptomatic men	30 (6-76)	189	y = 212 − 0.775 (age)	NA	NA
Sheffield	95	Men with CHD	39 (19-69)	176 ± 14	y = ± 216 − 0.88 (age)	−0.58	11‡
Bruce	1295	Men with CHD	52 ± 8	148 ± 23	y = 204 − 1.07 (age)	−0.36	25‡
Hammond	156	Men with CHD	53 ± 9	157 ± 20	y = 209 − 1.0 (age)	−0.30	19
Morris	244	Asymptomatic men	45 (20-72)	167 ± 19	y = 200 − 0.72 (age)	−0.55	15
Morris	1388	Men referred for evaluation for CHD	57 (21-89)	144 ± 20	y = 196 − 0.9 (age)	−0.43	21

*Åstrand used bicycle ergometry; all other studies performed on treadmill.
†Data compiled from graphs in reference cited.
‡Calculated from available data.
CHD, Coronary heart disease; HR max, maximal heart rate; NA, not able to calculate from available data.

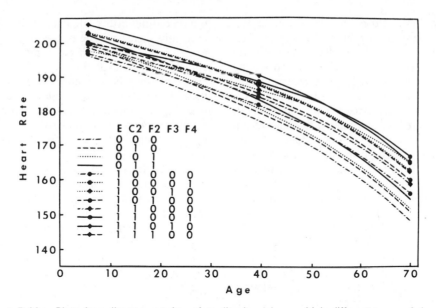

Figure 5-11   Plots from literature review of studies involving multiple different types of dynamic exercise by Londeree and Moeschberger. Under *E* (ergometer), *0* = bicycle and *1* = treadmill; under *C2* (European), *F2* (sedentary), *F3* (active), and *F4* (endurance trained), *1* = class inclusion (that is, a member of that category) and *0* = class excusion.

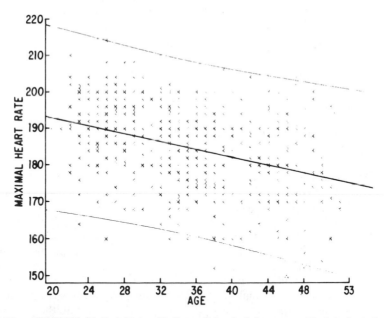

Figure 5-12   USAFSAM (United States Air Force School of Aerospace Medicine) study of healthy pilots showing each individual's datum point and illustrating the normal scatter.

dence interval, even when accounting for these factors, was 45 beats/minute (Figure 5-11). Heart rates at maximal exercise were lower on bicycle ergometry than on the treadmill and lower still with swimming. Their analysis revealed that trained individuals had a significant lowering of maximal heart rates.

At the USAFSAM, we compared the cardiovascular responses to maximal treadmill testing using three different popular treadmill protocols to evaluate reproducibility among tests.[36] The Bruce, Balke, and Taylor protocols were used in the evaluation of 15 healthy men; each man performed one test per week for 9 weeks repeating each protocol three times in randomized order. The maximal heart rates achieved were reproducible within each protocol, and there were no significant differences in heart rate achieved among the three protocols. Also, larger numbers of normals were studied as shown in Figure 5-12, which also shows the wide scatter. In general, these findings are in agreement with more recent data from our laboratory in Long Beach. Graettinger and co-workers from our laboratory recently presented clinical, echocardiographic, and functional determinants of maximal heart rate in preliminary form.[37] Despite controlling for age, activity status, sex, and hypertension, measures of cardiac size and function added little to the prediction of HR max. Most of the variance in HR max was accounted for simply by age. Given the large degree of individual variability in cardiac variables as well as the HR max/age relationship, HR max may always be a difficult variable to explain.

Bed rest. Another factor that affects maximal heart rate and is important to clinical medicine is bed rest. Convertino and colleagues examined the cardiovascular responses to maximal exercise in normal man after 10 days of bed rest. A significant increase in HR max was found after bed rest when compared to pre–bed rest tests. It was suggested that lack of gravitational forces on baroreceptor mechanisms may have played a role in this accentuated heart rate response. Measurements of VO_2 max in both the supine and upright positions revealed lower values with upright exercise. Oxygen consumption during maximal supine exercise was not impaired compared to pre–bed rest measurements. Since maximal heart rates increased significantly but VO_2 max decreased, changes in heart volume are likely involved and may reflect changes in plasma volume during prolonged bed rest.

Altitude. Altitude may affect the heart rate response to exercise. At sea level, atropine administration does not impair maximal heart rate, an indication that parasympathetic withdrawal may be complete at maximal exercise. Maximal heart rate decreases after prolonged exposure to hypoxia. Cunningham and colleagues have shown that catecholamine levels are elevated in plasma and urine at high altitudes.[39] Hartley and co-workers examined maximal heart rate before and after the administration of atropine in 5 normal untrained men who lived at sea level all their lives.[40] The subjects were studied with bicycle ergometry at sea level and at 15,000 feet of altitude. The maximal heart rates decreased a mean of 24 beats/min and the maximal oxygen uptake decreased 26% at this altitude. Atropine adminis-

tration did not affect HR max at sea level but significantly increased HR max at high altitude (165 to 176 beats/min). At high altitude there is an increased parasympathetic tone at maximal exercise. This may be secondary to increased sympathetic tone and the baroreceptor reflex. Mean HR max did not increase with the administration of supplemental oxygen, and so the impaired heart rate response was not attributable to hypoxia alone.

A final factor determining maximal exercise heart rate is motivation to exert oneself maximally. Older patients may be restrained by poor muscle tone, pulmonary disease, claudication, orthopedic problems, and other noncardiac causes of limitation. The usual decline in HR max with age is not so steep in people who are free from myocardial disease and stay active, but it still occurs.

Measures of maximal effort

Various objective measurements have been used to confirm that a maximal effort was performed. As maximal aerobic capacity is reached, the rate of oxygen consumption may plateau. An RQ (respiratory quotient) greater than 1.15, a decrease or failure to increase oxygen uptake by 150 cc/min with increased work loads historically marks the "plateau" and should accurately reflect maximal oxygen uptake when one is using interrupted protocols. However, a plateau is infrequently seen in continuous treadmill protocols in our experience and may actually be attributable to holding onto the handrails, incomplete expired air collection, the criteria used for plateau, differences in the sampling interval, or the equipment utilized. This controversy is discussed in more detail in Chapter 3. Indicators of maximal effort are listed in Table 5-8.

The Borg scale has been developed to subjectively grade levels of exertion. This method is best applied to match levels of perceived exertion during comparison studies. The linear scale ranges from 6 (very very light) to 20 (very very hard), the nonlinear scale ranges from 0 to 10, and both correlate with the percentage of maximal

Table 5-8 Indicators of maximal effort

Patient appearance and breathing rate
Borg scale
Age-predicted heart rate and exercise capacity
Systolic blood pressure
Expired gas measurements: anaerobic threshold, respiratory quotient, plateau, $\dot{V}E$
Venous lactate concentration

heart rate during exercise (Tables 5-9 and 5-10). The respiratory quotient, the ratio of carbon dioxide production to oxygen utilization, increases in proportion to exercise effort. Values of 1.15 are reached by most individuals at the point of maximal dynamic exercise. However, this varies greatly and requires gas-exchange analysis during exercise. Lactic acid levels have also been used (that is, >7 or 8 mmol) but they also require mixed venous samples and also vary greatly between individuals.

Type of dynamic exercise. Although steps, escalators, ladders, and other devices are used, the three predominant types of exercise testing used clinically are treadmill, supine bicycle, or upright bicycle ergometry. The position and the type of exercise influence the heart rate responses. We have found maximal heart rate to be fairly consistent in a wide range of patients with various treadmill and upright ergometer protocols. Supine bicycle ergometry is used for radionuclide studies or for cardiac catheterization studies. Because of changes in venous return and filling pressures, the supine position results in lower resting heart rate and higher end diastolic volumes. As exercise begins, there is little change in the stroke volume or the end-diastolic volume when compared to values obtained at rest. Because of the unusual position and positional disadvantage, there usually is an element of isometric exercise and a lower mechanical efficiency in the supine position. In general, patients are not as able to give maximal efforts in the supine position, and the HR max is usually significantly lower whereas the systolic blood pressure is higher. Patients with significant coronary heart disease may develop angina at

lower double products in the supine than in the upright position, and such angina also contributes to lower maximal heart rates.

A consistent finding in population studies has been a relatively poor relationship of maximal heart rate to age. Correlation coefficients of -0.4 are usually found with a standard error of the estimate of 10 to 25 beats/min. In general, this has not been "tightened" by consideration of activity status, weight, cardiac size, maximal respiratory quotient, or perceived exertion. An exercise program most likely has divergent effects on this relationship at the extremes of ages. Younger people may be able to achieve larger changes in cardiac dimensions than older people. This may affect maximal heart rate. Older individuals achieve a large learning effect whereby they are less afraid to give maximal effort and achieve higher HR max on later testing when they are less apprehensive. Indiscriminant use of age-predicted maximal heart rate in making exercise prescriptions or in setting goals for treadmill performance should be avoided.

The physiological limits on maximal heart rate in normal man are determined by the rapidity of sinus node recovery, cardiac dimensions, left ventricular filling, and contractile state. Systole has a relatively fixed time interval; when heart rate increases, relatively less time of the cardiac cycle is spent in diastole. It seems logical that a limit would be approached where an increase in heart rate would not effectively increase cardiac output because of decreased diastolic filling; not only would the heart receive less blood to pump thereby imposing mechanical limitations, but also the degree of coronary artery perfusion would decrease, imposing metabolic constraints. Although this theoretical limitation is reasonable, there is little experimental work to support it.

Table 5-9 Borg 20-point scale of perceived exertion

6	
7	Very, very light
8	
9	Very light
10	
11	Fairly light
12	
13	Somewhat hard
14	
15	Hard
16	
17	Very hard
18	
19	Very, very hard
20	

Table 5-10 Borg nonlinear 10-point scale of perceived exertion

0	Nothing at all	
0.5	Extremely light	(Just noticeable)
1	Very light	
2	Light	(Weak)
3	Moderate	
4	Somewhat heavy	
5	Heavy	(Strong)
6		
7	Very heavy	
8		
9		
10	Extremely heavy	(Almost maximal)
●	Maximal	

CHRONOTROPIC INCOMPETENCE (CI) OR HEART RATE IMPAIRMENT (HRI)

Ellestad and Wan analyzed the results from 2700 patients tested in their treadmill laboratory and defined a group below the 95% confidence limit for maximal heart rate regressed on age, as having "chronotropic incompetence."[41] Patients with no ST-segment depression who had CI had a four times greater incidence of coronary events than did those without CI in the 4 years after the test. The age-adjusted heart rate limits used for their study were published in Ellestad's text.

In a similar follow-up study of 1500 patients who underwent angiography and treadmill testing, McNeer and co-workers found that those with a maximal exercise heart rate less than 120 beats/min had a 60% survival rate at 4 years versus a 90% survival in those who exceeded a maximal heart rate of 160 beats/min.[42] Bruce and co-workers followed 2000 clinically healthy men after screening them with treadmill testing and found that the inability to achieve a maximal heart rate 90% of that predicted for age had a four times increased risk for coronary events after 5 years.[43]

None of these studies considered the prevalence of exercise test–induced angina or evaluated other factors in their patients with CI. From previous studies of normal subjects and in evaluating patients with coronary heart disease, we have noted no distinguishing features in those with heart rate impairment. Therefore Hammond and co-workers initiated a study to better characterize patients with CI.[44] These patients represented a cross section of patients with coronary heart disease, including those who had a myocardial infarction and coronary artery bypass surgery or angina pectoris, or both. Because the definition of CI required that patients have an impaired heart rate on two separate tests, our sample group was more rigidly defined than in previous studies. Patients who met the criteria for chronotropic incompetence had both significantly less prevalence of bypass surgery and a greater prevalence of exercise-induced angina than the other patients did. It appeared that the limited maximal heart rates were attributable to angina-limited effort; in addition, it appeared that patients who had bypass surgery had less heart rate impairment. Because of these differences, the 156 men were divided into subgroups based on whether they had angina and coronary bypass surgery. The mean heart rate of patients with CI at a submaximal work load (5% grade) was significantly lower than that of the other patients except for those in the angina group (Figure 5-13). Rate-pressure product, an estimate of myocardial oxygen consumption, was significantly lower in those patients with CI. There was a lower mean maximal oxygen consumption in all the patients with CI except for the surgical bypass group. This demonstrates that patients with CI are functionally impaired. This difference retained significance in the group without angina, and therefore symptom limitation is not the only explanation.

Although peripheral adaptations are believed to contribute to widening the arteriovenous oxygen difference in trained athletes, patients that are so quickly limited by their cardiovascular systems are not likely to benefit by this adaptation. Thus the differences in maximal oxygen consumption must be attributable to the heart rate or the stroke volume, or both. Because the degree of heart rate impairment is proportional to the degree of impairment in aerobic capacity, the most likely explanation for aerobic impairment is the limited heart rate. However, the mean level of aerobic impairment was above the 5 MET threshold, at which level most studies have found that patients have a poor prognosis.

Is exercise-induced angina or myocardial dysfunction the cause of chronotropic incompetence?

Much of what has been called "chronotropic incompetence" is related to early termination of exercise because of angina pectoris. Nevertheless, a significant number of patients are not limited by angina but have heart rate impairment. These patients also have significantly lower aerobic capacity than age-matched patients with a normal heart rate response have. Two groups of patients with CI were characterized: those limited by angina and those limited by other factors. From the radionuclide testing, it appears that the patients with CI with angina have good mechanical myocardial reserve with less scar, higher ejection fractions, and lower end-diastolic volumes. In contrast, the patients with CI without angina have more scarring, lower ejection fractions, and higher end-diastolic volumes. This difference in the state of the myocardium was not apparent from clinical features, such as history of congestive heart failure, myocardial infarction, or pathologic Q-waves but was apparent only from the results of radionuclide testing.

From previous studies, one would assume that patients defined as having CI during a treadmill test would have a poor prognosis. Therefore we expected abnormal radionuclide studies and poor prognostic features to be concentrated in our patients with CI. However, we were surprised to find that most patients with CI stopped testing because of angina; in those without angina, the extent of myocardial damage was correlated to their

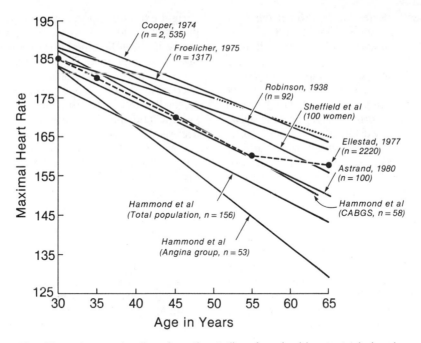

Figure 5-13   Plots of regression lines from the studies of maximal heart rate during dynamic exercise, including population size. See Table 5-7 for additional details.

impaired heart rate response. Previous studies overlooked the occurrence of angina and evidence for prior myocardial infarction in their examination of patients with so-called heart rate impairment. Patients with CI most likely represent a mixed group of patients with a variety of explanations for their impaired heart rate response, including angina, myocardial dysfunction, and simply normal variation.

BLOOD PRESSURE RESPONSE

Systolic blood pressure should rise with increasing treadmill work load. Diastolic blood pressure usually remains about the same, but the fifth Korotkoff sound can sometimes be heard all the way to zero in healthy young subjects. Although a rising diastolic blood pressure can be associated with coronary heart disease, more likely it is a marker for labile hypertension, which leads to coronary disease. The highest systolic blood pressure should be achieved at maximal work load. When exercise is stopped, approximately 10% of the people tested will abruptly drop their systolic blood pressure because of peripheral pooling. To avoid fainting, patients should not be left standing on the treadmill. The systolic blood pressure usually normalizes upon resumption of the supine position during recovery but may remain below usual values for several hours after the test. Despite studies showing discrepancies between non-

invasively and invasively measured blood pressure, the product of heart rate and systolic blood pressure, determined by cuff and auscultation, correlates with measured myocardial oxygen consumption during exercise. Usually an individual patient's angina pectoris will be precipitated at the same double product (systolic blood pressure times heart rate). This product is also an estimate of the maximal work load that the left ventricle can perform. It should be emphasized that the automated methods of measuring systolic blood pressure have not proved to be accurate. Although the available devices may correlate with manual methods, they have not yet been adequately validated, particularly for the detection of exertional hypotension.

Irving and colleagues examined variations in clinical noninvasive systolic pressure at the point of symptom-limited exercise on a treadmill in six groups of subjects: 5459 men and 749 women classified into three categories each.[45] Among the men, 2532 were asymptomatic healthy, 592 were hypertensive, and 1586 had clinical manifestations of coronary heart disease. Among the women, 244, 158, and 347 were in these respective clinical categories. None had had cardiac surgery; all had follow-up status ascertained by periodic mail questionnaires. Reported deaths were reviewed and classified by three cardiologists; 140 deaths were attributed to coronary heart disease, 118 of them in the men classified as having coronary heart disease. Retesting of 156 persons from 1 to 32 months later showed that pressure values agreed within 10% in two thirds, the overall mean difference was only 8.6 mm Hg, and the correlation at maximal exercise was superior to that of the resting observations just before exercise. The hypertensive patients had a significantly greater body weight than normotensive persons have. Among men, the lowest maximal systolic pressure was observed in the group with coronary heart disease; among women, the lowest mean pressure was found in the healthy group. Patients with coronary heart disease were slightly older, and only the women showed a significant correlation between maximal pressure and age. Only 5% of the variation in maximal systolic pressure in the patients with coronary heart disease was attributable to a shortened duration of exercise. Maximal systolic pressures correlated fairly well ($r = 0.46$ to 0.68 for the various groups) with resting systolic pressure, and this relation was independent of the diagnosis of cardiovascular disease in both men and women. Relations between pressure and the number of stenotic coronary arteries and impaired ejection fraction at rest were examined in 22 men without and 182 men with coronary artery disease. Lower maximal systolic pressures were often associated with two- or three-vessel disease or reduced ejection fraction, or both. The prognostic value of maximal systolic pressure for subsequent death from coronary heart disease was examined in the men with coronary heart disease. The annual rate of sudden cardiac death decreased from 97.9 per 1000 men to 25.3 and 6.6 per 1000 men as the range of maximal systolic pressure increased from less than 140 to 140 to 199 and to 200 mm Hg or more, respectively. Cardiomegaly, Q waves in the resting electrocardiogram and persistent postexertional ST-segment depression were more common in men with the lowest systolic pressure at maximal exercise.

Exertional hypotension

Exercise-induced hypotension (EIH) has been demonstrated in most studies to predict either a poor prognosis or a high risk of coronary angiographic disease. Although the prognosis of EIH has not been specifically examined in patients after myocardial infarction, an abnormal systolic blood pressure response has been found to indicate an increased risk for cardiac events in this population. In addition, EIH has been associated with cardiac complications during exercise testing and appears to be corrected by coronary artery bypass surgery.[46-48]

The normal blood pressure response to dynamic

upright exercise appears as a progressive increase in systolic blood pressure, no change or a decrease in diastolic blood pressure, and a widening of the pulse pressure.[49] Even when tested to exhaustion, normal individuals do not exhibit a reduction in systolic blood pressure of any kind.[50] Normally, after exercise, there is a drop in both systolic and diastolic pressure. Exercise-induced decreases in systolic blood pressure (EIH) can occur in patients with coronary artery disease, valvular heart disease,[51] cardiomyopathies, and arrhythmias. Occasionally, patients without clinically significant heart disease will exhibit exercise-induced hypotension during exercise because of antihypertensive therapy including beta blockers, prolonged strenuous exercise, and vasovagal responses, or it can occur in normal women. Pathophysiologically, EIH could be attributable to chronic ventricular dysfunction, exercise-induced ischemia causing left ventricular dysfunction, or papillary muscle dysfunction and mitral regurgitation. Rich and co-workers[52] described a patient in whom EIH was found to be caused by right ventricular ischemia.

Numerous studies have addressed the diagnostic and prognostic implications of EIH. Their important findings regarding definition, prevalence, high risk subgroups, intervention, and mortality are summarized in Table 5-11. One difficulty encountered in interpreting these previous studies is that although EIH has been consistently related to coronary artery disease and a poor prognosis, various criteria have been used to define it.

The Long Beach Veterans Affairs Medical Center Study of EIH

To further demonstrate the causes, definition, and predictive power of exercised-induced hypotension, we analyzed the experience at the LB-VAMC.[53] This prospective study included all patients referred for clinical reasons to the treadmill laboratory and then followed for a 2-year period for cardiac events. The population consisted of 2036 patients who underwent testing from April 1984 to May 1987, 131 (6.4%) of whom exhibited a drop below standing rest.

To clarify the uncertainty regarding the definition of EIH, the following criteria were applied: (1) a systolic blood pressure (SBP) drop of 20 mm Hg or more after an initial rise but without a fall below rest and (2) an SBP drop below the standing rest value. A drop of 20 mm Hg should be sufficient to avoid the technical limitations of determining blood pressure changes during treadmill testing. It was demonstrated that, in our population, the definition of a drop below rest was clearly a better criterion than a drop of 20 mm Hg

Table 5-11 Summary of studies addressing diagnostic and prognostic implications of exercise-induced hypotension

	Definition	Prevalence of EIH	Prevalence of LM/3VD	Predictive value of EIH for LM/3VD	Subgroups at high risk	EIH reversed by revascularization	Mortality MED	Mortality CABG/PTCA
Dubach et al (1988)	SBP drop below rest	5% (94/2022)	45%	61%	No deaths in those with either ischemia or MI	18/22	12/95	0/22
Hammermeister[55] (1983)	SBP drop below rest	7% (93/1241)	25%	50%	Angina, poor exercise capacity, LM/3VD with low EF			
Weiner[54] (1982)	SBP drop below rest	11% (47/436)	28%	55%	Ischemia, PVCs, poor exercise capacity		2/24	1/23
SanMarco et al (1980)	Failure of SBP to rise 10 mm Hg in first minute; or 20 mm Hg drop	24% (90/378)	39%	70%	None found			
Li et al[48] (1979)	SBP equal to or drop below rest	23% (55/234)	100%	100%		33/37		
Hakki et al (1986)	Decrease of SBP by 10 mm Hg	7% (127/1800)			3VD and LV dysfunction			
Thompson and Keleman[47] (1975)	SBP drop below rest	100% (17/17)	100%	100%		6/6	2/9	0/6
Levites et al (1978)	SBP drop below rest	3% (30/1105)	20%	20%	Women had false-positive results)			
Morris et al[46] (1978)	Decrease of SBP by 10 mm Hg	5% (23/438)	24%	78%	None found	6/6	0/12	
Mazzotta et al (1987)	Decrease of SBP by 5 mm Hg	20% (44/224)			None found			
Gibbons et al (1987)	Decrease in SBP by 10 mm Hg	3% (27/820)	—	—	Older age, LM, 3VD, LV dysfunction	—	—	—

From Dubach P et al: *Circulation* 78(6):1380-1387, 1988.
CABG/PTCA, Patients treated with revascularization; *EF*, ejection fraction; *EIH*, exercise-induced hypotension; *LM/3VD*, left main or three-vessel coronary artery disease; *LV*, left ventricular; *MED*, medically treated; *MI*, myocardial infarction; predictive value, percentage with EIH who had three-vessel disease or left main disease; *PVCs*, premature ventricular contractions; *SBP*, systolic blood pressure.

for predicting increased risk for deaths and myocardial infarctions. Therefore we calculated the odds (risk) ratio of EIH for death using only the criterion of a systolic blood pressure drop below rest.

There are several ways to classify a drop in SBP below rest. It could occur with or without an initial rise. When we classified our EIH patients in this way, no differences were found. Although other cutoff points for an inadequate systolic blood pressure response to exercise were found to generate odds ratios, particularly in patient subsets, only the results for this criteria for exertional hypotension are presented.

The average prevalence of EIH among the studies cited in Table 5-11 was 8% (553/6693), whereas the prevalence at LBVAMC was 5%. The prevalence and predictive value for left main and three-vessel disease together ranged from 20% to 100%, with an average of 48% for the prevalence and an average of 68% for the predictive value. In our study, the prevalence was 45% and the predictive value was 61%. The wide scatter of prevalences of EIH and of left main and three-vessel disease and consequently in the predictive value of EIH is the result of the variability in patient selection and methodologies used in the studies. In the reported studies, varying percentages of patients underwent cardiac catheterization, and it was not always possible to distinguish between left main and three-vessel disease or whether the right coronary artery was also involved when left main disease was present. Patients with valvular heart disease, cardiomyopathy, and women were not consistently included or excluded. Despite the above-mentioned limitations, a consistent finding was that slightly more than half of the patients with known or suspected coronary artery disease and EIH had left main or three vessel disease.

Fifteen percent of our patients with EIH had neither a history of myocardial infarction nor an ischemic response during treadmill testing. There was no bradycardia as is usually associated with a vasovagal reaction nor could we find a relationship between beta-blocker therapy and EIH. Our results therefore indicate that factors other than those mentioned above can cause EIH, such as an abnormal peripheral vasodilatation during exercise or exercise-induced mitral regurgitation.

All our patients with EIH who died had either a history of MI or an ischemic response during the exercise test. Since no deaths occurred in patients with EIH who had neither a prior MI nor ischemia, there could be two hypothetical mechanisms for EIH: (1) a primary cardiac cause, being left ventricular dysfunction or ischemia, which is associated with an increased risk of death, and (2) an unknown, noncardiac cause, being probably an abnormal but benign peripheral vascular response. Patients with EIH have an increased risk of death. In all subgroups in the present study, the risk of death was at least two times as great in patients with EIH as compared to those without EIH, except for patients recovering from a recent MI. The patients recovering from a recent MI had the highest death rate, an indication that the degree of left ventricular dysfunction must predominate over other predictors including EIH.

Weiner,[54] Thompson,[47] and Morris[46] along with their respective collaborators found a lower mortality in patients with EIH who received an intervention compared to those who were medically treated. The average death rate in the medically treated group of all studies was 4 out of 33 compared with 1 out of 41 in the intervention group. Our results are even more striking: 12 deaths in 95 medically treated and no deaths in 22 patients who had an intervention. This would indicate that PTCA (percutaneous transluminal coronary angioplasty) or CABS (coronary artery bypass surgery) in patients with EIH can reduce mortality. However, the patients were not randomized to surgery in any of those studies. Li,[48] Thompson,[47] and Morris[46] along with their respective collaborators reported a reversing of EIH with CABS. Eighteen of our patients had EIH that was reversed by revascularization.

In the Seattle Heart Watch,[55] exercise-induced hypotension was defined as a drop in systolic blood pressure below rest. The study was performed in 1241 patients who had treadmill testing and angiography. As defined, exercise induced hypotension had a limited sensitivity for severe forms of coronary heart disease and a risk ratio of 2 or less. However, the predictive value is high when it does occur—50% for three-vessel or left main coronary artery disease. Of course, the predictive value is directly related to the prevalence of left main disease in the population. It is interesting to note that it was equally accurate for diagnosing three-vessel disease, left main disease, or left ventricular dysfunction, but the difference in predictive value was attributable to the different prevalences of these abnormalities.

These results were confirmed by Weiner who found that a fall in SBP occurred in 23% of the patients with left main disease versus 17% of those with three-vessel disease and 6% of those with less disease. As an indicator of either left main or three-vessel disease, a fall in SBP had a predictive value of 66% and a sensitivity of 19%.[54] Irving and Bruce reported six men, clinically diagnosed as having coronary heart disease, with postexertional ventricular fibrillation after maximal exercise testing.[56] The common feature of their treadmill test was exertional hypotension, that is, a decrease or a limited increase (10 mm Hg) in systolic blood pressure. All six men were successfully cardioverted. They concluded that close monitoring of changes in systolic pressure during and shortly after exercise testing is as important as searching for ST-segment changes.

The limitations of our study included the following: invasive measurements were not made during exercise to clarify the causes of EIH; the reproducibility of EIH was not evaluated; inadequate numbers of patients had ventricular function data; and the pre-exercise SBP was the reference value rather than the usual SBP. In addition, left ventricular function was only indirectly assessed by a history of MI, and thallium scintigraphy was not available to confirm silent ischemia. Finally, as in other studies, patients with EIH were not randomized to interventions, and so conclusions regarding the impact of revascularization on survival need to be confirmed by a randomized trial. The results of this study are in accordance with previous studies in regard to the prevalence, prognosis, and predictive value of EIH. It is important to note that EIH has been noted to occur only during treadmill testing and does not appear to occur with bicycle ergometer testing.

The following conclusions can be made regarding EIH:

1. The definition of EIH is of crucial importance in the evaluation of the exercise test response. A drop in systolic blood pressure below pre-exercise values is the most ominous criterion, whereas a drop of 20 mm Hg or more without a fall below pre-exercise values has little if any predictive value.
2. The causes of EIH can be either left ventricular dysfunction (as reflected by MI status) or ischemia. In the 10% of patients in which EIH occurs without association with either of these two factors, EIH appears to be benign. Although speculative, other potential mechanisms of EIH that deserve further investigation include exercise-induced mitral regurgitation and a (noncardiac) peripheral vasodilatory mechanism.
3. As for the prognostic value of EIH, although the risk of death was increased in patients with EIH, two subgroups did not show this. EIH was not associated with an increased risk in those tested within 3 weeks after an MI or in those without a prior MI or ischemia during the exercise test.

Exercise-induced hypotension is usually related to myocardial ischemia or myocardial infarction, is best defined as a drop of systolic blood pressure during exercise below the standing pre-exercise value, and indicates a significantly increased risk for cardiac events. This increased risk is not found in those who did not have either a prior myocardial infarction or signs or symptoms of ischemia during the exercise test. It is usually associated with three-vessel or left main coronary artery disease. Although exercise-induced hypotension appears to be reversed by revascularization procedures, confirmation of a beneficial effect on survival requires a randomized trial.

Exercise/recovery systolic blood pressure ratio

Amon and colleagues have reported that the normal decline in SBP during the recovery phase of treadmill exercise does not occur in some patients with coronary artery disease whereas in others recovery SBP values exceed the peak exercise values.[57] To examine the diagnostic value of this observation, they studied 31 normal subjects and 56 patients undergoing a treadmill test before coronary cineangiography. Because of large differences in peak exercise pressures between the two groups, they derived recovery ratios by dividing the SBP at 1, 2, and 3 minutes after exercise by the peak exercise SBP. The 1-, 2-, and 3-minute ratios in the normal subjects declined steadily from 0.85 to 0.79 and to 0.73 respectively, whereas the ratios in the patients with coronary artery disease remained elevated at 0.97 to 0.93. Abnormal ratios were more frequent in patients with coronary artery disease than in those with ST-segment depression, angina, or both.

Normal heart rate and blood pressure values

The early emphasis placed on the exercise electrocardiogram tended to deemphasize other exercise responses. Measurements of these responses may improve the diagnostic value of exercise testing and may be useful for identifying the presence or the severity of coronary artery disease. The value of any measurement in providing diagnostic information from exercise testing depends on (1) the accuracy and completeness with which a measurement has been made in healthy individuals (reference values) and (2) the effectiveness with which certain limits of the measurement (discriminant values) separate healthy individuals from those subgroups with disease. The complete set of reference values presented in Figure 5-14 should help to determine discriminant values for separating patient groups. Many exercise test responses do not have a gaussian distribution and require that nonparametric statistical tests be used. There-

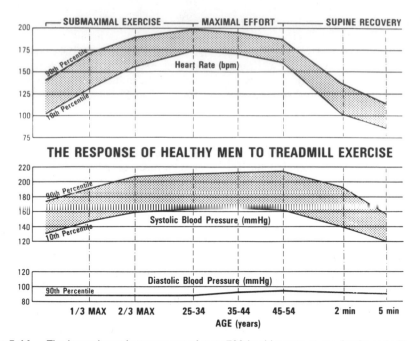

Figure 5-14   The hemodynamic responses of over 700 healthy men to maximal treadmill exercise. *Bands* represent 80% of the population with 10% having values exceeding the upper limit and 10% with lower values.

fore discriminant values should be determined as percentiles rather than as standard deviations or confidence limits.

Using hemodynamic measurements to estimate myocardial oxygen consumption

Although heart rate and stroke volume are important determinants of both maximal oxygen uptake and myocardial oxygen consumption, myocardial oxygen consumption has other independent determinants. It has been demonstrated that the relative metabolic loads of the entire body and those of the heart are determined separately and may not change in parallel with a given intervention. Although the heart receives only 4% of cardiac output at rest, it utilizes 10% of systemic oxygen uptake. The wide arteriovenous oxygen difference of 10 to 12 vol% at rest reflects the fact that oxygen in the blood passing through the coronary circulation is nearly maximally extracted. This value can be compared to the 4 vol% difference across the systemic circulation. When the myocardium requires a greater oxygen supply, coronary blood flow must be increased by coronary dilatation. During exercise, coronary blood flow can increase through normal coronary arteries up to five times the normal resting flow.

The increased demand for myocardial oxygen consumption required for dynamic exercise is the key to the use of exercise testing as a diagnostic

tool for coronary artery disease. Myocardial oxygen consumption cannot be directly measured in a practical manner, but its relative demand can be estimated from its determinants, such as heart rate, wall tension (left ventricular pressure and diastolic volume), contractility, and cardiac work. Although all these factors increase during exercise, increased heart rate is especially detrimental in patients who have obstructive coronary disease. Increases in heart rate results in a shortening of the diastolic filling period, the time during which coronary blood flow is the greatest. In normal coronary arteries, dilatation occurs. In obstructed vessels, however, dilatation is limited and flow is decreased by the shortening of the diastolic filling period. This situation results in both inadequate blood flow and oxygen delivery.

Variable threshold for exercise-induced ischemia

It has been taught that exercise-induced ischemia occurs at the same rate-pressure product (heart rate times systolic blood pressure), unless an intervention has been effective or the coronary artery obstructions have worsened. However, changes in this threshold have been suggested to be caused by coronary artery spasm. The effect of hyperventilation-induced alkalemia on angina was evaluated by Neil and co-workers in nine subjects with consistent exercise-induced chest pain and

ST-segment depression.[58] In five subjects who had arterial alkalemia while hyperventilating during exercise, the rate-pressure product during angina was 22,000 compared with 24,000 when they were breathing normally during exercise. The other four subjects appeared to hyperventilate but were not alkalemic, and their rate-pressure product was not significantly different during repeat testing to angina. Thus the threshold for angina during exercise was lowered in five patients in whom hyperventilation caused alkalemia. Was this effect from the coronary artery spasm or from changes in oxygen release from hemoglobin? A study by Waters and co-workers suggests that it is attributable to changes in coronary artery tone.[59]

SUMMARY

Because it can objectively demonstrate exercise capacity, exercise testing rather than reliance on functional classifications is now usually used for disability evaluation. A questionnaire or submaximal test cannot give the same results as a symptom-limited exercise test. Age-predicted maximal heart rate targets are relatively useless for clinical purposes, and it is surprising how much steeper the age-related decline in maximal heart rate is in referred populations as compared to age-matched normals or volunteers. The nomogram developed by Morris and co-workers greatly facilitates the description of exercise capacity relative to age and enables comparison between patients. Reporting exercise capacity as a percentage with 100% as normal for age has a lot to recommend it. Exertional hypotension, best defined as a drop in systolic blood pressure below standing rest, is very predictive of severe angiographic coronary artery disease and has a poor prognosis. A failure of systolic blood pressure to rise is particularly worrisome after a myocardial infarction. Until automated devices are adequately validated, we strongly recommend that blood pressure be taken manually with a cuff and stethoscope.

REFERENCES

1. Froelicher VF, Thompson AJ, Noquero I, et al: Prediction of maximal oxygen consumption: comparison of the Bruce and Balke treadmill protocols, *Chest* 68:331-336, 1975.
2. Patterson J, Naughton J, Pietras R, et al: Treadmill exercise in assessment of the functional capacity of patients with cardiac disease, *Am J Cardiol* 30:757, 1972.
3. Goldman L, Hashimoto B, Cook EF, Loscalzo A: Comparative reproducibility and validity of systems for assessing cardiovascular functional class: advantages of a new specific activity scale, *Circulation* 64:1227-1234, 1981.
4. Hlatky M, Boineau R, Higgenbotham M, et al: A brief, self-administered questionnaire to determine functional capacity (the Duke Activity Status Index), *Am J Cardiol* 64:651-654, 1989.
5. McKirnan D, Sullivan M, Jensen D, Froelicher VF: Treadmill performance and cardial function in selected patients with coronary heart disease, *J Am Coll Cardiol* 3:253-261, 1984.
6. Ehsani AA, Biello D, Seals DR, et al: The effects of left ventricular systolic function on maximal aerobic exercise capacity in asymptomatic patients with coronary artery disease, *Circulation* 70:552-560, 1984.
7. Weber KT, Kinasewitz GT, Janicki J, Fishman AP: Oxygen utilization and ventilation during exercise in patients with chronic cardiac failure, *Circulation* 65:1213-1222, 1982.
8. Litchfield RL, Kerber RE, Benge JW, et al: Normal exercise capacity in patients with severe left ventricular dysfunction: compensatory mechanisms, *Circulation* 66:129-134, 1982.
9. Higginbotham MB, Morris KG, Conn EH, et al: Determinants of variable exercise performance among patients with severe left ventricular dysfunction, *Am J Cardiol* 51:52-60, 1983.
10. Myers J, Froelicher VF: Hemodynamic determinants of exercise capacity in chronic heart failure, *Ann Intern Med* 115:377-386, 1991.
11. Sullivan MJ, Green HJ, Cobb FR: Exercise training in patients with severe left ventricular dysfunction: hemodynamic and metabolic effects, *Circulation* 78:506-515, 1988.
12. Pfeiffer MA, Pfeffer JM, Fishbein MC, et al: Myocardial infarction size and ventricular function in rats, *Circ Res* 44:503-512, 1979.
13. Carter CL, Amundsen LR: Infarct size and exercise capacity after myocardial infarction, *J Appl Physiol: Respirat Environ Exercise Physiol* 42:782-785, 1977.
14. Grande P, Pedersen A: Myocardial infarct size and cardiac performance at exercise soon after myocardial infarction. *Br Heart J* 47:44-50, 1982.
15. DePace NL, Iskandrian AS, Hakki A, et al: Use of QRS scoring and thallium-201 scintigraphy to assess left ventricular function after myocardial infarction, *Am J Cardiol* 50:1262-1268, 1984.
16. Jette M, Sidney K, Blumchen G: Metabolic equivalents (METS) in exercise testing, exercise prescription, and evaluation of functional capacity, *Clin Cardiol* 13:555-565, 1990.
17. Bruce RA, Kusumi F, Hosmer D: Maximal oxygen intake and nomographic assessment of functional aerobic impairment in cardiovascular disease, *Am Heart J* 85:546-562, 1973.
18. Morris C, Myers J, Kawaguchi T, et al: Nomogram for exercise capacity using METs and age, *J Am Coll Cardiol* 1993. (In press.)
19. Morris CK, Ueshima K, Kawaguchi T, et al: The prognostic value of exercise capacity: a review of the literature, *Am Heart J* 122:1423-1430, 1991.
20. Wolthuis RA, Froelicher VF, Fischer J, et al: New practical treadmill protocol for clinical use, *Am J Cardiol* 39:697-700, 1977.
21. American College of Sports Medicine: Guidelines for exercise testing and prescription, Philadelphia, 1991, Lea & Febiger.
22. Fletcher GF, Froelicher VF, Hartley LH, et al: Exercise standards: a statement for health professionals from the American Heart Association, *Circulation* 82:2286-2322, 1990.
23. Myers J, Buchanan N, Walsh D, et al: Comparison of the ramp versus standard exercise protocols, *J Am Coll Cardiol* 17:1334-1342, 1991.

24. Froelicher VF, Allen M, Lancaster MC: Maximal treadmill testing of normal USAF aircrewmen, *Aerospace Med* 45:310-315, 1974.

25. Dehn MM, Bruce RA: Longitudinal variations in maximal oxygen intake with age and activity, *J Appl Physiol* 33:805-807, 1972.

26. Hammond HK, Froelicher VF: Normal and abnormal heart rate responses to exercise, *Prog Cardiovasc Dis* 27:271-296, 1985.

27. Sullivan M, McKirnan D. Errors in predicting functional capacity for post-myocardial infarction patients using a modified Bruce protocol, *Am Heart J* 107:486-491, 1984.

28. Roberts JM, Sullivan M, Froelicher VF, et al: Predicting oxygen uptake from treadmill testing in normal subjects and coronary artery disease patients, *Am Heart J* 108:1454-1460, 1984.

29. McDonough JR, Danielson RA, Willie P.H, Vine R.L: Maximal cardiac output during exercise in patients with coronary artery disease, *Am J Cardiol* 33:23-29, 1974.

30. Hossack KF, Bruce RA, Kusumi F, Kannagi T: Prediction of maximal cardiac output in preoperative patients with coronary artery disease, *Am J Cardiol* 52(7):721-726, 1983.

31. Atwood JE, Myers J, Sandhu S, et al: Optimal sampling interval to estimate heart rate at rest and during exercise in atrial fibrillation, *Am J Cardiol* 63:45-48, 1989.

32. Sheffield LT, Malouf JA, Sawyer JA, et al: Maximal heart rate and treadmill performance of healthy women in relation to age, *Circulation* 57:79-84, 1978.

33. Bruce RA, Gey GO Jr., Cooper MN, et al: Seattle Heart Watch: initial clinical, circulatory and electrocardiographic response to maximal exercise, *Am J Cardiol* 33:459, 1974.

34. Cooper KH, Purdy JG, White SR, et al: Age-fitness adjusted maximal heart rates, *Medicine Sport* 10:78-88, 1977.

35. Londeree BR, Moeschberger ML: Influence of age and other factors on maximal heart rate, *J Cardiac Rehabil* 4:44-49, 1984.

36. Froelicher VF, Brammel H, Davis G, et al: A comparison of three maximal treadmill exercise protocols, *J Appl Physiol* 36:720-725, 1974.

37. Graettinger W, Smith D, Neupel J, et al: Influence of LV chamber size on maximal heart rate, *Circulation* 84:II-187, 1991.

38. Convertino V, Hung J, Goldwater D, et al: Cardiovascular responses to exercise in middle-aged man after 10 days of bedrest, *Circulation* 65:134-140, 1982.

39. Cunningham WL, Becker ES, Kreuzer F: Catecholamines in plasma and urine at high altitudes, *J Appl Physiol* 20:607-610, 1965.

40. Hartley LH, Vogel JA, Cruz JC: Reduction of maximal exercise heart rate at altitude and its reversal with atropine, *J Appl Physiol* 36:362-365, 1974.

41. Ellestad MH, Wan MKC: Predictive implications of stress testing: follow-up of 2700 subjects after maximal treadmill stress testing, *Circulation* 51:363-369, 1975.

42. McNeer JF, Margolis JR, Lee KL, et al: The role of the exercise test in the evaluation of patients for ischemic heart disease, *Circulation* 57:64-70, 1978.

43. Bruce RA, Fisher FD, Cooper MN, et al: Separation of effects of cardiovascular disease and age on ventricular function with maximal exercise, *Am J Cardiol* 34:757-763, 1974.

44. Hammond HK, Kelly TL, Froelicher V: Radionuclide imaging correlatives of heart rate impairment during maximal exercise testing, *J Am Coll Cardiol* 2(5):826-833, 1983.

45. Irving JB, Bruce RA, DeRouen TA: Variations in and significance of systolic pressure during maximal exercise (treadmill) testing, *Am J Cardiol* 39(6):841-848, 1977.

46. Morris SN, Phillips JF, Jordan JW, McHenry PL: Incidence of significance of decreases in systolic blood pressure during graded treadmill exercise testing, *Am J Cardiol* 41:221-226, 1978.

47. Thomson PD, Kelemen MH: Hypotension accompanying the onset of exertional angina, *Circulation* 52:28-32, 1975.

48. Li W, Riggins R, Anderson R: Reversal of exertional hypotension after coronary bypass grafting, *Am J Cardiol* 44:607-611, 1979.

49. Wolthuis RA, Froelicher VF, Fischer J, Triebwasser JH: The response of healthy men to treadmill exercise, *Circulation* 55:153-157, 1977.

50. Saltin B, Sternberg J: Circulatory response to prolonged severe exercise, *J Appl Physiol* 19:833-838, 1964.

51. Atwood JE, Kawanashi S, Myers J, Froelicher VF: Exercise and the heart: exercise testing in patients with aortic stenosis, *Chest* 93:1083-1087, 1988.

52. Rich MW, Keller A, Chouhan L, Fischer K: Exercise-induced hypotension as a manifestation of right ventricular ischemia, *Am Heart J* 115:184-186, 1988.

53. Dubach P, Froelicher VF, Klein J, et al: Exercise-induced hypotension in a male population: criteria, causes, and prognosis, *Circulation* 78:1380-1387, 1988.

54. Weiner DA, McCabe CH, Cutler SS, Ryan TJ: Decrease in systolic blood pressure during exercise testing: reproducibility, response to coronary bypass surgery and prognostic significance, *Am J Cardiol* 49:1627-1631, 1982.

55. Hammermeister KE, DeRouen TA, Dodge HT, Zia M: Prognostic and predictive value of exertional hypotension in suspected coronary heart disease, *Am J Cardiol* 51:1261-1265, 1983.

56. Irving JB, Bruce RA: Exertional hypotension and postexertional ventricular fibrillation in stress testing, *Am J Cardiol* 39(6):849-851, 1977.

57. Amon KW, Richards KL, Crawford MH: Usefulness of the postexercise response of systolic blood pressure in the diagnosis of coronary artery disease, *Circulation* 70:951-956, 1984.

58. Neill WA, Pantley GA, Nakornchai V: Respiratory alkalemia during exercise reduces angina threshold, *Chest* 80:149-153, 1981.

59. Waters DD, Chaitman BR, Bourassa MG, Tubau JF: Clinical and angiographic correlates of exercise-induced ST-segment elevation: increased detection with multiple ECG leads, *Circulation* 61:286, 1980.

6 Interpretation of ECG Responses

ELECTROCARDIOGRAPHIC RESPONSE TO EXERCISE

The first attempt to evaluate the response of the electrocardiogram to exercise was performed by Einthoven. In 1908, he made a number of accurate observations in a postexercise electrocardiogram, including an increase in the amplitude of the P- and T-waves and depression of the J-junction. In 1953, Simonson studied the electrocardiographic response to treadmill testing of a wide age range of normal subjects.[1] In 1965, Blomqvist reported his classic description of the response of the Frank vectorcardiographic leads to bicycle exercise using computer techniques.[2] Rautaharju and colleagues analyzed P-, ST-, and T-vector functions in the Frank leads at rest and during exercise.[3] All P-wave vector functions increased during exercise and were compatible with right atrial overload whereas T-wave vectors decreased slightly. The ST-segment vector shifted clockwise, to the right, and upward.

Simoons and Hugenholtz reported Frank lead waveform changes during exercise in normal subjects.[4] The direction and magnitudes of time-normalized P, QRS, and ST vectors and other QRS parameters were analyzed during and after exercise in 56 apparently healthy men, 23 to 62 years of age. The PR interval and the P-wave amplitude increased during exercise, but the direction of the P vectors did not change consistent with right atrial overload. No significant change in QRS magnitude was observed, and the magnitude in spatial orientation and the maximum QRS vectors remained constant. QRS onset to T-wave peak shortened. The terminal QRS vectors and the initial ST vectors gradually shortened and shifted to the right and superiorly. The T-wave amplitude lessened during exercise. In the first minute of recovery, the P and T magnitudes greatly increased,

and then all measurements gradually returned to the resting level. There was an increase in S-wave duration in leads X and Y. QRS right-axis shift was heart rate dependent. The ST-segment shifted toward the right superiorly and posteriorly, and the T-wave magnitude increased greatly in the first minute of recovery. Shortening of the QRS complex (3 msec) was found in some young individuals during exercise.

Riff and Carleton demonstrated in patients with atrioventricular dissociation that the duration of atrial repolarization (the atrial T-wave) can play a role in the normal rate-related depression of the J-junction in inferior leads (aV_F, II) and can increase S-wave amplitude.[5] The effect of atrial repolarization on the ST-segments in the lateral leads is less important, but it affects a bipolar lead such as CM_5, which contains anterior and inferior forces.

Morales-Ballejo and colleagues analyzed the response of Q-waves in lead CM_5 in 50 patients with coronary artery disease and in 50 normal subjects before and immediately after exercise.[6] The septal Q-wave in lead CM_5 was smaller in patients with coronary disease than it was in normal subjects at rest and immediately after exercise. Disappearance of the Q-wave in lead CM_5 along with ST-segment depression after exercise was 100% specific for coronary artery disease. They believed that low Q-wave voltage and its failure to increase after exercise indicated abnormal septal activation and reflected loss of contraction because of ischemia. Loss of the septal Q could also be attributable to septal fibrosis secondary to coronary disease.

R-wave changes

Exercise-induced R-wave amplitude changes were studied by Kentala and Luurela in healthy individuals and in patients with known coronary disease.[7] Physically active normal subjects and patients with coronary disease who responded well to an exercise program demonstrated an increased R-wave amplitude in lead V_5 relative to pre-exercise supine rest measurements both on assumption of an upright posture and in response to exercise. The R-wave amplitude then decreased in the supine position after exercise. Such changes were not found in patients who did not benefit from physical conditioning.

Bonoris compared exercise-induced R-wave amplitude changes and ST-segment depression in 266 patients, many of whom were specifically chosen as false-positive or false-negative responders.[8] With use of R-wave criteria the sensitivity was improved. In a second study, 45 subjects with angiographically normal coronary arteries were evaluated; 41 (91%) demonstrated a decrease in R-wave amplitude with exercise. Among 44 patients with angiographic coronary disease, R-wave amplitude increased in 26 patients (59%) with severe coronary disease and decreased in 18 patients (41%) with normal or minimally abnormal resting ventriculograms and less severe coronary artery disease.

Uhl and Hopkirk examined R-wave amplitude changes in 44 asymptomatic men with left bundle branch block.[9] Among the seven men with angiographically significant coronary artery disease, all demonstrated an increase in the amplitude of the R-wave from rest to maximal exercise. In only 10 of the 37 men with normal angiograms did exercise induce an increase in R-wave amplitude, resulting in a sensitivity of 100% and a specificity of 73%.

Yiannikas and colleagues used the sum of the change in R-wave amplitudes in V_4, V_5, and V_6 to investigate the response of 50 men with ST-T wave changes on their resting ECGs.[10] Four of six subjects who increased R-wave amplitude during exercise had angiographically significant coronary artery disease, and the other two had cardiomyopathies. Greenberg and co-workers were able to improve the sensitivity of the exercise test from 50% to 76% by including R-wave criteria in 50 patients without compromising specificity or predictive value.[11] Baron and co-workers, using the mean of the R-wave changes inferiorly and laterally, reported that, of 62 patients with coronary artery disease, 61 (98%) increased the amplitude of the R-wave with exercise.[12] The mean increase in R-wave amplitude was greatest among patients with multivessel disease and with either hypokinesia or akinesia. Nearly as many studies have been unable to demonstrate that changes in the R-wave amplitude during exercise are useful clinically. Van Eenige and co-workers were unable to improve sensitivity using R-wave amplitude changes as compared to ST-segment changes.[13] This was despite the use of several lead systems, clinical subsets of patients, and different criteria for abnormal.

R-wave amplitude changes and left ventricular function. Battler and co-workers at UCSD found poor correlations between ejection fraction and R-wave amplitude at rest and during exercise in 60 patients ($r = 0.50$ and 0.51 respectively).[14] Further, there was no significant relationship between changes in R-wave amplitude and changes in left ventricular ejection fraction during exercise in these patients or in 10 normals. Luwaert and co-workers studied 252 patients evaluated for chest pain and demonstrated a significant though low correlation between the sum of the orthogonal R-waves and resting ejection fraction ($r = 0.22$).[15] Van Eenige and co-workers studied the value of R-wave amplitude changes during exercise in determining ejection fraction, end diastolic pressures, and left ventricular wall motion. No useful diagnostic information was obtained when R-wave changes were used in this study.

Mechanism of R-wave amplitude changes. Brody's demonstration of a relationship between left ventricular volume and R-wave amplitude resulted in this being called the "Brody effect."[16] However, other investigators provide evidence against this concept. Battler and colleagues demonstrated a poor correlation between changes in R-wave amplitude and left ventricular volume. This has been corroborated by others. Talbot and colleagues have, in fact, reported an inverse association between end diastolic volume and R-wave voltage. Levken and colleagues reported that the endocardial QRS amplitude decreased during volume increases in dogs.[17] Deanfield and colleagues reported that R-wave amplitude was essentially unaffected by both increases or decreases in left ventricular volume.[18]

That cardiac enlargement secondary to congestive heart failure may cause a decrease in R-wave amplitude also contradicts the Brody hypothesis. Further, if R-wave amplitude changes were strictly the result of changes in volume, one would expect R-wave amplitude to increase when changing from standing to supine, since diastolic volume would increase. However, this change in R-wave amplitude does not necessarily occur. Since the R-wave has been shown to correlate with systolic volume and ejection fraction, an association with contractility has been suggested. Axis shifts have been implicated as the cause of changes in R-wave amplitude. However, the shift of the QRS and ST-segment vector toward the right and posteriorly is a normal response to exercise. David and co-workers performed an experi-

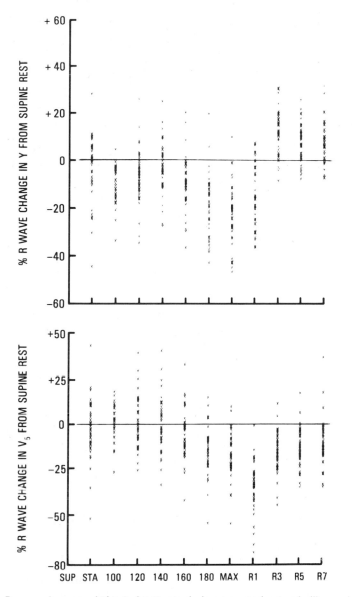

Figure 6-1 R-wave changes relative to heart rate during progressive treadmill exercise in a group of low-risk normals. Graph of percent change of R-wave amplitude for each individual compared with his R-wave at supine rest in V_5 and Y.

ment that was strongly against the concept that R-wave amplitude changes are attributable mainly to changes in ventricular volume.[19] After inducing ischemia in dogs, R-wave amplitude continued to increase despite clamping of the vena cava, which reduced ventricular volume.

If the R-wave-to-volume relationship does not explain the increase in R-wave amplitude that accompanies myocardial infarction, exercise, or coronary spasm, it could be attributable to ischemia-induced changes in the electrical properties of the myocardium. This is supported by the experimental data from David and co-workers. After

inducing myocardial ischemia in dogs, they demonstrated that biphasic R-wave changes directly correlated with changes in intramyocardial conduction times, whereas intracardiac dimensional changes and R-wave changes were unrelated.

UCSD R-wave study. The acquisition of exercise ECGs by computer offered an opportunity to relate R-wave changes with ischemic ST-segment shifts.[20] The ECG changes were analyzed spatially; that is, they were recorded in three dimensions, enabling optimal representation of global myocardial electrical forces. Patients were separated into groups achieving maximal heart rates higher and lower than the mean maximal heart rate achieved of 161 beats per minute. Data on asymptomatic normals has borne out that the R-wave amplitude typically increases from rest to submaximal exercise, perhaps to a heart rate of 140 beats/min, and then decreases to the maximal exercise end point (Figure 6-1). Therefore, if a patient were limited by exercise intolerance whether attributable to objective or subjective symptoms or signs, the R-wave amplitude would increase from rest to such an end point. Such patients may be demonstrating a normal R-wave response but be classified "abnormal," since the severity of disease causes a lower exercise tolerance and heart rate. Exercise-induced changes in R-wave amplitude have no independent predictive power but are associated with coronary artery disease because such patients are often submaximally tested and an R-wave decrease normally occurs at maximal exercise.

S-wave changes

During exercise there is an increase in the S-wave in the lateral precordial leads. It was hypothesized that this increase in the S-wave reflects the normal increase in cardiac contractility during exercise and that its absence is indicative of ventricular dysfunction. It is more likely, however, that the increase in S-wave is caused by exercise-induced axis shifts and conduction alterations.

U-wave changes

In a study by Gerson and co-workers, 248 patients underwent exercise testing using leads CC_5 and aV_L, 36 of whom had exercise-induced U-wave inversion.[21] Of 71 patients with significant left anterior descending or left main disease and no prior myocardial infarction, 35% had U-wave inversion compared to only 4% of 57 patients without left anterior descending or left main disease and only 1% of 82 patients who had no coronary artery disease. U-wave inversion was diagnosed if there was a discrete negative deflection within the TP segment relative to the PR segment, which occurred during or after exercise. Inverted U-waves were not diagnosed if the exercise heart rate increased to a level such that the QT interval could not be accurately measured. This has not been confirmed by other researchers, and McHenry now believes that it is an artifact of his bipolar ECG lead system.

Junctional depression

Mirvis and colleagues studied junctional depression during exercise using left precordial isopotential mapping.[22] During exercise, junctional depression was maximal along the left lower sternal border. In the early portion of the ST-segment they found a minimum isopotential along the lower left sternal border that was continuous with terminal QRS forces in both intensity and location. The late portion of the ST-segment had a minimum isopotential located in the same areas as that observed at rest (that is, the upper left sternal border). These observations indicated that junctional depression might be the result of competition between normal repolarization and delayed terminal depolarization forces. Junctional depression was most pronounced along the left lower sternal border; most subjects did not exhibit these changes in only V_5 and V_6. Also, the slope of the ST-segment varied from site to site and was directly correlated to magnitude and direction of the J-point deviation. Thus junctional depression is the result of the presence of negative potentials over the left lower sternal border during early repolarization. These negative potentials responsible for physiological junctional depression could be caused by delayed activation of basal areas of the left and right ventricles, which leads to accentuated depolarization-repolarization overlap.

Blood composition shifts

During exercise, there are elevations in plasma osmolality, potassium, sodium, calcium, phosphate, lactate, and proteinase. There is a constant and gradual increase for both males and females in these measurements regardless of environmental conditions. Sodium and potassium rapidly return to normal after exercise. During respiratory acidosis, there is a loss of potassium from the musculoskeletal system that is increased by muscular activity. Potassium enters the myocardium during acidosis and exits after exercise. The mechanism for this variance between myocardial and skeletal muscle is not known. Serum potassium increases immediately after exercise, and this increase may be related to postexercise T-wave changes. The increase in potassium during exercise contrasts with the decrease in T-waves during exercise, but there is no explanation as to why there should be a postexertional T-wave peak caused by hyperkalemia when there is no T-wave peak during exercise.

Coester and colleagues drew arterial samples for blood gases and electrolytes at rest, during the last minute of maximal bicycle exercise, and at recovery.[23] The amplitude of the T- and P-waves increased in bipolar lead CH_5 and reached a maximum in the first 2 minutes after exercise. All electrolytes measured were increased at the end of exercise, with potassium up 60% and phosphorus up 53%. Potassium dropped the most rapidly below resting values, along with plasma bicarbonate. ECG alterations were not closely related in time with any single factor such as potassium, but they appeared to reflect an interaction of the changes in mineral balance. The normal right-axis and posterior-axis deviation of the QRS complex and decreasing R-wave amplitude could be attributable to right ventricular overload, respiratory-induced descent of the diaphragm, changes in thoracic impedance, or changes in ventricular blood volume. Patients who develop left anterior hemiblock during exercise that responded in a normal rightward fashion after coronary artery bypass surgery have been noted. The decreased T-wave amplitude may be related to decreased end-systolic volume, changes in sympathetic tone, electrolyte concentration changes, or shifts in the T-wave vector. Other factors may also contribute to the changes in the exercise ECG, such as positional changes in the electrodes, changes in action potentials, electrolyte or hematocrit changes, changes in intracardiac blood volume, and augmentation of the atrial repolarization wave. The effect of age must be considered because there is extensive normal variation related to age. For example, greater ST-segment depression and greater right-axis deviation occur in older persons.

USAFSAM normal exercise ECG study

Using computer techniques, we analyzed data from 40 low-risk normal subjects utilizing measurements of amplitude, intervals, and slope that were then processed and analyzed for treadmill times on the basis of electrocardiographic component and lead.[24] Figure 6-2 shows the waveforms produced using median values of the measurements of all 40 subjects for leads V_5, Y, and Z. These illustrations demonstrate the specific waveform alterations that occur in response to maximal treadmill exercise. Supine, exercise to HR 120, maximal exercise, 1-minute recovery, and 5-minute recovery were chosen as representative times for presentation of these median-based simulated waveforms. There is depression of the J-junction and the tall-peaked T-waves at maximal exercise and at 1-minute recovery that can be an early sign of ischemia, but they are seen here in normal subjects. Along with the J-junction depression, rapid ST-segment upsloping is seen. J-junction depression did not occur in Z lead (which is equivalent to and of the same polarity as V_2). As the R-wave decreases in amplitude, the S-wave increases in depth. The QS duration shortens minimally, but the RT duration decreases in a larger amount.

Q-wave, R-wave, and S-wave amplitudes. In leads CM_5, V_5, CC_5, and Y, the Q-wave shows very small changes from the resting values; however, it does become slightly more negative at maximal exercise. Measurable Q-wave changes were not noted in the Z lead. Changes in median R-wave amplitude are not detected until near-maximal and maximal effort is approached. At maximal exercise and on into 1-minute recovery, a sharp decrease in R-wave amplitude is observed in CM_5, V_5, and CC_5. These changes are not seen in the Z lead. The lowest median R-wave value in lead Y occurred at maximal exercise, with R-wave amplitude increasing by 1-minute recovery. In leads CM_5, V_5, and CC_5 the lowest R-wave amplitude was seen at 1-minute recovery. This quite different temporal response in R-waves in the lateral versus inferior leads is unexplained. There is little change in S-wave amplitude in lead Z. In the other leads, however, the S-wave became greater in depth or more negative, showing a greater deflection at maximal exercise, and then gradually returning to resting values in recovery. A decrease in the QS interval occurred, and it was shortest at maximal exercise. By 3 minutes of recovery, QS interval returned to normal. A steadily decreasing RT-interval duration was observed as exercise increased. The shortest interval was seen at maximal exercise and 1-minute recovery. Changes in this interval followed changes in heart rate.

ST-slope, J-junction depression, and T-wave amplitude. The amplitude of the J-junction in lead Z was very little changed through exercise but was elevated slightly in recovery. The location of the J-junction (QRS end) in Z was determined by using the Z-lead signal alone, rather by a three-dimensional method, and so it is relatively inaccurate. It appears that the lead system affects the anteroposterior presentation of the ST vector more than anticipated. Careful studies applying spatial determination of QRS end are needed to see whether the J-junction shifts anteriorly or posteriorly. The J-junction was depressed in all other leads to a maximum depression at maximal exercise, and then it gradually returned toward but not to pre-exercise values slowly in recovery. There was very little difference between the three left precordial leads. A dramatic increase in ST-segment slope was observed in all leads and was greatest at 1-minute recovery.

These changes returned toward pretest values during later recovery. The greatest or steepest slopes were seen in lead CM_5, which did not show the greatest ST-segment depression. A gradual decrease in T-wave amplitude was observed in all leads during early exercise. At maximal exercise the T-wave began to increase, and at 1-minute recovery the amplitude was equivalent

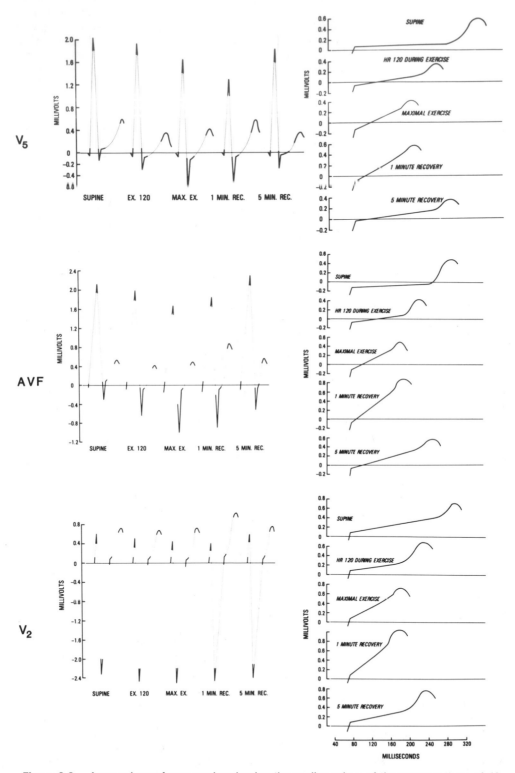

Figure 6-2 Averaged waveforms produced using the median values of the measurements of 40 low-risk normal subjects for leads V_5, aV_F, and V_2.

to resting values, except in leads Y and Z where they were greater than at rest. However, there was a great deal of overlap.

Percent R-wave changes. Figure 6-1 illustrates the percent change of R-wave amplitude for each individual compared with his R-wave at supine rest in V_5 and and Y. At lower exercise heart rates, the great variability of R-wave response was apparent and many normal individuals had significant increases in R-wave amplitude. Although most showed a decline at maximum exercise, some normal subjects had an increase, whereas others showed very little decrease. At 1-minute recovery there was a greater tendency toward a decline in lead V_5 but not in Y. Further into recovery, R-wave amplitude remained decreased in lead V_5 but increased in Y.

Abnormal ST-segment changes

Epicardial electrode mapping usually records ST-segment elevation over areas of severe ischemia and ST-segment depression over areas of lesser ischemia. ST-segment depression is the reciprocal of the injury effect occurring in the endocardium as viewed from an electrode overlying normal epicardium. ST-segment elevation seen from the same electrode reflects transmural injury or, less frequently, epicardial injury. On the surface electrocardiogram, exercise-induced myocardial ischemia can result in one of three ST-segment manifestations: elevation, normalization, or depression.

ST-segment elevation. Variant angina with its associated ST-segment elevation was first described by Prinzmetal and co-workers[25] in 1959 and explained as being secondary to coronary artery spasm. They reported 32 patients with rest angina and ST-segment elevation with reciprocal ST-segment depression. The chest pain spontaneously terminated, but often there were arrhythmias that could lead to ventricular fibrillation and death. Although many of these patients had normal coronary arteries on cardiac catheterization, subsequent studies showed that approximately half of them had significant fixed lesions in addition.[26-28] Patients with variant angina can also have typical ST depression during exercise testing.[29] Weiner[30] has reported 4 patients with Prinzmetal angina who developed ST-segment depression in recovery only after a treadmill test. Thus treadmill testing can be helpful in the diagnosis of such patients.

Prevalence of exercise-induced ST elevation. The most common electrocardiogram abnormality seen in the exercise laboratory is ST-segment depression, while ST-segment elevation is relatively rare (see Table 6-1, studies of exercise-induced ST elevation). Its prevalence depends on the population tested but occurs more frequently in patients who have had a myocardial infarction.

Fortuin and Friesinger reported the angiographic and clinical findings and 2-year follow-up study of 12 patients with 0.1 mV or more ST-segment elevation during or after exercise.[31] These patients were selected from 400 patients who had coronary angiography and exercise testing. Seven of them had previous myocardial infarctions, and 9 of the 10 with angina developed it during the exercise test. One patient with atypical chest pain had normal coronary arteries and improved during the follow-up period. Seven of eight with exercise-induced ST-segment elevation in lead V_3 had left anterior descending coronary disease. All four with inferior elevation had right coronary disease. None had ST-segment elevation at rest, but many had Q-waves or T-wave inversion, or both. Within 2 years, four of the patients died, one had a documented myocardial infarction, and two became unstable.

Hegge and co-workers found 11% of the patients they studied with maximal treadmill testing and coronary angiography to have exercise-induced ST-segment elevation in the postexercise 12-lead electrocardiogram.[32] This relatively high prevalence of ST-segment elevation is probably explained by inclusion of V_1 and V_2, leads not monitored in other studies. The ST-segment elevation was present in precordial leads only in 12 patients, in the inferior leads only in five patients, and in both in one patient. Seventeen patients had severe coronary artery disease in the arteries supplying the appropriate area and the remaining patient had a normal coronary angiogram.

Chahine and colleagues reported the prevalence of exercise-induced ST-segment elevation in 840 consecutive patients to be 3.5%.[33] CM_5 and CM_6 were the only leads monitored, and so lateral-wall ST-segment elevation was all that could be detected. Only about 20% of those who had coronary artery disease showed ST-segment elevation. Sixty-four percent of the patients with left ventricle dyskinesia displayed ST-segment elevation. Manvi and Ellestad presented results in 29 patients with coronary artery disease who had abnormal left ventriculograms.[34] ST-segment elevation occurred in 48%, 33% developed ST-segment depression, and the remaining 19% had no changes. ST-segment elevation occurred in 1.3% of 2000 exercise tests.

Simoons and colleagues investigated the spatial orientation of exercise-induced ST-segment changes in relation to the presence of dyskinetic areas, as demonstrated by left ventriculography.[35] In patients with an anterior infarct, the ST vectors

Table 6-1 Studies of exercise-induced ST-segment elevation during standard clinical testing

Study	Size of population tested	Type of population	Percent of population with prior MI	Number of leads measured for elevation	Criteria for elevation	Prevalence of abnormal elevation (%)	Percent prior MI in patients with elevation
Bruce (1988)	3050	Angina	47	11	1 mm	4	83
Bruce (1974)	1136	CHD	47	CB_5	>0 mV	5	57
Sriwattanakomen (1980)	1620	All referred	—	11	1 mm	4	47
Longhurst (1979)	6040	All referred	—	12 + XYZ	0.5 mm	8	79
Chahine (1976)	840	VAMC	—	V_5, V_6	1 mm	4	86
Dunn (1981)	190	No anterior Q-waves	0	aV_L and V_1	—	24	
Stiles (1980)	650	541 patients with ST depression versus 109 with ST elevation	10	11	1 mm	4	61
Waters (1980)	720	Mixed	1	12 ± CM_5	—	7	76

From Nosratian FJ, Froelicher VF: *Am J Cardiol* 63:986-987, 1989.
All, All patients referred to exercise lab; *CHD,* coronary heart disease; *MI,* myocardial infarction; *TMT,* treadmill test; *VAMC,* Veterans Affairs Medical Center.

were widely scattered but were most often directed to the left, anterior, and superior. Patients with an inferior myocardial infarction had ST-segment vectors rightward and anterior, and also inferiorly if inferior dyskinesia was present. Anteriorly orientated ST-segment changes were associated with anterior or apical scars in patients with anterior infarcts. Thus ST-segment vector shifts associated with dyskinesia resulted in ST-segment elevation over the dyskinetic area. In patients with dyskinetic areas, the direction of the ST-segment changes varied so widely that only the magnitude of the changes could be used as a criterion for exercise-induced ischemia.

Sriwattanakomen and colleagues reviewed 1620 exercise tests and found 3.8% to have ST-segment elevation when all leads except aV_R were evaluated.[36] They then correlated exercise-induced ST-segment elevation with the coronary arteriography and left ventriculograms of 38 patients, 37 of which had significant coronary disease. In 27 patients with Q-waves, 25 had significant disease and ventricular aneurysms, whereas among 11 patients with no Q-waves and significant disease, only two had ventricular aneurysms. One patient had a ventricular aneurysm but no coronary disease. The sites of ST-segment elevation correctly localized the area of ventricular aneurysm in 30 of 33 instances and determined the diseased vessels in 38 of 40 instances. They concluded that ST-segment elevation during exercise in the absence of Q-waves indicates significant proximal disease without ventricular aneurysm,

whereas with Q-waves, ST-segment elevation is indicative of ventricular aneurysm in addition to significant proximal disease. Ischemia and abnormal wall motion may independently or additively underlie the mechanism for ST-segment elevation during exercise.

Longhurst and Kraus reviewed 6040 consecutive exercise tests and found 106 patients (1.8%) without previous myocardial infarctions who had exercise-induced ST-segment elevation.[37] Their criterion was 0.5 mm elevation in a 15-electrode array. Forty-six of these patients with ST-segment elevation had ventriculography and coronary angiography. Coronary disease was detected in 40 of 46, with nearly equal numbers having one-, two-, and three-vessel disease. Ventriculograms were normal in 36 of 40 patients. Of 21 patients with anterior ST-segment elevation, 86% had left anterior descending obstruction. There was no anatomic correlation in those with lateral or inferoposterior exercise-induced elevation.

Dunn and colleagues performed exercise thallium scans on 35 patients with exercise-induced ST-segment elevation and coronary artery obstruction.[38] Ten patients developed exercise ST-segment elevation in leads that showed no Q-waves on the resting electrocardiogram. The site of elevation corresponded to a reversible perfusion defect and a severely obstructed coronary artery. Associated ST-segment depression in other leads occurred in seven patients, but only one had a second perfusion defect at the site of depression. Three of the 10 patients had a wall motion abnormality at the same site. Twenty-five patients developed exercise ST-segment elevation in leads with Q-waves. The site of the elevation corresponded to a severe stenosis and a thallium-perfusion defect that persisted on the 4-hour redistribution scan. Associated ST-segment depression in other leads occurred in 11 patients, and eight had a second perfusion defect at the site of the depression. In all 25 patients, there was a wall-motion abnormality at the site of the Q-wave. Therefore, without a previous infarct, ST-segment elevation indicates the site of severe transient ischemia; associated ST-segment depression is usually reciprocal. In patients with Q-waves, exercise-induced ST-segment elevation may be attributable to ischemia around the infarct, abnormal wall motion, or both. Association ST-segment depression may be attributable to a second area of ischemia rather than being reciprocal.

Braat has assessed the value of lead V_{4R} during exercise testing for predicting proximal stenosis of the right coronary artery.[39] In 107 patients, a Bruce exercise test with the simultaneous recording of leads I, II, V_{4R}, V_1, V_4, and V_6 was followed by coronary angiography. ST-segment changes were recorded in the conventional leads and in lead V_{4R}. Seventy-nine of the 107 patients were studied because of inadequate control of angina pectoris. In the 46 patients who had a previous MI, the infarct location was inferior in 28 and anterior in 18. Seven of the 14 patients without MI and significant proximal stenosis in the right coronary artery showed an ST-segment deviation of 1 mm or greater in lead V_{4R} during exercise. This was also observed in 11 of 18 patients with an old inferior wall infarction and proximal occlusion of the right coronary artery. None of the 53 patients without significant proximal stenosis in the right coronary artery showed exercise-related ST-segment changes in lead V_{4R}. Exercise-related ST-segment deviation in lead V_{4R} (elevation in 17 and depression in 4 patients) had a sensitivity of 56%, a specificity of 96%, and a predictive accuracy of 84% in recognizing proximal stenosis in the right coronary artery.

To determine if patterns of ST depression or elevation during exercise testing provide reliable information about the location of an underlying coronary lesion, Mark and co-workers studied 452 consecutive patients with one-vessel disease who underwent treadmill testing.[40] Exercise ST changes were classified as elevation or depression and by lead groups involved. The ST depression occurred most commonly in leads V_5 or V_6 regardless of which coronary artery was involved. In contrast, anterior ST elevation indicated left anterior descending coronary disease in 93% of cases, and inferior ST elevation indicated a lesion in or proximal to the posterior descending artery in 86% of cases. Furthermore, anterior ST elevation in leads without diagnostic Q waves usually indicated a high-grade, often proximal, left anterior descending stenosis, whereas anterior ST elevation in leads with Q-waves usually indicated a totally occluded left anterior descending coronary artery. Thus ST elevation during exercise testing, though uncommon, is a reliable guide to the location of the underlying coronary lesion, whereas ST depression is not. ST elevation means something different and has a different physiological basis when it occurs over pathological Q-waves (or an old transmural MI site) from when it occurs in a normal ECG. Unfortunately, many of the studies have not made that distinction or considered location.

Waters and co-workers[41] reported that 47 patients of 720 who underwent treadmill testing developed ST elevation. Chahine and colleagues[33] found 29 patients with ST-segment elevation among 840 patients who had an exercise test. Bruce and co-workers[42] reported a prevalence of 0.5% in the Seattle Heart Watch Study in 1974, but Bruce and Fisher[43] later reported a prevalence of 4.7% in 1136 patients observed in Seattle community practice. Part of this increase would be attributable to the quantitative measurements made using signal averaging. De Feyter and colleagues[44] in his study of 680 patients reported a prevalence of 1%, but a multilead system was not used. Bruce also analyzed the Coronary Artery Surgery Study registry data[45] and compared it to the results of the Seattle Heart Watch Study. He found that although the two groups were relatively matched, patients in the coronary artery surgery study had more left ventricular dysfunction and less ST elevation than in the Seattle study. However, the Coronary Artery Surgery Study used visual analysis of 12-lead electrocardiograms and the Seattle study used computer analysis of lead CB_5. In both groups, however, the 6-year survival for patients with ST elevation was significantly lower than patients with ST depression (71% versus 86%).

Methods of measurement. ST-segment depression is measured from the isoelectric baseline, or when ST-segment depression is present at rest, the amount of additional depression is measured. However, ST-segment elevation is always considered from the baseline ST level. Whether the elevation occurs over or adjacent to Q-waves or in non–Q wave areas is important. Unfortunately, many of the studies do not provide the methods of measurement or the condition of the underlying electrocardiogram. Table 6-2 lists some of the factors that should be considered when one is assessing studies of ST-segment elevation. Multiple causes for ST-segment elevation during treadmill testing have been suggested. These include left ventricular aneurysm, variant angina, severe ischemic heart disease, and left ventricular wall-motion abnormalities. Left ventricular aneurysm after myocardial infarction is the most frequent cause of ST-segment elevation on the resting electrocardiogram and occurs over Q-waves or in electrocardiographic leads adjacent to Q-waves. Early repolarization is a normal variant pattern of resting ST-segment elevation that occurs in normal individuals who do not have diagnostic Q-waves. This normally sinks to or below the isoelectric line.

Ischemia or wall-motion abnormality?

There is controversy regarding whether ischemia or wall motion abnormalities are the major cause of ST-segment elevation. Fortuin and co-workers[31] studied 12 patients and concluded that severe coronary artery disease found on angiography was the cause of ST-segment elevation. The location of elevation also correlated with the coronary obstruction. They noted that temporary ligation of an artery in dogs produced reversible ST-segment elevation and these changes do not occur unless the blood flow is decreased to at least 70%. Hegge and colleagues studied 158 patients, 18 of whom had ST-segment elevation on treadmill testing.[46] Seventeen of these patients were found to have significant coronary artery disease correlating anatomically with the area where ST-segment elevation occurred. Lahiri and colleagues reported five patients who presented with ST-segment elevation during exercise and chest pain at rest.[47] These patients also had positive thallium tests with reversible defects. Three of these patients subsequently had myocardial in-

Table 6-2 List of some factors that should be considered when ST-segment elevation studies are assessed

Population tested (prevalence of myocardial infarction patients, patients with varient angina or spasm)
Baseline (resting) electrocardiogram
Electrocardiographic leads monitored
Leads in which elevation occurs relative to Q-waves
Criteria for elevation
Methods of ST-shift detection (visual or computerized)

From Nosratian FJ, Froelicher VF: *Am J Cardiol* 63:986-987, 1989.

farction and two died. However, Caplin and Banim[48] and Hill and colleagues[49] have shown that such electrocardiograph changes can occur in patients with normal coronary arteries who develop spasm and have an excellent prognosis. Fox and co-workers[50] reported the results of coronary artery bypass surgery on 24 patients after myocardial infarction who had exercise-induced ST-segment elevation. Fifteen of these patients had loss of both symptoms and exercise-induced ST-segment elevation. Since this ST elevation was abolished by coronary bypass surgery, they believed that the underlying mechanism was myocardial ischemia.

Waters and co-workers[41] found that 36 of 47 patients who presented with ST-segment elevation on exercise testing had Q waves in inferior or anterior leads on their resting electrocardiogram. Ninety-four percent of their patients had evidence of wall-motion abnormality on cardiac catheterization. In the remaining 11 patients, 10 had Prinzmetal's angina and no Q-wave or wall-motion abnormalities. They concluded that ST-segment elevation was caused directly by a segmental wall-motion abnormality in patients with a previous myocardial infarction but by spasm in patients with variant angina. Gerwitz and co-workers[51] studied 28 patients with a previous anterior myocardial infarction with thallium exercise testing. Fifteen of the patients had evidence of ST elevation, whereas 13 did not. They found that patients with ST elevation had larger anterior lateral or septal thallium defects and lower ejection fractions. They concluded that myocardial ischemia was not required for exercise-induced ST-segment elevation to occur and that such ST elevation primarily reflects the extent of previous anterior wall damage and to a lesser extent an increase in heart rate.

Chahine and co-workers[33] arrived at similar conclusions after studying 29 patients who had ST elevation during exercise testing. Twenty-five of their patients had evidence of electrocardiographic anterior myocardial infarction. Eighteen of the 21 patients who had an angiogram showed left ventricular aneurysm, and 19 had critical left anterior descending lesions. They reviewed all patients with anterior myocardial infarction or critical left anterior descending disease and found that only 22% and 18% respectively showed exercise-induced ST-segment elevation, whereas 64% of the cases with left ventricular aneurysm displayed this phenomenon. They concluded that exercise-induced ST-segment elevation is usually attributable to left ventricular aneurysms.

Stiles and co-workers[52] and Longhurst and co-workers[37] reviewed a large number of patients with ST elevation during exercise. Their conclusion was that most of these patients had previous Q-wave infarcts and regional wall-motion abnormalities. If there was no previous myocardial infarction, ST-segment elevation was related to the severity of coronary artery disease. Dunn and co-workers[38] correlated thallium and angiography results and concluded that in patients without previous myocardial infarction the site of ST-segment elevation correlates with severe coronary artery disease. ST-segment depression in these patients represents either reciprocal changes or two areas of ischemia independent of each other. In patients with Q-wave infarcts, however, ST elevation was caused by wall-motion abnormality, peri-infarction ischemia, or both. They also found that ST elevation in V_1 and aV_L in patients without evidence of myocardial infarction correlates well with significant lesions in the left anterior descending artery and ischemia in the anterior wall. Shimokawa and co-workers[53] arrived at similar conclusions. They found that in patients with ST elevation the degree of perfusion defect may be larger on the thallium scan than in the patients with ST depression.

Retrospective studies by Arora and co-workers[54] and Sriwattanakomen and co-workers[36] found that the patients with ST-segment elevation on exercise testing and no previous Q-waves on the resting electrocardiogram usually stop because of angina, have reversible thallium defects, and have single-vessel disease on cardiac catheterization. On the other hand, patients with abnormal Q-waves had multivessel disease, fixed thallium defects, and stopped because of fatigue and shortness of breath.

These studies are summarized in Table 6-1. In conclusion, in patients with ST-segment elevation during exercise when no abnormal Q-wave is seen on the baseline electrocardiogram, there is a very high likelihood of a significant proximal narrowing in the coronary artery supplying the area where it occurs. It is also likely to be associated with serious arrhythmias. When elevation occurs in an electrocardiogram with abnormal Q-waves, it is usually attributable to a wall-motion abnormality and the elevation can conceal ST-segment depression because of ischemia. Figure 6-3 is an example of ST elevation in a normal baseline ECG (Patient had a tight left anterior descending artery lesion that responded to percutaneous trans-

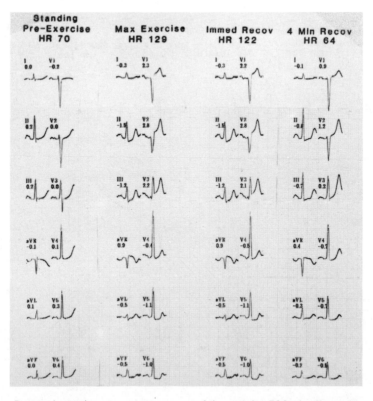

Figure 6-3 Rest and exercise computer averages of the exercise ECG of patient with normal resting ECG and elevation. Patient was found to have a tight left anterior descending lesion that responded very well to PTCA (percutaneous transluminal coronary angioplasty).

luminal coronary angioplasty), and Figure 6-4 illustrates the typical ST elevation over Q-waves that occurs after a myocardial infarction. This patient is unusual in that the elevation occurs in multiple areas.

ST-segment normalization or absence change. Another manifestation of ischemia can be no change or normalization of the ST-segment because of cancellation effects. Electrocardiographic abnormalities at rest, including T-wave inversion and ST-segment depression, have been reported to return to normal during attacks of angina and during exercise in some patients with ischemic heart disease. This cancellation effect is a rare occurrence, but it should be kept in mind. The ST-segment and T-wave represent the uncancelled portion of ventricular repolarization. Since ventricular geometry can be roughly approximated by a hollow ellipsoid open at one end, the widespread cancellation of the relatively slowly dispersing electrical forces during repolarization is understandable. Patients with severe coronary artery disease would be most likely to have cancellation occur, yet they have the highest prevalence of abnormal tests. Manvi and Ellestad reported that 20% of the patients with dyskinesia and coronary artery disease had normal tests, and Chahine and co-workers reported that about 25% of their patients with dyskinesia and coronary artery disease normalized or minimally elevated their ST-segments during exercise. Nobel and colleagues reported normalization of both inverted T-waves and depressed ST-segments in 11 patients during exercise-induced angina.[55] When exercise testing fails to produce ST-segment depression or elevation in a patient with known coronary artery disease, this could be attributable to two or more severely ischemic myocardial segments causing canceling ST-segment vectors. Sweet and Sheffield reported a patient with minor ST-segment depression and T-wave inversion in lead V_5 who normalized, or "improved," his electrocardiogram during treadmill testing only to have an acute infarction 10 minutes after the test.[56] This normalization of ST-segment depression should thus be considered ST-segment elevation.

Lavie and co-workers from the Mayo Clinic studied 84 consecutive patients with resting T-wave inversion.[57] Radionuclide angiography revealed significant new wall-motion abnormalities in 13 (28%) of the 47 patients with persistent T-wave inversion and in 23 (62%) of the 37 patients with T-wave pseudonormalization during exercise. The response of the ejection fraction to

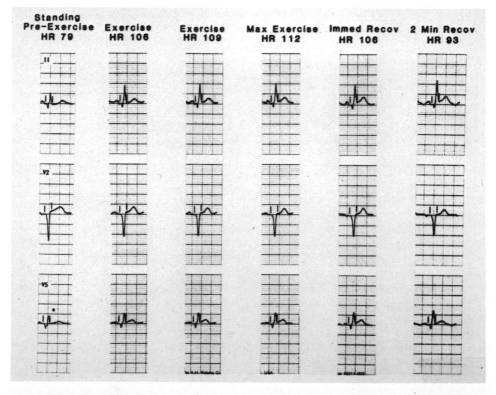

Figure 6-4   Average complexes from the exercise ECG of patient with inferior-lateral myocardial infarction.

exercise was better in patients with persistent T-wave inversion than in those with pseudonormalization. Mechanical evidence of ischemia was seen in 14 (61%) of the 23 patients with T-wave pseudonormalization but without ST-segment depression. In patients with resting T-wave inversion, pseudonormalization was slightly more sensitive but less specific than a positive exercise test for predicting significant new wall-motion abnormalities or decreases in the ejection fraction with exercise. The authors concluded that although pseudonormalization is not extremely useful alone, the presence or absence of this finding can increase the diagnostic accuracy of exercise electrocardiography in patients with resting T-wave inversion and suspected ischemic heart disease.

The prevalence of the canceling of surface ST-segment changes by multiple ischemic ST vectors is not known. The inability of patients to give an adequate effort are more likely explanations for the majority of false-negative exercise tests in patients with multivessel coronary artery disease. In those with single-vessel disease, the decreased sensitivity of exercise testing is most likely attributable to insufficient myocardial ischemia to cause surface ECG changes.

ST-segment depression

The most common manifestation of exercise-induced myocardial ischemia is ST-segment depression. The standard criterion for this type of abnormal response is horizontal or downward sloping ST-segment depression of 0.1 mV or more for 80 msec. It appears to be attributable to generalized subendocardial ischemia. A "steal" phenomena is likely from ischemic areas because of the effect of extensive collateralization in the subendocardium. ST-depression does not localize the area of ischemia as ST-elevation does or help to indicate which coronary artery is occluded. The normal ST-segment vector response to tachycardia and to exercise is a shift rightward and upward. The degree of this shift appears to have a fair amount of biologic variation. Most normal individuals will have early repolarization at rest, which will shift to the isoelectric PR-segment line in the inferior, lateral, and anterior leads with exercise. This shift can be further influenced by ischemia and myocardial scars. When the later portions of the ST-segment are affected, flattening or downward depression can be recorded. Both local effects and the direction of the spatial changes during repolarization cause the ST-segment to have a different appearance at the many surface sites that can be monitored. The more leads with these apparent ischemic shifts, the more severe is the disease.

The probability and severity of coronary artery disease are directly related to the amount of J-junction depression and are inversely related to the slope of the ST-segment. Downsloping ST-segment depression is more serious than horizontal depression is, and both are more serious than upsloping depression is. However, patients with upsloping ST-segment depression, especially when the slope is less than 1 mV/sec, probably are at increased risk. If a slowly ascending slope is utilized as a criterion for an abnormality, the specificity of exercise testing will be decreased (more false-positive results) though the test may become more sensitive. One electrode can show upsloping ST- depression, whereas an adjacent electrode shows horizontal or downsloping depression. If an apparently borderline ST-segment with an inadequate slope is recorded in a single precordial lead in a patient highly suspected of having coronary artery disease, multiple precordial leads should be scanned before the exercise test is called normal. An upsloping depressed ST-segment may be the precursor to abnormal ST-segment depression in the recovery period or at higher heart rates during greater work loads. It is preferable to call tests with an inadequate ST-segment slope but with ST-segment depression borderline response, but added emphasis should be placed on other clinical and exercise parameters. Examples of the various criteria for ischemic ST-depression are shown in Figure 6-5.

ST-segment depression in recovery. Because of technical limitations, the first diagnostic use of the exercise electrocardiography (ECG) involved observations made only after exercise. After ECG techniques were developed that made accurate ECG recording possible during activity, the emphasis in testing shifted to changes occurring during the exercise period itself. The diagnostic accuracy of ST changes limited to the period after exercise has been controversial. It has been proposed that such changes are more likely to represent false-positive responses[58] or are attributable to coronary artery spasm.[29] To facilitate imaging as soon as possible during recovery, studies[59] comparing nuclear procedures to the exercise ECG often do not even include an ECG evaluation done after exercise. Most exercise test scores involve consideration of only ST-segment changes occurring during exercise and excluding changes occurring during recovery alone. Although a cool-down walk is known to obscure recovery ST shifts,[60] such has been recommended for safety reasons.[61]

Patients were selected from a group of 3351 who underwent routine clinical exercise testing from 1985 to 1989. Thirty percent of this group underwent coronary angiography within 3 months

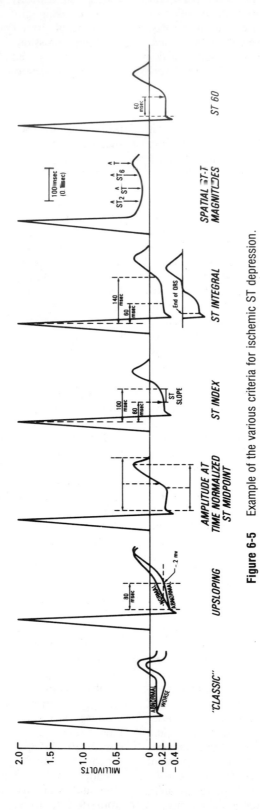

Figure 6-5   Example of the various criteria for ischemic ST depression.

of testing. After exclusion of females, patients with a myocardial infarction (by history or Q-wave presence), individuals with prior percutaneous transluminal coronary angioplasty or coronary artery bypass surgery, and those with left bundle branch block, 271 patients remained. Most were referred for testing because of chest pain syndromes; the remainder were tested for functional capacity evaluation or miscellaneous other reasons.

Abnormal responders were divided into "exercise only", "recovery only," and "abnormal in both exercise and recovery" as exclusive groups. In addition, "all abnormal" included those abnormal at any time (that is, all of the above), "abnormal in exercise" was defined as all tests that were abnormal during exercise (that is, "exercise only" plus "exercise and recovery") as if only the ECG

was monitored during exercise, and "abnormal in recovery" was defined as all tests that were abnormal in recovery (that is, "recovery only" plus "exercise and recovery") as if the ECG were monitored only during recovery. Our principle hypothesis was that the inclusion of ST-segment changes occurring during recovery improves diagnostic accuracy of the exercise test. This issue was addressed mainly by comparison of the "all abnormal" and "abnormal in exercise" groups.

Of the 271 patients, 107 had no coronary lesion of 75% or greater narrowing, 119 had one- or two-vessel disease, and 45 had left main or triple-vessel disease. The mean age of the total population was 59 years. Slightly more than half presented with typical angina pectoris. Overall, 21% were taking beta-blockers and 12% were taking digoxin. No significant differences were found

Table 6-3   Clinical and exercise variables in the Long Beach VAMC Study of the performance of temporal patterns of ST-segment depression for predicting angiographic coronary artery disease

	Normal responses (133 patients)	Abnormal responses					
		Exercise or recovery (138 patients)	Exercise without recovery considered (118 patients)	Recovery without exercise considered (122 patients)	Exercise and recovery (102 patients)	Exercise only (16 patients)	Recovery only (20 patients)
Age (years)	58 ± 9	61 ± 8	61 ± 8	61 ± 7	61 ± 7	62 ± 9	62 ± 7
Drugs used (%)							
Beta-blocker	19	23	22	24	23	19	30
Digoxin	14	10	12	10	12	13	0
Chest pain at presentation (%)							
Typical	42	61	63	62	63	56	50
Atypical	35	26	23	25	22	31	45
None or noncardiac	23	13	14	13	15	13	5
Chest pain during exercise (%)	21	53	53	52	53	56	50 ($p < 0.01$)
ST-segment depression (mm)							
Exercise	0.3 ± 0.7	2.1 ± 1.0	2.3 ± 0.9	2.2 ± 1.0	2.4 ± 1.0	1.7 ± 0.6	1.3 ± 0.8
Recovery	0.3 ± 0.6	1.9 ± 1.0	2.0 ± 1.0	2.1 ± 0.9	2.2 ± 0.9	0.7 ± 0.6	1.6 ± 0.6
Hemodynamic values							
METs	7 ± 3	7 ± 3	7 ± 3	7 ± 3	7 ± 3	8 ± 3	7 ± 3
Maximal heart rate (beats/min)	129 ± 24	129 ± 19	128 ± 18	129 + 18	128 + 17	132 + 22	135 ± 22
Maximal systolic blood pressure (mm Hg)	171 ± 30	167 ± 28	166 ± 28	167 ± 28	165 ± 28	167 ± 30	173 ± 27
Maximal double product (× 10^3)	22 ± 6	22 ± 5	21 ± 5	22 ± 5	21 ± 5	22 ± 6	24 ± 6
Cardiac catheterization values							
Vessels with ≥75% stenosis	1.5	1.7	1.7	1.8	1.8	1.0	1.5 ($p < 0.001$)
Ejection fraction (%)	67	66	66	65	65	72	67

between those with one- or two-vessel disease and those with three-vessel or left main disease; however, all parameters were significantly different between those with none and those with any disease. Table 6-3 describes the patterns of ST responses observed. Of the 271 patients, 138 (51%) patients had abnormal ST responses; 20 (7%) patients had abnormal ST-segment responses in recovery only, 16 (6%) had abnormal ST-segment responses during exercise only, and 102 (38%) had abnormal ST responses during both exercise and recovery.

As shown in Table 6-3, there are few meaningful differences in the clinical features associated with the five patterns of ST depression. Those with a normal response were the youngest. As expected, angina during the test was significantly more common in those with ST depression than in those without, but over half of the patients with ST depression exhibited silent ischemia. Differences in maximal ST depression during and after exercise were consistent with the criteria for each group. In the "recovery only" group, the mean value for ST depression during exercise was 1.3 mm, but the slopes were upward in those with 1 mm or more depression, and none were abnormal by standard criteria during exercise.

There was a tendency toward higher mean hemodynamic parameters in individuals with abnormal ST depression in exercise only. These values generally reflect a greater exercise capacity and were even higher than those obtained in patients with a normal exercise response. The number of vessels diseased was significantly lower for both those with a normal response and for those abnormal during exercise only. Patients with an abnormal ST response in "recovery only" had the highest maximal heart rate, systolic pressure, and double product despite the lowest exercise capacity. These findings support the conclusion that "recovery only" changes are not associated with submaximal effort but are associated with exercise intolerance from other factors such as poor physical conditioning.

Table 6-4 lists the performance of the temporal patterns of ST depression for predicting any coronary disease or left main/three-vessel coronary disease. As would be expected, the sensitivities become low for patterns that do not occur frequently. For comparison between patterns, the predictive value is the most important to consider because it is the percentage of all patients with the pattern who have disease. All the patterns have comparable predictive values, demonstrating that none is more likely to be associated with false-positive responses. The "exercise only" group had a higher predictive value for any disease and a lower predictive value for left main/three-vessel disease consistent with the smaller mean vessel score and higher hemodynamic parameters found in this group. When one compares "all abnormals" to "abnormal in exercise," the sensitivity was significantly greater in the former group without a change in predictive value.

Table 6-4   Sensitivity, specificity, and positive predictive value for temporal patterns of exercise-induced ST-segment depression in patients with any coronary artery disease or three-vessel and left main coronary artery or disease

Abnormal responses	Any significant coronary disease			Three-vessel or left main artery disease		
	Sensitivity	Specificity	Predictive value (95% confidence interval)	Sensitivity	Specificity	Predictive value (95% confidence interval)
Exercise or recovery (138 patients)	67	74	80 (73-86)	80	55	26 (19-33)
Exercise without recovery considered (118 patients)	57	77	79 (71-86)	73	62	28 (20-36)
Recovery without exercise considered (122 patients)	61	79	82 (75-89)	73	61	27 (19-35)
Exercise and recovery (102 patients)	51	82	81 (74-89)	67	68	29 (21-38)
Exercise only (16 patients)	6	94	63 (35-85)	6	94	19 (4-46)
Recovery only (20 patients)	10	97	85 (62-97)	6	94	15 (3-38)

Other studies evaluating "recovery only" changes. Several previous studies have considered ST-segment changes occurring in recovery only. The Program of Surgical Control of Hyperlipidemia (POSCH) data set was used for one such analysis as baseline evaluation included both treadmill exercise testing and coronary angiography. Karnegis and co-workers investigated hemodynamic, angiographic, and electrocardiographic variables in subjects whose diagnostic ECG changes appeared during exercise rather than during recovery.[62] Subjects were 30 to 64 years of age when entered, had one prior myocardial infarction, and had a serum cholesterol of at least 220 mg%. Out of 838 subjects enrolled in POSCH, the exercise test response was abnormal in 328 (39%). Of these abnormals, the test result was abnormal during exercise in 94% and during recovery in 6%. The authors concluded that the same clinical significance should be attributed to abnormal ST responses that occur during recovery and that electrocardiographic, hemodynamic, and cardiac catheterization variables do not distinguish between subjects who exhibit these two different temporal responses.

Savage et al[63] evaluated 2000 exercise tests and identified 62 patients (3.2%) who developed 1 mm or more horizontal or downsloping ST-segment depression in the recovery period despite a normal ST response during exercise. This report gave information only about the 62 patients with "recovery only" responses. They were largely male (39 out of 62) with a mean age of 58 years. Coronary artery disease was confirmed angiographically in 26 patients. The authors concluded that isolated postexercise ST-segment depression was usually associated with coronary artery disease often indicated multivessel disease and that men were more likely to have abnormal thallium scan results.

Froelicher and co-workers considered patterns of ST-segment depression in two groups of asymptomatic men undergoing screening exercise testing: one group who underwent coronary angiography and the other who were followed for 5 years for cardiac events.[64] Maximal treadmill testing was performed with only one bipolar CC_5 lead monitored with patients supine after exercise. ST interpretation was the same as in the current study. As is shown in Table 6-5, "recovery only" ST-segment depression had a similar predictive value as other patterns.

Ellestad commented on patients who do not have ST-segment depression with or immediately after exercise but who develop changes 3 to 8 minutes later.[65] In a follow-up study of 308 subjects he found this response to be a definite but weak predictor of subsequent coronary events. He contrasts them with a normal group who have ST-segment depression at rest, return to normal with exercise, and again develop ST-segment depression late in recovery.

Abnormal ST-segment depression occurring only in recovery provides clinically useful information and is not more likely to represent a false-positive response. When considered together with changes in exercise, changes in recovery increase the sensitivity of the exercise test without a decline in predictive value. A cool-down walk should be avoided after exercise testing, and one should consider recovery ST measurements in exercise test scores and nuclear testing. Avoidance of a cool-down walk has not resulted in an increased complication rate.

R-wave adjustment. The degree of exercise-induced ST-segment depression can be influenced by R-wave amplitude and perhaps should be normalized to a standard voltage. The average "gain factor" correction of R-wave amplitude should be approximately 25 mm (that is, average R-wave

Table 6-5 Analysis of the predictive value of various patterns of ST depression from screening asymptomatic aircrewmen. Recovery-only ST-segment depression had a predictive value similar to that of other patterns

ST depression occurrence time	140 men with abnormal treadmill response in a follow-up study			111 men with abnormal treadmill response in an angiographic study	
	Occurrence rate (%)	Risk ratio*	Predictive value (%)	Occurrence rate (%)	Predictive value (%)
Exercise only	9	7	23	11	8
Recovery only	36	4	12	42	28
Exercise and recovery	55	12	25	47	39
All abnormal responders	100	14	20	100	30

*Relative risk for cardiac events during follow-up observation compared to that for normal subjects.

voltage in V_5). In the studies by Hollenberg and co-workers the magnitude of ST-segment depression was calibrated to a standard R-wave amplitude of 12 mm in lead V_5 and 8 mm in lead aV_F.[66] Hakki and co-workers determined the influence of exercise R-wave amplitude on ST-segment depression in 81 patients with coronary disease.[67] Exercise thallium scintigraphy increased the sensitivity of the test in patients with low R-wave amplitude. We have not found R-wave adjustment to improve the diagnostic performance of the exercise test.

Exercise-induced ST-segment depression not attributable to coronary artery disease. Table 6-6 lists some of the conditions that can possibly result in false-positive responses. Simonson has suggested that in a population with a high prevalence of heart disease other than coronary artery disease, an abnormal exercise test would be as diagnostic for that disease as it would be for coronary artery disease in populations with a high prevalence of coronary artery disease. Digitalis and other drugs can cause exercise-induced repolarization abnormalities in normal individuals. Patients who have had abnormal responses and who have anemia, electrolyte abnormalities, or are taking medications should be retested when these conditions are altered. Meals and even glucose ingestion can alter the ST-segment and T-wave in the resting ECG and can potentially cause a false-positive response. To avoid this problem, all electrocardiographic studies should be performed after at least a 4-hour fast. This requirement is also important because of the hemodynamic stress put on the cardiovascular system by eating. After eating, functional capacity is decreased and angina occurs sooner.

WOMEN. Gender has an effect on the exercise ECG that is not explained by hormones alone. Estrogen given to men does not increase the rate of false-positive responses. Bruce has suggested that the lower specificity of exercise-induced ST-segment depression in women is attributable to hemodynamic or hemoglobin concentration differences. Table 6-7 summarizes the studies that were evaluations of the exercise ECG in women.[68]

Robert and co-workers assessed whether the diagnostic value of exercise testing could be enhanced in women by using multivariate analysis of exercise data.[69] Between 1978 and 1984, 135 infarct-free women underwent exercise testing and coronary angiography in Brussels. Significant coronary artery disease was present in 41% of the patients. In this first group, maximal exercise variables were submitted to a stepwise logistic analysis. Work load, heart rate, and ST60 in lead X were selected to build a diagnostic model. The model was tested in a second group of 115 catheterized women (significant coronary artery disease in 47%) and of 76 volunteers. They compared their model with conventional analysis of the exercise electrocardiogram, with ST changes adjusted for heart rate, and with a previously described analysis. In both groups, sensitivity was better with the present model (66% and 70%) than by conventional analysis (68% and 59%) and by the previously described analysis (57% and 44%) without a loss of specificity (85% and 93%). Receiver-operator characteristic curves showed also a better diagnostic accuracy with the

Table 6-6 Some conditions that can result in false-positive responses

Valvular heart disease	Left ventricular hypertrophy
Congenital heart disease	Wolff-Parkinson-White syndrome
Cardiomyopathies	
Pericardial disorders	Preexcitation variants
Drug administration	Mitral valve prolapse syndrome
Electrolyte abnormalities	
Nonfasting state	Vasoregulatory abnormality
Anemia	
Sudden excessive exercise	Hyperventilation repolarization abnormalities
Inadequate recording equipment	Hypertension
Bundle branch block	Excessive double product
Improper interpretation	Improper lead systems
	Incorrect criteria

Table 6-7 Results of some major diagnostic exercise testing studies performed in women

Principal investigator	Year	Number	Sensitivity (%)	Specificity (%)
Caru	1978	168	73	74
Cahen	1978	100	88	92
Sketch	1975	56	50	78
Detry	1977	45	89	63
Linhart	1974	98	71	78
Lesbre	1978	150	66	77
Broustet	1978	84	50	70
Barolsky	1979	92	60	68
Weiner	1979	580	76	64
Val	1982	112	79	66
Manca	1979	508	88	73
Bengtsson	1981	194	—	85

The last two conducted follow-up studies, whereas the others used angiography.

present model. They concluded that in women, logistic analysis of exercise variables improves the diagnostic value of exercise testing. It yields a significantly better sensitivity without a loss of specificity.

DIGOXIN. Sundqvist and co-workers studied the effect of digoxin on the electrocardiogram at rest and during and after exercise in 11 healthy subjects.[70] Exercise was performed on a heart rate–controlled bicycle ergometer with stepwise increased loads up to a heart rate of 170 beats/min. The subjects were studied after digoxin at 2 dose levels and after withdrawal of digoxin. Administration of digoxin induced significant ST-T depression at rest and during exercise even at the small dose. The ST-T changes were numerically small and dose dependent. There was usually junctional depression and no downsloping, but six individuals had as much as a millimeter of ST-segment depression. The most pronounced ST-segment depression occurred at a heart rate of 110 to 130 beats/min. At higher heart rates the ST depression was less pronounced but still statistically significant. During the first minutes after exercise no significant digitalis-induced ST T depression was seen. This type of reaction is not usually seen in myocardial ischemia. Fourteen days after withdrawal of the drug there were no significant digitalis-induced ST-T changes.

LEFT BUNDLE BRANCH BLOCK. Whinnery and associates reported 31 asymptomatic men who serially developed left bundle branch block and who were studied with both maximal treadmill testing and coronary angiography.[71] They demonstrated that there can be a pronounced degree of exercise-induced ST-segment depression in addition to that found at rest in healthy men with left bundle branch block. No difference was found between the ST-segment response to exercise in those with or those without significant coronary artery disease. Thus the ST-segment response to exercise testing cannot be used to make diagnostic decisions on patients with left bundle branch block.

RIGHT BUNDLE BRANCH BLOCK. Whinnery and associates also reported the response to maximal treadmill testing 40 asymptomatic men with acquired right bundle branch block.[72] There was no exercise-induced ST-segment depression in the inferior and lateral leads. Exercise-induced ST-segment depression in the anterior precordial leads is frequently noted in patients with right bundle branch block. This is most apparent in the right precordial leads with an rSR or a notched R-wave; these leads often show a downsloping ST-segment at rest, and such a finding is thus not indicative of myocardial ischemia. Figure 6-6 shows ST-segment depression in lateral leads in patients with angina, and Figure 6-7 shows no ST-segment depression in lateral leads in a patient without coronary heart disease, both with ST depression anteriorly.

Vasey reviewed the records of 2584 consecutive patients who underwent both treadmill testing and coronary angiography to determine the relation between exercise-induced acceleration-dependent left bundle branch block (LBBB) and the presence of coronary artery disease (CAD).[73] Rate-dependent LBBB during exercise was identified in 28 patients (1.1%), who were categorized according to their presenting symptoms: classic angina pectoris, atypical chest pain, symptomatic arrhythmias, and asymptomatic. Asymptomatic individuals were being screened for silent CAD. CAD was present in 7 of 10 patients who presented with classic angina pectoris, but 12 of 13 patients presenting with atypical chest pain had normal coronary arteries. All 10 patients in whom LBBB developed at a heart rate of 125 beats/min or higher were free of CAD, whereas 9 of 18 patients in whom LBBB developed at a heart rate of less than 125 beats/min had CAD. Normal coronary arteries were present in 3 patients who presented with angina and in whom both chest pain and LBBB developed during exercise. They concluded that (1) patients who presented with atypical chest pain and have rate-dependent LBBB are significantly less likely to have CAD than patients who presented with classic angina; (2) the onset of LBBB at a heart rate of 125 beats/min or higher is highly correlated with the presence of normal coronary arteries, regardless of patient presentation; and (3) patients with angina in whom both chest pain and LBBB develop during exercise may have normal coronary arteries.

OTHER CAUSES. Individuals with the left ventricular hypertrophy and strain pattern on their resting ECG are at high risk for coronary artery disease. Healthy individuals with the Wolff-Parkinson-White syndrome can have exercise-induced ST-segment depression. Some individuals with preexcitation, a short PR interval, and a normal QRS complex may have a false-positive exercise test. A group of patients with the prolapsing mitral valve syndrome were reported to have abnormal exercise tests but normal coronary angiograms. In individuals with this syndrome false-positive responses are apparently more common, occurring in approximately 25%.

Sapin and co-workers postulated that exaggerated atrial repolarization waves during exercise could produce ST-segment depression mimicking myocardial ischemia.[74] The P-waves, PR-seg-

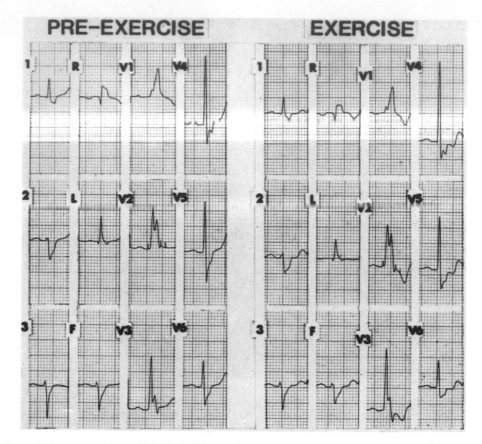

Figure 6-6   Example of exercise-induced ST depression in lateral leads in patient with right bundle branch block with coronary artery disease and ischemia.

ments and ST-segments were studied in leads II, III, aV$_F$, and V$_4$ to V$_6$ in 69 patients whose exercise ECG was suggestive of ischemia (100 µV horizontal or 150 µV upsloping ST-segment depression 80 msec after the J-point). All had a normal ECG at rest. The exercise test in 25 patients (52% male, mean age 53 years) were false positive based on normal coronary arteriograms and left ventricular function (5 patients) or normal-stress single-photon emission computed tomographic thallium or gated blood pool scans (16 patients), or both test results (4 patients). Forty-four patients with a similar age and sex distribution, anginal chest pain, and at least one coronary stenosis ≥80% served as a true-positive control group. The false-positive group was characterized by (1) sharply downsloping PR segments at peak exercise, (2) longer exercise time and more rapid peak exercise heart rate than those of the true positive group, and (3) absence of exercise-induced chest pain. The false-positive group also displayed significantly greater absolute P-wave amplitudes at peak exercise and greater augmentation

of P-wave amplitude by exercise in all six ECG leads than were observed in the true-positive group. Multivariable analysis revealed that exercise duration and downsloping PR segments in the inferior ECG leads were independent predictors of a false-positive test. The combination of downsloping PR-segments in two of three inferior leads and either exercise duration of ≥4 minutes or peak heart rate of ≥125 beats/min allowed identification of false-positive tests with a sensitivity of 84% and a specificity over 85%.

Individuals with vasoregulatory asthenia and orthostatic or vasoregulatory abnormalities can have abnormal exercise-induced ST-segment changes without coronary artery disease. The same can be said for those with hyperventilation repolarization changes before treadmill testing, or these maneuvers can be reserved only for patients who have an abnormal response. Such changes are unusual and have rarely been responsible for false-positive tests. Orthostatic and hyperventilation changes have been associated with the mitral valve prolapse syndrome. When they do occur with

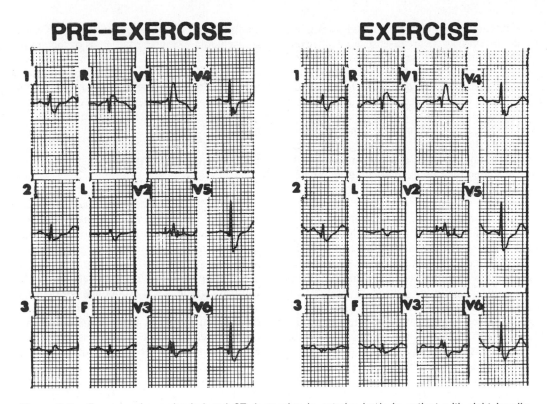

PRE-EXERCISE   **EXERCISE**

Figure 6-7   Example of exercise-induced ST depression in anterior leads in patient with right bundle branch block without evidence for ischemia.

exercise-induced changes, the interpretation of ischemia should be avoided and the clinician must rely on other parameters to make a diagnosis.

Persons with hypertension or an excessive double product (SBP × HR) during exercise could hypothetically have a physiologic imbalance between myocardial oxygen supply and demand. An excessive number of false-positive responses was were not found, however, in one reported population of mild hypertensives. Barnard and co-workers demonstrated that a sudden strenuous work load of treadmill exercise can yield ST-segment depression in healthy individuals on this basis.[75] Foster and associates could not reproduce the ST-segment depression with sudden strenuous bicycle exercise even though the ejection fraction dropped in their normal subjects.[76] A recorder with an inadequate frequency response can either artifactually induce ST-segment depression in normal subjects or show upsloping depression when horizontal depression is actually present. Use of the proper equipment should avoid this type of distortion. In conclusion, the conditions discussed above can be avoided and should not be the major causes of false-positive responses in a good exercise testing laboratory. The most common cause of a false-positive test should be the normal variant in a patient who has a physiological ST-segment vector that is similar to that produced by ischemia.

ST-segment shift location and ischemia. Many clinicians use the ST-segment shifts observed in different leads to infer that there was ischemia in the underlying areas of myocardium. Validating the localization of ischemia with coronary angiography has several limitations. First, collaterals may adequately perfuse areas of the heart served by an obstructed artery. Second, coronary angiography cannot quantify the degree to which an infarcted area of the heart remains ischemic. Finally, the validity of relating anatomic lesions visualized at rest to exercise-induced changes in the electrocardiogram so that only ischemia is inferred is questionable. These limitations partially explain the difficulty correlating electrocardiographic alterations with the specific number or location of coronary angiographic obstructions. With the advent of coronary artery bypass surgery, precise localization of critical ischemia has assumed more than academic interest. Localization could help to direct surgical intervention to the site of jeopardized myocardium or the source of angina pectoris.

Abouantoun and co-workers studied 54 patients with stable coronary heart disease all with exercise-induced thallium scintigraphic defects.[77] Their exercise ECG test results were compared to their thallium images and also to 14 low risk normal subjects. They analyzed exercise data for spatial ST vector shifts using a computer program to classify ST-segment depression and elevation most accurately. None of the scintigraphic ischemic sites or angiographic diseased areas could be specifically identified by exercise-induced ST vector shifts.

Fuchs and colleagues evaluated the 12-lead ECG for localizing the site of coronary artery disease in 134 patients with angiographically documented single-vessel coronary disease.[78] They reviewed 10 years of cardiac catheterization at Johns Hopkins Hospital to select these patients who had ECGs recorded during myocardial infarction, spontaneous rest angina, or treadmill exercise. Q-wave location allowed one to identify correctly the location of the coronary lesion in 98% of the cases, ST elevation in 91%, T-wave inversion in 84%, and ST depression in only 60%. No response could separate right from left circumflex coronary artery disease. ST-segment elevation was recorded in 20 of the 56 patients who underwent exercise testing. All 56 had angina during the test. An association was found only between elevation in limb lead III and right coronary artery disease.

Simoons and co-workers[35] studied the exercise-induced spatial ST vector shifts 30 and 80 msec after QRS end in 34 patients who had coronary angiography and thallium exercise scans because of clinically important chest pain. The electrocardiogram was normal at rest in 30. Twenty-two had significant coronary artery obstructions, and 12 had normal angiograms. Four of these "normals" (33%) had abnormal exercise tests as well as chest pain. They found that in patients with exercise thallium ischemia defects, the ST vectors were posteriorly oriented in 15 of 22 and anteriorly oriented in 9 of 12 of those without ischemia defects. However, they could find no systematic difference in the ST-vector direction of patients with anteroseptal compared to patients with posterolateral perfusion defects. These studies have been corroborated by the excellent angiographic study by Mark and co-workers from Duke.[40]

Localized transmural ischemia results in generalized subendocardial ischemia, which slows electrical conduction, changing the action potentials, as is seen in myocardial infarction. The ST-segment changes registered during exercise are partially dependent on the location of scar tissue. ST-segment elevation or depression, or various combinations of ST-segment shifts, do not localize ischemia to myocardial areas or the arteries inferred by these areas. For example, ST-segment depression in leads II and aV_F do not necessarily mean that there is inferior ischemia (or right coronary artery disease) nor does depression in V_5 mean that there is lateral ischemia (or left coronary artery disease).

SUBJECTIVE RESPONSES

Careful observation of the patient's appearance is necessary for the safe performance of an exercise test and is helpful in the clinical assessment of a patient. Patients who exaggerate their limitations or symptoms and those unwilling to cooperate are usually easy to identify. A drop in skin temperature during exercise can indicate an inadequate cardiac output with secondary vasoconstriction and can be an indication for not encouraging a patient to a higher work load. Neurological manifestations such as light-headedness or vertigo can also be indications of an inadequate cardiac output.

Findings on physical examination can be helpful, but their sensitivity and specificity have not been demonstrated. Gallop sounds, a mitral regurgitant murmur, or a precordial bulge could be attributable to left ventricular dysfunction. An S_3 can sometimes be heard in normals after exercise, but a new S_4 brought out by exercise has been said to be specific for coronary heart disease. The physical findings of congestive heart failure, including rales and neck vein distension, should be encountered rarely in patients referred for exercise testing. However, some exercise testing laboratories use the sitting position for the recovery period to avoid problems with the patient who develops orthopnea. It is preferable to have patients lie supine after exercise testing and allow those who develop orthopnea to sit up. Also, severe angina or ominous dysrhythmias after exercise can be lessened by allowing the patient to sit up. Attempts to make the findings of the physical examination less subjective include the use of phonocardiography, apexcardiography, and cardiokymography. Left ventricular ejection time can be determined by the ear densitigram and its first derivative more easily than by trying to obtain a carotid pulse tracing.

Chest pain

Weiner and co-workers reported 281 consecutive patients studied with treadmill testing and coronary angiography with the following responses: (1) 76 patients with ST-segment depression and treadmill test–induced chest pain, (2) 85 patients with ST-segment depression and no chest pain, (3) 40 patients with treadmill test induced–chest pain who had no ST-segment changes, and (4) 80 patients with neither chest pain nor ST-segment changes. They found that 91% of the first group, 65% of the second group, 72% of the third group, and only 35% of the fourth group had significant angiographically determined coronary artery disease.[79] Cole and Ellestad followed 95 patients with abnormal treadmill tests.[80] At 5-year of follow-up observation the incidence of coronary artery disease was 73% in those with both chest pain and an abnormal ST-segment response compared with 43% in those who only had an abnormal ST-segment response. Mortality was also twice as high in those with both ST-segment changes and chest pain induced by the treadmill test. The results of these studies indicate that ischemic chest pain induced by the exercise test may be predictive of the presence of coronary artery disease as well as ST-segment depression, and when they occur together, they are even more predictive of coronary artery disease than either is alone. It is important, though, that a careful description of the pain be obtained from the patient to ascertain that it is typical rather than atypical angina.

OBSERVER AGREEMENT IN INTERPRETATION

The complexity of not only the human body but also the human mind has created, in medicine, measurements that when applied to medical diagnosis lead to observations with great variability, that is, ST-segment displacement. The inherent subjective nature of these medical observations require questioning of the results of most diagnostic methods, not only in regard to accuracy or validity, but also in agreement (among different interpreters for a given test). Attempts at describing or assessing agreement have been complex and variable as evidenced in the literature by the numerous terms used: agreement, variability, consistency, within-observer correlation coefficients of disagreement, and many others. Agreement has two subgroupings: intraobserver, referring to agreement of the individual observer with himself on two separate occasions, and interobserver, referring to agreement among two or more persons.

Blackburn had 14 observers (from seven separate institutions) interpret 38 individual exercise electrocardiographic tests as to normal, abnormal, or borderline.[81] Five readers repeated the readings. In only nine of the 38 (24%) exercise ECGs was there complete agreement among the 14 readers, and only 22 ECGs (58%) were read in agreement. This low value may be attributed to the fact that Blackburn's study did not allow a dichotomous decision because there was the third interpretation of borderline. In terms of intraobserver agreement there was a wide range from 58% to 92% and an average still less than ours for a dichotomous decision. Blackburn attributed this wide variation in both intraobserver and interobserver agreement to (1) the absence of defined criteria, (2) technical problems such as noise, and (3) differences in opinion as to ST-segment upsloping. Strict criteria such as the Minnesota code and computer analysis have been recommended as a means to increase agreement in electrocardiography.

REPRODUCIBILITY OF TREADMILL TEST RESPONSES

Sullivan and co-workers studied 14 male patients with exercise test–induced angina and ST-segment depression with treadmill testing on three consecutive days to evaluate the reproducibility of certain treadmill variables.[82] Computerized ST-segment analysis and expired gas analysis, including anaerobic threshold, were evaluated for reproducibility using an intraclass correlation coefficient analysis (ICC). The ICC is a generalization of the Pearson product-moment correlation, which is not affected by the addition or multiplication of a given number of observations and provides a better indication of reproducibility than the coefficient of variation does. Oxygen uptake had a higher reliability coefficient ($r = 0.88$) and a smaller 90% confidence interval when compared to treadmill time ($r = 0.70$) consistent with a better correlation. The double product and heart rate were highly reproducible ($r = 0.90$ and 0.94 respectively). In addition, the 90% confidence interval for both double product and heart rate was small. The ST60 displacement in lead X and the lead of greatest displacement were very reproducible ($r = 0.83$).

Measured oxygen uptake displayed better reproducibility than treadmill time at peak exercise, the onset of angina, and the gas exchange anaerobic threshold. The double product, heart rate, and ST-segment displacement in lead X were found to be reproducible at peak exercise, the onset of angina, and the anaerobic-threshold gas exchange. Gas-exchange analysis provided accurate physiological determinants of exercise capacity in patients with angina pectoris. Noninvasive estimates of myocardial oxygen demand and ischemia were reproducibly determined. These findings are summarized in Table 6-8.

Table 6-8   Mean ± standard deviation of exercise test variables at maximal angina limited exercise

Variable	Mean and standard deviation			ANOVA $p < 0.05^*$	Intraclass correlation coefficient	
	Day 1	Day 2	Day 3		r	90% confidence interval
Time (sec)	503 ±72	516 ±85	526 ±66	0.35	0.70	0.48-0.86
VO₂ (L/min)	1.559 ±0.289	1.553 ±0.334	1.557 ±0.294	0.99	0.88	0.76-0.95
Double product × 10^3	18.9	19.6	18.9			
Heart rate (beats/min)	111 ±19	112 ±20	110 ±17	0.66	0.94	0.88-0.97
ST60 X (mV)	−0.14 ±0.11	−0.14 ±0.10	−0.14 ±0.10	0.99	0.83	0.63-0.92
ST60GD (mV)	−0.19 ±0.08	−0.17 ±0.11	−0.20 ±0.09	0.17	0.82	0.60-0.92

ANOVA, Analysis of variance model to determine time trends; *GD*, lead of greatest ST-segment depression; *ST60*, ST-segment depression 60 msec after QRS end; *VO₂*, volume of oxygen; *X*, lead X.
$P < 0.05$ would indicate a significant change over the three testing periods.

INTERPRETATION OF EXERCISE TEST–INDUCED PREMATURE VENTRICULAR CONTRACTIONS

Exercise-induced supraventricular dysrhythmias are unusual and have not been related to coronary artery disease. Of major concern are exercise-induced premature ventricular contractions. Premature ventricular contractions occur in approximately one third of asymptomatic men who perform a maximal treadmill test, and their prevalence is directly related to age. Premature ventricular contractions occur most frequently at maximal exercise and often are not reproducible on repeat testing. A subgroup of healthy men (approximately 2%) will have severe exercise-induced ventricular dysrhythmias. This group will have three times the normal risk of developing coronary artery disease, but only about 10% of them will actually do so. Only 7% of those who develop coronary artery disease will have had so-called ominous ventricular dysrhythmias, and their premature ventricular contractions often occur at lower heart rates than they do in healthy subjects.

Busby and co-workers studied 1160 subjects 21 to 96 years of age who underwent maximal exercise treadmill testing an average of 2.4 times.[83] Eighty (6.9%) developed frequent (≥10% of beats in any 1 minute) or repetitive (≥3 beats in a row) ventricular ectopic beats on at least one test. These 80 individuals were significantly older than the group without such arrhythmia (63.8 ± 12.5 versus 50.0 ± 16.1 years; $p < 0.001$). A striking age-related increase in the prevalence of frequent or repetitive exercise-induced ventricular ectopic beats was seen in men ($p < 0.0001$) but not in women. The prevalence of electrocardiographic abnormalities at rest, exercise-induced ST-segment depression, thallium perfusion defects, duration of treadmill exercise, maximal heart rate, systolic blood pressure, and rate-pressure product did not differ between these 80 study subjects with frequent exercise-induced ventricular ectopic beats and a control group matched for age and sex. Furthermore, the incidence of cardiac events (angina pectoris, nonfatal myocardial infarction, cardiac syncope, or cardiac death) (10% versus 12.5%) as well as noncardiac mortality (each 7.5%) was found to be similar for the study and control groups, respectively, over a mean follow-up period of 5.6 years. No study subjects required antiarrhythmic drugs over this time interval. Thus frequent or repetitive exercise-induced ventricular ectopic beats in these predominantly older, asymptomatic individuals without apparent heart disease are not predictive of increased cardiac morbidity or mortality and therefore do not require specific therapy.

Dysrhythmias suppressed by acute exercise do not rule out the presence of coronary artery disease. Ambulatory monitoring and isometric exercise can allow identification of premature ventricular contractions in more people than dynamic exercise testing can. The demonstration of the prognostic significance of exercise-induced ventricular dysrhythmias in coronary artery disease and the value of medical suppression will require careful follow-up studies. In addition, the total information from an exercise test may be more helpful in patient management and more cost effective than ambulatory monitoring.

In general, exercise-induced arrhythmias must be interpreted in relation to the medical condition of the individuals in whom they occur (that is, the company they keep). Exercise-induced ST-segment depression is related to subendocardial ischemia and is less arrhythmogenic than ST-segment elevation (not over Q-waves), which is associated with transmural ischemia. As pointed out by McHenry, the presence of premature ventricular contractions on the resting ECG should be used to classify patients as to their exercise response.[58] The methods of recording and capturing premature ventricular contractions greatly affects the prevalence data.

Prognostic studies

Sami and co-workers performed a retrospective study to examine the prognostic significance of exercise-induced ventricular arrhythmia in patients with stable coronary artery disease (CAD) who were included in the multicenter patient registry of the Coronary Artery Surgery Study.[84] The population included 1486 patients selected from 1975 to 1979 and followed an average of 4.3 years. All underwent a standard Bruce exercise test and had CAD by cardiac catheterization at entry. Patients were classified depending on whether they had minimal or significant CAD. They were further subclassified depending on whether they had exercise-induced ventricular arrhythmia (EIVA). Patients with minimal CAD and EIVA (16 patients) and 229 patients without those conditions had similar clinical and angiographic characteristics except for the average ejection fraction (EF), which was 50% for those with and 64% for those without premature ventricular contractions. One hundred thirty patients with significant CAD and EIVA had a higher prevalence of previous myocardial infarction, a lower mean EF, and a higher proportion with at least two coronary arteries significantly narrowed than those without EIVAs and significant CAD (1111 patients). The 5-year event-free survival was not influenced by the presence of EIVA; it was 76% and 88% in those with minimal CAD or with EIVA respectively and 71% and 76% in both groups with significant CAD, respectively. With use of a stepwise Cox regression analysis of selected clinical and angiographic risk factors, the only independent significant risk factors that were found for cardiac events were the number of coronary arteries diseased and the ejection fraction.

Califf and co-workers at Duke studied the prognostic information provided by ventricular ar-

rhythmias associated with treadmill testing in 1293 consecutive nonsurgically treated patients undergoing an exercise test within 6 weeks of cardiac catheterization.[85] The 236 patients with simple ventricular arrhythmias (at least one premature ventricular contraction, but without paired complexes or ventricular tachycardia) had a higher prevalence of significant CAD (57% versus 44%), three-vessel disease (31% versus 17%), and abnormal left ventricular function (43% versus 24%) than patients without ventricular arrhythmias had. Patients with paired complexes or ventricular tachycardia had an even higher prevalence of significant coronary artery disease (75%), three-vessel disease (39%), and abnormal left ventricular function (54%).

In the 620 patients with significant CAD, patients with paired complexes or ventricular tachycardia had a lower 3-year survival rate (75%) than patients with simple ventricular arrhythmias (83%) and patients with no ventricular arrhythmias (90%) had. Ventricular arrhythmias were found to add independent prognostic information to the noninvasive evaluation, including history, physical examination, chest x-ray film, ECG, and other exercise test variables ($p = 0.03$). Ventricular arrhythmias made no independent contribution once the cardiac catheterization data were known. In patients without significant coronary artery disease, no relation between ventricular arrhythmias and survival was found.

Weiner and co-workers investigated the determinants and prognostic significance of ventricular arrhythmias during exercise testing.[86] Eighty-six patients with such arrhythmias were identified from a consecutive series of 446 patients who underwent treadmill testing and cardiac catheterization. The prevalence of these arrhythmias was 19% in the total group but increased to 30% in the 120 patients with three-vessel or left main CAD. Patients with exercise-induced arrhythmias were more likely to have three-vessel or left main CAD, a lower resting ejection fraction, 0.2 mV of ST-segment depression, and more severe segmental wall-motion abnormalities than patients without this finding. Repeat exercise testing in 22 patients with exercise-induced arrhythmias after coronary artery bypass surgery revealed that persistence of these arrhythmias was associated with either severe wall-motion abnormalities preoperatively or residual ST-segment depression during the postoperative exercise testing. At a mean follow-up period of 5.3 years the presence of exercise-induced ventricular arrhythmias was not associated with increased cardiac mortality in the medically treated patients.

Marieb and co-workers analyzed the significance of exercise-induced ventricular arrhythmias in 383 patients who had undergone both exercise thallium exercise testing and cardiac catheterization.[87] Two hundred twenty-one patients (58%) had no EIVAs whereas 162 (42%) did. There was no difference between patients with and without EIVAs in terms of previous myocardial infarction, prevalence of fixed thallium-201 defects, number of diseased vessels, and resting ejection fraction. In contrast, evidence of provocable ischemia (redistribution on thallium-201 and ST-segment depression on the electrocardiogram) were more likely to be seen in patients with EIVAs. Discriminant function analysis revealed that these two variables best separated patients with and without EIVA. In a 4- to 8-year follow-up observation, 89 patients had adverse cardiac events. Of these 89, there were 41 deaths, 9 nonfatal myocardial infarctions, and 39 coronary revascularization procedures performed later than 3 months after catheterization. Patients with EIVAs were more likely to have these events than those without. These arrhythmias provided independent prognostic information beyond that provided by the thallium-201 stress test and coronary angiography. These studies are summarized in Table 6-9.

Exercise testing to evaluate ST depression during supraventricular tachycardia

Petsas and co-workers studied 16 patients who had manifested ST-segment depression during episodes of paroxysmal supraventricular tachycardia (PSVT) with exercise testing in order to detect coronary artery disease.[88] No ST-segment depression was observed during exercise testing in 15 of the 16 patients tested. Paroxysms of supraventricular tachycardia associated with ST-segment depression occurred during exercise testing in three cases. The ST-segment depression was immediately apparent, remained constant throughout the supraventricular tachycardia, and was almost instantly abolished after conversion to sinus rhythm. Patients with heart rates greater than 250 beats/min during PSVT had pronounced ST-segment depression associated with the tachycardia. These results are suggestive that coronary artery disease and myocardial ischemia are not involved in the genesis of ST-segment depression during PSVT. Tachycardia itself may be the cause of ST-segment depression by altering the slope of phase 2 of the ventricular action potential. Retrograde atrial activation may also induce ST-segment shifts in some of the cases.

Ventricular tachycardia during exercise testing

Fleg and Lakatta studied the prevalence of ventricular tachycardia (VT) associated with maximal treadmill exercise in 597 male and 325 female volunteers 21 to 96 years of age from the Baltimore Longitudinal Study on Aging who were without apparent heart disease.[89] Ten subjects, 7 men and 3 women, with exercise-induced VT were identified, representing 1.1% of those tested; only 1 was younger than 65 years. All episodes of VT were asymptomatic and nonsustained. In 9 of 10 subjects, VT developed at or near peak exercise. The longest run of VT was 56 beats; multiple runs of VT were present in 4 subjects. Two subjects had exercise-induced ST-segment depression, but subsequent exercise thallium results were normal in each. Compared with a group of age- and sex-matched control subjects, those with asymptomatic, nonsustained VT displayed no difference in exercise duration, maximal heart rate, or the prevalence of coronary risk factors of exercise-induced ischemia as measured by the ECG and thallium scintigraphy. Over a mean follow-up period of 2 years, no subject developed symptoms of heart disease or experienced syncope or sudden death. Exercise-induced VT in apparently healthy subjects occurred mainly in the elderly, was limited to short, asymptomatic runs of 3 to 6 beats usually near peak exercise, and did not predict increased cardiovascular morbidity or mortality over a 2-year follow-up period.

Long Beach VAMC study. On a retrospective re-

Table 6-9 Four major studies evaluating the prognostic value of exercise-induced ventricular arrhythmias in patients with coronary artery disease

Study	Number	Follow-up (years)	Mortality	
			With EIVA (%)	Without EIVA (%)
Nair	280	3.9	No difference	
Weiner	446	5.3	14 (any)	10
			20 (complex)	
Califf	1293	3	17 (simple)	10
			25 (complex)	
Sami	1486	4.3	29 (any)	24

view of 3351 patients who had undergone routine clinical exercise testing between September 1984 and June 1989, we identified 55 patients with exercise-induced ventricular tachycardia[90] (Figure 6-8). The mean follow-up period was 26 months (range 2 to 58 months). Fifty patients had nonsustained ventricular tachycardia during exercise testing, and one of these patients died because of congestive heart failure during the follow-up period. Five patients had sustained ventricular tachycardia during exercise testing, and one died suddenly 7 months after the test. Ventricular tachycardia was reproduced in only two of the 29 patients who underwent repeat exercise testing. Nonsustained ventricular tachycardia was defined as greater or equal to three consecutive ventricular ectopic beats. Sustained ventricular tachycardia was defined as ventricular tachycardia longer than 30 seconds or requiring intervention.

There was a total of 58 episodes of exercise-induced ventricular tachycardia in 55 patients. The patients had a mean age of 62 years with a range of 39 to 76. Of the 55 patients, 50 had exercise-induced nonsustained ventricular tachycardia (range 3 to 21 beats). The mean (± 1 SD) and median number of consecutive ventricular ectopic beats per episode were 4.5 (± 3.6) and 3 beats respectively. Thirty of the patients with nonsustained exercise-induced ventricular tachycardia exhibited only three consecutive ventricular ectopic beats. Of the 50 episodes of nonsustained ventricular tachycardia, 26 episodes occurred during exercise and 24 occurred in recovery; only 10 occurred at peak exercise and led to cessation of the exercise test. Five patients had exercise-in-

duced sustained ventricular tachycardia; two patients had their bouts of ventricular tachycardia during exercise and three during recovery. Of these five patients, only two patients required intervention: one was given lidocaine intravenously and one was cardioverted because of hypotension. The only other episode of serious ventricular arrhythmia to occur in this time period occurred in a patient without prior cardiac history who developed ventricular fibrillation during exercise that required electrical defibrillation.

Prior disease. Of the 55 patients with exercise-induced ventricular tachycardia, 45 had clinical evidence of coronary artery disease; this included 19 with a prior myocardial infarction, 5 patients who had undergone percutaneous transluminal coronary angioplasty, and 9 patients with prior coronary artery bypass surgery. Two patients had cardiomyopathy, and three patients had valvular heart disease. Five patients had no clinical evidence of heart disease.

The major findings of this study were that the occurrence of nonsustained exercise-induced ventricular tachycardia during routine treadmill testing was not associated with complications during testing or with increased cardiovascular mortality within 2 years after testing. Both the prevalence and the reproducibility of exercise-induced ventricular tachycardia were low (1.2% and 6.9% respectively), despite a high prevalence of structural heart disease (mostly coronary artery disease) in the study population. The annual mortality among patients with exercise-induced ventricular tachycardia was 1.7% compared to 2.4% (171 deaths in 3351 patients) in the study population. Thus

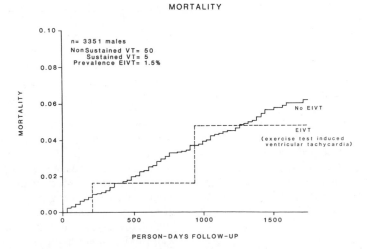

Figure 6-8   Kaplan-Meier survival curve illustrating mortality with ventricular tachycardia (VT) during standard treadmill testing in a referred clinical population. *EIVT,* Exercise test–induced ventricular tachycardia.

exercise-induced ventricular tachycardia during treadmill testing did not portend a worsened prognosis even among our patients with coronary artery disease. This statement cannot be extended to the five patients with sustained ventricular tachycardia because of their small number and because they were treated.

Mokotoff and co-workers selectively examined 26 of 45 consecutive patients with ventricular tachycardia during exercise testing, 18 of whom had organic heart disease (mostly coronary artery disease).[91] One half of the patients exhibited the minimum of three consecutive ventricular ectopic beats. Condini and co-workers described 47 patients with ventricular tachycardia occurring during exercise testing (a prevalence of 0.8% in 5730 treadmill tests).[92] Forty of the 47 patients had heart disease, mostly coronary artery disease. Ventricular tachycardia was brief and self-terminated in all but one instance. No follow-up data were provided. Milanes and co-worker reported a 4.0% prevalence of ventricular tachycardia in 900 treadmill tests performed in patients with coronary artery disease compared to a 0.07% prevalence in 1700 tests among patients without coronary artery disease.[93] They reported a 4-year mortality of 38% for patients with ventricular fibrillation or ventricular tachycardia of four beats or more. Of note, 79% of patients within this combined group of ventricular fibrillation and tachycardia had an abnormal ST response as well.

In general during exercise, transmural ischemia as indicated by ST-segment elevation is arrhythmogenic, whereas subendocardial ischemia associated with ST-segment depression is not. In our study, none of the patients with nonsustained ventricular tachycardia had ST-segment elevation with their exercise test, and 20 had abnormal ST depression. Of the five patients with sustained ventricular tachycardia, none had ST-segment elevation, and two patients had abnormal ST-segment depression before the onset of ventricular tachycardia. Detry and co-workers reported six patients without myocardial infarction specifically referred to them for spontaneous angina known to be associated with ST-segment elevation.[94] During exercise testing, five of them exhibited elevation, three of whom developed ventricular tachycardia and one of whom developed ventricular fibrillation. We have subsequently seen one such patient who developed ST-segment elevation and then ventricular tachycardia (20 beats) at maximal exercise.

SUMMARY

The interpretation of the exercise test is not a simple skill but requires the understanding of physiology and pathophysiology. One should not accept that all medical professionals can adequately interpret an exercise test. Certification is extremely important now that this technology is rapidly spreading beyond the subspeciality of cardiology. Training and experience are required because they are in other diagnostic procedures. In part for these reasons, the American College of Physicians has recently published guidelines on clinical competence for physicians performing exercise testing.[95]

All the results of the test must be considered. One should make the interpretation reliable by using good methods and following the above suggestions. When properly interpreted, the exercise test is one of the most important diagnostic and clinically helpful tests in medicine.

Observer agreement is best when one is using dichotomous interpretations and worst (most variable) when one is using more complex descriptions such as those involved in specifying location or overlapping areas. Reproducibility can be improved by (1) simple dichotomous decisions, (2) standardized report forms such as the one used in the study described above, (3) multiple observers or one very experienced reader, (4) multiple blinded or unbiased interpretations, and (5) computer analysis. Computer analysis of the exercise electrocardiogram and measurement of gas exchange variables can be highly reproducible. However, as long as human judgment with all its complexities remains the basis for the final interpretation, there will always be some variation, and the human element will always be needed in medical diagnosis.

ST-segment depression is a representation of global subendocardial ischemia, with a direction determined largely by the placement of the heart in the chest. ST-segment depression does not localize coronary artery lesions. ST-segment depression in the inferior leads (II, aV_F) is most often attributable to the atrial repolarization wave, which begins in the PR segment and can extend to the beginning of the ST segment. Severe transmural ischemia, resulting in wall-motion abnormalities, causes a shift of the vector in the direction of the wall-motion abnormality. However, preexisting areas of wall-motion abnormality (such as a scar), usually indicated by a Q-wave, also cause such a shift resulting in ST elevation without ischemia being present. When the resting ECG shows Q-waves of an old myocardial infarction, ST elevation is attributable to ischemia or wall-motion abnormalities, or both, whereas accompanying ST-segment depression can be attributable to a second area of ischemia or reciprocal changes. When the resting ECG is normal, however, ST-segment elevation is attributable to severe ischemia (spasm or a critical lesion) though accompanying ST-segment depression is reciprocal. Such ST-segment elevation is uncommon and very arrhythmogenic, and it localizes.

Exercise-induced R-wave and S-wave amplitude changes do not correlate with changes in left ventricular volume, ejection fraction, or ischemia. The consensus of many studies is that such changes do not have diagnostic value. ST-segment segment depression limited to the recovery period does not generally represent a "false-positive" response. Inclusion of analysis during this period increases the diagnostic yield of the exercise test. The use of exercise test scores has not been adequately validated and should be used with caution. Performing exercise ECG analysis with scintigraphy or performing a cool-down walk can falsely lower the sensitivity of the exercise ECG because they obscure ST-segment changes occurring in recovery. Other criteria including downsloping ST changes in recovery and prolongation of ST-segment depression can improve test performance.

As with resting ventricular arrhythmias, the significance of exercise-induced ventricular arrhythmias is related to the disease processes they are associated with (history of syncope, sudden death, physical examination of a large heart, murmurs, ECG showing prolonged QT, preexcitation, Q-waves). If there are no signs or symptoms of associated diseases, you can usually ignore exercise-induced ventricular arrhythmias (don't behave as you would in a coronary care unit). Exercise-induced ventricular arrythmias most likely do not have an independent association with death in most patients with coronary disease; that is, you can get better prediction from other variables. There most likely is a small percentage of patients in whom exercise-induced ventricular arrythmias are independently predictive of death. Nonsustained ventricular tachycardia is uncommon during routine clinical treadmill testing, is well tolerated, and is associated with a relatively good prognosis. Outcome is primarily determined by concomitant clinical features such as ventricular function, ischemia, and the presence or absence of symptoms. Treatment should be directed toward these signs and symptoms rather than the episode of arrhythmia.

The same exercise test responses can have different meanings from one population or clinical subset to another, and so interpretation depends on the application of the test.

REFERENCES

1. Simonson E: Electrocardiographic stress tolerance tests, *Prog Cardiovasc Dis* 13:269-292, 1970.

2. Blomqvist G: The Frank lead exercise electrocardiogram, *Acta Med Scand* 178:1-98, 1965.

3. Rautaharju PM, Punsar S, Blackburn H, et al: Waveform patterns in frank-lead rest and exercise electrocardiograms of healthy elderly men, *Circulation* 48:541-548, 1973.

4. Simoons ML, Hugenholtz PG: Gradual changes of ECG waveform during and after exercise in normal subjects, *Circulation* 52:570-577, 1975.

5. Riff DP, Carleton RA: Effect of exercise on the atrial recovery wave, *Am Heart J* 82:759-763, 1971.

6. Morales-Ballejo H, Greenberg P, Ellestad M, et al: Septal Q wave in exercise testing: angiographic correlation, *Am J Cardiol* 48:247-253, 1981.

7. Kentala E, Luurela O: Response of R wave amplitude to posterior changes and to exercise, *Ann Clin Res* 7:258-263, 1975.

8. Bonoris PE, Greenberg PS, et al: Evaluation of R wave amplitude changes versus ST segment depression in stress testing, *Circulation* 57:904-910, 1978.

9. Uhl GS, Hopkirk AC: Analysis of exercise-induced R wave amplitude changes in detection of coronary artery disease in asymptomatic men with left bundle branch block, *Am J Cardiol* 44:1247-1250, 1979.

10. Yiannikas J, Marcomichelakis J, Taggart P, et al: Analysis of exercise induced changes in R wave amplitude in asymptomatic men with electrocardiographic ST-T changes at rest, *Am J Cardiol* 47:238-243, 1981.

11. Greenberg PS, Ellestad MH, Berg R, et al: Correlation of R wave and EF changes with upright bicycle stress testing, *Circulation* 62:111-200, 1980.

12. Baron DW, Lisley C, Sheiban I, et al: R-wave amplitude during exercise: relation to left ventricular function coronary artery disease, *Br Heart J* 44:512-517, 1980.

13. van Eenige MJ, de Feyter PJ, Jong JP, Roos, JP. Diagnostic incapacity of exercise-induced QRS wave amplitude changes to detect coronary artery disease and left ventricular dysfunction, *Eur Heart J* 3:9-16, 1982.

14. Battler A, Froelicher VF, Slutsky R, et al: Relationship of QRS amplitude changes during exercise to left ventricular function and volumes and the diagnosis of coronary artery disease, *Circulation* 60:1004-1013, 1979.

15. Luwaert R, Cosyns J, Rousseau M, et al: Reassessment of the relation between QRS forces to the orthogonal electrocardiogram and left ventricular ejection fraction, *Eur Heart J* 4:103-109, 1983.

16. Brody DA: A theoretical analysis of intracavitary blood mass influence on the heart-lead relationship, *Circ Res* 54:731-738, 1956.

17. Levken J, Chatterjee K, Tyberg JV, et al: Influence of left ventricular dimensions on endocardial and epicardial QRS amplitude and ST segment elevations during acute myocardial ischemia, *Circulation* 61:679-689, 1980.

18. Deanfield JE, Davies G, Mongiadi F, et al: Factors influencing R wave amplitude in patients with ischaemic heart disease, *Br Heart J* 49:8-14, 1983.

19. David D, Naito M, Michelson E, et al: Intramyocardial conduction: a major determinant of R wave amplitude during acute myocardial ischemia, *Circulation* 65:161-167, 1982.

20. Myers J, Ahnve S, Froelicher V, Sullivan M: Spatial R wave amplitude during exercise: relation with left ventricular ischemia and function, *J Am Coll Cardiol* 6:603-608, 1985.

21. Gerson MC, Morris SN, McHenry PL: Relation of exercise induced physiologic ST segment depression to R wave amplitude in normal subjects, *Am J Cardiol* 46:778-782, 1980.

22. Mirvis DM, Ramanathan KB, Wilson JL: Regional blood flow correlates of ST segment depression in tachycardia-induced myocardial ischemia, *Circulation* 2:363-373, 1986.

23. Coester N, Elliott JC, Luft UC: Plasma electrolytes, pH, and ECG during and after exhaustive exercise, *J Appl Physiol* 34:677, 1973.

24. Wolthuis RA, Froelicher VF, Hopkirk A, et al: Normal electrocardiographic waveform characteristics during treadmill exercise testing, *Circulation* 60:1028-1035, 1979.

25. Prinzmetal M, Kennamer R, Merliss R, Wach T, Bor N: Angina pectoris: a variant form of angina pectoris, *Am J Med* 27:375, 1959.

26. Endo M, Kanda I, Hosoda: Prinzmetal's variant form of angina pectoris: re-evaluation of mechanisms, *Circulation* 52:33, 1975.

27. Shubrooks SJ, Bete JM, Hutter AM: Variant angina pectoris: clinical and anatomic spectrum and results of coronary bypass surgery, *Am J Cardiol* 36:142, 1975.

28. Higgins CB, Wexler L, Silverman JF, Schroeder JS: Clinical and arteriographic features of Prinzmetal's variant angina: documentation of etiologic factors, *Am J Cardiol* 37:831, 1976.

29. Maseri A, Severi S, Nes MD, et al: "Variant" angina: one aspect of continuous spectrum of vasospastic myocardial ischemia, *Am J Cardiol* 42:1019-1025, 1978.

30. Weiner DA, Schick EC Jr, Hood WB Jr, Ryan TJ: ST segment elevation during recovery from exercise, *Chest* 74:133, 1978.

31. Fortuin NJ, Friesinger GC: Exercise-induced ST segment elevation: clinical, electrocardiographic and arteriographic studies in twelve patients, *Am J Med* 49:459, 1970.

32. Hegge FN, Tuna N, Burchell HB: Coronary arteriographic findings in patients with axis shifts or ST segment elevations on exercise testing, *Am Heart J* 86:603, 1973.

33. Chahine RA, Raizner AE, Ishimori T: The clinical significance of exercise-induced ST-segment elevation, *Circulation* 54:209, 1976.

34. Manvi KN, Ellestad MH: Elevated ST segments with exercise in ventricular aneurysm, *J Electrocardiol* 5:317-323, 1972.

35. Simoons ML, Withagen A, Vinke R, et al: ST-vector orientation and location of myocardial perfusion defects during exercise, *Nucl Med* 17:154-156, 1978.

36. Sriwattanakomen S, Ticzon AR, Zubritzky SA, et al: ST segment elevation during exercise: electrocardiographic and arteriographic correlation in 38 patients, *Am J Cardiol* 45:762-768, 1980.

37. Longhurst JC, Kraus WL: Exercise-induced ST elevation in patients without myocardial infarction, *Circulation* 60:616, 1979.

38. Dunn RF, Freedman B, Kelly DT, et al: Exercise-induced ST-sgement elevation in leads V_1 or AV_L: a predictor of anterior myocardial ischemia and left anterior descending coronary artery disease, *Circulation* 63:1357, 1981.

39. Braat SH, Kingma H, Brugada P, Wellens HJJ: Value of lead V4R in exercise testing to predict proximal stenosis of the right coronary artery, *J Am Coll Cardiol* 5:1308-1311, 1985.

40. Mark DB, Hlatky MA, Lee KL, et al: Localizing coronary artery obstructions with the exercise treadmill test, *Ann Intern Med* 106:53-55, 1987.

41. Waters DD, Chaitman BR, Bourassa MG, Tubau JF: Clinical and angiographic correlates of exercise-induced ST-segment elevation: increased detection with multiple ECG leads, *Circulation* 61:286, 1980.

42. Bruce RA, Gey GO Jr, Cooper MN, et al: Seattle Heart Watch initial clinical, circulatory and electrocardiographic response to maximal exercise, *Am J Cardiol* 33:459, 1974.

43. Bruce RA, Fisher LD: Unusual prognostic significance of exercise-induced ST elevation in coronary patients, *J Electrocardiol* 20(suppl):84-88, 1987.

44. de Feyter PJ, Majid PA, van Eenige MJ, et al: Clinical significance of exercise-induced ST segment elevation, *Br Heart J* 46:84-92, 1981.

45. Bruce RA, Fisher LD, Pettinger M, et al: ST segment elevation with exercise: a marker for poor ventricular function and poor prognosis: Coronary Artery Surgery Study (CASS) confirmation of Seattle Heart Watch results, *Circulation* 4:897-905, 1988.

46. Hegge FN, Tuna N, Burchell HB: Coronary arteriographic findings in patients with axis shifts or S-T-segment elevations on exercise-stress testing, *Am Heart J* 5:603-615, 1973.

47. Lahiri A, Subramanian B, Millar-Craig M, et al: Exercise-induced ST-segment elevation in variant angina, *Am J Cardiol* 45:887, 1980.

48. Caplin JL, Banim SO: Chest pain and electrocardiographic ST-segment elevation occurring in the recovery phase after exercise in a patient with normal coronary arteries, *Clin Cardiol* 8:228, 1985.

49. Hill JA, Conti CR, Feldman RL, Pepine CJ: Coronary artery spasm and its relationship to exercise in patients without severe coronary obstructive disease, *Clin Cardiol* 11:489-494, 1988.

50. Fox KM, Jonathan A, England D, Selwyn AP: Significance of exercise-induced ST-segment elevation in patients with previous myocardial infarction, *Am J Cardiol* 49:933, 1982 (abstract).

51. Gerwitz H, Sullivan M, O'Reilly G, et al: Role of myocardial ischemia in the genesis of exercise-induced ST segment elevation in previous anterior myocardial infarction, *Am J Cardiol* 51:1293, 1983.

52. Stiles GL, Tosati RA, Wallace AG: Clinical relevance of exercise-induced ST-segment elevation, *Am J Cardiol* 46:931, 1980.

53. Shimokawa H, Matsuguchi T, Koiwaya Y, et al: Variable exercise capacity in variant angina and greater exertional thallium-201 myocardial defect during vasospastic ischemic ST segment elevation than with ST degression, *Am Heart J* 103:142, 1982.

54. Arora R, Ioachim L, Matza D, Horowitz SF: The role of ischemia and ventricular asynergy in the genesis of exercise-induced ST elevation, *Clin Cardiol* 11:127-131, 1988.

55. Nobel RJ, Rothbaum DA, Koebel SB, et al: Normalization of abnormal T waves in ischemia, *Arch Intern Med* 136:391, 1976.

56. Sweet RL, Sheffield LT: Myocardial infarction after exercise-induced electrocardiographic changes in a patient with variant angina pectoris, *Am J Cardiol* 33:813, 1974.

57. Lavie CJ, Oh JK, Mankin HT, et al: Significance of T-wave pseudonormalization during exercise: a radionuclide angiographic study, *Chest* 94:512-516, 1988.

58. McHenry PL, Morris SN: Exercise electrocardiography—current state of the art. In Schlant RC, Hurst JW, editors: *Advances in electrocardiography*, vol 2, New York, 1976, Grune & Stratton, pp 265-304.

59. Detrano R, Janosi A, Lyons KP, et al: Factors affecting sensitivity and specificity of a diagnostic test: the exercise thallium scintigram, *Am J Med* 84:699-710, 1988.

60. Gutman RA, Bruce R: Delay of ST depression after maximal exercise by walking for 2 minutes, *Circulation* 42:229, 1970.

61. Gibbons L, Cooper K: The safety of maximal exercise testing, *Circulation* 80:846, 1989.

62. Karnegis JN, Matts J, Tuna N, Amplatz K, The Posch Group: Comparison of exercise-positive with recovery-positive treadmill graded exercise tests, *Am J Cardiol* 60:544-547, 1987.

63. Savage MP, Squires LS, Hopkins JT, et al: Usefulness of ST-segment depression as a sign of coronary artery dis-

ease when confined to the post exercise recovery period, *Am J Cardiol* 60:1405-1406, 1987.

64. Froelicher VF, Thompson AJ, Longo MR, et al: Value of exercise testing for screening asymptomatic men for latent coronary artery disease, *Prog Cardiovasc Dis* 18:265-276, 1976.

65. Ellestad M: Stress testing: principles and practice, ed 3, Philadelphia, 1986, F.A. Davis Co.

66. Hollenberg M, Mateo GO, Massie BM, et al: Influence of R wave amplitude on exercise-induced ST depression: need for a "gain factor" correction when interpreting stress electrocardiograms, *Am J Cardiol* 56:13-17, 1985.

67. Hakki A, Iskandrian AS, Kutalek S, et al: R wave amplitude: a new determinant of failure of patients with coronary heart disease to manifest ST segment depression during exercise, *J Am Coll Cardiol* 3:1155-1160, 1984.

68. Val PG, Chaitman BR, Waters D: Diagnostic accuracy of exercise ECG lead system in clinical subsets of women, *Circulation* 65:1465-1472, 1982.

69. Robert AR, Melin JA, Detry JM: Logistic discriminant analysis improves diagnostic accuracy of exercise testing for coronary artery disease in women, *Circulation* 83(4):1202-1209, 1991.

70. Sundqvist K, Atterhög JH, Jogestrand T: Effect of digoxin on the electrocardiogram at rest and during exercise in healthy subjects, *Am J Cardiol* 57:661-665, 1986.

71. Whinnery JE, Froelicher VF, Stuart AJ: The electrocardiographic response to maximal treadmill exercise in asymptomatic men with left bundle branch block, *Am Heart J* 94:316, 1977.

72. Whinnery JE, Froelicher VF, Stuart AJ: The electrocardiographic response to maximal treadmill exercise in asymptomatic men with right branch bundle block, *Chest* 71:335, 1977.

73. Vasey CG, O'Donnell J, Morris SN, McHenry, P: Exercise-induced left bundle branch block and its relation to coronary artery disease, *Am Heart J* 56:892-895, 1985.

74. Sapin PM, Koch G, Blauwet MB, et al: Identification of false positive exercise tests with use of electrocardiographic criteria: a possible role for atrial repolarization waves, *J Am Coll Cardiol* 18:127-135, 1991.

75. Barnard R, MacAlpin R, Kattus A, et al: Ischemic response to sudden strenuous exercise in healthy men, *Circulation* 48:936, 1973.

76. Foster C, Dymond DS, Carpenter J, Schmidt DH: Effect of warm-up on left ventricular response to sudden strenuous exercise, *J Appl Physiol* 53:380-383, 1982.

77. Abouantoun S, Ahnve S, Savvides M, et al: Can areas of myocardial ischemia be localized by the exercise electrocardiogram? A correlative study with thallium-201 scintigraphy, *Am Heart J* 108:933-941, 1984.

78. Fuchs RM, Achuff SC, Grunwald L, et al: Electrocardiographic localization of coronary artery narrowings: studies during myocardial ischemia and infarction in patients with one-vessel disease, *Circulation* 66:1168-1175, 1982.

79. Weiner DA, McCabe C, Hueter DC, et al: The predictive value of anginal chest pain as an indicator of coronary disease during exercise testing, *Am Heart J* 96:458-462, 1978.

80. Cole JP, Ellestad, MH: Significance of chest pain during

treadmill exercise: correlation with coronary events, *Am J Cardiol* 41:227-232, 1978.

81. Blackburn H and the Technical Group on Exercise ECG: The exercise electrocardiogram: differences in interpretation, *Am J Cardiol* 29:871-880, 1968.

82. Sullivan M, Genter F, Savvides M, et al: The reproducibility of hemodynamic, electrocardiographic, and gas exchange data during treadmill exercise in patients with stable angina pectoris, *Chest* 86:375-382, 1984.

83. Busby MJ, Shefrin EA, Fleg JL: Prevalence and long-term significance of exercise-induced frequent or repetitive ventricular ectopic beats in apparently healthy volunteers, *J Am Coll Cardiol* 14:1659-1665, 1989.

84. Sami M, Chaitman B, Fisher L, et al: Significance of exercise-induced ventricular arrhythmia in stable coronary artery disease: a coronary artery surgery study project, *Am J Cardiol* 54:1182, 1984.

85. Califf RM, McKinnis RA, McNeer M, et al: Prognostic value of ventricular arrhythmias associated with treadmill exercise testing in patients studied with cardiac catheterization for suspected ischemic heart disease, *J Am Coll Cardiol* 2:1060-1067, 1983.

86. Weiner DA, Levin SR, Klein MD, Ryan TJ: Ventricular arrhythmias during exercise testing: mechanism, response to coronary bypass surgery and prognostic significance, *Am J Cardiol* 53:1553, 1984.

87. Marieb MA, Beller GA, Gibson RS, et al: Clinical relevance of exercise-induced ventricular arrhythmias in suspected coronary artery disease, *Am J Cardiol* 66:172-178, 1990.

88. Petsas AA, Anastassiades LC, Antonopoulos AG: Exercise testing for assessment of the significance of ST segment depression observed during episodes of paroxysmal supraventricular tachycardia, *Eur Heart J* 11:974-979, 1990.

89. Fleg JL, Lakatta EG: Prevalence and prognosis of exercise-induced nonsustained ventricular tachycardia in apparently healthy volunteers, *Am J Cardiol* 54:762, 1984.

90. Yang JC, Wesley RC, Froelicher VF: Ventricular tachycardia during routine treadmill testing: risk and prognosis, *Arch Internal Med* 151:349-353, 1991.

91. Mokotoff D, Quinones M, Miller R: Exercise-induced ventricular tachycardia, clinical features, relating to chronic ventricular ectopy, and prognosis, *Chest* 77:10-16, 1980.

92. Condini M, Sommerfeldt L, Eybel C, Messer J: Clinical significance and characteristics of exercise-induced ventricular tachycardia, *Cathet Cardiovasc Diagn* 7:227-234, 1981.

93. Milanes J, Romero M, Hultgren HN, Shettigar U: Exercise tests and ventricular tachycardia, *West J Med* 145:473-476, 1986.

94. Detry JR, Mengeot P, Rousseau MF, et al: Maximal exercise testing in patients with spontaneous angina pectoris associated with transient ST segment elevation: risks and electrocardiographic findings, *Br Heart J* 37:897-905, 1975.

95. Schlant RC, Friesinger GC, Leonard JL: Clinical competence in exercise testing, *Circulation* 5:1884-1888, 1990.

7 | Diagnostic Application of Exercise Testing

Exercise can be considered the true test of the heart because it is the most common everyday stress that humans undertake. The exercise test is the most practical and useful procedure in the clinical evaluation of cardiovascular status. The common clinical applications of exercise testing to be discussed in this book are listed in the first box. Four applications that require extensive review, diagnostic exercise testing, prognostic exercise testing, exercise testing of post–myocardial infarction patients, and screening of apparently healthy individuals, are covered in separate chapters. Other specific uses, some of which are touched upon in Chapter 11, are listed in the second box.

DIAGNOSIS OF CHEST PAIN AND OTHER CARDIAC FINDINGS

To evaluate a test for a disease, one must demonstrate how well the test distinguishes between those individuals with and those without the disease. Evaluation of exercise testing as a diagnostic test for coronary artery disease depends on the population tested, which must be divided into those with and those without coronary artery disease by independent techniques. Coronary angiography and clinical follow-up study for coronary events are two methods of separating a population into those with and those without coronary disease.

Limitations of coronary angiography

It has been demonstrated in studies comparing angiographic and pathological findings that coronary angiography usually underestimates the pathologic severity of coronary artery disease. Coronary angiography can be interpreted as normal when severe coronary artery disease is present. This can be attributable to total cut-off of an artery at its origin, to diffuse atherosclerotic narrowing of an artery, and to failure to use axial views to visualize proximal left coronary artery lesions. Another limitation of coronary angiography is that coronary artery spasm as a cause of ischemia may be missed because it is often transient. Also, coronary angiographic interpretation is subject to variability because of observer error, as has been previously described. Recent studies using Doppler flow techniques and videodensitometric techniques have shown a wide discrepancy between angiographic lesions and coronary flow reserve.

Coronary reserve. To determine the accuracy of the exercise electrocardiography in detecting a physiologically significant coronary stenosis, Wilson and co-workers studied 40 patients with one-vessel, one-lesion coronary artery disease, a normal resting electrocardiogram, and no hypertrophy or prior infarction.[1] Each patient underwent exercise electrocardiography that was interpreted as abnormal if the ST-segment developed 0.1 mV or greater depression 80 msec after the J point. The physiological significance of each coronary stenosis was assessed by measurement of the coronary flow reserve (peak divided by resting blood flow velocity) in the stenotic artery using a Doppler catheter and intracoronary papaverine (normal, 3.5 or greater ratio of peak-to-resting velocity). The percent diameter and percent area stenosis produced by each lesion were determined by use of quantitative angiography. Of the 17 patients with reduced coronary flow reserve in the stenotic artery, 14 had an abnormal exercise electrocardiogram (sensitivity, 82%; 95% confidence interval, 70% to 94%). On the other hand, 20 of 23 patients with normal coronary flow reserves had normal exercise tests (specificity, 87%; 95% confidence interval, 77% to 97%). The exercise electrocardiogram was abnormal in each of 11 patients with greatly reduced coronary flow reserve (less than 2.5 peak/resting velocity) and in three of six patients with moderately reduced reserve (2.5 to 3.4 peak/resting velocity). The products of systolic blood pressure and heart rate at peak exercise were significantly correlated with coronary reserve in patients with truly abnormal exercise tests. In comparison, the sensitivity (61%; 95% confidence interval, 46% to 76%) and specificity (73%; 95% confidence interval, 60% to 86%) of exercise electrocardiography in detecting a 60% or greater diameter stenosis was significantly lower. Exercise electrocardiography, therefore, was a good predictor of the physiological significance (assessed by coronary flow reserve) of a coronary stenosis but less so of angiographically classified disease.

Collateral coronary vessels. The occurrence and influence of coronary collateral circulation and obstruction of the supplying coronary arteries on left ventricular contractility, prevalence of myocardial infarction, and bicycle ergometry were studied by Pellinen and co-workers in a random sample of 286 patients with angiographically documented coronary artery disease.[2] Collateral vessels appeared increasingly in all three main coronary arteries in proportion to the grade of obstruc-

tion. The highest prevalence of collaterals occurred in stenosis of the right coronary artery (60%), followed by the left descending artery (45%); they occurred least in the left circumflex artery (21%). The frequency of intra-arterial collateral circulation was 42%, 11%, and 12% respectively. The presence or absence of collaterals had no obvious influence on ST-segment response during the exercise test. In three-vessel disease, peak work capacity was better when collaterals to the left anterior descending artery were not jeopardized than when jeopardized.

Limitations of other end points

There are some important limitations of using clinical events and pathological end points to separate patients with coronary artery disease from disease-free groups. Coronary disease events and symptoms can be caused by relatively minor lesions. Hemorrhage into nonobstructive plaques or thrombosis can cause symptoms or even death. Spasm has been demonstrated to occur proximally to relatively minor lesions. Pathological studies have shown that approximately 7% of people dying from a clinically diagnosed myocardial infarction have insignificant or no coronary atheroma. Coronary angiographic studies have shown that some patients with classic angina pectoris and myocardial infarction can have normal coronary angiograms. Despite these limitations, coronary angiography and the observation of clinical symptoms or coronary events are at present the most practical end points that distinguish between those with and without coronary artery disease.

Predictive accuracy definitions

Sensitivity and specificity are the terms used to define how reliably a test distinguishes diseased from nondiseased individuals. *Sensitivity* is the percentage of total patients in whom a test gives an abnormal result when those with the disease are tested. *Specificity* is the percentage of patients in whom a test gives a normal result when those without the disease are tested. This is quite different from the colloquial use of the word "specific." The method of calculating these terms is shown in Table 7-1.

A basic step in applying any testing procedure for the separation of normals from patients with disease is to determine a value measured by the test that best separates the two groups. A problem is that there is usually a considerable overlap of measurement values of a test in the groups with and without disease. Two bell-shaped normal distribution curves, one for the test variable in a population of normals and the other for this variable in a population with disease are illustrated in

Table 7-1 Definitions and calculation of terms used to demonstrate the diagnostic value of a test

$$\text{Sensitivity} = \frac{TP}{TP + FN} \times 100 \qquad\qquad \text{Relative risk} = \frac{\dfrac{TP}{TP+FP}}{\dfrac{FN}{TN+FN}}$$

$$\text{Specificity} = \frac{TN}{FP + TN} \times 100 \qquad\qquad \text{Predictive value of abnormal test} = \frac{TP}{TP + FP} \times 100$$

TP = true positives or those with abnormal test results and disease; *FN* = false negatives or those with normal test results and with disease; *TN* = true negatives or those with normal test results and no disease; *FP* = false positives or those with abnormal test results and no disease.

Predictive value of an abnormal response is the percentage of individuals with an abnormal test result who have disease.

Relative risk, or risk ratio, is the relative rate of occurrence of a disease in the group with an abnormal test result compared to those with a normal test result.

Figure 7-1. Along the vertical axis is the number of patients, and along the horizontal axis could be the value for such measurements as Q-wave size, exercise-induced ST-segment depression, or creatine phosphokinase (CPK). Notice that there is considerable overlap between the two curves. The optimal test would be able to achieve the clearest separation of these two bell-shaped curves minimizing the overlap. Unfortunately, most of the tests currently used for the diagnosis of coronary artery disease, including the exercise test, have a considerable overlap of the range of measurements for the normal population and for those with heart disease. Therefore problems arise when a certain value is used to separate these two groups (that is, 0.1 mV of ST-segment depression, a 10 mm Hg drop in systolic blood pressure, less than 5 MET exercise capacity, and 3 consecutive premature ventricular contractions). If the value is set far to the right (that is, 0.2 mV of ST-segment depression) to allow identification of

nearly all the normals as being free of disease, giving the test a high *specificity,* then a substantial number of those with the disease are called normal. If a value is chosen far to the left (that is, 0.5 mV of ST-segment depression) to allow identification of nearly all those with disease as being abnormal, giving the test a high *sensitivity,* then many normals are identified as abnormal. If a value is chosen that equally mislabels the normals and those with disease, the test will have its highest predictive accuracy. However, there may be reasons for wanting to adjust a test to have a relatively higher sensitivity or relatively higher specificity than possible when predictive accuracy is optimal. But remember that sensitivity and specificity are inversely related. That is, when sensitivity is the highest, specificity is the lowest and vice versa. Any test has a range of inversely related sensitivities and specificities that can be chosen by specifying a certain discriminant or diagnostic value.

Further complicating the choice of a discriminant value is that many diagnostic procedures do not have values established that best separate normals from those with disease. Even the Q-wave on the standard resting electrocardiogram or exercise-induced ST-segment depression have uncertainty regarding what is the best discriminant value (or cut-off point) and what the sensitivity and specificity of the currently used criteria are.

Once one chooses a discriminant value to determine a test's specificity and sensitivity, the population tested must be considered. If the population is skewed towards individuals with a greater severity of disease, the test will have a higher sensitivity. For instance, the exercise test has a higher sensitivity in individuals with three-vessel disease than in those with single-vessel disease. Also, a test can have a lower specificity if it is used in individuals more likely to give false positive results. For instance, the exercise test has a

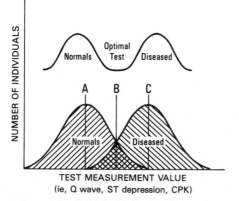

Figure 7-1 Bell-shaped curves illustrating the distribution of individuals with test results expressed as continuous variables.

lower specificity in individuals with mitral valve prolapse and in women.

The sensitivity and specificity of exercise-induced ST-segment depression can be demonstrated by analysis of the results obtained when exercise testing and coronary angiography have been used to evaluate patients. From these studies, the exercise test cut point of 0.1 mV horizontal or downsloping ST-segment depression has approximately an 84% specificity for angiographically significant coronary artery disease; that is, 84% of those without significant angiographic disease had a normal exercise test.

These studies demonstrated a mean 66% sensitivity of exercise testing for angiographic coronary artery disease with a range of 40% for one-vessel disease to 90% for three-vessel disease. Most of these studies, however, used only the criterion of 0.1 mV horizontal or downsloping ST-segment depression to indicate an abnormal exercise test, and in many of them only a single lead was recorded. Sensitivity decreased for the milder degrees of coronary artery disease, but it is likely that some patients with single-vessel coronary disease do not have myocardial ischemia.

Two additional terms that help to define the diagnostic value of a test are its relative risk and predictive value. Table 7-1 also shows how these terms are calculated. The relative risk is the relative chance of having disease if the test shows abnormal results as compared with the chance of having disease if the test shows normal results. The predictive value of an abnormal test is the percentage of those persons with an abnormal test result who have disease. Predictive value cannot be estimated directly from a test's demonstrated specificity or sensitivity. Predictive value is dependent on the prevalence of disease in the population tested. Table 7-4 illustrates how a test with a 70% sensitivity and a 90% specificity performs in a population with a 5% prevalence of disease. Since 5% of 10,000 men have disease, 500 men have disease. In the middle column are the number of men with abnormal test results, and in the far right column are the number with normal test results. Since the test is 70% sensitive, 350 of those with disease have abnormal test results and are true positives. The remaining 150 have normal test results and are false negatives. Since the test is 90% specific, 90% of the 9500 without disease are true negatives, whereas the remainder are false positives. To calculate the predictive value, the number of true positives is divided by the number of those with an abnormal test result. Table 7-2 also shows the performance of a test with the same 70% sensitivity and 90% specificity in a

Table 7-2   Test performance versus predictive value and risk ratio: a model in a population of 10,000

Disease prevalence	Subjects	Number with abnormal test results	Test performance	Number with normal test results
5%	500 diseased	450 (TP)	90% sensitivity	50 (FN)
		350 (TP)	70% sensitivity	150 (FN)
	9500 nondiseased	2850 (FP)	70% specificity	6650 (TN)
		950 (FP)	90% specificity	8550 (TN)
50%	5000 diseased	4500 (TP)	90% sensitivity	500 (FN)
		3500 (TP)	70% sensitivity	1500 (FN)
	5000 nondiseased	1500 (FP)	70% specificity	3500 (TN)
		500 (FP)	90% specificity	4500 (TN)

	Predictive value of abnormal test		Risk ratio*	
Disease prevalence	5	50	5	50
Sensitivity/specificity				
70%/90%	27%	88%	27	3
90%/70%	14%	75%	14	5
90%/90%	32%	90%	64	9
66%/84%	18%	80%	9	3

*Times that for normal subjects.
TP = true-positive test result; *FP* = false-positive test result; *FN* = false-negative test result; *TN* = true-negative test result.

population with a 50% prevalence of disease. The predictive value of an abnormal response is directly related to the prevalence of the disease in the population tested. There are more false positive responses when exercise testing is used in a population with a low prevalence of disease than when it is used in a population with a high prevalence of disease. This fact explains the greater number of false positive results found when using the test as a screening procedure in an asymptomatic group as opposed to when using it as a diagnostic procedure in patients with symptoms most likely attributable to coronary artery disease. Also, in Table 7-2 are the calculations for a test with a sensitivity and specificity of 90% and for a test with a sensitivity of 90% and a specificity of 70%.

Range-of-characteristic (ROC) curves

Plots of sensitivity versus specificity for a range of measurement cut points provides an efficient way to compare test performance. They are particularly helpful when optimal cut points for discriminating those with disease from those without disease are not established. A straight diagonal line indicates that the measurement or test has no discriminating power for the disease being tested. The greater the area of the curve beyond the diagonal line, the greater is its discriminating power. Care must be taken that scores are not compared at cut points that are impossible in clinical practice. True Epistat software makes it possible to perform ROC analysis on a standard personal computer. ROC curves make it possible to determine and then chose the appropriate cut points for the desired sensitivity or specificity and demonstrate the respective specificity and sensitivity. An example of an ROC curve is given in Figure 7-2.

Probability analysis

The information most important to a clinician attempting to make a diagnosis is the probability of the patient having the disease once the test result is known. Such a probability cannot be accurately estimated from the test result and the diagnostic characteristics of the test alone. It also requires knowledge of the probability of the patient having the disease before the test is administered. Bayes' theorem states that the probability of a patient having the disease after a test is performed will be the product of the disease probability before the test and the probability that the test provided a true result.

The probability of a test result being true can be shown as the likelihood ratio, which is the ratio of true results to false results. In the case of an

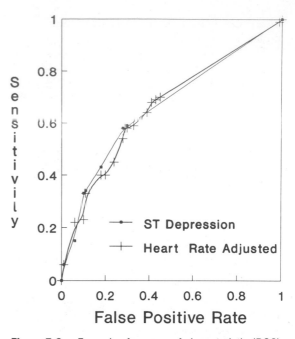

Figure 7-2   Example of a range-of-characteristic (ROC) curve plot comparing two different methods of measuring ST-segment depression during exercise testing for diagnosing coronary disease. Symbols are plotted at various cut points for the measurements.

abnormal test result, the positive likelihood ratio equals

$$\frac{\text{Percent with disease with abnormal test}}{\text{Percent without disease with abnormal test}} \text{ or } \frac{\text{Sensitivity}}{1 - \text{Specificity}}$$

In the case of a normal test result the negative likelihood ratio equals

$$\frac{\text{Percent without disease with normal test}}{\text{Percent with disease with normal test}} \text{ or } \frac{\text{Specificity}}{1 - \text{Sensitivity}}$$

By analyzing the statements in the equations on the left side, it can be seen that they are equivalent to the numerators and denominators in the equations on the right.

The likelihood ratio is an indicator of the diagnosticity of a test; the higher it is, the greater the diagnostic clarity of the test. Using conventional techniques of analyzing ST-segment depression with a cut point of 0.1 mV, the maximal or near-maximal exercise test has a sensitivity of approximately 66% and a specificity of 84%. Therefore the likelihood ratio for an abnormal test result is as follows:

Positive likelihood ratio $= \dfrac{0.66}{1 - 0.84} = 4.0$

and the likelihood ratio for a normal test result equals

Negative likelihood ratio $= \dfrac{0.84}{1 - 0.66} = 2.5$

Bayes's theorem may be expressed in the following fashion:

$$\begin{array}{c}\text{Post test odds} \\ \text{of disease}\end{array} = \begin{array}{c}\text{Pretest odds} \\ \text{of disease}\end{array} \times \begin{array}{c}\text{Likelihood ratio} \\ \text{of test results}\end{array}$$

The clinician often makes this calculation intuitively when he suspects as a false result the abnormal exercise test result of a 30-year-old woman with chest pain (low prior odds or probability). The same abnormal response would be accepted as a true result in a 60-year-old man with angina who had a previous myocardial infarction (high prior odds or probability).

Angiographic studies have been used to investigate the prevalence of significant coronary artery disease in patients with different chest pain syndromes. Because chest pain is the presenting complaint in the majority of patients referred for a diagnostic exercise test, the nature of the pain would seem a practical basis for estimating the prior probability of coronary artery disease. Approximately 90% of the patients with true angina pectoris have been found to have significant an-

giographic coronary disease. In patients presenting with atypical angina pectoris, approximately 50% have been found to have significant angiographic coronary disease. Atypical angina refers to pain that has an unusual location, prolonged duration, or inconsistent precipitating factors or that is unresponsive to nitroglycerin. Figure 7-3 demonstrates the calculation of the probability of coronary artery disease in such patients.

The 50-year-old male patient with typical angina pectoris has a 90% probability or 9:1 chance of having significant coronary artery disease. An abnormal exercise test result increases these odds from 9:1 to 36:1. Such an impressive change in odds represents a relatively small increase in the probability of disease from 90% to 98%. Because such a patient still has a 75% probability of disease after a negative test, coronary angiography may yet be required to rule out coronary disease definitely. The greatest diagnostic impact of such a circumstance would be in patients with atypical angina. An abnormal test result would increase the odds from 1:1 to 4:1 (the probability of disease to 80%) and, for practical purposes, establish the diagnosis. With a normal test result, the probability of coronary disease would be reduced to 25%.

An important but often neglected assumption in using Bayes' theorem is that the sensitivity and specificity do not depend on the variables that de-

	PRE-TEST ODDS	LIKELIHOOD RATIO	POST-TEST ODDS	POST-TEST PROBABILITY
ANGINAL	9 : 1	ABNORMAL TEST (x4)	36:1	(36/37)=98%
		NORMAL TEST (x2.5)	9:2.5	(9/12)=75%
ATYPICAL ANGINA	1 : 1	ABNORMAL TEST (x4)	4:1	(4/5)=80%
		NORMAL TEST (x2.5)	1:2.5	(1/4)=25%
NON-ANGINAL	1 : 9	ABNORMAL TEST (x4)	4:9	(4/13)=31%
		NORMAL TEST (x2.5)	1:23	(1/24)=4%
ASYMPTOMATIC	1 : 19	ABNORMAL TEST (x4)	4:19	(4/23)=17%
		NORMAL TEST (x2.5)	1:48	(1/49)=2%

Figure 7-3   Influence of clinical presentation and exercise test results on probability of disease.

termine the pretest probability. For example, if one determines the pretest probability by using knowledge of the patient's sex, the theorem will not be completely valid if the specificity of the test depends on sex, as many investigators have found for exercise testing. Likewise, if the pretest probability is based on the character of the chest pain reported, any dependence of specificity on this symptom will invalidate the application of the theorem. Since there is evidence that exercise test results (ST-segment depression) are more sensitive in patients with typical angina pectoris, this would appear to invalidate the theorem's application. Actually, this problem is not as serious as one might imagine as long as the number of variables determining the pretest probability is relatively small. Perhaps more caution is needed when one is attempting to apply the theorem to the results of tests and populations of patients that are very different from those used to determine sensitivity and specificity. Detrano and co-workers have produced results that are suggestive that such an erroneous application can produce relatively large errors in posttest probabilities.

An example will help illustrate these principles. If a 50-year old woman without prior myocardial infarction and atypical angina and 0.15 mV ST-segment depression has a pretest probability of 0.40, the posttest probability can be calculated from Bayes' theorem.

$$\text{Posttest probability} = \frac{0.40\text{Se}}{0.40\text{Se} + 0.60\,(1 - \text{Sp})}$$

Now, if one uses a sensitivity of 0.90 and a specificity of 0.90 from a study done on men with severe typical angina, the result would be:

$$\frac{\text{Posttest}}{\text{probability}} = \frac{0.40 \times 0.90}{0.40 \times 0.90 + 0.60 \times 0.20} = 0.75$$

However, if a more appropriate study done on women with atypical chest pain produced a sensitivity of 0.70 and a specificity of 0.65, then using these appropriate values:

$$\frac{\text{Posttest}}{\text{probability}} = \frac{0.40 \times 0.70}{0.40 \times 0.70 + 0.60 \times 0.35} = 0.57$$

A clinician who refers patients with greater than 70% disease probability by coronary angiography would mistakenly refer this patient if he had used the inappropriate sensitivity and specificity. The clinician who does not calculate disease probabilities but instead uses intuition might also be in error if he assumed the test to be as accurate for his 50-year-old woman patient as it is for men with severe angina.

Bayesian versus multivariate analytic techniques

To compare the relative accuracy of bayesian versus discriminant function, Detrano and co-workers analyzed 303 subjects referred for coronary angiography who also had exercise testing, thallium scintigraphy, and cinefluoroscopy.[3] Angiographic disease was defined as at least one greater than 50% occlusion of a major vessel. Four calculations were done: (1) bayesian analysis using literature estimates of pretest probabilities, sensitivities, and specificities was applied to the clinical and test data of a randomly selected subgroup (group I with 151 patients) to calculate posttest probabilities; (2) bayesian analysis using literature estimates of pretest probabilities (but with sensitivities and specificities derived from the remaining 152 subjects [group II]) was applied to group I data to estimate posttest probabilities; (3) a discriminant function with logistic regression coefficients derived from the clinical and test variables of group II was used to calculate posttest probabilities of group I; and (4) a discriminant function derived with the use of test results form group II, and pretest probabilities from the literature were used to calculate posttest probabilities of group I. Receiver operating characteristic curve analysis showed that all four calculations could equivalently rank the disease probabilities for our patients. A goodness-of-fit analysis was suggestive of the following relationship between the accuracies of the four calculations: (1) < (2) = (4) < (3). These results are suggestive that data-based discriminant functions are more accurate than literature-based bayesian analysis if one assumes independence in predicting coronary disease based on clinical and noninvasive test results. The accuracy of the bayesian method is degraded by the assumption of independence and perhaps more importantly by the use of sensitivities and specificities derived from other patient populations with different testing protocols. Morise and Duval have also written on this subject.[4]

Even though a test may not have an important influence on disease probability in a patient, the test can be used for other purposes, such as demonstrating the severity or prognosis of a disease or the result of a therapeutic intervention. In addition, we should remember that any test gives only a probability statement and how this affects an individual patient is greatly dependent on the physician's clinical judgment.

Methodological problems with diagnostic studies

To determine why exercise testing remains controversial as a diagnostic test for coronary artery disease, Philbrick and co-workers undertook a methodological review of 33 studies comprising

7501 patients who had undergone both exercise tests and coronary angiography.[5] These studies were published betweeen 1976 and 1979 and had to include at least 50 patients (Table 7-3). Seven methodological standards were declared necessary: (1) adequate identification of the groups selected for study, (2) adequate variety of anatomic lesions, (3) adequate analysis for relevant chest pain syndromes, (4) avoidance of a limited challenge group, (5) avoidance of work-up bias, (6) avoidance of diagnostic review bias (the result of the exercise test is allowed to influence the interpretation of the coronary angiogram), and (7) avoidance of test review bias (occurring when the result of the coronary angiogram is allowed to influence the interpretation of the exercise test). Of these seven methodological standards for research design, only the requirement for an adequate variety of anatomic lesions received general compliance. Less than half of the studies complied with any of the remaining six standards: adequate identification of the groups selected for study; adequate analysis for relevant chest pain syndromes; avoidance of a limited challenge group; and avoidance of bias attributable to work-up method, diagnostic review bias, or test review. Only one study met as many as five standards.

These methodological problems help explain the wide range of sensitivity (35% to 88%) and specificity (41% to 100%) found for exercise testing. The variations could not be attributed to the usual explanations: definition of anatomic abnormality, exercise test technique, or definition of an abnormal test. Determining the true value of exercise testing requires methodologic improvements in patient selection, data collection, and data analysis. Another important consideration is the exclusion of patients after myocardial infarction. These patients most often have obstructive coronary artery disease and should not be included in diagnostic studies of any coronary artery disease but can be included when disease severity is evaluated.

Detry and colleagues evaluated modern approaches to exercise testing including computer averaging of the ECG, multivariate analysis of results, compartmental diagnostic approach, and probabilistic interpretation of the results.[6] These methods were tested in a group of 387 patients who had computer assisted maximal exercise tests. Because of the problems of including patients with prior myocardial infarction in such studies, they were carefully excluded. In 284 symptomatic patients, the diagnosis was made by arteriography, and 103 healthy men were included. The computer-averaged ECG signals of leads X, Y, and Z recorded at maximal exercise, maximal heart rate, blood pressure, and work load, and the onset of angina pectoris during exercise were entered into a multivariate stepwise discriminant analysis. The pretest likelihood for coronary artery disease was calculated from age and history; the posttest likelihood was calculated from Bayes' theorem and the average information content of several diagnostic methods was assessed in categorical and compartmental models. By multivariate analysis, five variables collected at maximal exercise were selected; they included the heart rate, the ST-segment level, the onset of angina during the test, the work load, and the slope of the ST-segment in lead X. The average information content of the analysis using five variables was 44% in a categorical model versus

Table 7-3 Angiographic studies evaluating the diagnostic value of exercise testing

Investigator	Year	Number of cases	Sensitivity (%)	Specificity (%)
Hultgren	1967	55	66	100
Eliasch	1967	65	84	81
Demany	1967	75	64	49
Mason	1967	84	78	89
Kassenbaum	1968	68	47	97
Roitman	1970	100	73	82
Newton	1970	52	57	81
Fitzgibbon	1971	160	48	80
Cohn	1971	110	86	73
McConahay	1971	100	35	100
Ascoop	1971	96	59	94
Martin	1972	100	62	89
McHenry	1972	166	81	95
Kellerman	1973	74	54	96
Bartel	1974	465	65	92
Piessens	1974	70	65	83
Rios	1974	50	83	89
Sketch	1975	251	53	88
Borer	1975	89	49	41
Jelinek	1976	153	45	89
Goldschlager	1976	153	45	89
Santinga	1976	283	73	78
Detry	1977	98	55	85
Chaitman	1978	100	88	82
McNeer	1978	1222	53	91
Balnave	1978	70	81	100
Berman	1978	164	84	67
Weiner	1978	302	76	76
Chaitman	1979	200	84	72
Weiner	1979	2045	79	69
Aldrich	1979	181	40	92
Raffo	1979	100	91	96
Borer	1979	75	63	95
AVERAGES			66	84

Modified from Philbrick et al: *Am J Cardiol* 46:807, 1980.

55% in a compartmental model. For comparison the information content of the analysis using the ST-segment alone was only 16% and 27% respectively. The classification provided by the analysis of the ST-segment changes was barely better than one provided by the simple history. The probabilistic use of a multivariate and compartmental analysis of the data led to a significantly better and more accurate classification of the patients (83% correct classification).

Another problem with determining specificity is including enough normals and the problem of the definition of normals. Should they be low-risk individuals or patients without significant angiographic disease? The decline of specificity in other forms of exercise testing may well be attributable to pretest and posttest reference bias.[7] Analysis of the ST-segments in Detry's study achieved results similar to that in the literature. The best cut-off point was 0.095 mV, a value very close to the commonly used diagnostic criterion of 0.10 mV. Computer analysis was not an improvement over visual reading. Detry concluded that the value of exercise testing for the diagnosis of coronary artery disease is limited if one persists in using the classic univariate and categorical interpretation of ST-segment changes only. To be clinically relevant, diagnostic exercise testing requires firstly the consideration of other exercise test responses and secondly the analysis of these parameters in a compartmental and probabilistic way. This approach is facilitated by computer quantification and processing of the data.

Other investigators have attempted to combine exercise ECG variables in a nonlinear fashion. Usually this involves an intuitively derived or empirical scale such as requirement of greater ST-segment depression when ST-segments are upsloping or calculation of the rate of change of ST-segment shifts with heart rate. Detrano and co-workers have compared some of these rules for modifying the ST-segment response in a group of 303 consecutive subjects without prior myocardial infarction who were referred for angiography to the Cleveland Clinic.[8]

A basic step in applying any test for the separation of those without from patients with disease is to determine a value measured by the test that best separates the two groups (that is, discriminate value or cut point). Cut points cannot allow absolute discrimination because those with and without disease have overlapping values. This overlapping explains why sensitivity and specificity are inversely related; that is, if you increase one with use of a certain cut point, you decrease the other. Although other ECG responses (such as

R-wave amplitude, QT or QRS duration, ST-segment elevation) have been reported as useful in the analysis of ECG results for separation of those with disease, ST-segment depression has received the most attention. Experts agree concerning the importance of ST-segment depression in the diagnosis of coronary disease; however, there are disagreements as to how to make the ST-segment measurements. Furthermore, differences occur as to the number and type of leads used, type of exercise, computerization scores, and treatment of equivocal results.

Gianrossi and co-workers recently investigated the variability of the reported diagnostic accuracy of the exercise electrocardiogram by applying metanalysis.[9] One hundred forty-seven consecutively published reports involving 24,074 patients who underwent both coronary angiography and exercise testing were summarized, and the results were entered into a computer spreadsheet. Details regarding population characteristics and methods were entered including publication year, number of ECG leads, exercise protocol, pre-exercise hyperventilation, definition of an abnormal ST response, exclusion of certain subgroups, and blinding of test interpretation. Wide variability in sensitivity and specificity was found (the mean sensitivity was 68% with a range of 23% to 100% and a standard deviation of 16%; the mean specificity was 77% with a range of 17% to 100% and a standard deviation 17%).

Sensitivity was found to be significantly and independently related to four study characteristics:

1. The method of dealing with equivocal or nondiagnostic tests: Sensitivity decreased when these tests were considered having normal results.
2. Comparison with a "better" test (that is, thallium scintigraphy): The sensitivity of the exercise ECG was lower when the study compared it with another testing method being reported as "superior."
3. Exclusion of patients on digitalis: Exclusion of patients taking digitalis was associated with improved sensitivity.
4. Publication year: An increase in sensitivity and decrease in specificity were noted over the years that the exercise test has been used. The reason may be that as clinicians become more familiar with a test and increasingly trust its results, they allow its results to influence the decision to perform angiography.

Specificity was found to be significantly and independently related to four variables:

1. Treatment of upsloping ST-segment depression: When upsloping ST-segment depression was classified as abnormal, specificity was lowered significantly (73% versus 80%).
2. Exclusion or inclusion of subjects with prior infarction: The exclusion of patients with prior myocardial infarction was associated with a decreased specificity.
3. Exclusion or inclusion of patients with left bundle branch block: The specificity increased when patients with left bundle branch block were excluded.
4. Pre-exercise hyperventilation: The use of pre-exercise hyperventilation was associated with a decreased specificity.

Stepwise linear regression explained less than 35% of the variance in sensitivities and specificities reported in the 147 publications. This wide variability in the reported accuracy of the exercise ECG is not explained by the information available in the published reports. Although this variability could be explained by unsuspected technical, methodological, or clinical variables that affect test performance by poorly understood mechanisms, it is more likely that the authors of the 147 reports did not disclose important information or did not consider the key points that are known to affect test performance when they were performing and analyzing their studies.

This wide variability in test performance makes it important that clinicians apply rigorous control of the methods they use for testing and analysis. Individuals with truly nondiagnostic or equivocal tests should be retested or offered other testing methods and ST-segment analysis should not be used to make a diagnosis in patients receiving digoxin, those with resting ST-segment depression, or those with left bundle branch block. Upsloping ST-segment depression should be considered borderline or negative, and hyperventilation should not be performed before testing.

"Believability" criteria for diagnostic test

Guyatt recommends that certain criteria must be applied to judge the credibility and applicability of the results of studies evaluating diagnostic tests.[10] First, the evaluation must include clearly defined comparison groups, at least one of which is free of the disease of interest. The studies should include consecutive patients or randomly selected patients for whom the diagnosis is in doubt. Any diagnostic test appears to function well if obviously normal subjects are compared with those who obviously have the disease in question. In most cases we do not need sophisti-

cated testing to differentiate the normal population from the sick. Rather, we are interested in examining patients who are suspected but not known to have the disease of interest and in differentiating those who do from those who do not. If the patients enrolled in the study do not represent this "diagnostic dilemma" group, the test may perform well in the study, but it may well not perform well in clinical practice. Another problem is including patients who most certainly have the disease (that is, post-MI patients) in this diagnostic sample. They may be included in studies to predict disease severity but should not be included in studies attempting to distinguish those with disease from those without disease.

The second "believability" criterion requires an independent, "blind" comparison of the test with the performance of a reliable standard. Such a standard really should measure a clinically important state. For example, for coronary artery disease an invasive test, such as catheterization, is used as the standard rather than symptoms of chest pain alone. The result from this standard should not be available to those interpreting the test. Also, if this standard requires subjective interpretation (as would be the case even for coronary angiography), the interpreter should not know the test result. Blinding the interpreters of the test to the standard and vice versa minimizes the risk of bias.

If these two criteria are met, the study can be used as a basis for performance of the test in clinical practice. To apply the test properly to patients the following must be considered. Most tests merely indicate an increase or decrease in the probability of disease. To apply imperfect tests appropriately, you must estimate the probability of disease before the test is done ("pretest probability") and then revise this probability according to the test result.

The clinician's estimation of pretest probability is based on the patient's history (including age, sex, chest-pain characteristics), physical examination and initial testing, and the clinician's own experience with this type of problem. Although forming accurate estimations from examination and experience may sound difficult, it is what we implicitly do; we just do not usually make the estimates explicit. Lack of symptoms makes the pretest probability so low that a positive test result is most likely to be associated with no disease. Typical angina makes the pretest probability of disease so high that the test result does not affect it much. Atypical angina is a 50/50 probability, and the test result really affects the outcome. The pretest probability is the basis for incorporating the test result. You can use the pretest probability from the study as a guide, especially if the patients were randomly selected from a defined group or a consecutive series and the clinical setting was similar to the reader's. Even then, the findings from the patient must be taken into account.

Sensitivity (the proportion of diseased in whom the test shows a positive result) and specificity (the proportion of nondiseased in whom the test show a negative result) must be appreciated. Applying the concepts of sensitivity and specificity is still the best way of using tests that yield yes or no results. The mathematics of taking a patient from pretest probability to posttest probability has been presented earlier. For tests in which there are more than two possible results, a strongly positive test increases the probability more than a moderately positive test. This information is presented in likelihood ratios, but a simple nomogram (Figure 7-4) can be used to avoid calculations.[11]

SIGNIFICANCE AND EFFECT OF RESTING ST-SEGMENT DEPRESSION

Additional modalities to complement exercise testing have been developed to increase the diagnostic accuracy of exercise testing, especially in subsets of patients in whom standard exercise electrocardiography is compromised such as those with resting ST-segment depression. However, the additional expense of these modalities limits their widespread applicability. Resting ST-segment depression has been identified as a marker for adverse cardiac events in patients with and without known coronary artery disease. To correlate this with exercise testing, coronary angiography, and how it affects long-term prognosis, Miranda and colleagues reported a retrospective study of 476 patients of which 223 had no clinical or electrocardiographic evidence of prior myocardial infarction whereas 253 were survivors of an infarction.[12] Exclusions were women, left bundle branch block, left ventricular hypertrophy, use of digoxin, previous revascularization procedures, or significant valvular or congenital heart disease. Long-term follow-up observation was carried out for an average of 45 months.

Of the patients without prior infarction, 23 (10%) had persistent resting ST-segment depression, and of those with a prior history of infarction, 37 (15%) also had resting ST-segment depression. Patients with resting ST-segment depression and no prior myocardial infarction had a higher prevalence of severe coronary disease (three vessel or left main, or both) than those without resting ST-segment depression (16%).

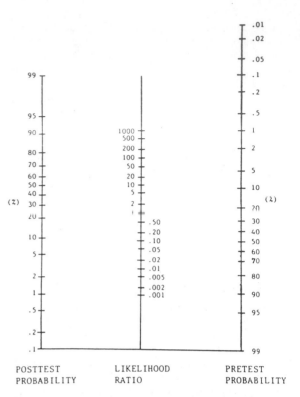

Figure 7-4   Nomogram developed by Fagan for Bayes theorem (MKSAP VIII, Part D, Book 3, Figure 14) allows calculation of posttest probability when a line is drawn through pretest probability and the likelihood ratio of the test.

The criteria of 2 mm of additional exercise-induced ST-segment depression was a particularly useful marker in these patients for the diagnosis of any coronary disease. Patients with resting ST-segment depression and a prior myocardial infarction had a 2.5 times higher prevalence of severe coronary artery disease compared to patients without resting ST-segment depression (43% versus 17% prevalence respectively) and also had larger left ventricles after infarction. To allow identification of severe coronary artery disease in postinfarction patients with persistent resting ST-segment depression, the criterion of ≥2 mm of additional exercise-induced ST-segment depression (likelihood ratio 3, 95% confidence interval 1.1 to 7.9, $p = 0.02$) or having the additional exercise-induced ST-segment depression persist ≥4 minutes into recovery (likelihood ratio 3.6) was in either case a better marker than the standard criterion of ≥1 mm of additional ST-segment depression (likelihood ratio 1.7). Receiver-operating-characteristic curve analysis revealed that additional exercise-induced ST-segment depression continued to discriminate between those with or without any or severe coronary disease despite having baseline ST-segment depression at rest. After a cumulative follow-up study of 4.4 years, patients with resting ST-segment depression, with or without prior myocardial infarction, had a lower infarct-free survival rate than those without it.

OTHER PROGNOSTIC STUDIES

Resting ST-segment depression on the baseline electrocardiogram, not caused by left bundle branch block, left ventricular hypertrophy, or drug effect, in patients of appropriate age may be caused by ischemia. It has been shown that resting ST-segment abnormalities have been a marker for adverse cardiac events in patients without known coronary disease. Blackburn reported the results of a study analyzing risk factors for coronary disease and noted that men with 0.5 to 0.9 mm of ST-segment depression on their initial resting were 4.3 times more likely to die in a 5-year follow-up period.[13] Men with ≥ 1.0 millimeter ST-segment depression were 10 times more likely to die. The Busselton study followed subjects for 13 years and noted that cardiovascular mortality was over two times greater in those who had 0.5 to 1 mm of resting ST-segment depression.[14] Aronow followed 1106 unselected elderly patients for a mean of 37 months.[15] In patients with no significant resting ST-segment depression, 23% of them suffered cardiac events during follow-up study. Patients with 0.5 to 0.9 mm of ST-segment depression had a 43% cardiac event rate, and those with 1 mm of ST-segment depression had a 71% cardiac event rate. Califf and co-workers analyzed 2946 patients with a Cox regression model to identify clinical variables that were independently predictive of prognosis.[16] The presence of resting ST-T changes suggestive of ischemia on the baseline electrocardiogram was found to be the strongest negative predictor for infarction-free survival and was correspondingly weighted the most in their final angina score.

There have also been numerous studies that have correlated persistent ST-segment depression in patients with known coronary artery disease to a poorer outcome. Harris and associates followed 1214 symptomatic, medically treated patients with coronary artery disease.[17] Resting ST-T changes were found to be an independently significant predictor of survival over 7 years ($p <$ 0.01). Schlant and colleagues for the Coronary Drug Project Research Group studied the natural history of coronary artery disease in 2789 men who were recovering from a recent myocardial infarction, were in New York Heart Association functional class I or II, and were randomized to placebo medication during a 5-year follow-up period.[18] ST-segment depression on the baseline electrocardiogram was strongly related to all-cause mortality. Lembo and associates studied 43 consecutive patients with an acute inferior transmural myocardial infarction, 10 of whom had persistent anterior precordial ST-segment depression of 1 mm or greater.[19] This latter group with persistent ST-segment depression had a higher morbidity and mortality over a 1-year follow-up period compared to those without persistent ST-segment depression. These patients also had less residual myocardial function after infarction. Schechtman and co-workers for the Diltiazem Reinfarction Study Research Group followed 515 survivors of a non–Q wave myocardial infarction for 1 year.[20] The strongest predictor of mortality was persistent ST-segment depression even after adjustment for left ventricular function. Wong and colleagues studied 251 survivors of a Q-wave myocardial infarction, from the Framingham study, and followed them for a mean of greater than 10 years to ascertain the prognostic importance of abnormalities on the baseline electrocardiogram.[21] They found that ST-segment changes were a powerful predictor of coronary death.

Miranda's study documents a relationship between persistent resting ST-segment depression after infarction and a higher prevalence of three-vessel and left main coronary artery disease. It has been shown previously, in agreement with the above studies, that the severity of coronary arterial lesions is an independent predictor of survival after myocardial infarction.[22,23] Therefore patients with resting ST-segment depression (not attributable to drugs, conduction defects, or left ventricular hypertrophy) have a high pretest probability for coronary disease or cardiac events, and an abnormal exercise test response in this subgroup of patients would lead to a high posttest probability as well.

Severity of coronary disease

Humphries and colleagues found more severe coronary disease to be associated with ST-T abnormalities,[24] and Mirvis and colleagues, in an analysis of 9801 patients, found a relative risk of 2.1 for severe coronary disease if resting ST-segment depression were present.[25] Perhaps of even more clinical significance may be the finding that patients with postinfarction resting ST-segment depression have larger ventricular volumes compared to those without resting ST-segment depression. White and colleagues studied 605 male patients under 60 years of age at 1 to 2 months after a myocardial infarction.[26] Using multivariate analysis they showed that left ventricular end-systolic and end-diastolic volumes had the greatest predictive value for survival over a mean of 78 months of follow-up time.

One additional millimeter of ST-segment depression during exercise testing

Kansal and colleagues evaluated 37 patients with chest pain and resting ST-segment depression of 0.5 mm or greater (not attributable to left ventricular hypertrophy or drugs) with exercise testing and coronary angiography; patients with Q-waves were not excluded.[27] An additional 1 mm of ST-segment depression during exercise was found to be 92% sensitive and 75% specific for the diagnosis of at least one significant coronary artery obstruction. Harris and associates studied 80 patients with at least 0.5 mm of resting horizontal ST-segment depression or T-wave inversion with exercise testing and coronary angiography.[28] Patients with diagnostic Q-waves, conduction defects, and left ventricular hypertrophy and those receiving digoxin were excluded. They found a sensitivity of 75% for an additional 1 mm of ST-segment depression for the diagnosis of coronary artery disease, but the specificity was only 53%. These two studies lend support to our results: the standard criterion of an additional 1 mm of exercise-induced ST-segment depression in the patient with resting ST-segment depression often represents a highly sensitive indicator of coronary artery disease and not necessarily a false positive finding.

Other studies have found decreased sensitivity and specificity in patients with resting ST-segment depression.[29,30] However, these studies included bundle branch blocks, previous infarction, and "nonspecific" ST-T changes such as T-wave inversions or flattening, and they did not isolate left ventricular hypertrophy and resting ST-segment depression groups. Detrano and colleagues performed a metanalysis on 150 studies of exercise electrocardiography from the previous 22 years to analyze factors affecting its diagnostic accuracy.[31] They found that resting ST-segment depression does not invalidate the exercise electrocardiogram, since the sensitivity and specificity were virtually unchanged whether patients with resting ST-segment depression were excluded from the studies reviewed.

Two additional millimeters of ST-segment depression

In Harris's study of 80 patients, he also investigated the criterion of an additional 2 mm of exercise-induced ST-segment depression and found it to have a sensitivity of only 48% but a specificity of 95%. This differs from Miranda's study, which reported a higher sensitivity. Harris's study included women and "nonspecific T-wave changes" on the baseline electrocardiogram (not only resting ST-segment depression as in our study), an inclusion that would increase the false-positivity rate.

ST-segment depression persisting late into recovery

Although previous studies have not specifically evaluated patients with resting ST-segment depression with this criterion, data have been presented supporting a correlation between prolonged ST-segment depression during recovery and more severe coronary artery disease. Goldschlager and associates noted that although the patients with rapid normalization of their ST-segments during recovery had a 58% prevalence of two- or three-vessel coronary artery disease, patients who had ischemic changes persisting 8 minutes or greater into recovery had a 67% prevalence of three-vessel or left main disease.[32] Callaham and co-workers studied 290 patients and noted that prolonged ST-segment depression during recovery was a highly specific marker for proximal left anterior descending, multivessel, and left main coronary disease.[33] These data corroborate the present study in that the patients who had three-vessel or left main disease and resting ST-segment depression were all identified with a prolonged recovery of their additional exercise-induced ST-segment depression.

Downsloping ST-segment depression during recovery

Goldschlager and associates studied 330 patients with both exercise testing and coronary angiography. Seventy-six patients had their non-upsloping ST-segment depression confined to the recovery period. Of these 76 patients, 47 (62%) developed downsloping depression during recovery, and only one of these patients was a false-positive finding. This is supportive of the present study in that this criterion was a specific marker for coronary artery disease in patients with resting ST-segment depression not associated with left ventricular hypertrophy, conduction defects, or drug effect.

Patients who had resting ST-segment depression on their baseline electrocardiogram, not attributable to left ventricular hypertrophy, conduction defects, or drug effect, had a higher prevalence of severe coronary artery disease and a poorer long-term prognosis than patients without resting ST-segment depression. Exercise-induced ST-segment depression continued to have discriminatory power for the diagnosis of coronary artery disease in these same patients. For the diagnosis of coronary artery disease in patients without a prior myocardial infarction, the criteria of 2 mm of additional exercise-induced ST-segment depression and the appearance of downsloping ST-segment depression during recovery were particularly effective in these patients. For the diagnosis of severe coronary disease in patients who had survived a prior myocardial infarction, the criteria of 2 mm of additional exercise-induced ST-segment depression and prolonged recovery ST-segment depression were better markers than standard criteria. Other criteria in addition to the standard criterion of 1 mm of additional ST-segment depression appear to improve upon the diagnostic accuracy of standard exercise testing in this group of patients.

Clinical implications in survivors of a myocardial infarction

It is clear now why postinfarction patients with persistent resting ST-segment depression have a poorer prognosis than patients without this abnormality: they have a higher prevalence of severe coronary artery disease along with decreased ventricular function. How does this finding affect clinical decision making? An argument can be made that if these patients already have a higher prevalence of severe coronary artery disease they should proceed directly to diagnostic coronary angiography, which allows identification of those who could benefit from a revascularization procedure. This is a possible option but may lead to unnecessary catheterizations and not be cost effective.[34] However, utilizing the criterion of an additional 2 mm of exercise-induced ST-segment depression or prolonged ST-segment depression during recovery more than doubles the odds of selecting those patients who actually have severe coronary artery disease. In patients whose clinical situation dictates conservative treatment, these exercise test criteria may offer a more logical strategy for postinfarction risk stratification.

ALTERNATIVE CRITERIA FOR PATIENTS USING DIGOXIN

When a patient is identified as using digoxin, he or she is usually considered to undergo exercise testing in concert with another imaging modality to eliminate false-positive exercise electrocardiograms, or that patient has his or her digoxin held several days before testing. However, some patients' heart failure may clinically decompensate off digoxin or lose heart rate control from an underlying atrial dysrhythmia (such as, atrial fibrillation). Furthermore, the improvement in diagnostic accuracy offered by these additional imaging modalities may be minimal whereas their cost is substantial.

Digoxin use at the time of exercise testing has been believed to invalidate the predictive value of exercise electrocardiography as a marker for coronary artery disease. Miranda and co-workers performed an analysis to ascertain if alternative methods of interpreting the exercise electrocardiogram could improve its clinical utility in these patients.[35] A retrospective study of 224 patients was undertaken, 200 patients not receiving digoxin and without resting ST-segment depression and 24 patients receiving digoxin at the time of exercise testing. Exclusions were women, left ventricular hypertrophy, left bundle branch block, prior myocardial infarction or revascularization procedures, or significant valvular or congenital heart disease.

Receiver-operating-characteristic curve analysis revealed that standard criteria of exercise-induced ST-segment depression had no discriminatory power in the patients receiving digoxin as a marker for coronary artery disease (area = 0.64, $z = 1.220$, $p = NS$). However, the criteria of exercise-induced ST-segment depression persisting 4 minutes or more into recovery (likelihood ratio 2.4) and the development of downsloping ST-segment depression during recovery of any magnitude (likelihood ratio 3.6) could allow better prediction of coronary artery disease in patients while receiving digoxin than the standard criterion of 1 mm exercise-induced ST-segment depression (likelihood ratio 1.6). Therefore alternative criteria to help in evaluation of the exercise electrocardiogram can improve its utility in patients taking digoxin.

An additional 1 millimeter of ST-segment depression was required in patients with baseline ST-segment depression. Three additional criteria for abnormality were considered in this study: an additional 2 mm of ST-segment depression, the persistence of abnormal ST-segment depression 4 minutes or longer into the recovery period, and the appearance of downsloping ST-segment depression during the recovery period. To fulfill this last criterion, no absolute amount of ST-segment depression was required, just the appearance of a downward slope. A standard criterion of exercise-induced ST-segment depression cannot discriminate between patients with and without coronary disease while they are taking digoxin. However, the alternative criterion of having the exercise-induced ST-segment depression persist to 4 or more minutes into recovery or exhibiting downsloping ST-segment depression during recovery were more likely to identify patients with coronary disease.

A metanalysis of 150 exercise testing studies over the past 22 years was performed by Detrano and associates to identify factors that affected the test's diagnostic accuracy.[31] There were 64 studies that included patients on digoxin during exercise testing, and 21 studies that specifically excluded patients on digoxin; both the mean sensitivity and the mean specificity were higher in the latter group of studies. A study by Meyers and co-workers also showed a decreased diagnostic accuracy of exercise testing in patients on digoxin.[10] These results agree with the present study in that the standard criterion of exercise-induced ST-segment depression is inadequate in the patient receiving digoxin to allow identification of coronary artery disease.

Data corroborate the Miranda study in that the patients receiving digoxin who do not have significant coronary artery disease do not have prolonged ST-segment depression in recovery (very specific). This is in agreement with previous observations by Tonkon and associates who studied 15 normal subjects, before and after the administration of digoxin, with exercise testing.[36] Fourteen subjects developed 0.1 to 0.5 mV of ST-segment depression with exercise, but the ST-segments normalized at maximal stress and remained normal throughout recovery. Sketch and co-workers studied 98 healthy males, 22 to 70 years of age, who were administered digoxin at 0.25 mg per day for 14 days and then underwent daily exercise testing until it was interpreted as normal.[37] Twenty-four subjects had an abnormal ST-response to exercise, and in 20 of them the ST-segment depression resolved less than 4 minutes into recovery. Sundqvist and colleagues studied 11 healthy people with a mean age of 28 years with bicycle ergometry while they were receiving digoxin.[38] Six subjects developed ST-segment depression that resolved quickly upon cessation of exercise and was not present in the first 2 minutes of recovery. Some subjects though apparently did redevelop ST-segment depression later in recovery, and the authors believed that this differed from the typical ischemic response.

BETA-BLOCKER THERAPY

Herbert and co-workers have demonstrated how the ST-segment response and diagnostic testing is affected by beta-adrenergic receptor blocker therapy.[39] In their sample of 200 middle-aged men referred for exercise testing to evaluate possible or definite coronary artery disease, no differences were found in test performance with the use of classical ST-segment criteria or the ST/heart rate index. With patients subgrouped according to beta-blocker administration as initiated by their referring physician, no differences in test performance were found. Therefore for routine exercise testing in the clinical setting it appears unnecessary for physicians to accept the risk of stopping beta-blockers before testing when a patient is showing possible symptoms of ischemia. Their results are illustrated in Figure 7-5.

INFERIOR LEAD ST-SEGMENT DEPRESSION

Miranda and co-workers found exercise-induced ST-segment depression in inferior limb leads to be a poor marker for coronary artery disease in and of itself,[40] as illustrated in Figure 7-6. Precordial lead V_5 alone consistently outperformed the inferior lead and the combination of leads V_5 with II because lead II had such a high false-positive rate. Blackburn and Katigbak studied 100 consecutive patients and found that lead V_5 alone detected 89% of ischemic ST-segment re-

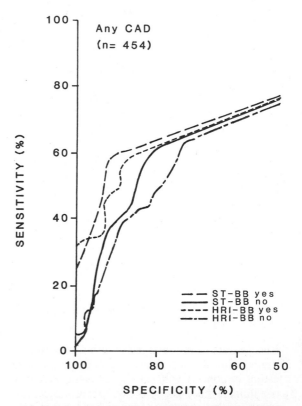

Figure 7-5   Range-of-characteristic curves comparing standard ST criteria (ST) to ST/HR index (HRI) for diagnosing any significant angiographic coronary disease in patients receiving or not receiving beta-blocker therapy (BB).

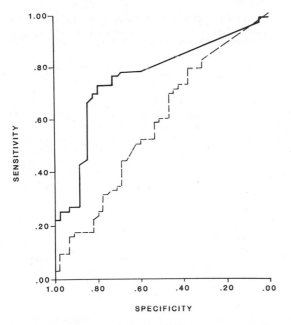

Figure 7-6 Range-of-characteristic curves comparing ST measurements using inferior leads (the dashed line is nearly straight) to lateral leads *(solid line)* for diagnosing any significant angiographic coronary disease.

sponses.[41] Miller and colleagues evaluated 44 consecutive patients who had both abnormal responses to exercise tests and perfusion defects on thallium-201 scintigraphy.[42] Thirty patients (68%) had ST-segment changes in the inferior leads, but all these patients had concomitant ST-segment changes in leads V_4 or V_5 as well, leading to Miller and colleagues[3] conclusion that monitoring of the inferior leads rarely provides additional diagnostic information. Mason and colleagues found that in 67 patients with angina who underwent exercise testing, 19 of them showed an abnormal ECG response in one lead only (a total of seven leads were monitored) and of these only two were isolated to lead II alone.[43] Miranda and co-workers had seven patients manifest ST-segment depression in lead II only, without concomitant electrocardiographic changes in lead V_5, and only three of these responses were true positives. Sketch and associates studied 203 men with both exercise testing and coronary angiography and found that lead II had a sensitivity of only 34%.[44] In evaluating body-surface potential distributions in 50 subjects with normal baseline electrocardiograms, of which 25 had documented coronary artery disease, Simoons and Block concluded that a single bipolar V_5 lead was adequate to diagnose ischemia in patients without a prior myocardial infarction and normal electrocardiograms at rest.[45]

These studies are all supportive of the findings that exercise-induced ST-segment depression in lead V_5 is an excellent marker for coronary disease and any inferior lead provides little additional diagnostic information. Riff and Carleton studied patients in atrioventricular dissociation and demonstrated that atrial repolarization can cause J-point depression in the inferior leads,[46] and this may produce the false-positive responses. It should be remembered that even though the inferior-lead ST-segment depression is not a reliable, independent marker for the diagnosis of coronary artery disease it is helpful for diagnosis of severe ischemia because multiple-lead involvement has been associated with multivessel[47] and left main coronary disease.[48] However, concomitant exercise-induced inferior-lead ST-segment depression may be an indicator of multivessel ischemia, but it does not localize right coronary involvement.[49] In patients without prior myocardial infarction and normal resting electrocardiograms precordial lead V_5 alone is a reliable marker for coronary artery disease, and the monitoring of inferior limb leads adds little additional diagnostic information. Exercise-induced ST-segment depression confined to the inferior leads is of little value for the identification of coronary disease.

SUMMARY

In studies that took into account the number of coronary arteries involved, all found increasing sensitivity of the test as more vessels were involved. The most false-negative responses have been found among patients with single-vessel disease, particularly if the diseased vessel was not the left anterior descending artery. No matter what techniques are used, there is a reciprocal relationship between sensitivity and specificity. The more specific a test is (that is, the more able it is to determine who is disease free), the less sensitive it is and vice versa. The values for sensitivity and specificity can be altered by adjustment of the criterion used for abnormal. For instance, when the criterion for an abnormal exercise-induced ST-segment response is altered to 0.2 mV depression, making it more specific for coronary artery disease, the sensitivity of the test will be reduced by half. For unknown reasons, the specificity of the ST-segment response is decreased when the test is used in women and in patients who have ST-segment depression at rest, left ventricular hypertrophy, vasoregulatory abnormalities, and mitral valve prolapse and when ST depression is isolated to the inferior leads. Standard criteria of exercise-induced ST-segment depression fail to distinguish between patients with or without coronary artery disease if they are taking digoxin at the time of exercise testing. However, persistence of exercise-induced ST-segment depression to four or more minutes into recovery or the development of downsloping ST-segment depression during recovery are better markers for coronary artery disease in these same patients. Patients who had resting ST-segment depression on their baseline electrocardiogram that was not attributable to left ventricular hypertrophy, conduction defects, or drug effects have a higher prevalence of severe coronary artery disease and a poorer long-term prognosis than patients without resting ST-segment depression. Exercise-induced ST-segment depression continues to have discriminatory power for the diagnosis of coronary artery disease in these patients. For the diagnosis of coronary artery disease in patients without a prior myocardial infarction, the criterion of 2 mm of additional exercise-induced ST-segment depression and the appearance of downsloping ST-segment depression during recovery are particularly effective. For the diagnosis of severe coronary disease in patients who had survived a prior myocardial infarction, the criterion of 2 mm of additional exercise-induced ST-segment depression and prolonged recovery ST-segment depression are better markers than standard criteria. An understanding of predictive modeling (the effect of disease prevalence or positive predictive value) and bayesian statistics (pretest and posttest probability and likelihood ratios) is important for the clinician. In addition, the rules by Feinstein and Guyatt outlined in this chapter are important for assessing new diagnostic techniques.

REFERENCES

1. Wilson RF, Marcus ML, Christensen BV, et al: Accuracy of exercise electrocardiography in detecting physiologically significant coronary arterial lesions, *Circulation* 83:412-421, 1991.
2. Pellinen TJ, Virtanen KS, Toivonen L, et al: Coronary collateral circulation, *Clin Cardiol* 14:111-118, 1991.
3. Detrano R, Leatherman J, Salcedo EE, et al: Bayesian analysis versus discriminant function analysis: their relative utility in the diagnosis of coronary disease, *Circulation* 73:970-977, 1986.
4. Morise AP, Duval RD: Comparison of three Bayesian methods to estimate posttest probability in patients undergoing exercise stress testing, *Am J Cardiol* 64:1117-1122, 1989.
5. Philbrick JT, Horwitz RI, Feinstein AR: Methodologic problems of exercise testing for coronary artery disease: groups, analysis and bias, *Am J Cardiol* 46:807, 1980.
6. Detry JMR, Luwaert RJ, Rousseau MF, et al: Diagnostic value of computerized exercise testing in men without previous myocardial infarction: a multivariate, compartmental and probabilistic approach, *Eur Heart J* 6:227-238, 1985.
7. Rosanski A, Diamond GA, Berman DS, et al: The declining specificity of exercise radionuclide ventriculography, *N Engl J Med* 309:518-522, 1983.
8. Detrano R, Yiannikas J, Salcedo EE, et al: Bayesian probability analysis: a prospective demonstration of its clinical utility in diagnosing coronary disease, *Circulation* 69:541-550, 1984.
9. Gianrossi R, Detrano R, Mulvihill D, et al: Exercise-induced ST depression in the diagnosis of coronary artery disease: a meta-analysis, *Circulation* 80:87-98, 1989.
10. Guyatt GH: Readers' guide for articles evaluating diagnostic tests: what ACP Journal Club does for you and what you must do yourself, *ACP Journal Club* 115:A-16, 1991.
11. Fagan TJ: Nomogram for Bayes theorem, *N Engl J Med* 293:257, 1975.
12. Miranda CP, Lehmann KG, Froelicher VF: Correlation between resting ST segment depression, exercise testing, coronary angiography, and long-term prognosis, *Am Heart J* 122:1617-1626, 1991.
13. Blackburn H: Canadian Colloquium on Computer-Assisted Interpretation of Electrocardiograms. VI. Importance of the electrocardiogram in populations outside the hospital, *Can Med Assoc J* 108:1262-1265, 1973.
14. Cullen K, Stenhouse NS, Wearne KL, Compston GN: Electrocardiograms and 13 year cardiovascular mortality in Brusselton study, *Br Heart J* 47:209-212, 1982.
15. Aronow WS: Correlation of ischemic ST-segment depression on the resting electrocardiogram with new cardiac event rates in 1,106 patients over 62 years of age, *Am J Cardiol* 64:232-233, 1989.
16. Califf RM, Mark DB, Harrell FE, et al: Importance of clinical measures of ischemia in the prognosis of patients with documented coronary artery disease, *J Am Coll Cardiol* 11:20-26, 1988.
17. Harris PJ, Harrell FE, Lee KL, et al: Survival in medically treated coronary artery disease, *Circulation* 60:1259-1269, 1979.
18. Schlant RC, Forman S, Stamler J, Conner PL, for the Coronary Drug Project Research Group: The natural history of coronary heart disease: prognostic factors after recovery from myocardial infarction in 2,789 men: the 5-year findings of the Coronary Drug Project, *Circulation* 66:401-414, 1982.
19. Lembo NM, Starling MR, Dell'Italia LJ, et al: Clinical and prognostic importance of persistent precordial (V_1-V_4) electrocardiographic ST-segment depression in patients with inferior transmural myocardial infarction, *Circulation* 74:56-63, 1986.
20. Schechtman KB, Capone RJ, Kleiger RE, et al, and the Diltiazem Reinfarction Study Research Group: Risk stratification of patients with non Q-wave myocardial infarction: the critical role of ST-segment depression, *Circulation* 80:1148-1158, 1989.
21. Wong ND, Levy D, Kannel WB: Prognostic significance of the electrocardiogram after Q-wave myocardial infarction: the Framingham Study, *Circulation* 81:780-789, 1990.
22. DeFeyter PJ, van Eenige MJ, Dighton DH, et al: Prognostic value of exercise testing, coronary angiography and left ventriculography 6-8 weeks after myocardial infarction, *Circulation* 66:527, 1982.
23. Sanz G, Castaner A, Betriu A, et al: Determinants of prognosis in survivors of myocardial infarction: a prospective clinical angiographic study, *N Engl J Med* 306:1065-1070, 1982.
24. Humphries JO, Kuller L, Ross R, et al: Natural history of ischemic heart disease in relation to arteriographic findings, *Circulation* 49:489-497, 1974.

25. Mirvis DM, El-Zeky F, Vander Zwaag R, et al: Clinical and pathophysiologic correlates of ST-T-wave abnormalities in coronary artery disease, *Am J Cardiol* 66:699-704, 1990.

26. White HD, Norris RM, Brown MA, et al: Left ventricular end-systolic volume as the major determinant of survival after recovery from myocardial infarction, *Circulation* 76:44-51, 1987.

27. Kansal S, Roitman D, Sheffield LT: Stress testing with ST-segment depression at rest, *Circulation* 54:636-639, 1976.

28. Harris JF, DeMaria AN, Lee G, et al: Value and limitations of exercise testing in detecting coronary disease with normal and abnormal resting electrocardiograms, *Adv Cardiol* 22:11-15, 1978.

29. Roitman D, Jones WB, Sheffield LT: Comparison of submaximal exercise ECG test with coronary cineangiocardiogram, *Ann Intern Med* 72:641-647, 1970.

30. Meyers DG, Bendon KA, Hankins JH, Stratbucker RA: The effect of baseline electrocardiographic abnormalities on the diagnostic accuracy of exercise-induced ST-segment changes, *Am Heart J* 119:272-276, 1990.

31. Detrano R, Gianrossi R, Froelicher VF: The diagnostic accuracy of the exercise electrocardiogram: a meta-analysis of 22 years of research, *Prog Cardiovasc Dis* 33:173-205, 1989.

32. Goldschlager N, Selzer A, Cohn K: Treadmill stress tests as indicators of presence and severity of coronary artery disease, *Ann Intern Med* 85:277-286, 1976.

33. Callaham PR, Thomas L, Ellestad MH: Prolonged ST-segment depression following exercise predicts significant proximal left coronary artery stenosis, *Circulation* 76(suppl IV):IV-253, 1987 (abstract).

34. Dittus RS, Roberts SD, Adolph RJ: Cost-effectiveness analysis of patient management alternatives after uncomplicated myocardial infarction: a model, *J Am Coll Cardiol* 10:869-878, 1987.

35. Miranda C: Alternate criteria for interpretation of the exercise test for patients receiving digoxin. (Submitted 1992.)

36. Tonkon MJ, Lee G, DeMaria AN, et al: Effects of digitalis on the exercise electrocardiogram in normal adult subjects, *Chest* 72:714-718, 1977.

37. Sketch MH, Moss AN, Butler ML, et al: Digoxin-induced positive exercise tests: their clinical and prognostic significance, *Am J Cardiol* 48:655-659, 1981.

38. Sundqvist K, Atterhög JH, Jogestrand T: Effect of digoxin on the electrocardiogram at rest and during exercise in healthy subjects, *Am J Cardiol* 57:661-665, 1986.

39. Herbert WG, Dubach P, Lehmann KG, Froelicher VF: Effect of β-blockade on the interpretation of the exercise ECG: ST level versus ST/HR index, *Am Heart J* 122:993-1000, 1991.

40. Miranda CP, Liu J, Kadar A, et al: Usefulness of exercise-induced ST-segment depression in the inferior leads during exercise testing as a marker for coronary artery disease, *Am J Cardiol* 69:303-308, 1992.

41. Blackburn H, Katigbak R: What electrocardiographic leads to take after exercise? *Am Heart J* 67:184-188, 1964.

42. Miller TD, Desser KB, Lawson M: How many electrocardiographic leads are required for exercise treadmill tests? *J Electrocardiol* 20:131-137, 1987.

43. Mason RE, Likar I, Biern RO, Ross RS: Multiple-lead exercise electrocardiography: experience in 107 normal subjects and 67 patients with angina pectoris, and comparison with coronary cinearteriography in 84 patients, *Circulation* 36:517-525, 1967.

44. Sketch MH, Nair CK, Esterbrooks DJ, Mohiuddin SM: Reliability of single-lead and multiple-lead electrocardiography during and after exercise, *Chest* 74:394-401, 1978.

45. Simoons ML, Block P: Toward the optimal lead system and optimal criteria for exercise electrocardiography, *Am J Cardiol* 47:1366-1374, 1981.

46. Riff DP, Carleton RA: Effect of exercise on the atrial recovery wave, *Am Heart J* 81:759-763, 1971.

47. Weiner DA, McCabe CH, Ryan TJ: Prognostic assessment of patients with coronary artery disease by exercise testing, *Am Heart J* 105:749-755, 1983.

48. Weiner DA, McCabe CH, Ryan TJ: Identification of patients with left main and three vessel coronary disease with clinical and exercise test variables, *Am J Cardiol* 46:21-27, 1980.

49. Mark DB, Hlatky MA, Lee KL, et al: Localizing coronary artery obstructions with the exercise treadmill test, *Am Intern Med* 106:53-55, 1987.

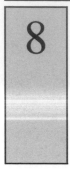

8 Prognostic Applications of the Exercise Test

RATIONALE

There are two principal reasons for estimating prognosis. First is to provide accurate answers to patient's questions regarding the probable outcome of their illness. Although discussion of the prognosis is inherently delicate and probability statements can be misunderstood, most patients find this information useful in planning their affairs regarding work, recreational activities, personal estate, and finances. The second reason to determine prognosis is to identify those patients in whom interventions might improve outcome. This is becoming even more important since the exercise test has been demonstrated to be of value in new subsets of patients including those with uncompleted infarcts because of thrombolytic therapy,[1] those with non–Q wave myocardial infarctions,[2] and those after unstable angina.[3,4]

Although improved prognosis equates with increased quantity of life, quality of life issues must also be taken into account. In that regard, it is apparent that in certain clinical settings, catheter or surgical interventions provide better therapy than medication. However, these interventions when misapplied can have a negative effect on the quality of life (inconvenience, complications, and discomfort), as well as creating a financial burden to the individual and to society.

Patients with known or suspected coronary disease are usually evaluated initially with exercise testing. It can be performed safely and inexpensively in the physician's office. In addition to diagnostic information, the test gives practical and clinically valuable information regarding exercise capacity and response to therapy. Patients with responses considered abnormal are frequently evaluated further by coronary arteriography. A study evaluating the appropriateness of the performance of coronary angiography in clinical practice con-

sidered angiography to be inappropriate 17% of the time mainly because of the failure to obtain an exercise test.[5] As will be reviewed, numerous investigators have indicated that responses to exercise testing allow prediction of the severity of underlying coronary disease and prognosis. However, exercise testing cannot allow one to predict angiographic findings or a poor prognosis with absolute certainty. Also, patients with certain known coronary pathoanatomic patterns are conferred a survival benefit from bypass surgery.[6] For these reasons, coronary arteriography has been considered the proper standard for evaluating patients for the presence of coronary disease and determining which patients might benefit from surgical therapy. Although understandable, it is unfortunate that determination of coronary anatomy has become emphasized to such a great extent over the functional correlates of this anatomy. Angiographic interpretation is subject to significant intraobserver variability and quantitative error. Angiography defines static anatomy since it is performed at rest and does not quantitate coronary blood flow.[7]

Why not perform coronary angiography on everyone? It is quite natural that when a cardiologist sees lesions in the coronary arteries there is a tendency to want to do something. An intervention is done under the assumption that an unnatural alteration in the blood supply is an improvement on nature. However, only patients with certain anatomic patterns have improved survival with coronary artery bypass surgery. They are those with moderately depressed ventricular function (from 30% to 50%) and angiographic lesions including left main occlusion greater than 50%, three-vessel disease, and left main equivalents. Left main equivalent specifically means those with 75% or greater lesions in the proximal circumflex and in

148

the left anterior descending artery before the first septal perforator. Since it is only patients with these anatomic subsets who have improved survival, it is important to select patients carefully for catheterization in whom intervention can improve the quality and quantity of life. Patients may be considered for interventions who do not meet the criteria if they judge the quality of their life to be unsatisfactory with medical management.

To deliver cost-effective health care, an effort has been made to use decision analysis to decide who should undergo cardiac catheterization.[8,9] Decision analysis depends on having accurate information regarding the predictive accuracy of the exercise test. This chapter begins with the pathophysiological basis of the exercise test responses and then follows with a discussion of the pertinent studies.

PATHOPHYSIOLOGY

The basic pathophysiological features of coronary artery disease that determine prognosis include arrhythmic risk, amount of remaining myocardium (reflected by left ventricular function), and the amount of myocardium in jeopardy. Arrhythmic risk does not appear to be independent but is closely related to left ventricular abnormalities. What exercise test responses are caused by myocardial ischemia or dysfunction? The exercise responses from ischemia include angina, ST-segment depression, and ST-segment elevation over ECG areas without Q-waves. Predicting the amount of ischemia (that is, the amount of myocardium in jeopardy) is difficult. It appears to be inversely related to the double product at the onset of signs or symptoms of ischemia. The responses attributable both to ischemia or left ventricular dysfunction include chronotropic incompetence or heart rate impairment,[10] systolic blood pressure abnormalities,[11] and a poor exercise capacity.[12] Their combined causality explains why they are so important in predicting prognosis. Exercise-induced dysrhythmias indicate electrical instability most often because of left ventricular dysfunction rather than ischemia (except for an ST-segment elevation in a normal ECG, which is very arrhythmogenic) and do not appear to have independent predictive power.

The only response specifically associated with left ventricular dysfunction is ST-segment elevation over Q-waves. This carries an increased risk in patients with Q-waves and indicates that they have lower left ventricular function and possibly larger aneurysms as compared to those with Q-waves without elevation.[13] If ST-segment elevation decreases with subsequent exercise tests, such patients are believed to have a better prognosis. Those with elevation over Q-waves have poorer resting left ventricular function than those without elevation.[14]

Previous studies have shown that exercise capacity poorly correlates with left ventricular function in patients without signs or symptoms of right-sided failure.[15] Exercise testing is not very helpful in identifying patients with moderate left ventricular dysfunction, which is part of the requirement for improved survival with surgery. This is better recognized by a history of congestive heart failure with use of a physical examination, resting ECG,[16] echocardiogram, or radionuclide ventriculography.

Can we answer the question, Who needs to undergo cardiac catheterization among patients with stable coronary artery disease? This is easy to decide when symptoms cannot be controlled, but otherwise it is often difficult to decide who should be considered for intervention to prolong life. Can we identify low-risk patients who do not need catheterization and high-risk patients who may benefit when it is feasible to attempt intervention?

STATISTICAL METHODS

To answer these questions follow-up studies must be performed and special statistical methods called "survival analysis" applied. Survival analysis comprises a group of univariate and multivariate mathematical techniques that involve consideration of the exposure time of each person and use that to calculate hazard or risk. The key difference between it and other statistical methods is censoring or removal from exposure. Censoring is done at the time of "lost to follow-up," removal from risk (that is, by CABS, PTCA), or termination of the study. The two most commonly used technique are Kaplan-Meier survival curves for univariate analysis and the Cox hazard model for multivariate analysis. Multivariate analysis is necessary because many of the variables interact. Univariately, variables can be associated with death, but the association may be through other variables. For instance, digoxin use associates through congestive heart failure, and exercise-induced ST-segment elevation associates with death most often through the underlying Q-waves.

The patient groups that have been studied to determine their prognosis using exercise testing include (1) patients after myocardial infarction, (2) patients with stable coronary heart disease, and (3) asymptomatic individuals. Patients after myocardial infarction and asymptomatic individuals are discussed in separate chapters.

PREDICTION OF HIGH RISK IN PATIENTS WITH STABLE CORONARY HEART DISEASE

This chapter is a discussion of studies using exercise testing in patients with stable coronary heart disease involving prediction of the following:

1. Angiographic findings
2. Cardiovascular disease end points
3. Improved survival with coronary artery bypass surgery

In addition, a special group of follow-up studies including variables from clinical assessment and the resting ECG, the exercise test, and cardiac catheterization that used multivariate statistical models to determine which variables best predict prognosis will be subjected to simple metanalysis.

Predicting angiographic findings

Which clinical characteristics obtained by a physician during an initial clinical examination are important for estimating the likelihood of three-vessel or left main coronary artery disease? To answer this question and determine whether estimates based on these characteristics remain valid when applied prospectively and in different patients groups, Pryor and co-workers examined clinical characteristics predictive of severe disease in 6435 consecutive symptomatic patients referred for suspected coronary artery disease between 1969 and 1983.[17] Eleven of 23 characteristics were important for estimating the likelihood of severe angiographic disease. These included chest pain type, previous myocardial infarction, age, gender, duration of chest pain symptoms, risk factors, carotid bruit, and chest pain frequency. A model using these characteristics accurately estimated the likelihood of severe disease in an independent sample of 2342 patients referred to Duke University School of Medicine since 1983. The model also accurately estimated the prevalence of severe disease in large series of patients reported in the literature. A similar study was performed by Hubbard and colleagues from the Mayo Clinic.[18] Five variables were found to be predictive of severe disease: age, sex, diabetes, typical angina, and history of prior myocardial infarction. An international cross-validation study was performed by Detrano and colleagues concluding that use of their algorithm could avert at least 10 angiograms on patients with less severe disease for every missed case of severe disease.[19] These studies demonstrate that the clinician's initial evaluation can identify patients at high or low risk of anatomically severe coronary artery disease. These important studies emphasizes that cost-conscious quality care can be accomplished by consideration of simple clinical variables to identify patients at higher risk for severe coronary artery disease who are most likely to benefit from further evaluation.

Table 8-1 includes some of the angiographic studies that have tried to predict left main disease using exercise testing.[20-22] Different criteria have been used with varying results. Predictive value here refers to the percentage of those with the abnormal criteria that actually had left main disease. Naturally, most of the "false positives" actually had coronary artery disease but less severe forms. Sensitivity here refers to the percentage of only those with left main disease that are detected. These criteria have been refined over time, and the last study by Weiner using the Coronary Artery Surgery Study data deserves further mention.[23] Weiner defined a strongly positive exercise test, as shown in the box. This was from a study of 436 consecutive patients referred for suspected or known coronary artery disease who were able to undergo both exercise testing and coronary angiography. All patients underwent treadmill testing using the Bruce protocol, and 12-lead electrocardiograms were obtained during exercise. A lesion of the left main coronary artery was considered significant if it had greater than 50% diameter narrowing and this criterion was 70% in other vessels. Fifty-five patients were excluded because of left ventricular hypertrophy, digoxin therapy, left bundle branch block, and the attainment of less than 85% maximal predictive heart rate (of these 55, two had left main coronary artery disease, and four had three-vessel disease; therefore the exclusion criterion had a predictive value of 10%). Four patient groups were defined by angiographic findings: (1) 35 with left main coronary artery disease, (2) 89 with three-vessel disease without left main disease, (3) 188 patients with either one- or two-vessel disease, and (4) 124 patients with no significant coronary disease. Of the 35 patients with left main disease, most had disease of other coronary arteries and nearly

---

THE STRONGLY POSITIVE RESPONSE OF WEINER FROM CORONARY ARTERY SURGERY STUDY

More than 0.2 mV downsloping ST-segment depression
Involving 5 or more leads
Occurring at less than 5 METs
Prolonged late into recovery

Table 8-1 Left main disease and exercise testing: studies evaluating the predictive value and sensitivity of the exercise test for identifying patients with left main coronary artery disease

Principle investigator	Year	Number with left main disease (total)	Criterion	Predictive value (%)	Sensitivity (%)
Cheitlin	1975	11 (106)	0.2 mV depression	24	100
Goldschlager	1976	15 (410)	0.1 mV downsloping	8	67
McNeer	1978	108 (1472)	0.1 mV in stage I and II	23	47
Nixon	1979	26 (115)	Angina or 0.1 mV depression at low work load	19 26	96 54
Levites, Anderson	1978	11 (75)	0.2 mV depression abnormal in stage I	50 24	82 63
Morris	1978	18 (460)	Exertional hypotension	14	17
Weiner	1981	35 (436)	Strongly positive Exertional hypotension	32 23	74 23
Blumenthal	1981	14 (40)	0.2 mV depression Anterior and inferior depression Exertional hypotension	38 57 75	100 93 21
Sanmarco	1980	29 (378)	0.3 mV only Exertional hypotension Both	15 15 27	24 28 35

Predictive value = % of those with abnormal response who have left main disease as defined by criteria; *sensitivity* = % of those with left main disease who have an abnormal response as defined by the investigators.

half had three-vessel disease. Exercise test responses that were considered included the amount of ST-segment depression, configuration, onset, and duration, and the number of leads in which it occurred. Hemodynamic responses included treadmill time, systolic blood pressure, and maximal heart rate. Other measurements included angina, premature ventricular contractions, and abnormal R-wave response in lead V_5.

Ninety-seven percent of patients with left main disease had at least 0.1 mV of ST-segment depression, and 91% had 0.2 mV or more of ST-segment depression. Patients with left main disease as a group were distinguished from patients with three-vessel disease by an early onset and longer persistence of ST-segment depression, as well as by a greater number of leads in which the depression occurred. A fall in systolic blood pressure occurred in 23% of the patients with left main disease versus 17% of those with triple-vessel disease and 6% of those with single or double-vessel disease. As an indicator of either left main or three-vessel disease, a fall in systolic blood pressure had a predictive value of 66% and a sensitivity of 19%. The criterion of 0.3 mV or more of

ST-segment depression occurred in 44% of such patients and had only a slightly lower predictive value (64%). Combined analysis of test variables (that is, a strongly abnormal response) disclosed that the development of 0.2 mV or more of downsloping ST-segment depression beginning at 4 METs, persisting for at least 6 minutes into recovery, and involving at least five ECG leads had the greatest sensitivity (74%) and predictive value (32%) for left main coronary disease. This abnormal pattern identified either left main or three-vessel disease with a sensitivity of 49%, a specificity of 92%, and a predictive value of 74%.

It appears that individual clinical or exercise test variables are unable to detect left main coronary disease because of their low sensitivity or predictive value. However, a combination of the amount, pattern, and duration of ST-segment response was highly predictive and reasonably sensitive for left main or three-vessel coronary disease. The question still remains of how to identify those with abnormal resting ejection fractions, those who will benefit the most with prolonged survival after coronary artery bypass surgery. Perhaps those with a normal resting ECG will not need surgery for increased longevity because of the associated high probability of normal ventricular function.

Blumenthal and co-workers validated the ability of a strongly positive exercise test to predict left main coronary disease even in patients with minimal or no angina.[24] The criteria for a strongly positive test included (1) early ST segment depression, (2) 0.2 mV or more of depression, (3) downsloping ST-segment depression, (4) exercise-induced hypotension, (5) prolonged ST-segment changes after the test, and (6) multiple areas of ST-segment depression.

Lee, Thomas, and Goldman used excellent statistical methods and included many clinical and exercise test variables.[25] A learning set and a test set of patients were studied. Only three variables were found to help predict left main disease: angina type, age, and the amount of exercise-induced ST-segment depression. Using a bayesian approach, the pretest likelihood of left main disease was best determined by the type of angina and age. Despite the many clinical markers considered, such as unstable angina, history of myocardial infarction, and others, only age and the angina type were found best to predict pretest probability of disease, as shown in Figure 8-1. The only exercise test variable that was found to then improve the posttest probability was the amount of ST-segment depression. As shown in Figure 8-1, there is a low pretest probability of left main disease in 40-year-old men with atypical angina and a high pretest probability of left main disease in older men with typical angina. Figure 8-2 shows how the amount of ST-segment depression affects probability. Given a pretest probability of, for example, 50%, the posttest probability could range from 20% to 75% according to the degree of ST-segment depression.

The problem with using the amount of depression as a predictor is that in many exercise labs an exercise test is stopped at 2 mm of ST-segment depression for safety reasons or because of severe angina. Also, some physicians stop the test at an age-predicted maximal heart rate. Surprisingly, exercise-induced hypotension and exercise duration did not affect posttest probability in their analysis.

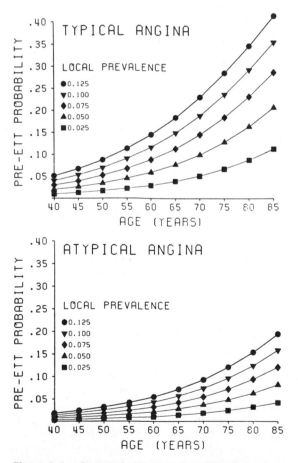

Figure 8-1 Range-of-characteristic curves for pretest probability of left main coronary artery disease by age, type of angina, and the prevalence of left main disease. (From Lee TH, Cook EF, Goldman L: *Med Decision Making* 6:136-144, 1986.)

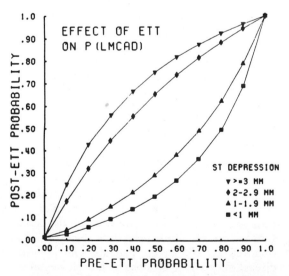

Figure 8-2 Range-of-characteristic curves for posttest probability of left main coronary artery disease by the amount of ST-segment depression. (From Lee TH, Cook EF, Goldman L: *Med Decision Making* 6:136-144, 1986.)

Metanalytic studies predicting angiographic severity

To evaluate the variability in the reported accuracy of the exercise ECG for predicting severe coronary disease, Detrano and co-workers applied metanalysis to 60 consecutively published reports comparing exercise-induced ST-segment depression with coronary angiographic findings.[26] The 60 reports included 62 distinct study groups comprising 12,030 patients who underwent both tests. Both technical and methodologic factors were analyzed. Wide variability in sensitivity and specificity was found (mean sensitivity 86% [range 40% to 100%, SD 12%]; mean specificity 53% [range 17% to 100%, SD 16%]) for left main or three-vessel disease. All three variables found to be significantly and independently related to sensitivity were methodological (the exclusion of patients with right bundle branch block, the comparison with another exercise test believed to be superior in accuracy, and the exclusion of patients taking digitalis). Exclusion of patients with right bundle branch block and comparison with a "better" exercise test were both significantly associated with sensitivity for the prediction of three-vessel or left main coronary artery disease. Unfortunately, this study did not consider the effect of the ST-segment criteria used.

Hartz and colleagues compiled results from the literature on the use of the exercise test to identify patients with severe coronary artery disease.[27] Pooled estimates of sensitivity and specificity were derived for the ability of the exercise test to identify three-vessel or left main coronary artery disease. One-millimeter criteria averaged a sensitivity of 75% and a specificity of 66%, whereas 2 mm criteria averaged a sensitivity of 52% and a specificity of 86%. There was great variability among the studies examined in the estimated sensitivity and specificity of a given criterion for severe coronary artery disease. This variability could not be explained by reported variations in study design. The findings indicate that the accuracy of the exercise test and other tests cannot be properly interpreted without much greater detail presented in the literature on patient selection and test administration.

Statistical methods for predicting disease severity. Controversy currently exists regarding the most appropriate statistical methods for predicting severe coronary artery disease. The most common methods employed include bayesian statistics and discriminant function analysis. The bayesian approach, which considers pretest clinical variables, is a logical method in clinical practice and helps one decide which tests are appropriate. However, most statisticians believe that discriminant function analysis permits a more robust prediction of disease. Since a previous study by Lee and co-workers using the bayesian approach found that the only pretest clinical variable with predictive power for left main disease was the type of chest pain and the only exercise test variable with predictive power was the amount of ST-segment depression, we decided to apply discriminant function analysis to determine if similar results would be obtained. The results of the Lee study were controversial, since pretest factors such as prior myocardial infarction and other exercise test variables, including exercise capacity and systolic blood pressure response, are considered important predictors of severe disease.[28] We also investigated the effect of various anatomic patterns of severe coronary disease that can affect the responses to exercise.

In a Veterans Affairs medical center, Ribisl studied 607 male patients to determine whether patterns and severity of coronary artery disease could be predicted using standard clinical and exercise test data.[29] We found significant differences in clinical, hemodynamic, and electrocardiographic measurements among patients with progressively increasing disease severity determined by angiography. Left main coronary artery disease produced responses significantly different from those of three-vessel disease only when accompanied by a 70% or greater narrowing of the right coronary artery. Discriminant function analysis revealed that the maximum amount of horizontal or downsloping ST-segment depression in exercise or recovery was the most powerful predictor of disease severity, with 2 mm ST-segment depression yielding a sensitivity of 55% and specificity of 80% for prediction of severe coronary artery disease (3VD plus LMD). Patients with increasingly severe disease also demonstrated a greater frequency of abnormal hemodynamic responses to exercise. Our findings also indicate that the exercise test will best distinguish left main or left main equivalent disease only when there is significant disease in the right coronary artery (that is, similar to three-vessel disease). Otherwise, the exercise responses are similar to patients with two-vessel disease. This data set was examined further to consider several other issues: correlation with a coronary jeopardy score, the effect of dividing the ST-segment shift by the heart rate change (the ST/HR index), and the effect of beta-blockers. Figure 8-3 illustrates the correlation of the maximal amount of abnormal ST-segment depression during exercise or recovery with the coronary disease score. It shows that

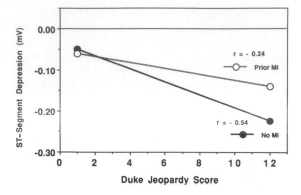

Figure 8-3 Relationship of Duke Coronary Artery Jeopardy Score (CAJS) with ST-segment depression in patients with and without prior myocardial infarction.

viable ischemic myocardium (no MI patients) "correlates" better with ST-segment depression than in patients with diseased vessels to dead myocardium (MI patients). Figure 8-4 illustrates that the exercise test does not function worse in patients selected for beta-blocker adminstration and that standard ST-segment analysis (ST) outperforms the ST/HR index (HRI) in either situation.[30] The ST/HR index findings are in agreement with the report of Bobbio and colleagues with 10 centers involved.[31]

Predicting cardiac end points

Summarized in Table 8-2 are two of the many studies that predicted prognosis in chronic stable coronary heart disease. The first study is from Duke University School of Medicine by McNeer and co-workers[22] and the other study is from the Coronary Artery Surgery Study (CASS) data by Weiner and co-workers.[23] Both contained over 1000 patients and had at least a 1-year follow-up period. Those at high risk in the Duke study had more than 1 mm of ST-segment depression at less than 7 METs; the risk was even higher if the maximal heart rate was less than 120. Those at

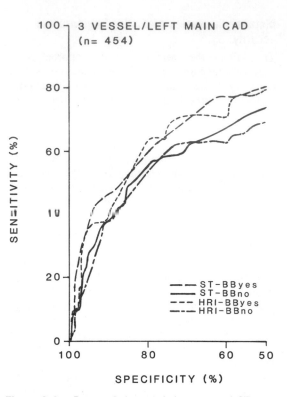

Figure 8-4 Range-of-characteristic curves of ST-segment depression and the ST/HR index in patients by their beta-blocker administration.

low risk did not have ST-segment depression, were able to exceed 13 METs, or had a maximal heart rate of over 160. CASS patients at high risk had markers of either congestive heart failure or ST-segment depression at a low work load. Patients able to exceed 13 METs were at low risk regardless of their other responses.

The study by Podrid and colleagues has placed some doubt on the use of exercise testing to identify high-risk patients.[32] They contend that the prevailing view "that patients with marked amounts of ST depression have far advanced mul-

Table 8-2 Two studies using the exercise test to predict prognosis in patients with stable coronary artery disease

	Patients	Follow-up period	High risk	Low risk
McNeer	1472	1 year	1 mm of ST depression at <7 METs (higher if MHR <120)	no ST depression or >13 METs or MHR >160
Weiner	4083	4 years	CHF or 1 mm of ST depression at <5 METs	>13 METs

CHF, Congestive heart failure; *MET,* metabolic equivalents; *MHR,* maximal heart rate.

tivessel disease and that CABS is the only way to improve their outlook" is in error. In their select group of patients with normal ventricular function who were referred because of profound ST-segment depression, they did not find a bad prognosis. In 142 patients with coronary artery disease and severe ST-segment depression with a mean follow-up of 59 months, there was only a 1.4% mortality and only 1.3% had coronary artery bypass surgery per year. This study points out that it is necessary to consider multiple variables when one is predicting the risk of ischemic heart disease. A relatively low-risk group can be found in any population identified using one risk predictor, by excluding patients with other risk predictors.

Dagenais and co-workers analyzed the factors influencing the 5-year survival rate in 220 patients with at least 0.2 mV of ST-segment depression during exercise testing.[33] They confirmed previous observations that survival was directly related to the duration of exercise: all patients who achieved 10 METs survived, and the patient survival rate declined in relation to exercise capacity.

Bruce and colleagues added to their analysis of the Seattle Heart Watch by applying noninvasive criteria, in a learning set for exercise enhanced-risk assessment for events attributable to coronary heart disease, to a test series in a later population sample.[34] In this series, subsequent follow-up study of 5308 men enrolled in the learning series of the Seattle Heart Watch during 1971 to 1974 were compared with findings from 3065 men enrolled from 1975 to 1981. Of the 8373 men, 4105, or almost half, were classified before exercise testing as asymptomatic healthy individuals. Another 1374 men had hypertension and 2894 had prior clinical manifestations of coronary heart disease including angina, myocardial infarction, cardiac arrest, or cardiac death. Men in the same age and risk groups for each pretest clinical classification showed similar gradients of risk. Age-standardized event rate showed a reduction longitudinally in healthy men and in patients who underwent coronary bypass surgery. It is important to realize that the majority of events occurred in men with only increased risk rather than high risk. The two exercise predictors of survival were duration of exercise and the ST-segment response.

Predicting improved survival with coronary artery bypass surgery

Which exercise test variables indicate those patients who would have an improved prognosis if they underwent coronary artery bypass surgery? The problem with the studies available is that the patients were not randomized to surgery according to their exercise test results, and the analysis is retrospective.

Bruce and colleagues demonstrated noninvasive screening criteria for patients who had improved 4-year survival after coronary artery bypass surgery.[35] Their data have come from 2000 men with coronary heart disease enrolled in the Seattle Heart Watch who had a symptom-limited maximal treadmill test; these subjects received usual community care, which resulted in 16% of them having coronary artery bypass surgery in nonrandomized fashion. The diagnosis of coronary heart disease was based on a history of angina, myocardial infarction, or cardiac arrest. Cardiomegaly was determined by physical and chest x-ray examinations. The patients were divided into three groups. One group had only myocardial ischemia manifested by exercise test–induced ST-segment elevation or depression or angina or both. The second group could have myocardial ischemia but had to have "left ventricular dysfunction" manifested by at least two of the following: cardiomegaly, less than 4 METS exercise capacity, and less than 130 mm Hg maximal systolic blood pressure. A third group had none of the above. Comparisons were then made within each group between the operated and unoperated patients, and surprisingly little difference was found. However, life table analysis showed a significantly higher survival rate of 94% at 4 years among the operated patients, as compared with the 68% survival of the unoperated patients in the group with left ventricular dysfunction. If the 4.6% death rate attributable to surgery in those with "ischemia only " was reduced, perhaps the patients who were operated on in that group would have had a significantly improved survival as well. Thus Bruce and colleagues demonstrated that patients with cardiomegaly, less than 5 MET exercise capacity, or a maximal systolic blood pressure of less than 130 would have a better outcome if treated with surgery. Two or more of the above parameters present the highest risk and the greater differential for improved survival with bypass. Four-year survival in this group would be 94% for those who had surgery versus 67% for those who received medical management (in those who had 2 or more of the above factors). In the European surgery trial,[36] patients who had an exercise test response of 1.5 mm of ST-segment segment depression had improved survival with surgery. This also extended to those with baseline ST-segment depression and those with claudication.

From the CASS study group,[37] in more than 5000 nonrandomized patients, though there were definite differences between the surgical and nonsurgical groups, this could be accounted for by stratification in subsets. The surgical benefit regarding mortality was greatest in the 789 patients with 1 mm of ST-segment depression at less than 5 METs. Among the 398 patients with three-vessel disease with this exercise test response, the 7-year survival was 50% in those medically managed versus 81% in those who underwent coronary artery bypass surgery. There was no difference in mortality in patients able to exceed 10 METs exercise capacity. From the Veterans Affairs surgery randomized trial, Hultgren and co-workers[38] reported a 79% survival rate with coronary artery bypass surgery versus 42% for medical management in patients with two or more of the following: 2 mm or more of ST depression, heart rate of 140 or greater at 6 METs, or exercise-induced premature ventricular contractions, or all three types. The results from those four studies are summarized in Table 8-3.

SPECIAL FOLLOW-UP STUDIES OF STABLE CORONARY ARTERY DISEASE

Clinical evaluation, exercise testing, and coronary angiography are routinely used by physicians to decide whether interventions are needed in patients with coronary artery disease. Since the pioneering studies from the University of Alabama,[39,40] numerous investigators have utilized clinical, exercise test, and catheterization data to predict prognosis in patients with coronary artery disease. Implicit in these studies has been the issue of which variables are predictive, and whether exercise testing or coronary angiography improve prediction sufficiently over clinical information to merit their performance despite their expense and risk.

Using discriminant function analysis, Oberman and co-workers found cardiac enlargement on chest x-ray film and a history of congestive heart failure to be the two most predictive independent clinical variables and that angiography improved prediction of death. They did not consider exercise test results because of incomplete data but found that those unable to perform the test had a poorer prognosis. Ellestad and co-workers[41] reported the predictive implications of maximal exercise testing in 2700 individuals followed from 6 months to 9 years. Both ST-segment depression and prior myocardial infarction were associated with subsequent higher mortality. This study did not require coronary angiography, and so work-up bias was not a problem.

From the Seattle Heart Watch, Hammermeister and co-workers[47] assessed 733 medically treated patients by going stepwise first through clinical markers and then through the exercise test. Congestive heart failure was the most important clinical variable, and the maximal double product was the most important treadmill variable. Maximal systolic blood pressure, heart rate, and exercise capacity were far less important. Cox's regression analysis showed ejection fraction, age, number of diseased vessels, and resting ventricular arrhythmias in that order to be most predictive. From Bad Krozingen (Mülheim), Gohke and co-workers[43] followed 1034 patients with coronary artery disease specifically to answer the question, can exercise testing provide additional prognostic information when angiographic information was available? They found exercise work load, angina during the exercise test, and maximal heart rate to independently predict risk of death. Exercise-induced ST-segment depression was only independently predictive in the subgroup with three-vessel disease and normal ventricular function.

From the Italian Multicenter Study, Brunelli and co-workers[44] reported their findings in 1083 patients less than 65 years of age followed for a mean of 66 months. They found clinical markers to stratify risk and that coronary angiography added prognostic information only in patients

Table 8-3   Studies evaluating exercise test responses indicate improved survival with coronary artery bypass surgery

Study	Markers of improved survival with surgery
Seattle Heart Watch	Cardiomegaly, <5 METs, and/or maximal systolic blood pressure less than 130
European Surgery Trial	ST-segment depression at rest, 1.5 mm of ST-segment depression with exercise, or claudication
Coronary Artery Surgery Study (CASS)	1 mm of ST-segment depression at less than 5 METs; no difference if 10 METs exceeded
Veterans Affairs Coronary Artery Bypass Surgery Study	Two or more of the following: 2 mm of ST-segment depression, HR >140 at 6 METs, exercise-induced premature ventricular contractions

with moderately severe disease. Q-wave presence and history of infarction were the most important clinical predictors (congestive heart failure was not considered). Exercise-induced ST-segment depression was not considered independently but rather was combined with angina and exercise capacity in order to create a marker associated with cardiovascular death.

From the Coronary Artery Surgery Study (CASS), Weiner and co-workers[45] analyzed 30 exercise test, coronary angiographic, and clinical variables in 4083 patients to identify predictors of mortality in medically treated patients with symptomatic coronary artery disease. This study was based on analysis of 16% of the registry of patients with no previous coronary artery bypass surgery who were able to undergo a standard or modified Bruce protocol within 1 month of their catheterization. During the mean follow-up period of 4 years, 212, or 5%, died. This represents a very low annual mortality, and approximately 40% of the patients had a prior myocardial infarction and 36% underwent coronary artery bypass surgery during a 3-year minimal follow-up period. Standard clinical variables including chest pain, congestive heart failure, physical exam, family history, risk factor index, drugs, and cardiac catheterization findings were included. Exercise test variables included limiting symptoms, premature ventricular contractions, peak heart rate, peak systolic blood pressure, ST-segment response, and final exercise stage. Thirty variables were analyzed in 4000 patients. Regression analysis demonstrated that seven variables were independent predictors of survival. A high-risk subgroup (annual mortality about 5%) was identified consisting of patients with either congestive heart failure or ST-segment depression and a final exercise stage in the Bruce protocol of one or less (5 METs or less). When all 30 variables were analyzed jointly, the left ventricular contraction pattern and the number of diseased vessels were the best predictors of survival. In a subgroup of 572 patients with three-vessel disease and good left ventricular function, the probability of survival at 4 years ranged from 53% for patients able to achieve only stage ½ to 100% for patients able to exercise into stage 5 (MET level of 10). Thus in patients with defined coronary pathoanatomy, clinical and exercise variables primarily relating to left ventricular function are helpful in assessing prognosis. The following are some of the univariate risk ratios generated by some of the variables: age greater than 60, 2.5×; prior myocardial infarction, 2.4×; congestive heart failure, 5×; cardiac enlargement, 9×; digoxin, 4×; less than stage 1, 2×; more than 0.1 mV ST-segment depression, 1.4×. The presence of congestive heart failure was the most potent clinical predictor of survival when the clinical and exercise test variables were analyzed. Two other significant clinical variables, prior myocardial infarction and cardiac enlargement, were also related to ventricular dysfunction. These results confirmed two other large studies involving multivariate analysis of clinical data. Hammermeister and co-workers identified the clinical variables of cardiac enlargement, use of diuretics, S_3 gallop, and congestive heart failure as predictive of survival among 47 variables analyzed from the Seattle Heart Watch study.

Mark and colleagues studied 2842 consecutive patients who underwent cardiac catheterization and exercise testing and whose data were entered into the Duke computerized medical information system.[46] The median follow-up period for the study population was 5 years and 98% complete. All patients underwent a Bruce protocol exercise test and had standard ECG measurements recorded. A treadmill angina index was assigned a value of 0 if angina was absent, 1 if typical angina occurred during exercise, and 2 if angina was the reason the patient stopped exercising. Before the test, 54% of the patients had taken propranolol and 11% had taken digoxin. ST measurements considered were the sum of the largest net ST-segment depression and elevation, the sum of the ST-segment displacements in all 12 leads, the number of leads showing ST-segment displacement of 0.1 mV or more, and the product of the number of leads showing ST-segment displacement and the largest single ST-segment displacement in any lead. To make the score apply to other treadmill protocols, it is necessary to convert minutes in the Bruce protocol to METs with the equation:

$$\text{METs} = 1.3 \text{ (minutes)} - 2.2, \text{ or minutes in the}$$
$$\text{Bruce protocol} = \text{METs} + 2.2 \div 1.3$$

Patients with ST-segment segment elevation in ECG leads with pathological Q-waves were excluded because this ST-segment response has a different meaning.

Six steps were used to derive the prognostic treadmill score. First, the patient population was randomly split into two groups: a training sample of 1422 patients and a validation sample of 1420 patients. Second, the Cox proportional hazards regression model was used in the training sample to assess the strength of association between the primary study end point (death of cardiovascular cause) and treadmill responses. Treadmill responses were then ranked using the likelihood ratio derived from the Cox model. Third, the most important treadmill response was entered into a Cox regression model, and the remaining responses were then entered in order until the model represented the independent prognostic information available from the exercise test. Fourth, the regression coefficients from this regression model were used to form a linear treadmill score. Fifth, the new score was tested to determine if patients with different levels of scores had a survival pattern similar to that seen in the training sample. Finally, the score was recalculated based on variables derived from the test results in all patients. Kaplan-Meier life table estimates were used to generate cumulative survival curves. Subgroup rates were not calculated beyond the point in the follow-up study when fewer than 15 patients remained at risk. All patients were considered to have been initially treated nonsurgically. In the 24% of the patients who had coronary artery surgery, the follow-up time was measured to the time of surgery. Data from these patients were then censored from calculations of survival rates. Seventy percent of the study patients were men, and the median age was 49 years. Two thirds had stable angina, and one third had progressive anginal symptoms. A history of myocardial infarction was present in 29%, and 22% had pathological Q-waves. At catheterization, 27% had three-vessel or left main coronary artery disease, and the mean ejection fraction was 60%.

The largest net ST-segment deviation recorded during exercise in any one of the 12 leads proved to be the single most important variable for predicting prognosis. After adjustment for maximum net ST-segment deviation using the Cox model, only two other variables contained additional prognostic information: the treadmill angina index and the exercise time. The results did not change substantially when patients taking beta-blockers or digoxin were excluded. The results also remained unchanged when patients treated surgically were excluded from the study. A score was calculated as: Exercise time − (5 × ST maximum net deviation) − (4 × Angina index), where exercise time is measured in minutes and ST deviation in millimeters. Patients at high risk with a score of −11 or lower had a 5-year survival of 72%. Patients at moderate risk with a score of −10 to +4 had a 5-year survival of 91%, and patients with a low risk score of +5 or greater had a 5-year survival of 97%. When total cardiac events were considered, the high-risk group had a 5-year survival of 65%, the moderate-risk group 86%, and the low-risk group 93%. The treadmill score contained prognostically important information even after the information provided by clinical and catheterization data was considered. The

prognostic stratifying power of the treadmill score was greatest in patients with three-vessel disease and lowest in those with one-vessel disease. Patients at highest risk have the greatest potential to increase their survival duration by having coronary artery bypass surgery. Patients with three-vessel disease and a treadmill score of −11 or less had a 5-year survival rate of 67%. Patients with three-vessel disease and a risk of this magnitude appear to gain a survival advantage through surgery. Those patients with three-vessel disease and a treadmill score at or greater than 7 have an excellent prognosis.

From the VA randomized trial of CABS, Peduzzi and co-workers[47] reported on the 7-year follow-up results of the 245 patients randomized to medical management who had a baseline treadmill test. Univariately and with Cox analysis, ST-segment depression (≥2 mm), exercise-induced premature ventricular contractions, and final heart rate greater than 140 beats/min were significant predictors. Unfortunately, they did not censor on interventions. These results are in distinct contrast to ours and other studies, since PVCs have not had independent predictive power, high heart rates have been protective rather than associated with risk, and they did not find a poor exercise capacity to be predictive; these unusual results might be explained by their failure to censor on interventions.

In Buenos Aires, Lerman and colleagues[48] reported 190 patients with exercise test and coronary angiograms who were followed for 6 years. Their study began in 1978; patients had a high annual mortality and a low rate of interventions yet exercise-induced ST-segment depression failed to allow one to predict prognosis. Maximal systolic blood pressure of less than 130 mm Hg was the strongest predictor.

Wyns and co-workers evaluated the independent prognostic information provided by exercise testing by calculating the survival rates with the life table method in 372 men referred for coronary arteriography.[49] A previous myocardial infarction was noted in 146, and 248 had typical angina. During a mean follow-up time of 29 months, 32 patients died and 27 patients had nonfatal events. Both typical angina pectoris or an old myocardial infarction and an abnormal exercise test (angina or ST-segment shifts occurred) had a significant prognostic value. In patients with a myocardial infarction or angina or both, the 5-year cumulative survival rate was 76% if the exercise test was abnormal versus 94% if it was normal. Cox regression analysis was performed, and by univariate analysis the age and the maximal work load were the only noninvasive predictive variables for survival or cardiac events. Exercise capacity provided prognostic information that was not available either from the history or from cardiac catheterization. Unfortunately, the ST-segment response was confused when both elevation and depression were confounded since angina and elevation over Q-waves was not excluded.

A second study from Saint-Luc Hospital in Brussels is worthy of discussion because patients with a prior myocardial infarction were excluded.[50] From 1978 to 1985, 470 consecutive male patients with complaints of chest pain underwent a maximal exercise test with a thallium scan and coronary angiography. During follow-up study (1 to 8 years) 32 patients died of cardiovascular causes and 30 had a nonfatal myocardial infarction. The average annual cardiovascular death rate was 2%. Of historical variables, only age was chosen as significant multivariately, whereas angina and pretest likelihood were chosen univariately. A maximal exercise test score based on maximal heart rate, ST60 at maximal exercise, angina during the test, maximal work load, and ST slope in lead X was chosen in multivariate analysis. This combined score is similar to the ischemic index used in the Italian study, which made a test abnormal if one or more of the following occurred: angina, ST-segment depression, or poor exercise capacity. These combined scores make it impossible to calculate the weight of individual measurements such as ST-segment depression or exercise capacity.

In a Veterans Affairs medical center, 588 male patients who underwent exercise testing and cardiac catheterization were followed to determine whether cardiovascular mortality could be predicted by clinical and exercise test data.[51] Over a mean follow-up period of 3.8 years (±1.4 years) there were 39 cardiovascular deaths and 45 nonfatal myocardial infarctions. The Cox proportional hazard model demonstrated the following characteristics to have a significant independent hazards ratio: history of congestive heart failure (relative risk = 4), ST-segment depression on the resting ECG (relative risk = 3), and a drop of systolic blood pressure below rest during exercise (relative risk = 5). Exercise-induced ST-segment depression was not associated with either death or nonfatal myocardial infarction. From cardiac catheterization, only the ejection fraction added independent information to the model. A simple score based on one item of clinical information (history of congestive heart failure), a resting electrocardiogram finding (ST-segment depression), and an exercise test response (exertional hypotension) stratified our patients for 4 years after testing,

from 75% with a low risk (annual cardiac mortality of 1%) to 17% with a moderate risk (annual mortality of 7%) and 1% with a high risk (annual cardiac mortality of 12%; hazard ratio of 20, 95% confidence interval 6× to 70×). This study demonstrated that variables available from the usual noninvasive work-up study of patients with known or suspected coronary artery disease enable prediction of risk of cardiovascular death. Three fourths of those usually undergoing cardiac catheterization could be identified by simple noninvasive variables as being at such low risk that invasive intervention is unlikely to improve prognosis.

Again from the Duke data base, Califf and co-workers[52] applied clinical measures of ischemia (exercise test results not considered) to predict infarct-free survival in 5896 patients with angina and angiographic (>75% lesions) coronary artery disease. The Cox regression model chose the following variables in descending order: more than 1 mm of resting ST-segment depression or T-wave inversion, frequency of angina, unstable angina, typical angina, and duration of symptoms. An angina score was derived from the Cox coefficients, and when entered into a model with catheterization data the following variables were chosen in descending order predicting survival: ejection fraction, number of diseased vessels, left main stenosis, angina score, age, and sex. This score helped predict prognosis even when the catheterization data were considered.

Detre and co-workers developed a multivariate risk function from the 508 patients randomized to medical treatment in the Veterans Affairs (VA) randomized study of coronary artery bypass surgery.[53] The variables, in order of importance, were ST-segment depression on resting ECG, history of myocardial infarction, history of hypertension, and New York Heart Association functional classification III or IV. Applying the risk function to medical and surgical patients of the 1972-1974 cohort yielded a 5-year probability of dying for each patients. Investigation of treatment effects in approximate tertiles obtained by collapsing the probability distribution into low-, middle-, and high-risk groups showed that surgery was beneficial for patients in the high-risk tertile even after removal of patients with left main coronary artery disease (17% surgical versus 34% medical mortality at 5 years; $p < 0.01$). This finding was accentuated when patients in the 10 hospitals with the lowest operative mortality (3.3%) were compared. Mortality results in the low-risk tertile favored medical treatment (medical versus surgical mortality 7% versus 17%; $p < 0.05$). The risk function predicted mortality well, not only for the

Table 8-4 Population descriptors including clinical variables and results from exercise testing and coronary angiography in the follow-up studies of multivariate prediction of cardiac events

Descriptors	LB VAMC (no cath)	LB VAMC	VA CABS	CASS	Duke
Clinical					
Years entered	1984-1990	1984-1990	1970-1974	1974-1979	1969-1981
Population size	2546	588	245	4083	2842
Age	59	59 (mean)	51 (mean)	50	49 (median)
Males (%)	100	100%	100%	80%	70%
Congestive heart failure	5%	8%	9%	8%	4%
Myocardial infarction	23%	45%	54%	40%	29%
Q-waves (at least one)	21%	37%	38%	22%	22%
Digoxin	8%	8%	NA	11%	11%
Beta-blockers	22%	35%	14%	40%	54%
Typical angina	21%	52%	100%	50%	47%
Exercise test					
% with 1 mm ST-segment depression	22%	58%	72%	44%	35%
% angina	4%	35%	66%	80%	50%
Maximal heart rate (beats/min)	137	124	125	138	134
Maximal systolic blood pressure (mm Hg)	175	159	156	171	160
METs	8.4	6.6	5.7	NA	7
Premature ventricular contractions	5%	12%	19%	12%	6%
Cardiac catheterization findings					
Three-vessel disease (%)	NA	14%	55%	23%	22%
Left main artery disease (%)	NA	7%	13%	7%	5%
No significant lesion (%)	NA	26%	0%	34%	40%
Ejection fraction	NA	60 (mean)		57%	60 (median)
Significant lesion criteria	NA	70%	50%	70%	75%
Follow-up					
Years	5	5	7	5	5
Coronary artery bypass surgery	2%	20%	24%	36%	24%
Annual cardiovascular mortality	1.5%	2.7%	NA	1.0%	1.6%
Annual total mortality	2.8%	3.5%	4.0%	1.6%	1.8%
Independent predictors of mortality by priority					
	CHF/digoxin	CHF	E-I PVCs	CHF	E-I−ST depression
	METs	SBP drop	MHR >140	Treadmill stage	Angina index
	Max SBP	Resting ST depression	E-I−ST dep >2 mm	E-I−ST depression	Treadmill time
	E-I−ST depression				

AP, Angina pectoris; *CABS*, coronary artery bypass surgery; *CASS*, Coronary Artery Surgery Study; *CHF*, congestive heart failure; *Dep*, depression; *E-I*, exercise-induced; *LB*, Long Beach; *METs*, metabolic equivalents; *MHR*, maximal heart rate; *MI*, myocardial infarction; *PVCs*, premature ventricular contractions; *SBP*, systolic blood pressure; *VA*, Veterans Affairs; *VAMC*, Veterans Affairs Medical Center.

Italian	Belgian	Belgian (no MI)	German	Seattle	Buenos Aires
1976-1979	1972-1977	1978-1985	1975-1978	1971-1974	1972-1982
1083	372	470	1238	733	180
49 (mean)	48	52	50 (mean)	52 (mean)	51 (mean)
90%	100%	100%	90%	80%	96%
Excluded	1%		Excluded	13%	Excluded
42%	39%	Excluded	>50%	40%	64%
37%	39%	Excluded	50%	45%	
	0%	Excluded	8%	18%	
	0%				
95%	67%	75%	95%	86%	71%
42%	27%	54%	56%		65%
60%	49%	44%	61%		60%
130	148	140	118	145	128
171	NA	186	182	160	151
5.4	9	8	5	6.5	5.2
15%	2%	NA		18%	21%
5%	34%	26%	33%	12%	44%
5%	8%	8%	0%		8
26%	18%	22%	0%	39%	0%
60	NA	65	60	60	
75%	50%	50%	50%	70%	75%
5.5	5	5	5	3.5	6
15%	28%	29%			9%
1.5%	1.8%	2.0%		2.6%	4.6%
2.0%	2.4%		2.4%	3.1%	
Q-wave	Age	Age	Exercise capacity	CHF	Max SBP <130
Prior MI	Exercise capacity	Max exercise score (−2 to +2)	Angina	Max double product	ST elevation
Effort ischemia		(MHR, ST60, AP, watts, ST slope)	MHR	Max SBP Angina frequency Resting ST dep	<4 METs Inappropriate dyspnea
Exercise capacity					

VA medical group, but also for an independent symptomatic coronary heart disease population from the University of Alabama arteriographic registry.

Why do these excellent studies fail to agree?

These nine studies have utilized clinical, exercise test, and catheterization data to predict prognosis in patients with coronary artery disease. Implicit in these studies has been the issue of which variables are predictive and whether exercise testing and coronary angiography improve prediction sufficiently to merit their performance despite their expense and risk. A careful literature search has yielded the nine studies in Table 8-4 for comparison. All used multivariate survival analysis techniques, and the variables chosen are listed in order of predictive power. Some investigators combined variables, whereas others did not consider key variables or excluded patients with certain clinical features (that is, those with congestive heart failure, those receiving digoxin). Nevertheless, two of the nine found a history of congestive heart failure, two found exercise systolic blood pressure, and one found resting ST-segment depression to be associated with death as we did. In contrast to our study though, three found exercise-induced ST-segment depression, and six of the nine found poor exercise capacity to be predictive of death. Unfortunately, for comparison sake, the Duke study did not have maximal systolic blood pressure collected for consideration. The choice of variables in the Cox hazard models from these studies is tabulated in Table 8-5. Age is not chosen by most of the studies, including ours, because of the narrow age range for patients submitted to cardiac catheterization. Exertional hypotension has previously been examined in our population and in the other studies reviewed. Notice, however, that this is the first time it was chosen by a Cox model rather than just observed univariately. Still not resolved though is the issue of whether the standing pretreadmill systolic blood pressure is representative of the patient's usual blood pressure.

Because of the differences in the variables chosen to have independent predictive power in the reported studies, we have presented their key characteristics in Table 8-4. Other than that the Duke population and the VA CABS study patients appeared to be more "ischemic," no obvious population, methodological, or test characteristics explain the different results. All studies had to deal with interventions that alter the natural history, but each censored on them as we did, except for the earlier VA CABS study. The first explanation that comes to mind for the failure of ST-segment depression to predict prognosis in ours and five of the other nine studies might be that the clinical process was highly effective in selecting high-risk patients with exercise-induced ST-depression for interventions. However, all patients were censored at the time of their CABS or PTCA and the same variables were chosen when the patients who received these interventions during follow-up study were excluded. Also, in the five comparable studies that did not find ST-segment segment depression to be predictive, this did not appear to be related to surgical intervention rates.

Ischemic exercise test variables clearly are related to ischemic events during follow-up study (that is, nonfatal myocardial infarction, CABS, PTCA). This is logical but of little help in clinical decision making, since the clinician has no trouble in justifying these procedures for patients whose symptoms accelerate after adequate medical management, given the established symptomatic benefit from interventions. The problem lies in justifying intervention to improve survival for patients whose symptoms are satisfactorily managed medically. Our study demonstrates that simple clinical indicators can stratify these patients with stable coronary artery disease into high- or low-risk groups. Cardiac catheterization is not needed to do so in the majority of such patients. Surprisingly, exercise-induced ischemic variables commonly believed by physicians to identify high risk did not do so in this veteran population, nor were they predictive in five of the nine comparable studies.

The following discussion of end points is an attempt to explain why the studies available for making clinical prediction rules do not agree. Cardiac death occurs in a spectrum between patients with myocardial damage who die of congestive heart failure (or pump failure) and those with normal ventricles in whom ischemia precipitates death. The clinical and test markers would thus be expected to be quite different for patients who die at the extremes of this spectrum. Although

Table 8-5 Metanalysis of prognosis in stable coronary artery disease studies requiring exercise test and catheterization ($n = 9$)

Poor exercise capacity	6/9
Congestive heart failure	3/9
ST-segment depression	
Resting	2/9
Exercise	3/9
Exercise systolic blood pressure	3/9

markers of myocardial damage (history of congestive heart failure, Q-waves) track the former, markers of ischemia (angina, ST-segment depression) better track the latter. Arrhythmias, poor exercise capacity, and exertional hypotension are associated with both. Further complicating prediction algorithms, "damage" markers predict short-term deaths, whereas "ischemic" markers predict deaths occurring 2 or more years later.

Given this etiological milieu, associating clinical and test markers with death as an outcome becomes quite difficult. We believe that our other ischemic events (that is, unstable angina, hospitalization for chest pain) were too soft for consideration. In addition, interventions, even if considered only an end point if they occur months after testing, are clearly related to the test response (that is, patients are submitted for interventions because of abnormal tests). Since nonfatal myocardial infarction most likely is an ischemic event, infarct free survival is another way of including more ischemic end points, but we had similar results when this was considered the end point in the Cox model. Differences in populations may have a higher proportion of one or the other type of mortality (pump failure versus ischemia). This may explain why ischemic variables are more predictive in one population and "myocardial damage" variables are more predictive in another. One could argue that our population included a majority of patients who died from congestive heart failure, however the same results were obtained after removal of patients who either carried that diagnosis or were taking digoxin at entry into our study; most of the other studies had a similar proportion of patients with congestive heart failure.

Work-up bias

All the aforementioned studies selected patients by requiring that they also underwent coronary angiography. To evaluate the effect of this selection process, the Duke group repeated their analysis in an outpatient population that did not undergo cardiac catheterization.[54] The same variables were chosen in their Cox model, and the same equation was derived. Similarly, we analyzed 2546 male patients who underwent noninvasive evaluation for coronary artery disease including exercise testing. Over a mean follow-up period of 2.8 years there were 119 cardiovascular deaths and 44 nonfatal myocardial infarctions. The Cox proportional hazard model demonstrated the following characteristics to have a significant independent hazard ratio: history of congestive heart failure or taking digoxin, exercise-induced ST-segment depression, exercise capacity in

METs, and the response of systolic blood pressure during exercise. A simple score based on these four factors stratified patients from low risk (annual cardiac mortality of less than 1%) to high risk (annual cardiac mortality of 7%).

The first Duke study used "inpatients" all of whom had a catheterization, whereas the second report included only outpatients evaluated before the decision for cardiac catheterization. Their score based on treadmill time, exercise-induced ST-segment depression, and angina score during the test performed as well for prognostication as it did in the first paper. Therefore "work-up" bias did not affect their prognostication model. We have attempted the same type of validation in this study. In contrast to the Duke group, we included exercise systolic blood pressure and clinical data in our model. Although history of CHF/digoxin was the most powerful variable in both of our VA studies, surprisingly, different exercise test variables were chosen. The model from our first VA study in patients selected for catheterization involved the choice of only exertional hypotension, whereas the model from this second VA study (only noninvasive clinical evaluation) found exercise-induced ST-segment depression, exercise SBP, and exercise capacity to have predictive power.

The "work-up" bias inherent in choosing patients for cardiac catheterization in our first study resulted in a sicker, older, more disabled group with a higher annual cardiac mortality (2.6% versus 1.5%). This second study included a population with a near normal age adjusted exercise capacity, whereas the first study population had an average age-adjusted exercise capacity 75% of normal. Age is not chosen by most of the studies, including ours, because of the narrow age range for patients referred for evaluation of coronary artery disease and its relationship to other variables.

Using stepwise selection, the Cox model was allowed to build on each variable group to arrive at the final model that chose history of congestive heart failure/digoxin, the change in SBP score, METs, and exercise-induced ST-segment depression. A score using the coefficients from the Cox model was then formed as follows:

5 × (CHF/Dig [yes = 1,no = 0]) +
(Exercise-induced ST depression in millimeters) +
(Change in SBP score) − (METs)

Three groups were formed using the score: <−2 (low risk), −2 to +2 (moderate risk), and >2 (high risk). The Kaplan-Meier survival curves are illustrated in Figure 8-5. This score enabled identification of a low-risk group (80% of the population) with an annual mortality of less than

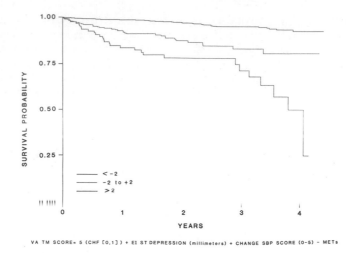

Figure 8-5   Kaplan-Meier survival curve for the Veterans Affairs prognostic score.

1% over the first 3 years after their exercise test, a moderate-risk group (14% of the population) with a 7% annual mortality, and a high-risk group (6% of the population) with a 15% annual mortality over the 3 years after their exercise test.

In addition, the Duke treadmill score was calculated. The treadmill angina index was modified because we did not have angina coded as the reason for stopping but was coded as "0" for not present and "1" as occurring during the test, and we used METs instead of minutes of exercise (DTMS = METs − 5 × [mm ST depression during exercise] − 4 × [Treadmill angina index]). In Figure 8-6 are the ROC curves for the Duke score and the VA score predicting cardiovascular deaths in the total group ($n = 3134$). The area under the VA score curve (0.76) was significantly greater ($Z = 2.34$, $p < 0.01$) than the area under the Duke score curve (0.68). Similar results were also obtained in the population presented in this study ($n = 2546$). These scores are summarized in the box.

Enthusiasm for a new technique (that is, car-

diac catheterization) may well have led to an acceptance of invasive measurements as superior to clinical variables for prognostication in patients with coronary artery disease. Although clinical variables were mentioned in the early studies, often key ones were not considered and they were not considered together or defined as accurately as they are today. It was assumed that laboratory methods and images were more accurate and precise than simple clinical data. Also, the importance of clinical data could have been underestimated because of the nonavailability of modern survival analysis techniques. A further consideration is that the decline in mortality by vessel score recently noted is not actually attributable to disease treatment but by patient selection (that is, excluding patients with congestive heart failure because of a better recognition of it).

On the basis of clinical and exercise test data, patients with signs and symptoms of coronary heart disease can be classified into low- and high-risk categories. The latter clearly should be considered for cardiac catheterization, whereas the

---

PROGNOSTIC SCORES

Duke score = METs − 5 × (mm E-I ST depression) − 4 × (TM AP index)

VA score = 5 × (CHF/Dig) + mm E-I ST depression + Change in SBP score − METs

Treadmill angina pectoris (TM AP) score: 0 if no angina, 1 if angina occurred during test, 2 if angina was the reason for stopping

Change in systolic blood pressure (SBP) score: from 0 for rise greater than 40 mm Hg to 5 for drop below rest

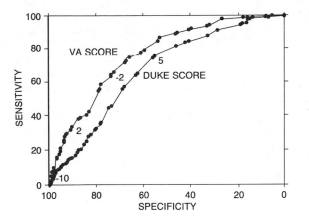

Figure 8-6   Range-of-characteristic curve for the Veterans Administration score and the Duke score for predicting cardiovascular death.

former should not, unless their symptoms dictate otherwise. The problem lies in justifying intervention to improve survival for patients whose symptoms are satisfactorily managed medically. Our study demonstrates that simple clinical indicators can stratify these patients with stable coronary artery disease into high- or low-risk groups. Cardiac catheterization is not needed to do so in the majority of such patients. In our VA population, we consider a history of congestive heart failure or digoxin administration and responses of three exercise tests as the most important predictors of cardiovascular death. Clinical judgment must be applied to decide whether intervention is likely to improve survival in our high-risk patients.

With the number of excellent outcome studies that have been completed but with divergent results to predict outcome, one must conclude that patient population as well as selection has a great effect upon results. Our results once again indicate that physicians may need to guide their practice based on studies of populations more similar to their own practices than previously believed and that populations selected for cardiac catheterization may not represent the populations seen in clinical practice.

Comparison to radionuclear techniques

Skeptics may say that the standard exercise test must be augmented by either radionuclide ventriculography or thallium scintigraphy. Most of the studies including these techniques have not compared them to clinical and routine exercise test results. Simari and co-workers[55] evaluated the ability of supine exercise ECG and radionuclide ventriculography to allow prediction of subsequent cardiac events in 265 patients with a normal resting ECG and not receiving digoxin who had undergone cardiac catheterization. The Cox model chose ST depression, exercise heart rate, and patient gender as equivalent to the radionuclide ventriculography data. They concluded that exercise radionuclide ventriculography was not justified for use over standard exercise variables. This is countered by Lee and colleagues[56] in 571 patients; radionuclide ventriculography provided more prognostic information than clinical variables. In an elegant review by Brown,[57] the prognostic value of thallium imaging was presented. Of the studies reviewed, the most comparable are those by Kaul and co-workers[58] and Melin and co-workers.[59] They concluded that the change in heart rate and other exercise test variables were superior to thallium defects for prognostication.

A limitation of these follow-up studies is an assumption of the Cox model that censoring is a random event. Interventions on which we censor are not random but linked to exercise-induced ST-segment depression as well as other variables. The effect of this on the reliability of the prediction model is unknown. However, all the other studies have had this same problem, and a true natural history study is not ethically possible. A multicenter observational study is needed to validate our findings, but it should also consider quality of life issues, including cost of treatment of ischemic events.

PROGNOSTIC STUDIES OF SILENT ISCHEMIA DURING EXERCISE TESTING

The preoccupation of many physicians with silent ischemia (that is, ST-segment depression without anginal symptoms) has come about because of four clinical observations: (1) the increased risk of coronary events when asymptomatic men are screened, (2) the frequency of painless ST-segment depression during exercise testing in patients with coronary heart disease, (3) episodes of painless ST-segment depression noted during Holter monitoring, and (4) the apparent high risk of painless ST-segment depression in patients with unstable ischemic syndromes. Its potential dangers include sudden death because of the lack of a warning mechanism and myocardial fibrosis because of chronic ischemia leading to congestive heart failure.

As for many other clinical syndromes, dividing into subsets can be very helpful. The types of silent ischemia described by Cohn are particularly useful:

Type I: occurring in asymptomatic apparently healthy individuals

Type II: occurring in patients after a myocardial infarction

Type III: occurring in patients with known coronary artery disease

Preliminary studies led to the hypothesis that "silent" myocardial ischemia had a worse prognosis than angina pectoris, since patients with it do not have an intact "warning system." However, in studies of patients referred for diagnostic purposes or with stable coronary syndromes, silent myocardial ischemia detected by exercise testing has been associated with either a lesser or a similar prognosis compared to patients with angina pectoris. Since exercise testing has advantages over ambulatory monitoring in regard to the leads monitored, chest pain description, and fidelity of the recording apparatus, confirmation of these findings would help resolve the controversy over the relative prognostic effect of silent myocardial ischemia. Exercise testing studies give us one means of evaluating the risk of silent ischemia. Unfortunately these exercise test studies do not evaluate patients with true silent ischemia. The patients are being tested because of some symptoms, usually angina. It's just that they do not have angina at the time of their test. However, patients with only silent ischemia are rare. Therefore the following data from exercise test studies gives us a good idea of how the usual patients seen in clinical practice with silent ischemia are likely to do.

For an evaluation of the significance of ischemic ST-segment depression without associated chest pain during exercise testing, data were analyzed from 2982 patients from the Coronary Artery Surgery Study (CASS) registry who underwent coronary arteriography and exercise testing and were followed for 7 years.[60] Patients with proved coronary artery disease (CAD) (at least 70% diameter narrowing) were grouped according to whether they had at least 1 mm of ST-segment depression or angina pectoris during exercise testing. Four hundred twenty-four had ischemic ST-segment depression without angina (+ST−AP or SI); 232 had angina but no ischemic ST depression (+AP−ST); 456 had both ischemic ST-segment depression and angina (+ST+AP); and 471 had neither ischemic ST-segment depression nor angina (−ST−AP). Sixty-three percent of +ST−AP (SI) patients and 55% +AP−ST patients had multivessel CAD (difference not significant). The 7-year survival rates were similar for patients in all groups (77%) except for −ST−AP patients (88%). Among patients with silent ischemia (SI), survival was related to severity of CAD. The 7-year survival rate was significantly worse

than that in a separate group of 282 patients with ischemic ST-segment depression without angina during exercise testing who had no CAD (95% survival). In patients with silent myocardial ischemia during exercise testing, the extent of CAD and the 7-year survival rate were similar to those of patients with angina during exercise testing. Prognosis is determined primarily by the severity of CAD. In patients without CAD, the survival rate is excellent.

At Duke, Marks and co-workers evaluated the clinical correlates and long-term prognostic significance of silent ischemia during exercise.[61] They analysed 1098 consecutive symptomatic patients with coronary artery disease who had both treadmill testing and cardiac catheterization. These patients were classified into three groups: group 1, patients with no exercise ST deviation (n = 856); group 2, patients with painless exercise ST deviation (n = 242); group 3, patients with both angina and ST-segment segment deviation during exercise (n = 600). Patients with exercise angina had a history of a longer and more aggressive anginal course (with a greater frequency of angina, with nocturnal episodes or a progressive symptom pattern) and more severe coronary artery disease (almost two thirds had three-vessel disease). The 5-year survival rate among the patients with painless ST-segment deviation was similar to that of patients with ST-segment deviation (86% and 88% respectively) and was significantly better than that of patients with both symptoms and ST-segment deviation (5-year survival rate 73% in patients with exercise-limiting angina). Similar trends were obtained in subgroups defined by the amount of coronary artery disease present. In the total study group of 1698 patients, silent ischemia on the treadmill was not a benign finding (average annual mortality 2.8%) but, compared with symptomatic ischemia, did indicate a subgroup of patients with coronary artery disease who had a less aggressive anginal course, less coronary artery disease, and a better prognosis. Thus silent ischemia during exercise testing in patients with symptomatic coronary artery disease represents an intermediate risk response in the spectrum of exercise-induced ischemia.

To evaluate whether patients with silent myocardial ischemia (SI) during exercise testing are at increased risk for developing a subsequent acute myocardial infarction or sudden death, the data on 424 such patients with proved CAD from the CASS registry were analyzed.[62] These patients were compared with 456 other patients with CAD who had both ischemic ST-segment depression and angina pectoris during exercise testing and with

1019 control patients without CAD. The probability of remaining free of a subsequent acute myocardial infarction or sudden death at 7 years was 80% and 91% respectively for SI patients; 82% and 93%% respectively for +ST+AP patients (difference not significant); and 98% and 99% respectively for the control patients. Among SI patients, the probability of remaining free of myocardial infarction and sudden death at 7 years was related to the severity of CAD and presence of left ventricular (LV) dysfunction and ranged from 90% for patients with one-vessel CAD and preserved LV function to 38% for patients with three-vessel CAD and abnormal LV function. Thus patients with either silent or symptomatic ischemia during exercise testing have a similar risk of developing an acute myocardial infarction or sudden death, except in the three-vessel CAD subgroup, where the risk is greater in silent ischemia. The risk of patients with silent myocardial ischemia is based primarily on angiographic variables.

Callaham and co-workers performed a study to determine the effect of silent ischemia on prognosis in patients undergoing exercise testing. In addition, this data set provided the opportunity to demonstrate if differences in the prevalence of silent ischemia and its effect on the prognosis of patients with silent ischemia could be explained by age or by their myocardial infarction and diabetes mellitus status. The design was retrospective with a 2-year mean follow-up period. The patient population was inpatient and outpatient referrals for exercise testing at a 1000-bed Veterans Affairs hospital. Exercise test responses were analyzed separately for the four subgroups: angina plus ST depression, silent ischemia, angina only, and no ischemia. Mean maximal heart rate, maximal systolic blood pressure, and maximal MET level attained were significantly higher for patients with silent ischemia than for patients with angina plus ST depression. Mean maximal ST-segment depression was significantly greater among angina plus ST depression patients than patients with silent ischemia. The prevalence of silent ischemia increased with age, whereas the prevalence of angina plus ST depression did not. There was a 7% prevalence of silent ischemia among patients less than 50 years of age, 17% prevalence in patients 50 to 59 years of age, 20% prevalence in the patients 60 to 69 years of age, and 36% prevalence for patients 70 or greater (Figure 8-7). Among 326 patients undergoing cardiac catheterization, the mean number of vessels diseased (two) and left ventricular ejection fraction (58%) were not significantly different according to ischemia status. During a 2-year follow-up period, 71 patients died, 68 patients underwent coronary artery bypass surgery, 51 patients underwent percutaneous transluminal coronary angioplasty as their sole revascularization procedure, and 13 patients underwent both coronary artery bypass surgery and percutaneous transluminal coronary angioplasty. Patients in the angina plus ST depression and silent ischemia groups had significantly higher overall 2-year mortality than patients without ST-segment depression. Overall mortality in the patients with angina plus ST depression and patients with silent ischemia was not significantly different.

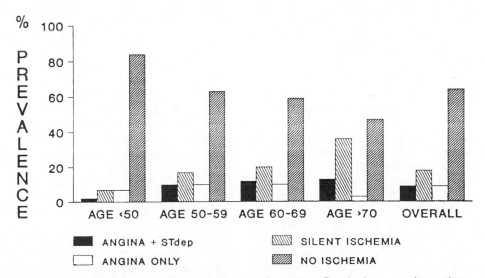

Figure 8-7   Prevalence of silent ischemia according to age. Results from exercise testing.

Maximal exercise capacity in METs as estimated from the work load achieved was not found to be independently associated with mortality. However, patients able to attain an exercise capacity of 8 METs or greater during the exercise test had a 1% 2-year mortality. On the hand, patients unable to perform 5 METs had a 9% 2-year mortality, and patients unable to exceed 2 METs had a 13% 2-year mortality.

We investigated whether prior myocardial infarction influenced silent ischemia and prognosis. Patients having recently suffered a myocardial infarction (within 2 weeks), and patients having suffered a myocardial infarction in the past (greater than 2 weeks) were grouped separately. No significant difference was seen in the prevalence of silent ischemia versus angina plus ST depression among the three groups. Prognosis was significantly worse among patients with a recent myocardial infarction particularly when ischemic ST-segment depression was present.

There were 93 insulin dependent and 87 non–insulin dependent patients with diabetes mellitus tested. Of those with ischemic ST-segment depression, 64% of insulin dependent and 61% of non–insulin dependent diabetic patients had silent myocardial ischemia. The prevalence of silent ischemia among the nondiabetic patients (60%) and that of the diabetic patients (62%) were not significantly different.

Mortality was significantly greater among patients with abnormal ST-segment depression compared to those without ST-segment depression. The presence or absence of angina pectoris during exercise testing was not significantly related to death. The prevalence of silent ischemia is not statistically different during exercise testing in patients with recent, remote, or no myocardial infarction, or insulin dependent or non–insulin dependent diabetes mellitus. Thus silent ischemia is associated with a similar prognosis as ST-segment depression associated with angina pectoris. These findings demonstrate that silent ischemia occurring with treadmill testing does not confer an increased risk for death relative to patients experiencing angina. Thus therapy should not be guided by the false hypothesis that patients with silent ischemia are at higher risk for death than those with angina and ST-segment depression.

Dagenais and co-workers[33] reported the 6-year cumulative survival in 298 moderately treated patients with exercise-induced ST-segment depression equal or greater than 2 mm. In those with silent myocardial ischemia, survival was 85%, whereas it was significantly lower (80%) in those with angina pectoris. Patients with silent myocardial ischemia reached a greater heart rate and

higher MET level than those with painful ischemia. Cumulative survival was very much related to the MET level achieved. Those who reached 10 METs had very few deaths, whereas those with less than 5 METs had approximately a 50% survival.

From these studies we would conclude that silent myocardial ischemia during treadmill testing does not predict increased risk for death. It appears that the concern that patients with silent myocardial ischemia were at higher risk than their peers with angina because of failure of their warning mechanism is not substantiated.

Coronary artery surgery study registry. To evaluate the significance of ischemic ST-segment depression without angina pectoris during exercise testing among patients with diabetes mellitus, Weiner and co-workers analyzed the data on 45 such patients from the Coronary Artery Surgery Study Registry.[63] These patients with silent ischemia were compared with 37 diabetic patients with both ischemic ST-segment depression and chest pain (symptomatic ischemia), with 31 diabetic patients without ischemic ST-segment depression or chest pain (no ischemia), and with 429 patients without diabetes who had silent ischemia during exercise testing. All patients had documented coronary artery disease (CAD) (>70% diameter narrowing). The 6-year survival among patients with silent ischemia was worse in diabetic than nondiabetic patients (59% versus 82% respectively). By contrast, the 6-year survival among patients without ischemia was similar among diabetic and nondiabetic patients. Among diabetic patients, survival at 6 years with medical treatment was 59% for silent ischemia 66% for symptomatic ischemia, and 93% for those with no ischemia. Survival among subsets of patients with diabetes and silent ischemia based on the extent of CAD and left ventricular function ranged from 100% to 32%. The survival of the 45 patients with diabetes mellitus and silent ischemia treated medically was compared with that of 28 patients receiving coronary artery graft bypass surgery. Survival at 6 years was enhanced by surgery compared with medical treatment among diabetic patients with silent ischemia and three-vessel CAD and either preserved left ventricular function (85% versus 52% respectively) or impaired left ventricular function (100% versus 32% respectively). These data indicate that, among patients with diabetes and CAD, silent myocardial ischemia during exercise testing may adversely affect survival and that coronary artery bypass graft surgery may improve the survival of diabetic patients with silent myocardial ischemia and three-vessel CAD.

Angiographic studies of silent ischemia

Visser and co-workers from the Netherlands studied 280 patients with anginal complaints, without prior myocardial infarction and with a positive exercise test response.[64] They were divided into those with exercise-induced silent myocardial infarction ischemia ($n = 67$) and those with exercise-induced angina pectoris ($n = 213$). Both underwent coronary angiography and were compared with each other with respect to various exercise and angiographic parameters. Patients with exercise-induced silent ischemia exercised longer and reached a higher peak exercise heart rate and a higher peak exercise rate pressure product than patients with exercise-induced angina pectoris. In the latter group, more patients showed exercise-induced ST-segment depression greater than 2 mm. The group of patients with silent ischemia encompassed more individuals with normal coronary arteries. More patients with exercise-induced angina pectoris had three-vessel disease. The exclusion of patients with normal coronary arteries (23% in those with silent ischemia and 6% in those with exercise-induced angina had no influence on the level of significance for peak heart rate, mean exercise duration, and exercise duration greater than 10 minutes. As in most other studies, exercise-induced silent myocardial ischemia is associated with better exercise performance and less extensive coronary arterial pathosis than exercise-induced angina pectoris is.

Miranda and co-workers performed a retrospective analysis of 416 male veterans referred for exercise testing who were selected for cardiac catheterization.[65] We found that exercise-induced ST-segment depression was a better marker for CAD than exercise test–induced angina and that symptomatic ischemia (ST depression plus angina) was a better indicator of severe angiographic disease than silent ischemia.

In the Program on the Surgical Control of the Hyperlipidemias (POSH), 838 subjects with hyperlipidemia who had one healed myocardial infarction were studied and followed for 6 to 13 years (mean 8.6).[66] Of the 417 control subjects, 279 had a treadmill test result that was definitely positive or negative. Angina was also included by exercise in 30% (45/150) and 8% (10/129) of those with a positive and a negative test result respectively. The data showed no difference between subjects with a positive or a negative test result with or without angina as regards levels of blood lipids, type of myocardial infarction (Q- or non-Q wave), left ventricular function, or prognosis as defined by death, atherosclerotic coronary heart disease death, or myocardial infarction.

The angiographic studies of silent ischemia reviewed by Miranda are summarized in Table 8-6.

In this review encompassing almost 6000 patients, a consistent finding was that patients with symptomatic ischemia had a higher prevalence of severe angiographic disease than patients with silent ischemia did.

Comparison of treadmill testing to ambulatory monitoring

In one of only a few studies comparing the prognostic value of the treadmill test and ambulatory monitoring, Tzivoni[67] followed 224 low-risk postinfarction patients for a mean of 28 months (range 12 to 58). Seventy-four patients developed ischemic changes during daily activity, of which 44 (60%) were silent, 14 (19%) were symptomatic, and 16 (21%) were both. All 74 patients had ischemic responses to treadmill testing, but, in addition, of the 150 patients with ischemic changes on the Holter monitor, 44 did show ischemia with the treadmill test. The incidence of cardiac events (that is, cardiac death, nonfatal myocardial infarction, development of unstable angina, coronary artery bypass grafting, or angioplasty) was significantly greater in patients with positive Holter and treadmill test results (38/74 = 51%) compared to positive exercise test results but negative Holter results (9/44 = 20%). As might be expected, the group with the least cardiac events had negative Holter and exercise test results (9/106). Interestingly, of the 74 patients with ischemic events on the Holter monitor, there was no correlation between symptoms (silent or symptomatic) and prognosis.

Most studies have used cardiac event surrogates such as angiographic findings or the need for coronary artery bypass surgery or percutaneous transluminal coronary angioplasty. Some studies have suggested that the standard exercise test for patients with coronary disease is just as effective as ambulatory monitoring, whereas others have not. Two representative studies that make an interesting comparison are those of Mody[68] and Mulcahy.[69] Mody studied 97 patients not taking antianginal medications. Sixty-three patients had no ischemia (poor sensitivity), 22 patients had 1 to 60 minutes of ischemia during 24 hours, and 12 patients exceeded 60 minutes for 24 hours. There was no correlation with exercise duration or time to ST-segment depression. However, prolonged ischemia on the Holter monitor correlated with the severe angiographic disease. On the other hand, Mulcahy found that in patients whose exercise test results were negative or who do not develop ST-segment depression before 5 METs rarely had silent myocardial ischemia during ambulatory monitoring. They found that ST-segment depression occurs at a lower heart rate with am-

Table 8-6 Studies of silent ischemia during exercise testing with angiographic correlation

Study	Number of patients	Exclusions	NOISCH MVD (%)	NOISCH 3V/LM (%)	APO MVD (%)	APO 3V/LM (%)	SI MVD (%)	SI 3V/LM (%)	STAP MVD (%)	STAP 3V/LM (%)
Amsterdam	92	No CAD, coronary stenoses <70%, normal ET	—	—	62	—	77	—	82	—
Deligonul	390	No CAD, coronary stenoses <50%, digoxin, LBBB, LM, LVH, failed PTCA	49	10	50	5	64	18	71	23
Erikssen	103	Coronary stenoses <50%, previously known CAD, other heart disease, HTN, DM, malignancy, musculoskeletal disorders, any other advanced disease	50	—	45	—	45	—	75	—
Falcone	473	No CAD, coronary stenoses <50%, digoxin, LBBB, CHF, valvular disease, variant angina, no exercise ST depression	—	—	—	—	85	56/5	84	55/7
Mark	1698	No CAD, coronary stenoses <75%, LBBB, exercise ST elevation, USA, valvular disease, congenital heart disease, cardiac surgery	—	27	—	37	79	48/12	88	60/12
Miranda	200	Digoxin, coronary stenoses <75%, LVH, LBBB, CABG/PTCA, women, prior MI, resting ST depression	16	6	13	9	50	20	51	30
Miranda	216	Digoxin, coronary stenoses <75%, LVH, LBBB, CABG/PTCA, women, resting ST depression	36	10	33	9	58	23	64	32
Ouyang	60	Coronary stenoses <70%, no exercise ST depression	—	—	—	—	74	29/11	81	54/6
Stern	480	No CAD, coronary stenoses <70%, no exercise ST depression, digoxin, "baseline ECG changes," valvular disease, cardiomyopathy	—	—	—	—	66	33	72	36
Visser	280	No CAD, coronary stenosis <50%, no exercise ST depression, LVH, LBBB, CHF, valvular disease, cardiomyopathy, prior MI, congenital heart disease	—	—	—	—	38	13	74	38
Weiner	1583	No CAD, coronary stenoses <70%	42	13	55	23	63	29	74	38

Table 8-6   Studies of silent ischemia during exercise testing with angiographic correlation—cont'd

Study	Number of patients	Exclusions	NOISCH MVD (%)	NOISCH 3V/LM (%)	APO MVD (%)	APO 3V/LM (%)	SI MVD (%)	SI 3V/LM (%)	STAP MVD (%)	STAP 3V/LM (%)
Weiner	302	Coronary stenoses <70%, digoxin, LBBB, LVH, valvular disease, patients without exercise angina or ST depression that did not achieve 85% of submaximal heart rate	21	—	67	—	51	—	94	—
TOTAL:	**5877**	**MEANS:**	**36**	**13**	**46**	**17**	**63**	**31**	**76**	**41**

APO, Angina pectoris only during exercise test; *CABG*, coronary artery bypass graft; *CAD*, coronary artery disease; *DM*, diabetes mellitus; *ET*, exercise test; *HTN*, hypertension; *LBBB*, left bundle branch block; *LM*, left main coronary artery disease is >50% narrowing; *LVH*, left ventricular hypertrophy; *MI*, myocardial infarction; *MVD*, multivessel disease (two-, three-vessel, or LM CAD); *NOISCH*, normal exercise test; *PTCA*, percutaneous transluminal coronary angioplasty; *SI*, ST-segment depression only during exercise test; *STAP*, ST-segment depression and angina pectoris during exercise test; *3V/LM*, three-vessel/left main coronary artery disease; *USA*, unstable angina pectoris.

bulatory monitoring than with exercise testing, but the results were highly correlated. Thus controversy remains whether ambulatory monitoring is superior to the standard treadmill test for evaluating silent myocardial ischemia.

Stern found that in 544 patients (299 with abnormal angiograms and 241 after myocardial infarction all of whom had abnormal treadmill tests) 47% had silent myocardial ischemia whereas 53% had chest pain.[70] The age, prior myocardial infarction, medications, number of vessels diseased, heart rate, blood pressure, and maximal ST-segment depression were similar in both groups. At 1 mm of ST-segment depression, patients with silent ischemia had a higher heart rate and exercise level, reached a higher double product, and had a faster recovery after exercise. However, if the ST-segment depression exceeded 2 mm, there were no differences between the two groups.

Flugelman studied painless persistent ST-segment depression after exercise testing.[71] There were 31 patients with angina and ST-segment depression. The angina pectoris disappeared at 3 minutes, whereas the ST-segment depression disappeared at 6 minutes in recovery. There was no change in this with nitroglycerin, and the persistence was longer in more elderly people. They found that silent myocardial ischemia persists after the disappearance of exercise induced angina pectoris.

The most important study is that of Hedblad and co-workers performed in the "'men born in 1914', from Malmö, Sweden."[72] It essentially shows that pretest probability (that is, chest pain symptoms) affects ambulatory monitoring for screening as it does for exercise testing.

SUMMARY

Why do the various studies fail to get the same results? Most likely the explanation lies in the fact that cardiac patients die in a pathophysiological spectrum ranging from those who die because of congestive heart failure (CHF) with little myocardium remaining to those who die from an ischemia-related event with ample myocardium remaining. Clinical and exercise test variables most likely associated with CHF deaths (CHF markers) include a history or symptoms of CHF, prior myocardial infarction, Q-waves, and other indicators of left ventricular dysfunction. Variables most likely associated with ischemic deaths (ischemic markers) are angina and rest-and-exercise ST-segment depression. Some variables can be associated with either extremes of the type of cardiovascular death; these include exercise capacity, maximal heart rate, and maximal systolic blood pressure, which may help explain why they are reported most consistently in the available studies. There is a problem that ischemic deaths occur later in the follow-up period and are more likely to occur in those lost to follow-up study whereas CHF deaths are more likely to occur early (within 2 years) and are more likely to be classified. Work-up bias probably explains why exercise-induced ST-segment depression fails to be a predictor in most of the angiographic studies. Ischemic markers are associated with a later and lesser risk, whereas CHF or left ventricular dysfunction markers are associated with a sooner and greater risk of death.

Rather than the differences perhaps it is better to stress the consistencies. One can assess risk by considering simple clinical variables. Greater than 5 METs exercise capacity, no evidence or history of CHF or ventricular damage (Q-waves and so on), no ST-segment depression, or only one of these clinical findings are associated with a very low risk. These patients are low risk in exercise programs and need not be considered for coronary artery bypass surgery (CABS) to prolong their life. High-risk patients can be identified by groupings of the clinical markers, that is, two or more. Exertional hypotension is particularly ominous. Identification of high risk implies that such patients in exercise training programs should have lower goals and should be monitored. Such patients should also be considered for CABS to improve their longevity. Intervention may not always be feasible, but it should at least be considered.

The mathematical models for determining prognosis are usually more complex than those used for identifying severe angiographic disease. Diagnostic testing can utilize multivariate discriminant function analysis to determine the probability of severe angiographic disease being present or not. Prognostic testing must utilize survival analysis, which includes censoring for patients with uneven follow-up study because of "lost to follow-up" or other cardiac events (that is, CABS, PTCA) and must account for time-person units of exposure. Survival curves must be developed and the Cox proportional hazards model is often preferred. How to test these models for confidence, accuracy, reproducibility, and power is controversial.

As shown by Stone and co-workers, the status of the right coronary artery greatly affects the hemodynamic and ST-segment responses to exercise testing in patients with multivessel coronary disease.[73] Left main coronary artery disease or left main coronary artery disease equivalents cannot be distinguished from 2-vessel disease when the right coronary artery is not diseased.

From this perspective, it is obvious that there is much information supporting the use of exercise testing as the first noninvasive step after the history, physical exam, and resting ECG in the prognostic evaluation of coronary artery disease patients. It accomplishes both of the purposes of prognostic testing: to provide information regarding the patient's status and to help make recommendations for optimal management. The exercise test results help us make reasonable decisions for selection of patients who should undergo coronary angiography. Perhaps some of the newer computerized ST-segment scoring techniques will enable an even more accurate prediction of high-risk patients. Since the exercise test can be performed in the doctor's office and provides valuable information for clinical management in regard to activity levels, response to therapy, and disability, the exercise test is the reasonable first choice for prognostic assessment.

REFERENCES

1. Topol EJ, Juni JE, O'Neill WW, et al: Exercise testing three days after onset of acute myocardial infarction, *Am J Cardiol* 60:958-962, 1987.
2. Benjamin ST, MacDonald PS, Horowitz JD, et al: Usefulness of early exercise testing after non-Q-wave myocardial infarction in predicting prognosis, *Am J Cardiol* 57:738-744, 1986.
3. Butman S, Piters K, Olson H, et al: Early exercise testing in unstable angina: angiographic correlation and prognostic value, *J Am Coll Cardiol* 1:638, 1983.
4. Swahn E, Areskog M, Berglund U, et al: Predictive importance of clinical findings and a predischarge exercise test in patients with suspected unstable coronary artery disease, *Am J Cardiol* 59:208-214, 1987.
5. Chassin MR, Kosecoff J, Solomon DH, Brook RH: How coronary angiography is used: clinical determinants of appropriateness *JAMA* 258:2543-2547, 1987.
6. Bolli R: Bypass surgery in patients with coronary artery disease: indications based on the multicenter randomized trials, *Chest* 91:760-764, 1987.
7. Marcus ML, Wilson FR, White CW: Methods of measurement of myocardial blood flow in patients: a critical review, *Circulation* 76:245-251, 1987.
8. Pauker SG, Kassirer JP: Decision analysis, *N Engl J Med* 316(5):250-272, 1987.
9. Knoebel SB: What we can't explain can hurt us and our patients, *J Am Coll Cardiol* 10:879-881, 1987.
10. Hammond HK, Kelly TL, Froelicher VF: Radionuclide imaging correlatives of heart rate impairment during maximal exercise testing, *J Am Coll Cardiol* 2:826-833, 1983.
11. Dubach P, Froelicher VF, Klein J, et al: Exercise-induced hypotension in a male population: criteria, causes, and prognosis, *Circulation* 78:1380-1387, 1988.
12. Morris CK, Ueshima K, Kawaguchi T, et al: The prognostic value of exercise capacity: a review of the literature, *Am Heart J* 122:1423-1430, 1991.
13. Stone PH, Turi ZG, Muller JE, et al: Prognostic significance of the treadmill exercise test performance 6 months after myocardial infarction, *J Am Coll Cardiol* 8:1007-1017, 1986.
14. Haines DE, Beller GA, Watson DD, et al: Exercise-induced ST segment evaluation 2 weeks after uncomplicated myocardial infarction: contributing factors and prognostic significance, *J Am Coll Cardiol* 9:996-1003, 1987.
15. McKirnan MD, Sullivan M, Jensen D, Froelicher VF: Treadmill performance and cardiac function in selected patients with coronary heart disease, *J Am Coll Cardiol* 3:253-261, 1984.
16. Bounous EP, Califf RM, Harrell FE Jr, et al: Prognostic value of the simplified Selvester QRS score in patients with coronary artery disease, *J Am Coll Cardiol* 11:35-41, 1988.

17. Pryor DB, Shaw L, Harrell FE, et al: Estimating the likelihood of severe coronary artery disease, *Am J Med* 90:553-562, 1991.

18. Hubbard BL, Gibbons RJ, Lapeyre AC III, et al: Identification of severe coronary artery disease using simple clinical parameters, *Arch Intern Med*, 152(2):309-312, 1992.

19. Detrano R, Janosi A, Steinbrunn W, et al: Algorithm to predict triple-vessel/left main coronary artery disease in patients without myocardial infarction: an international cross validation, *Circulation* 83(5 suppl III):III-89-96, 1991.

20. Cheitlin MD, Davia JE, de Castro CM, et al: Correlation of "critical" left coronary artery lesions with positive submaximal exercise tests in patients with chest pain, *Am Heart J* 89(3):305-310, 1975.

21. Goldschlager N, Selzer A, Cohn K: Treadmill stress tests as indicators of presence and severity of coronary artery disease, *Ann Intern Med* 85:277-286, 1976.

22. McNeer JF, Margolis JR, Lee KL, et al: The role of the exercise test in the evaluation of patients for ischemic heart disease, *Circulation* 57:64-70, 1978.

23. Weiner DA, McCabe CH, Ryan TJ: Identification of patients with left main and three vessel coronary disease with clinical and exercise test variables, *Am J Cardiol* 46:21-27, 1980.

24. Blumenthal DS, Weiss JL, Mellits ED, Gerstenblith G: The predictive value of a strongly positive stress test in patients with minimal symptoms, *Am J Med* 70:1005-1010, 1981.

25. Lee TH, EF Cook, Goldman L: Prospective evaluation of a clinical and exercise-test model for the prediction of left main coronary artery disease, *Med Decision Making* 6:136-144, 1986.

26. Detrano R, Gianrossi R, Mulvihill D, et al: Exercise-induced ST segment depression in the diagnosis of multi vessel coronary disease: a meta-analysis, *J Am Coll Cardiol* 14:1501-1508, 1989.

27. Hartz A, Gammaitoni C, Young M: Quantitative analysis of the exercise tolerance test for determining the severity of coronary artery disease, *Int J Cardiol* 24:63-71, 1989.

28. Schlant RC, Blomqvist CG, Brandenburg RO, et al: Guidelines for exercise testing: a report of the joint American College of Cardiology/American Heart Association Task Force on Assessment of Cardiovascular Procedures (Subcommittee on Exercise Testing), *Circulation* 74:653A-667A, 1986.

29. Ribisl PM, Morris CK, Kawaguchi T, et al: Angiographic patterns and severe coronary artery disease, *Arch Intern Med* 152:1618-1624, 1992.

30. Herbert, Dubach P, Lehmann KG, Froelicher VF: Effect of beta-blockade on the interpretation of the exercise ECG: ST level versus ΔST/HR index, *Am Heart J* 122(4 Pt 1):993-1000, 1991.

31. Bobbio M, Detrano R, Schmid JJ, et al: Exercise-induced ST depression and ST/heart rate index to predict triple-vessel or left main coronary disease: a multicenter analysis, *J Am Coll Cardiol* 19:11-18, 1992.

32. Podrid PJ, Graboys T, Lown B: Prognosis of medically treated patients with coronary artery disease with profound ST segment depression during exercise testing, *N Engl J Med* 305:111, 1981.

33. Dagenais GR, Rouleau JR, Christen A, Fabia J: Survival of patients with a strongly positive exercise electrocardiogram, *Circulation* 65:452-456, 1982.

34. Bruce RA, Fisher LD, Hossack KF: Validation of exercise-enhanced risk assessment of coronary heart disease events: longitudinal changes in incidence in Seattle community practice, *J Am Coll Cardiol* 5:875-881, 1985.

35. Bruce RA, Hossack KF, DeRouen TA, Hofer V: Enhanced risk assessment for primary coronary heart disease events by maximal exercise testing: 10 years' experience of Seattle Heart Watch, *J Am Coll Cardiol* 2:565-573, 1983.

36. European Cooperative Group: Long-term results of prospective randomized study of coronary artery bypass surgery in stable angina pectoris, *Lancet* 1:1173-1180, 1982.

37. Weiner DA, Ryan TJ, McCabe CH, et al: The role of exercise testing in identifying patients with improved survival after coronary artery bypass surgery, *J Am Coll Cardiol* 8(4):741-748, 1986.

38. Hultgran HN, Peduzzi P, Detre K, Takaro T: The 5 year effect of bypass surgery on relief of angina and exercise performance, *Circulation* 72:V79-V83, 1985.

39. Oberman A, Jones WB, Riley CP, et al: Natural history of coronary artery disease, *Bull NY Acad Med* 48:1109-1025, 1972.

40. Reeves TJ, Oberman A, Jones WB, Sheffield LT: Natural history of angina pectoris, *Am J Cardiol* 33:423-430, 1974.

41. Ellestad M, Wan M: Prediction implications of stress testing, *Circulation* 51:363-369, 1975.

42. Hammermeister KE, DeRouen TA, Dodge HT: Variables predictive of survival in patients with coronary disease: selection by univariate and multivariate analyses from the clinical, electrocardiographic, exercise, arteriographic, and quantitative angiographic evaluation, *Circulation* 59:421-430, 1979.

43. Gohike H, Samek L, Betz P, Roskamm H: Exercise testing provides additional prognostic information in angiographically defined subgroups of patients with coronary artery disease, *Circulation* 68:979-985, 1983.

44. Brunelli C, Cristofani R, L'Abbate A, for the ODI Study Group: Long-term survival in medically treated patients with ischemic heart disease and prognostic importance of clinical and electrocardiographic data (the Italian CNR Multicenter Prospective Study OD1), *Eur Heart J* 10:292-303, 1989.

45. Weiner DA, Ryan T, McCabe CH, et al: Prognostic importance of a clinical profile and exercise test in medically treated patients with coronary artery disease, *J Am Coll Cardiol* 3:772-779, 1984.

46. Mark DB, Hlatky MA, Harrell FE, et al: Exercise treadmill score for predicting prognosis in coronary artery disease, *Ann Intern Med* 106:793-800, 1987.

47. Peduzzi P, Hultgren H, Thomsen J, Angell W: Prognostic value of baseline exercise tests, *Prog Cardiovasc Dis* 28:285-292, 1986.

48. Lerman J, Svetlize H, Capris T, Perosio A: Follow-up of patients after exercise test and catheterization, *Medicina* (Buenos Aires) 46:201-211, 1986.

49. Wyns W, Musschaert-Beauthier E, van Domburg R, et al: Prognostic value of symptom limited exercise testing in men with a high prevalence of coronary artery disease, *Eur Heart J* 6:939-945, 1985.

50. Detry JM, Luwaert J, Melin J, et al: Non-invasive data provide independent prognostic information in patients with chest pain without previous myocardial infarction: findings in male patients who have had cardiac catheterization, *Eur Heart J* 9:418-426, 1988.

51. Brown M, Thomas R, McDonald T, et al: Risk stratification of cardiovascular mortality in patients with stable coronary artery disease, *Circulation* 86(4 suppl I):I-138, 1992.

52. Califf RM, Mark DB, Harrell FE, et al: Importance of clinical measures of ischemia in the prognosis of patients with documented coronary artery disease, *J Am Coll Cardiol* 11:20-26, 1988.

53. Detre K, Peduzzi P, Murphy M, et al: Effect of bypass

surgery on survival in patients in low- and high-risk subgroups delineated by the use of simple clinical variables, *Circulation* 63:1329-1338, 1981.

54. Mark DB, Shaw L, Harrell FE Jr, et al: Prognostic value of a treadmill exercise score in outpatients with suspected coronary artery disease, *N Engl J Med* 325:849-853, 1991.

55. Simari RD, Miller TD, Zinsmeister AR, Gibbons RJ: Capabilities of supine exercise electrocardiography versus exercise radionuclide angiography in predicting coronary events, *Am J Cardiol* 67:573-577, 1991.

56. Lee KL, Pryor DB, Pieper KS, et al: Prognostic value of radionuclide angiography in medically treated patients with coronary artery disease: a comparison with clinical and catheterization variables, *Circulation* 82:1705-1717, 1990.

57. Brown KA: Prognostic value of thallium-201 myocardial perfusion imaging: a diagnostic tool comes of age, *Circulation* 83:363-381, 1991.

58. Kaul S, Lilly DR, Gasho JA, et al: Prognostic utility of the exercise thallium-201 test in ambulatory patients with chest pain, *Circulation* 77:745-748, 1988.

59. Melin JA, Robert A, Luwaert R, et al: Additional prognostic value of exercise testing and thallium-201 scintigraphy in catheterized patients without previous myocardial infarction, *Int J Cardiol* 27:235-243, 1990.

60. Weiner DA, Ryan TJ, McCabe CH, et al: Significance of silent myocardial ischemia during exercise testing in patients with coronary artery disease, *Am J Cardiol* 59:725-729, 1987.

61. Mark DB, Hlatky MA, Califf RM, et al: Painless exercise ST deviation on the treadmill: long-term prognosis, *J Am Coll Cardiol* 14:885-892, 1989.

62. Weiner DA, Ryan TJ, McCabe CH, et al: Risk of developing an acute myocardial infarction or sudden coronary death in patients with exercise-induced silent myocardial ischemia: a report form the Coronary Artery Surgery Study (CASS) Registry, *Am J Cardiol* 62:1155-1158, 1988.

63. Weiner DA, Ryan TJ, Parsons, L, et al: Significance of silent myocardial ischemia during exercise testing in patients with diabetes mellitus: a report from the Coronary Artery Surgery Study (CASS) Registry, *Am J Cardiol* 68:729-734, 1991.

64. Visser FC, van Leeuwen FT, Cernohorsky B, et al: Silent versus symptomatic myocardial ischemia during exercise testing: a comparison with coronary angiographic findings, *Int J Cardiol* 27:71-78, 1990.

65. Miranda C, Lehmann K, Lachterman B, et al: Comparison of silent and symptomatic ischemia during exercise testing in men, *Ann Intern Med* 114:649-656, 1991.

66. Karnegis JN, Matts JP, Tuna N, Amplatz K, and the POSCH Group: Positive and negative exercise test results with and without exercise-induced angina in patients with one healed myocardial infarction: analysis of baseline variables and long-term prognosis, *Am Heart J* 122:701-708, 1991.

67. Tzivoni D, Gavish A, Zin D, et al: Prognostic significance of ischemia episodes in patients with previous myocardial infarction, *Am J Cardiol* 62:661 664, 1988.

68. Mody FV, Nademanee K, Intarachot V, et al: Severity of silent myocardial ischemia on ambulatory electrocardiographic monitoring in patients with stable angina pectoris: relation to prognostic determinants during exercise stress testing and coronary angiography, *J Am Coll Cardiol* 12:1169-1176, 1988.

69. Mulcahy D, Keegan J, Crean P, et al: Silent myocardial ischemia in chronic stable angina: a study of its frequency and characteristics in 150 patients, *Br Heart J* 60:417-423, 1988.

70. Stern S, Weisz G, Gavish A, et al: Comparison between silent and symptomatic ischemia during exercise testing in patients with coronary artery disease, *J Cardiopulmonary Rehabil* 12:507-512, 1988.

71. Flugelman MY, Halon DA, Shefer A, et al: Persistent painless ST-segment depression after exercise testing and the effect of age, *Clin Cardiol* 11:365-369, 1988.

72. Hedblad B, Juul-Möller S, Svensson K, et al: Increased mortality in men with ST segment depression during 24 h ambulatory long-term ECG recording: results from prospective population study 'Men born in 1914', from Malmö, Sweden, *Eur Heart J* 10:149-158, 1989.

73. Stone PH, LaFollette LE, Cohn K: Patterns of exercise treadmill test performance in patients with left main coronary artery disease: detection dependent on left coronary dominance or coexistent dominant right coronary disease, *Am Heart J* 104:13-19, 1982.

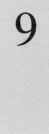

9 Exercise Testing of Patients Recovering from Myocardial Infarction

POINTS FOR CONSIDERATION

Although the death rate for coronary heart disease (CHD) has been decreasing steadily since the mid-1960s, it still remains the leading cause of death in the United States. Four deaths in every 10 are attributable to cardiac disorders and, of these, 90% can be attributed to coronary heart disease. The three distinct clinical manifestations of CHD are primary cardiac arrest, angina pectoris, and acute myocardial infarction (MI). MI has been carefully studied because most patients with this manifestation are admitted to coronary care units. Also, MI has a definable onset and can be diagnosed by objective means with established criteria (that is, pain syndrome, ECG changes, enzyme patterns). The case death rate in MI patients is temporally related to onset. The risk of death is highest within the first 24 hours of onset of signs or symptoms and declines throughout the following year. After the onset of a first MI in middle-aged males, 30% are dead within 30 days, and 85% of these deaths occur within the first 24 hours.

Those patients with a first MI who actually reach a hospital alive have a 10% to 18% risk of dying before discharge. The mortality thereafter falls from an annualized rate of 9% over months 2 through 6, to 4% for months 7 through 30, to 3% over the next 3 years. Other studies have suggested a mortality of 11% in the first 3 months after hospital discharge and then lower rates thereafter. Thus, after a short critical period, survivors of MI stabilize at a risk of dying that has been estimated as 2 to 5 times that of a comparable healthy peer group. Most return to work, particularly since physician and public attitudes have become more encouraging.

The pathophysiological determinates of prognosis are (1) the amount of viable myocardium and (2) the amount of myocardium in jeopardy. Inferences can be made regarding these two determinates clinically if a patient has had congestive heart failure (CHF) or cardiogenic shock and continued chest pain or ischemia. Utilizing cardiac catheterization, they can be assessed by ejection fraction and the number of vessels occluded. The clinical findings mainifested by abnormalities of these two determinates are the basis for several indices that have been used to predict risk. Clinical data have also been very useful in sorting patients in regard to the necessary length of stay in the hospital. The criteria for a complicated MI are listed in the box. Patients without these criteria, that is, those with uncomplicated MIs, are able to be discharged within 3 to 5 days, whereas those with these criteria require longer hospitalization and closer observation.

Health care professionals must be able to advise post-MI patients as to what they should or should not do to improve their prognosis. One strategy has been to identify high-risk patients by using various clinical markers and test results. Clinical markers that have indicated high-risk include prior MI, congestive heart failure, cardiogenic shock, tachycardia, continued chest pain, older age, stroke or transient ischemic attack, and complicating illnesses. Procedures used to determine risk with some success have included the chest x-ray film, routine ECG, ambulatory monitoring, radionuclide cardiac tests, high-frequency averaged ECGs, electrophysiological studies, and exercise testing. The assumption has been that patients at high risk should be considered for intervention; the interventions are coronary artery bypass surgery (CABS) and percutaneous transluminal coronary angioplasty (PTCA).

May and co-workers from the National Institutes of Health reviewed the clinical trials per-

---

CHARACTERISTICS THAT LEAD TO CLASSIFICATION OF A MYOCARDIAL INFARCTION AS BEING COMPLICATED

Congestive heart failure
Cardiogenic shock
Large myocardial infarction as determined by creatine phosphokinase or ECG, or both
Pericarditis
Dangerous arrhythmias, including conduction problems (including atrial fibrillation and bundle branch block)
Concurrent illnesses
Pulmonary embolus
Continued ischemia (angina, ST shifts)
Stroke or transient ischemia attack

---

formed to see if mortality can be altered in patients for a long term after an MI.[1] There have been no randomized trials demonstrating CABS to be effective in the post-MI population for preventing recurrent MI or death. Despite the lack of proof that CABS alters prognosis after MI, strategies have been proposed based on exercise test results delineating which patients should have coronary angiography and should be considered for CABS or PTCA. This proposal appears reasonable since there are many more studies using exercise testing after MI to evaluate risk than studies performed with other techniques. Basic clinical questions remain unanswered. What exercise test responses indicate an increased risk for subsequent cardiac events? Do the clinical parameters associated with MI (that is, CHF, prior MI, MI location and type, shock, continued ischemia) have adequate predictive power making the exercise test unnecessary? Which patients require coronary angiography?

This chapter begins with a summary of early studies and methodological studies that have provided useful information regarding the use of exercise testing after an MI. The studies that have compared exercise test results with coronary angiography are also presented. The main part is devoted to a critique of the follow-up studies.

Safety of exercise testing early after myocardial infarction

The risk of death and major arrhythmias when an exercise test is performed early after an MI is very small. However, the major experience is based on clinically selected MI patients: those without major complications such as heart failure, severe arrhythmias or ischemia, left ventricular

dysfunction, or other severe diseases. Risk is highest in those rejected for testing for these clinical reasons.

Submaximal testing

The exercise test can determine the possible risk the patient may incur with exercise. It is certainly safer that adverse reactions be observed in controlled circumstances. The risk-benefit ratio of this procedure can be improved by several considerations. Although maximal exercise testing soon after MI has been reported, until approximately 1 month after MI, a submaximal limited test is more clinically appropriate. Arbitrarily, a heart rate limit of 140 beats/min and a MET level of 7 is used for patients under 40, and 130 beats/min and a MET level of 5 for patients over 40. Particularily for patients receiving beta-adrenergic receptor blockers, a Borg perceived exertion level in the range of 16 is used to end the test. In addition, conservative clinical indications for stopping the test should be applied. The physician providing medical care for the patient can gain valuable information about the patient by being there during the test and interacting with the patient.

Early and methodological studies

Torkelson[2] reported results in 10 patients after an uncomplicated MI. During the sixth week of an inhospital rehabilitation program, a low-level treadmill test was performed using 1.7 mph at a 10% grade. He concluded that the treadmill test was valuable for discerning the exercise responses of MI patients. Ibsen and colleagues reported the results of a maximal bicycle test in the third week after MI in 209 patients.[3] Niederberger presented the values and limitations of exercise testing after MI in a monograph published in Vienna in 1977.[4] From his review and experience he recommended a bicycle test beginning with a work load of 25 watts increasing 25 watts every 2 minutes. Markiewicz and colleagues studied 46 men under 70 years of age using treadmill testing at 3, 5, 7, 9, and 11 weeks after their MI.[5] The test at 3 to 5 weeks and the test at 7 to 11 weeks appeared to provide most of the information obtained in all five tests performed. In selected low-risk patients, they performed maximal treadmill testing at 3 weeks after MI and found that a low heart rate response was associated with a poor prognosis.

Sivarajan and colleagues evaluated 41 post-MI patients.[6] They assessed symptoms, signs, and hemodynamic and ECG responses during and after three activities: sitting upright, walking to an adjacent toilet, and walking on a treadmill. These activities were studied at 3, 6, and 10 days, respectively, after infarction. They concluded that successful performance of these three activities provided useful criteria for discharge of a patient with a MI.

Effect on patient and spouse confidence

Taylor and co-workers evaluated the effects of the involvement of the wife in her husband's performance of a treadmill test 3 weeks after an uncomplicated acute MI.[7] They compared 10 wives who did not observe the test 10 who observed the test, and 10 who observed and performed the test themselves. In a counseling session after the treadmill test, wives were fully informed about the patient's capacity to perform activities. Perceived confidence in their husbands' physical and cardiac capabilities were significantly greater among those wives who also performed the test than in the other two groups. In a similar study, Ewart demonstrated that the patients' confidence was enhanced by the test also.[8]

Protocol comparisons

Handler and Sowton compared the Naughton and modified Bruce treadmill protocols in 20 patients 6 weeks after an MI.[9] Estimated exercise capacity and ischemic responses were similar using both protocols. The only significant difference was the relatively long mean maximal exercise duration in the Naughton protocol. Starling and co-workers evaluated 29 uncomplicated post-MI patients with heart-rate limited and symptom-limited modified Naughton treadmill test and 31 similar patients with a symptom-limited modified Naughton and standard Bruce test at 6 weeks after an MI.[10] Predischarge, the symptom-limited Naughton test allowed identification of a greater number of patients with ST-segment depression or angina than the heart rate limited test did (21 versus 13 patients). At 6 weeks after MI the standard Bruce test allowed identification of significantly more ischemic abnormalities than the symptom-limited modified Naughton test did (20 versus 13 patients). During the Bruce test, a higher double product was reached in a shorter time. It is more logical that the post-MI test protocol be individualized to the patient and that the initial level should begin at 2 METs and be followed by 1 or 2 MET incremental stages.

Reproducibility

Starling and co-workers evaluated the comparative predictive value of ST-segment depression or angina in 93 post-MI patients tested predischarge and 36 tested again at 6 weeks.[11] They concluded that angina alone, irrespective of the presence of ST-segment depression, was a better predictor of

multivessel disease than ST-segment depression alone. Repeat testing was helpful for confirming this likelihood. Handler and Sowton evaluated the diurnal variation and reproducibility of abnormalities occurring during predischarge treadmill testing in 41 patients.[12] Each patient was exercised using a symptom-limited Naughton protocol in the morning and the afternoon on 2 consecutive days. Ischemic abnormalities were poorly reproducible in any patient, but no significant diurnal variation occurred. The reproducibility of an ischemic result in all four tests was 66%. Starling and co-workers evaluated 89 patients with predischarge and sixth-week treadmill tests to determine the importance of doing repeat tests to identify abnormalities of known prognostic value.[13] Nineteen patients completed only a predischarge exercise test, nine of whom experienced an early cardiac event precluding repeat testing. All nine had prognostically important treadmill abnormalities during the predischarge test. ST-segment depression was highly reproducible between the early and the sixth-week test. Angina, inadequate blood pressure response, and ventricular arrythmias showed limited reproducibility and substantial individual variability.

Spontaneous improvement after myocardial infarction

Wohl and colleagues studied 50 patients after an acute MI.[14] They found that in stable patients, at 3 weeks there was an improvement of the relationship between myocardial oxygen supply and demand as detected by ST-segment changes. There was a delayed improvement between 3 and 6 months in functional capacity associated with increased stroke volume and cardiac output. Haskell and DeBusk[15] reported the cardiovascular responses to repeated treadmill testing at 3, 7, and 11 weeks after an acute MI. Two symptom-limited tests were performed on 24 males (mean age 54 years) several days apart. All test variables measured at maximum effort increased significantly between 3 and 11 weeks. Other studies have documented that exercise capacity increases spontaneously after an MI even in patients not in a formal exercise program.

Effect of Q-wave location on ST-segment shifts

Castellanet and co-workers studied 97 patients with a prior transmural MI who underwent coronary angiography and treadmill testing.[16] In patients with a previous inferior wall infarction, the ST-segment response had a high degree of sensitivity and specificity (approximately 90%) in detecting additional coronary disease. However, in patients with a previous anteroseptal MI, the ST

Table 9-1 Exercise testing studies of post–myocardial infarction patients requiring coronary angiography for correlation

Investigator	Year published	Patients tested	Exercise test characteristics				Angiography time after MI
			End points for testing	ECG leads	Protocol	Time after MI	
Weiner	1978	154	SS, SBPd, >4 mm, RVA	12LD	Bruce	2-36 mo	2-36 mo
Paine	1978	100	90% MHR, SS, IVCD, 1 mm	V$_{4-6}$	Bruce	4 mo	4 mo
Dillahunt	1979	20	SS, 1 mm, 3 PVC/min, 5 min	CM$_5$, V$_2$	Naughton	10-18 days	4-20 wk
Sammel	1980	77	SS, 6 METs	12LD	Green Lane	1 mo	1 mo
Fuller	1981	40	HR 120, SS, 1 mm, >5 PVCs	12LD	low Bruce	9-18 days	5-12 wk
Starling	1981	57	SS, VT, SBPd, HBP	12LD	Naughton	9-21 days	3-12 wk
Boschat	1981	65	85% MHR, 1 mm	12LD	Bruce	2-12 mo	2-12 mo
Schwartz	1981	48	SS, SBPd VT, 2 mm, 75% MHR	12LD	low Bruce	18-22 days	3 wk
De Feyter	1982	179	SS, VT	12LD	Bruce	6-8 wk	6-8 wk
Akhras	1984	119	SS	12LD	Bruce	2 wk	6 wk
Morris	1984	110	SS	12LD	UPR Bike	>6 wk	<3 mo
van der Wall	1985	176	SS	12LD	Bruce/TH	6-8 wk	6-8 wk

Exercise test characteristic columns: CM$_5$, A bipolar lead; *HBP,* high blood pressure; *HR,* heart rate; *IVCD,* intraventricular conduction defect; *MET,* a maximal exercise level allowed to be reached as estimated from work load; *MHR,* heart rate at maximal effort; *mm,* amount in millimeters of ST shift taken as an end point; *(percent heart rate),* percentage of age-predicted maximal heart rate chosen as a limit; *SBPd,* systolic blood pressure drop; *SS,* signs or symptoms, or both; *12LD,* the full set of 12 leads; V$_5$, fifth precordial lead; *VT,* ventricular tachycardia.

Protocol, Type of exercise study done: *Bruce,* Bruce protocol stopped at 85% of the age-predicted maximal heart rate; *low Bruce,* Bruce protocol with 0 and ½ stages, which are 0% and 5% grade at 1.7 miles per hour before stage 1 (10% grade at 1.7 miles per hour); *Bruce/TH,* Bruce protocol with thallium imaging; *Green Lane,* Green Lane Hospital treadmill protocol; *Naughton,* Naughton treadmill test; *UPR,* upright bicycle combined with radionuclide testing.

Time after MI, Mean time after myocardial infarction that the exercise test or angiography was done.

response had much less sensitivity. In this group, a positive test result indicated the probable presence of ischemia in the lateral or inferior posterior region. It was believed that the aneurysm generated an ST vector canceling ischemic ST-segment changes and producing a false-negative test result. If the anterior infarction extended beyond V$_4$, the sensitivity rate of treadmill testing dropped even further.

Ahnve and co-workers used thallium scintigraphy and computerized ST vector shifts to evaluate the effect of Q-wave location on the relationship of ST shifts to ischemia.[17] Anterolateral MIs had large ST-segment spatial shifts that did not indicate ischemia, whereas when shifts occurred in patients with inferior or subendocardial MIs, ischemia was detected by thallium defects. It appeared that large anterior MIs behave as if left bundle branch block were present and the ST

shifts have a very low specificity for ischemia. However, a subsequent study by Miranda demonstrated that severe angiographic disease could be recognized despite Q-waves using ST depression.[18]

RESULTS OF EXERCISE TESTING AND CORONARY ANGIOGRAPHY

Exercise testing results would be clinically most helpful in deciding about CABS if the exercise test could permit prediction of which patients have anatomic findings associated with improved survival if CABS were performed, that is, left main or three-vessel disease along with an ejection fraction of 30% to 50%. However, the end point usually predicted has been multivessel disease (MVD). Angiographic studies are thought of as "instant epidemiology," since the investigator

Population characteristics

Age/% women	Exclusions	MI % Transmural				% with angina	Meds	% MVD	ST depression		Angina	
		PR	SE	A	IP				Sens	Spec	Sens	Spec
25-65/12%	<85% MHR, BBB	0	27	33	41	45	No Dig	59	91	65		
48/7%	USA, CHF	22	4	48	48	59	18% BB, 23% Dig	66	41	88		
42-69/21%	>Killip 2, HTN	?	21	50	29		7% Dig	61	23	100	29	100
<60/0%	>60, prMI, LBBB	0	27	33	43	30	25%, BB, 12% Dig	33	48	89		
54/0%	>65, CHF	25	23	25	53	25	22% BB, 10% Dig	50	65	ST &/or Ang		90
56/7%	USA, CHF, HTN	19	25	37	39		25% Dig, 33% BB	72	54	75	68	81
50/2.5%	CHF, ANYM, USA	0	0	24	41	50	Stopped	65	60	?		
50/10%	CHF, USA	25	31	54	35	15		71	56	ST %/or Ang		86
28-65/10%	>65, BBB	8	12	35	45	29	Stopped	54	67	ST &/or Ang		67
50/6%	Complic, BBB	?	?	?	?		Stopped	73	94	94		
56/12%	Complic	0	0	53	47	31	Stopped	88	30	84	44	95
54/11%	>70, BBB	0	0	43	57	30	Stopped	44	64	70	20	63
							AVERAGES	59	58	82	40	83

Rest of table: *A*, Transmural (Q-wave) anterior-wall MI; *Age/% women*, mean age of patients and the percentage of women included in the study; *ANYM*, aneurysm; *BB*, beta-blocker; *BBB*, bundle branch block; *CHF*, congestive heart failure; *complic*, complications; *Dig*, digoxin; *Exclusions*, > (greater-than symbol) excludes patients above a certain age; *HTN*, hypertension; *IP*, transmural inferior or posterior MIs, or both types; *LBBB*, left bundle branch block; *Meds*, percentage of patients receiving digoxin (Dig) or a beta-blocker (BB) at the time of treadmill testing and often through the follow-up period; *MI %*, percentage of types of MIs included in the study; *% with angina*, percentage of population with classical angina; *%MVD*, percentage of population with multivessel disease; *PR* (or *prMI*), prior MI; *SE*, subendocardial or non–Q wave MIs; *Sens*, sensitivity; *Spec*, specificity; *ST*, abnormal ST-segment depression; *ST &/or Ang*, abnormal ST-segment depression or angina, or both, induced by the exercise test as the criterion for an abnormal response; *USA*, unstable angina pectoris.

does not need to wait upon end points. However, those who undergo this invasive procedure are highly selected. The angiographic studies are summarized in Table 9-1 and below.

Weiner and co-workers reported 154 patients with a single MI who had exercise testing and coronary angiography.[19] The patients averaged 1 year after MI. Eighty-three patients developed ST-segment depression only, 22 had elevation with depression in other leads, 19 had elevation only, and 30 had no changes. Respectively, multivessel disease was present in 76%, 91%, 21%, and 13% of the above groups. Left ventricular aneurysms were present respectively in 31%, 68%, 79%, and 40%. ST depression (with or without ST elevation) was predictive of multivessel disease; ST elevation alone or no ST shift was suggestive of single-vessel involvement; and elevation was predictive of left ventricular aneurysm.

Paine and co-workers studied 100 consecutive patients with exercise testing and cardiac catheterization at a median of 4 months after MI.[20] Of 31 patients with 0.1 mV of ST depression, 87% had two- or three-vessel disease, whereas of 21 patients with no depression, 38% had two- or three-vessel disease. Fourteen patients had ST elevation, and they had more left ventricular damage.

Dillahunt and Miller exercise tested 28 patients from 10 to 18 days after MI and catheterized the same patients 4 to 20 weeks later.[21] Among 11 patients with no symptoms, ST-segment changes, or arrhythmias during the treadmill test, eight had single-vessel disease (73%) and three had two-vessel disease. In contrast, among the 17 patients with any abnormality, 14 (82%) had three- or four-vessel disease. The ejection fraction was significantly lower in the 17 patients with an abnormal test.

Sammel and co-workers reported the results of exercise testing and coronary arteriography in 77 men under 60 years of age studied 1 month after MI.[22] The 22 patients with exercise-induced angina had a greater proportion of myocardium supplied by significant lesions compared to the 55 patients free of angina. The combination of ST-segment changes (0.1 mV or more depression or 0.2 mV or more elevation) and angina was 91% predictive of three-vessel disease. All four patients with significant left main disease (>75% stenosis) had both angina and ST-segment changes. It is difficult to compare their results to the other studies, since a scoring system that used the estimated muscle in jeopardy and the number of vessels diseased was not given.

Fuller and co-workers performed submaximal exercise tests on 40 MI patients before discharge and performed catheterization 5 to 12 weeks after MI.[23] Among the 15 patients with an abnormal treadmill test (angina with or without ST-segment depression of 0.1 mV or more), 13 (87%) had significant multivessel disease versus seven of 25 patients (28%) with a negative test. In a subgroup of 30 patients with a first MI, 89% with an abnormal test had multivessel disease, whereas 19% of those with a negative test had multivessel disease, and among 18 patients with a first inferior MI the test was even more predictive. The abnormal treadmill response before discharge was predictive for later angina both within the first month and later during a seventh-month follow-up observation. Among the 15 patients with an abnormal test, 73% later had angina compared to 16% among the 25 patients with a negative test.

Boschat and co-workers from France have reported their results in 65 patients who sustained their first transmural MI and within 4 months had undergone coronary angiography and treadmill testing.[24] These 65 who had a treadmill test were out of a group of 80 patients (81%) who had coronary angiography. Approximately one third of the 65 had post-MI angina. No patients were receiving drugs that would interfere with heart rate or ST-segment analysis. Care was taken to see which patients had ST-segment elevation over Q-waves associated with depression in the opposite direction. Only half of the vessels supplying the infarcted areas remained occluded meaning that half had undergone spontaneous recanalization. Multiple vessel and diffuse disease was more common in inferior than anterior wall MIs. Only 28 (43%) had an abnormal test by ST-segment depression criteria, and abnormals were more common in the inferior MIs (54%). The clinical severity of the angina was directly related to abnormal tests, whereas functional aerobic impairment closely correlated with the number of diseased vessels. ST-segment elevation was observed in patients with wall-motion abnormalities in the leads facing the areas of infarction and was associated with a lower ejection fraction but was a poor indicator of multivessel disease (MVD). ST-segment depression was only about 60% sensitive for MVD. The occurrence of ST-segment elevation in the leads facing the infarcted zone along with significant depression in the opposed leads always indicated that another major vessel was involved, but this occurred in only 25% of the cases presented. Patients who had both angina and exercise-induced ST-segment depression usually had MVD.

Schwartz and co-workers reported 48 patients studied with an exercise test and coronary angiography 3 weeks after their MI.[25] Among the 21 patients with an abnormal responses (>0.1 mV ST-segment depression or angina) 90% had MVD versus 55% among the 27 patients with a normal test. Exercise-induced ST-segment elevation in 24 patients was associated with a significantly lower ejection fraction (EF) and more abnormally contracting segments.

Starling and co-workers evaluated 57 uncomplicated patients with a symptom-limited Naughton treadmill test 9 to 21 days after MI and with coronary arteriography within 12 weeks.[26] They found that ST-segment depression (0.1 mV or more) and/or angina during the exercise test had a superior sensitivity (88%) for detection of MVD compared to ST-segment depression alone (54%). Patients with inadequate blood pressure response had frequent MVD (12 of 13), and they had significantly reduced EF (mean EF of 39%) compared with patients with a normal systolic blood pressure response (mean EF of 58%).

De Feyter and co-workers found that the prevalence of MVD was 63% in inferior and 42% in anterior MIs.[27] Left ventricle impairment was more severe in anterior and prior MIs and more prevalent than in inferior or nontransmural MIs. When they considered an abnormal exercise response to be ST-segment depression and/or angina for diagnosing MVD, the sensitivity and specificity for MVD was low for anterior and inferior MIs but an 80% sensitivity and a 91% specificity were obtained in 21 patients with non–Q wave MIs. With the definition of an abnormal test as depression and/or angina and elevation, they analyzed the diagnostic value for combined MVD and advanced left ventricular wall-motion abnormalities. A sensitivity of 41% and a specificity of 87% were obtained. In the whole group, the post-test risk for MVD with an abnormal exercise test (angina and/or ST depression) was 71% and for those with a negative test, it was 37%.

Akhras have reported results that are very different from those of other studies.[28] Of their 119 patients with an uncomplicated MI, it is not clear what percentage had prior MI nor did they specify non–Q wave and Q-wave MIs. Ischemic area criteria (ST-segment depression) were applied in the leads not affected by the MI. Incomplete information makes it impossible to compare their results to other studies.

Morris and co-workers compared the results from ECG and radionuclide ventriculography during upright bicycle testing in 110 patients undergoing coronary angiography after a single transmural MI.[29] Patients with ECG evidence of combined anterior and inferior/posterior MIs were excluded as well as patients with normal coronary angiograms, valvular disease, or a coronary artery bypass graft. Testing took place between 6 weeks and 3 months after MI. Combining exercise test–induced chest pain, ST-segment depression, and hypotension yielded a sensitivity of 44% and a specificity of 80% for MVD. An abnormal EF response (less than a 5% rise) had a sensitivity of 76% and a specificity of 65%, or if a fall in EF equal or greater than 5% was considered abnormal, the sensitivity was 43% and the specificity 95%. Wall-motion abnormalities had a specificity of 75% or less for MVD. The authors pooled the medical literature for prediction of MVD in 963 patients from a total of 21 studies of post-MI patients and found that, during exercise testing, chest pain had a sensitivity of 57% and a specificity of 86% and that ST-segment depression had a sensitivity of 59% and a specificity of 74%.

Van der Wall and co-workers from Amsterdam reported their findings in 202 patients 70 years of age or less admitted to their critical care unit with a definite first transmural MI.[30] Fifteen patients died and 11 patients refused to undergo angiography. All the remaining 176 patients underwent a Bruce treadmill combined with thallium scintigraphy 1 to 3 days before coronary angiography. They concluded that thallium scintigraphy or ECG or both, were not effective for clinical decision making.

Veenbrink and colleagues from Utrecht have attempted to answer an important question: Is there an indication for coronary angiography in patients under 60 years of age with no or minimal angina pectoris after a first MI? They defined high-risk coronary artery disease as three-vessel disease, proximal stenosis to the left anterior descending, or stenosis of the left main.[31] In addition to horizontal or downsloping ST-segment depression, criteria for an abnormal exercise ECG response included U-wave inversion and upsloping ST-segment depression. ST-segment depression was not considered abnormal if it accompanied ST-segment elevation over the infarcted area.

Only patients with transmural MIs were included and were roughly equally divided between anterior and inferior MIs. Cardiac catheterization was done approximately 2 months after the event. Ten percent of their patients had "high-risk" lesions; 11 patients had an abnormal exercise test including 8 of the 9 with high-risk disease. They concluded that coronary angiography in patients under 60 with no or minimal angina can be restricted to patients with an abnormal exercise test by their criteria, thus obviating the need for about 80% of coronary angiograms performed in this age group. Although this study had an admirable purpose, it is difficult to compare it to the other angiographic studies or to generalize their results because of the unusual exercise test criteria they used. No numerical data regarding patients with ST-segment depression alone or with other exercise findings were given.

Sia and co-workers in Australia evaluated an early symptom-limited maximal exercise test in predicting coronary anatomy and left ventricular ejection fraction and hemodynamics in 64 patients after an acute non–Q wave MI.[32] Ten of the patients were women, 28% had prior MIs, 11% were receiving beta-blockers, and 83% were receiving calcium antagonists. Exercise tests and cardiac catheterization were performed at a median of 6 and 7 days, respectively, after the MI. Forty-one percent of the patients had a negative exercise test response (no angina, less than 1 mm of ST-segment depression, and normal blood pressure responses). Twenty-five percent had a positive response (1 to 1.9 mm of ST-segment depression or angina); 34% had a "strongly positive" exercise test response (at least 2 mm of ST-segment depression or a 10 mm Hg drop in systolic blood pressure).

Cost efficacy

The cost effectiveness of the strategy of a routine predischarge exercise test (followed by coronary angiography and coronary artery bypass surgery if indicated) in patients with an uncomplicated myocardial infarction was compared with a policy of no routine exercise testing by Laupacis and colleagues.[33] Using data from the literature, a decision tree was developed to estimate the number of lives saved by the routine exercise test strategy (12 lives saved per 1000 tests), as well as the number of angiograms and coronary artery bypass procedures that would be performed. It was assumed that surgery decreases 1-year mortality by 25%. The resources consumed by bypass surgery were obtained from a chart review, and the costs were estimated by use of a method of fully allocated costing. Both direct and indirect costs were included. The average cost of coronary artery bypass surgery was $15,000. The cost of routine exercise testing was $260,000 per life saved. With sensitivity analyses this varied from $140,000 (coronary bypass surgery 50% effective) to (1,000,000 (bypass surgery 7.5% effective). They concluded that a routine post–myocardial infarction exercise test is an example of how a relatively inexpensive technology, by leading to other expensive clinical actions, can consume a significant amount of resources.

Summary of angiographic studies

For clinical purposes, it would be ideal if exercise testing would allow identification of patients with the angiographic lesions associated with improved survival after coronary artery bypass surgery (CABS). Given the current state of knowledge, such lesions would be three-vessel or left main disease accompanied by an ejection fraction from 30% to 50%. The angiographic studies have mainly been aimed at recognizing patients with any more vessels occluded than the vessel supplying the infarct site. These studies have had limited sensitivity and specificity for recognizing MVD, which includes patients with two-vessel disease and patients with normal left ventricular function. The high-risk subset is approximately only 20% to 30% of those with MVD.

What can our expectations be for identifying these patients? The exercise test can be expected to identify patients with much muscle in jeopardy because of lesions causing ischemia. However, it cannot be expected to recognize individuals with decreased ventricular function. Such patients are best recognized by a combination of prior history of MI or congestive heart failure, an abnormal ECG, and physical examination and chest x-ray findings. Many of the angiographic studies have attempted to use ST-segment elevation to identify patients with left ventricular aneurysm and have inferred that those with left ventricular aneurysms have decreased ventricular function.

These studies involve populations that are very selected, often containing a higher prevalence of patients with angina than the usual post-MI population, since they are more likely to undergo angiography. In some studies, ST depression and/or angina is considered an abnormal test result, and the results for each response cannot be separated. Few of these studies consider the other exercise test responses that have been associated with a poor prognosis, that is, a low exercise capacity, premature ventricular contractions, or an abnormal systolic blood pressure. However, review of the studies demonstrates a limited sensitivity and specificity for MVD. Certainly the sensitivity for detecting those with left main and triple vessel disease is higher but not 100%.

PROGNOSTIC STUDIES

This portion is based upon the analysis of published reports of longitudinal studies utilizing exercise testing in the early post-MI period with a follow-up study for cardiac events. We have chosen the most commonly cited studies and those of particular instructive value. These studies have been carefully analyzed for their: (1) methodology, (2) sample selection, (3) detailed description of sample, and, (4) description of statistical methods, in order to permit identification of differences that might show their lack of agreement or commonality. The cardiac event end points chosen are reinfarction and death. Some studies combine these two end points to predict outcome. Some investigators combine reinfarction and death with soft end points such as angina, worsening of symptoms, or CABS. The last is especially worrisome, since the results of the test can influence who will have CABS and CABS may affect mortality. These studies are summarized in Table 9-2. The studies are grouped and combined for metanalysis by the institution at which they were performed. Each column is explained in the legend.

In the first study reviewed, Ericsson and colleagues reported their results of treadmill testing 3 weeks after an acute MI in 100 out of 228 MI patients.[34] Ventricular dysrhythmias were classified as occurring during monitoring, during rest before the test, and during and after the treadmill test. They considered PVCs if equal or greater than 5 per minute and specifically as unifocal, multifocal, couplets, triplets, ventricular tachycardia, and ventricular fibrillation. During rest before the treadmill test 2 had unifocal and multifocal PVCs. During and after the treadmill test, 6 had unifocal, 8 had multifocal, 7 had 2 or 3 in a row, and one had 4 or more PVCs in a row. The exercise ECG or other exercise responses were not considered.

Kentala and associates have reported their findings in consecutive male patients discharged after acute MI in 1969 from the University of Helsinki Hospital.[35] During this period, 298 males less than 65 years of age were treated. Forty-five died in the hospital, and the patients were selected for follow-up study because of their availability and willingness to participate in a randomized trial of cardiac rehabilitation. The prognostic power of clinical and ECG variables recorded soon after MI and in connection with the exercise test were analyzed by stepwise multiple discriminant analysis. In this analysis, 18 clinical and electrocardiographic variables were chosen. They included the following: maximal exercise systolic BP, paradoxical apical pulsation, PVCs during hospital admission, forced vital capacity, T-wave negativity after exercise, age, terminal forces of the P-wave at rest, relative weight, resuscitated or not, physical work capacity, social classification, clinical cardiac failure, chest x-ray manifestations, PVCs during exercise, relative heart volume, ST-segment depression after exercise, initial and terminal notching of the QRS complex, and number of previous MIs. Based on the changes in discriminatory power of the variables during the 2-, 4-, and 6-year follow-up periods, they proposed a natural history for their patients. Patients dying within 2 years had a low exercise systolic blood pressure. With a longer follow-up period, the exercise blood pressure had a weaker influence. At the 4- and 6-year points, an abnormal resting terminal P-wave was the best predictor of poor prognosis. This probably identified a group with mild heart failure. Sudden death was defined as when a patient expired within 1 hour of symptoms, and such patients were more common late in the follow-up period. Patients with a high level of physical activity before infarction were less likely to die suddenly. Exercise-induced ST-segment depression did not identify a high-risk group at any point during the follow-up period and had very little power in the discriminant function. Of the many factors considered, an abnormal apical impulse, T-wave inversion after exercise, prior resuscitation, sedentary life-style before infarction, and occurrence of PVCs during exercise were of discriminatory value in relation to sudden death.

Granath and colleagues performed exercise tests at 3 and 9 weeks after an acute MI in 205 patients and followed them for 2 to 5 years.[36] There was a relatively high mortality of 25% but that rate was unadjusted for varying lengths of follow-up time. The end points of exercise testing were angina pectoris, dyspnea, and tachycardia. Tachycardia was judged to be a heart rate equal or greater than 130 at 33 watts at the third-week test or a heart rate equal or greater than 130 at 65 watts during the bicycle test at the third week. The criterion for ventricular dysrhythmias is not given. The investigators chose not to evaluate the ST-segments because of the accepted difficulties of evaluating ST shifts after MI and because of medications. The appearance of tachycardia at low work loads, major ventricular dysrhythmias, or anginal complaints during these early exercise tests was associated with a significantly increased mortality during the observation period. Exercise-induced PVCs proved to be of greater prognostic significance than those recorded at rest. They found the test valuable for evaluating the response to antidysrhythmic agents. Analysis of clinical data in the critical care unit failed to produce any differences between the survivors and those who died. However, there were more deaths among

those patients who had a previous infarction (17/37) as compared to those with a first infarction (40/168). During exercise testing, 9 weeks after infarct, PVCs were seen in 23% of the patients. During follow-up study, 16 of these died as compared to 25 of 134 without arrhythmias. Tachycardia during a submaximal work load (greater than 130 beats/min), which was 33 watts at 3 weeks and 65 watts at 9 weeks, identified a high-risk group at both time periods. Angina pectoris at the time of the 3-week test was not associated with an increased mortality, but there was a twofold risk for those who reported it at the 9-week test.

Smith and colleagues from Arizona did treadmill tests on 62 patients 18 days after admission for acute MI.[37] They considered the standard exercise predictors including ST-segment elevation and ST-segment depression but not their location. Death and MI were similarly high both in the group with elevation and in the group with depression. There was no difference in the mean Norris index for those exercise tested and those not tested. Thirty percent (6 of 20) of the patients who developed ST-segment depression either died or had another MI after discharge from the hospital versus only two (5%) of the 42 patients who did not have ST-segment depression during exercise.

The Royal Melbourne Hospital studies

Hunt and colleagues reported their findings in 75 patients under 70 years of age.[38] They selected their patients on the basis of having survived an MI complicated by arrhythmias or mechanical abnormalities. Only 56 were exercised to 70% of age-predicted heart rate on a bicycle 6 weeks after MI. Significant cardiac arrhythmias to gain entry into the study were ventricular, atrial, or junctional arrhythmias occurring at a rate of more than 1 per 10 beats; transient second- or third-degree atrioventricular block; or left bundle branch block. Mechanical abnormalities included rales, shock, enlarged heart, or x-ray signs of congestive heart failure. They were selected from 633 patients with MIs who met age and logistic criteria and were followed for 1 year. Of 11 patients with ST-segment depression of 1 mm or more, 36% died, whereas 4 of the 45 (11%) without depression died.

Srinivasan, Hunt, and colleagues reported a second study of exercise testing in patients with electrical or mechanical complications during their acute MI.[39] Criteria to gain entry into the study were the same as the previous study. They prospectively selected 154 patients who underwent an exercise test 4 to 6 weeks after discharge. The patients exercised on a bicycle until they

Table 9-2   Summary of the 28 prospective studies evaluating the ability of the exercise test after acute myocardial infarction to allow prediction of reinfarction and mortality

| | | | Exercise tested | | | | | Weeks after MI | Age/% of women | | MI % — Transmural | | | | |
| | | MI pop. size | | | | | | | | | PR | SE | A | IP | Meds (Dig or BB) |
Investigator	Year		n	%	End points	ECG leads	Protocol			Exclusions					
1 Ericsson	73	184	100	54	HR 140, SS	PC	TM	3	59/7	>65	25	?	51	43	
2 Kentala	75	298	158	53	Max	CH$_{1-6}$	Bike	6-8	53/0	>65, Rehab	28	13	42	58	35%D,1%BB
3 Granath	77	430	205	48	HR 140, SS	12LD	TM/Bike	3&9	59/11	>65	18	?	48	33	66%D
4 Smith	79	109	62	57	60% HR	12LD	GXT	3	60/?	?	?	5	?	?	10%BB
5 Hunt	79	633	56	9	70%HR, SS	7LD	Bike	6	57/11	No complic	?	0	47	53	?
Srinivasan	81		154			7LD					?	?	?	?	?
6 Saunul	71		200		SS	12LD	Naughton	3-52	57/10	CHF, USAP	8	9	29	62	8%D
Davidson	80	461	195	42	HR/SS	12LD	Stanford	3	53/0	>70, drgs, CHF	8	10	29	61	None
DeBusk	83	702	338	48	SS	12LD	Naughton	3	54/0	>70, CHF, USAP	?	?	?	?	3%D
7 Theroux	79	326	210	64	5 METs, 70%HR	CM5	Naughton	1.6	52/0	>70CHF, USAP	34	18	31	50	40%BB,1%D
Waters	85	330	225	68					53/16		25	21	43	55	6%D,32%BB
8 Koppes	80	410	108	26	Submax/Max	12LD	Bruce	3&8	52/13	CHF, drgs, ANG	?	24	28	48	None
9 Starling	80	190	130	68	HR130/SS	V$_{1,5,6}$	Naughton	2	53/14	USAP, CHF	24	29	34	37	26%D,16%BB
10 Weld	81	325	236	73	4 METs, SS	V5	low Bruce	2	54/12	>70	21	?	?	?	12%BB,41%D
11 Saunamaki	81	404	317	78	SS	PC	Bike	3	57/20	Age, CHF, ANG	10	?	32	?	20%D,2%BB
12 Velasco	81	958	200	21	30w, SS	PC	SupBike	2.5	60/22	>66, se, w	3	0	46	55	11%D,9%BB
13 De Feyter	82	222	179	81	SS	12LD	Bruce	6-8	52/0	>65, referrals	8	12	35	45	Stopped
14 Jelinek	82		188		Symptoms	V$_{4,5,6}$	Bike	1.5	52/10	ANG, CHF	18	28	29	42	?
15 Madsen	83	886	456	52	SS	9LD	Bike	2.6	51/?	>75, CHF, USAP	31	6	35	?	12%D,2%BB
16 Gibson	83	229	140	61	HR 120, SS	3LD	Naughton	1.6	63/13	>65, CHF	19	26	35	53	2%D,61%BB
17 Norris	84	395	315	80	SS	?	2.5 mph	4	51/13	>60	0	27	29	42	30%BB
18 Williams	84	226	205	91	6 METs	3LD	Bruce	1.7	50/0	>70	23	22	33	46	16%D,19%BB
19 Jennings	84	503	103	20	5 METs, SS	V$_5$	2 mph	1.7	56/18		?	?	51	49	4%D,10%BB
20 Fioretti	84	293	214	72	Symptoms	XYZ	Bike	2	54/13	>66, CHF, ANG		?			40%BB
	85	405	300	74					54/16	CHF, ANG	27		36	?	18%D,52%BB
21 Krone	85	1417	667	47	5 METs	3LD	low Bruce	2	?/20	>70	22	22	31	42	28%D,31%BB
Dwyer	85								60% < 60						
22 Handler	85	296	222	75	5 METs, 70%HR	3LD	Naughton	1.4	54/16	>65, CABS, BBB	?	21	42	37	1%D,17%BB
23 SCOR	85	1469	295	20	75%HR, SS	12LD	Mixed TM	1.7	58/18	MD judgment	21	18	38	44	26%D,53%BB
24 Jespersen	85		126		Max, SS	II, V$_{4,6}$	Bike	3.4	57/14	>71, CHF, USAP	0	36	31	33	13%D,20%BB
25 Paolila	85	362	263	73	Max	12	Bike	7	50/0	>65, CHF, USAP, w	3	11	32	57	2%D,2%BB
26 Murray	86	350	300	86	Sub		TM	2	53/17	>66, CHF	?	?	?	?	20%BB
27 Cleempoel	86	202	198	98	Sub	4	TM	1.6	58/0	>70, w, CHF	?	?	?	?	10%D,50%BB
28 Stone	86	719	473	66	Max	12	TM	24	54/21	>75, USAP, CHF, PVCs	22	28	?	?	26%D,39%BB
TOTAL			7029												

Investigator, The first author; *SCOR,* Specialized Center of Organized Research; **year,** year of publication; **MI Pop. size,** number of patients admitted to the hospital with myocardial infarction over the period of the study; **Exercise tested:** *n,* number, and %, percentage, of patients out of this MI population who underwent exercise testing.

Exercise test characteristics: *SS,* signs or symptoms, or both; *HR* with a heart rate value—a heart rate limit; *max,* maximal effort; *(percent heart rate),* percentage of age-predicted maximal heart rate chosen as a limit; *MET,* a maximal exercise level allowed to be reached as estimated from work load; *Symptoms,* symptoms alone were the end point. **PC,** Precordial leads; *12LD,* the full set of 12 leads; *CM$_5$,* a bipolar lead; *V$_5$,* fifth precordial lead (among others); *XYZ,* Frank vector leads. **Protocol,** Type of exercise study done: *TM,* treadmill; *GXT,* Bruce protocol stopped at 85% of the age-predicted maximal heart rate; *Stanford,* Stanford version of the Naughton test; *low Bruce,* Bruce protocol with 0 and ½ stages, which are 0% and 5% grade at 1.7 miles per hour before stage 1 (10% grade at 1.7 miles per hour). The Norris study at Green Lane used a 2.5 mph treadmill protocol with increasing grade. **Weeks after MI,** Mean time after MI that the exercise test or tests were done.

Population characteristics including age, sex, exclusions, MI mix, and medications: Age/% of women, Mean age of patients and the percentage of women included in the study. **Exclusions,** > (greater-than symbol) excludes patients above a certain age; other exclusion factors were *CHF,* congestive heart failure; *USAP,* unstable angina pectoris; *drgs,* cardiac drugs; *ANG,* angiography; *se,* subendocardial MI; *w,* women; *complic,* complications; *Rehab,* not in a rehabilitation program; *PVCs,* abnormal premature ventricular contractions; **MI %,** percentage of the types of infarctions included in the study; **PR,** prior MI; **SE,** subendocardial or non-Q wave MIs; **A,** transmural (Q-wave) anterior wall MI; **IP,** transmural inferior and/or posterior MI; **Meds,** percentage of patients on digoxin *(Dig, D)* or a beta-blocker *(BB)* at the time of treadmill testing and often through the follow-up period. *CABS,* coronary artery bypass surgery. **Mortality,** in those patients included in the study who underwent exercise testing *(ET) (yes)* and in those who were excluded from exercise testing for clinical reasons *(no);* **RE MI,** recurrent MI, the percentage who had a repeat MI if exercise tested *(yes,* left of /) or if not exercise tested *(no,* right of /).

Table 9-2   cont'd

Investigator	Mean or median	Range	% CABS	Mortality if ET performed yes/no	RE MI if ET performed yes/no	SBP	PVC	ExCap	Angina	ST	Statistical method
Ericsson	3 mo	3mo-?	?	5%/		NR	4×	?	?	NR	Descriptive
Kentala	6 yr	?	0%	32%/	?	+	+	NR	NR	+*	UV; some DF
Granath	2-5 yr	2-5 yr	?	25%/		NR	2×*	2×	2×	NR	UV
Smith	1.5 yr	?	?	10%/17%	?	NR	—	NR	NR	6×*	UV
Hunt	1 yr	?	?	14%/18%	?	NR	1	NR	4×*	3×*	Descriptive, UV
Srinivasan	1.25 yr	1-2 yr	?	8%	?	NR	?	NR	3×*	7×*	Not cited (UV)
Sami	19 mo	2-51 mo	10%	2%/	5%/	NR	—	1	NR	3×*	UV
Davidson	26 mo	1-60 mo	10%	1.5%/	6%/	?	?	+*	1	+*	MV-LR, LT, K-M est
DeBusk	34 mo	?	6%	2.1%/5.5%	2%/	NR	NR	NR	NR	8×*	UV; Cox to select some variables
Théroux	1 yr	1 yr	5.7%	9.5%/	6%/	NR	2×	NR	—	13×*	UV
Waters	2 yr	5-7 yr	16%	11%-3%		+*	+	+	NR	8×*	UV (Cox), MV-Cox/ conditional with regard to time
Koppes	2 yr	?		2%/		?	?	?	?	?	UV
Starling	11 mo	6-20 mo	?	8%/	9%/	5×	2×	NR	4×	4×	UV
Weld	1 yr	?	?	9%/		5×*	2×*	19×*	2×	2×	MV-LR; UV est
Saunamaki	5.7 yr	5-6 yr	?	35.6%/	?	3×*	2×*	NR	NR	1	LT w/in clinical subsets
Velasco	3 yr	3 mo-6 yr	?	11%/	3%/	3×	2×	NR	3×*	4×*	UV
De Feyter	28 mo	13-40 mo	13%	6%/	7%/	NR	3×	+	2×	1	UV
Jelinek	2.3 yr	10d-62 mo	?	7%/	19%/	—	NR	+	2×*	1	UV
Madsen	1 yr		0%	6.6%/28%	4%/12%	+*	+*	+*	?	1	MV-DF, Cox; algorithm
Gibson	1.3 yr	1-3 yr	14%	5%/	6%/	NR	NR	NR	+	+	UV
Norris	3.5 yr	1-6 yr	24%	13%/33%	12%/	NR	NR	?	?	1	UV-LT; Cox cited
Williams	1 yr	1 yr	12%	6%/31%	6.8%/	2×	—	2×*	2×	1	MV-DF; UV est
Jennings	1 yr	?	5%	9%/21%	3%/	8×*	1	8×*	?	1	UV
Fioretti	1.2 yr		8%	9%/23%		+*	2×	+	1	2×	UV
	1 yr	1 yr	8%	7%/28%	4%/	+*	+	+*	1	—	MV-DF, algorithm
Krone	1 yr	1 yr	12%	5%/14%		8×*	2×	3×*	3×*	1	UV;MV-LR
Dwyer					5%/10%	NR	?	?	?	?	UV;MV-LR
Handler	1.2 yr	6-36 mo	9%	7%/	4%/	5×*	1	8×*	1	2×	UV
SCOR	1 yr	?	?	7%/15%		1	2×	9×*	2×	3×	UV,MV-DF
Jespersen	1 yr	1 yr	<1%	7%	2%	1	1	1	1	3×*	UV, K-M
Paolila	2.6 yr	3-57 mo	6%	4.1%/	8.3%/	1	1	1	1	4×	UV
Murray	13 mo	6 mo-?	?	18%/	30%/	NR	NR	NR	+	1	UV
Cleempoel	0.16 yr	2 mo	?	5%/	?	NR	NR	+	NR	1	UV, MV DF
Stone	1 yr	?	?	3/16	5%/	5×	6×	6×	1	1	UV, MV, LT

			*Number of studies demonstrating significant risk predictor	**SBP RR** 9	**PVC RR** 5	**ExCap RR** 9	**Ang RR** 5	**ST RR** 9
			Number with positive risk	13	14	14	12	15
			Number with reported effect	18	23	18	20	24

Exercise test risk markers: SBP, abnormal systolic blood pressure response; **PVC,** abnormal premature ventricular contractions seen; **ExCap,** abnormally low exercise capacity tolerance; **Angina** *(Ang),* angina induced by test; **ST,** abnormal ST-segment response (usually only depression). These are the responses to exercise testing that have been most commonly reported as having prognostic value. *RR,* Risk ratio—univariate *(UV)* or multivariate *(MV)* analysis risk ratio. If significant statistically, the risk ratio has an asterisk.* Nonsignificant risk ratios permit trends across studies to be detected. The risk ratio means that if the cut point value for this abnormality was reached, those with that abnormality have a certain times (×) risk of death (high risk) as opposed to those without the abnormality. Only the hard end points of death (and in some studies, reinfarction) are considered. *NR,* Results of prediction with the exercise test marker were not reported; *LT,* clinical life table, usually stratified; *LR,* logistic regression; *K-M,* Kaplan-Meier; *est,* estimates; *w/in,* within; *DF,* discriminant function analysis; *?,* insufficient data to test significance; *1,* null effect; *+,* a positive nonsignificant association of usual high risk with death; *−,* a negative nonsignificant association of usual high-risk level with death; *Cox,* proportion hazard regression model for survival analysis; *algorithm,* detailed specific algorithm displayed for clinical use.

were unable to continue or had reached 70% of age-predicted maximal heart rate. Patients were excluded if CHF, hypertension, chest pain, or unstable ECG changes persisted, or if they were more than 70 years of age. There was no modification of their medication treatment because of the test, but specifics were not given, nor was a discription of their MI mix or other clinical features provided.

The Stanford studies

Sami and colleagues studied the prognostic value of treadmill testing in 200 males who were tested serially approximately five times each from 3 to 52 weeks after a MI.[40] None of these patients had congestive heart failure or unstable angina, and they were a relatively low-risk group, since only 2% died over the 2 years of follow-up time. At 3 weeks, 100% of those who subsequently had an episode of cardiopulmonary resuscitation and 60% of those who required CABS had 0.2 mV of ST-segment depression during treadmill testing. Only 35% of those without an event had a similar amount of ST-segment depression. At 5 weeks and beyond, recurrent PVCs during serial treadmill testing occurred in 90% of those who had a recurrent MI and in only 47% of those without an event. Exercise-induced PVCs or ischemic ST-segment depression 11 weeks after infarction identified patients with an increased risk of subsequent coronary events, whereas the absence of either identified a group of patients who were free of problems. The major emphasis concerned events 2 years after MI, though only half had been followed for that time. Differences were compared by chi-square and t-tests.

Davidson and DeBusk reported results of treadmill testing in 195 men tested 3 weeks after acute MI.[41] Stepwise logistic analysis on a subset of 92 with at least a 2-year follow-up time showed ST-segment depression equal or greater than 0.2 mV, angina, and a work capacity of less than 4 METs to be risk markers. These results were confirmed in the 195 men using stratified life table analysis with log rank tests. The patients were followed for 1 to 64 months, and the 150 followed for at least 1 year had a 19% event rate; however, more than half of these end-point events were coronary artery bypass surgery. The exercise test clearly could have biased this group of patients toward angiography and subsequent surgery. PVCs on a single treadmill test 3 weeks after MI had no independent prognostic value.

DeBusk and co-workers applied a stepwise risk stratification procedure sequentially combining historical and then clinical characteristics and finally treadmill test results in a study population of

702 consecutive men less than 70 years of age and alive 21 days after an acute MI.[42] Prior MI or angina or recurrence of pain in the critical care unit identified 10% of the patients with the highest rate of reinfarction and death within 6 months (18%). Clinical contraindications to exercise testing identified another 40% with an intermediate risk (6.1%). Exercise test results included ST-segment shifts, the MET level, angina pectoris, peak heart rate, peak systolic BP, exertional hypotension, and PVCs. In the patients who underwent treadmill testing, an abnormal test (≥ 0.2 mV depression and a heart rate less than 136) identified a high-risk group (9.7%), whereas those with a negative test had a 3.9% incidence of hard medical events. No other treadmill responses were predictive. A proportional hazards regression model was used to identify characteristics that significantly discriminated risk.

The Montreal Heart Institute studies

Théroux and colleagues studied the prognostic value of a limited treadmill test performed 1 day before hospital discharge after an MI in 210 consecutive patients.[43] These patients were followed for end points of heart disease for 1 year. Functional capacity and the blood pressure response were not considered. Sixty-five percent (28 of 43) who had angina during treadmill testing reported the onset of angina subsequently, according to the authors. This was statistically different from the 36% occurrence rate in those without chest pain during exercise testing. In those with a normal ECG response to exercise testing, there was a 2% mortality and a 0.7% sudden death rate; in those with ST-segment depression, there was a 27% mortality (17 of 64) and a sudden death rate of 16%. Statistical tests were performed by use of chi-square analysis.

Waters and co-authors have reported an expansion of the initial study from the same institution.[44] During 1976 to 1977, 12% of all patients admitted died in the hospital, 28% were excluded from the study, and 60% were included and underwent exercise testing. Mortality data was not reported on the 28% excluded from the study. Over the 5- to 7-year follow-up study of the 225 patients tested, 16% had CABS. They considered clinical and exercise test variables. ST-segment elevation and depression were similar risk predictors, and so they were combined. PVCs were classified by any appearance during or immediately after exercise, the blood pressure response was considered abnormal if the systolic BP failed to increase by 10 mm Hg or more, and functional capacity was considered abnormal if the patient failed to achieve the target heart rate or work load. The target heart rate was considered to be 70% of predicted maximal heart rate, and the maximal work load was 5 METs. Clinical variables included age, sex, previous MI, type and ECG location of the MI, recurrence of pain in the hospital, treatment with beta-blocking drugs or digitalis at discharge, and a QRS score. In the first year, overall mortality was 11%, and it was 3% per year afterwards. Exercise-induced ST-segment depression was present in 31% and generated a risk ratio of 7.8 for a 1-year mortality; 12% had ST-segment elevation in CM_5 and the risk ratio was slightly less than with ST-segment depression; 28% had PVCs; and 9% had a flat systolic blood pressure response. Predictors by the Cox regression model differed from the first year to the second year of follow-up study. During the first year, ST-segment shift in either direction, a flat systolic blood pressure response, or angina within the 48 hours after admission were predictors. During the second year, a history of prior MI, the QRS score, or PVCs were independent risk predictors.

Koppes and co-workers have presented their results in a highly selected group of 108 patients with MI out of a group of 410 admitted to Wilford Hall Air Force Medical Center from 1975 to 1978.[45] Starling and colleagues have reported their results using treadmill testing in 130 patients after an uncomplicated MI.[46]

Saunamaki and Andersen in Copenhagen reported the prognostic value of the exercise test 3 weeks after MI.[47] Clinical predictors were not considered, and a maximal bicycle test was used. They considered the general prognostic importance of ventricular arrhythmias associated with the exercise test, left ventricular function, and ST-segment changes. There was no significant difference in survival between patients with an ST-segment deviation of at least 0.1 mV and those without ST-segment deviation. The change of rate-pressure product (HR × SBP) from rest to maximal exercise adjusted for age was empirically found to be discriminating. Mortality increased among patients with major PVCs. Those with a small increase in rate pressure product or arrythmias, or both types, had a 5-year survival of 55% versus 80% in the others. In their 1982 study, they considered clinical parameters as well.[48] Clinical subgroups were defined as (1) patients with clinical heart failure during hospitalization or previous MI and (2) patients with anterior MI versus inferior or indefinite MI. Within each clinical group, exercise tests still determined a high-risk and low-risk group. The probability of survival in different risk strata was calculated according to Peto and the death rate according to

Nelson, and log rank testing was used to compare survival curves. Follow-up study was complete as maintained for a mean of 5.7 years.

Velasco and co-workers, from Spain, reported their findings using exercise testing after an uncomplicated transmural MI.[49] From 1973 to 1978, 958 patients with a preliminary diagnosis of MI were admitted to their critical care unit. Men less than 66 years of age with a transmural MI who survived were considered for the studies. This study is flawed by the large dropout rate (over 50% of those tested chose not to be followed) and by the use of only univariate analysis.

Weld and colleagues reported the results of low level exercise testing on 236 of 250 patients who had diagnosed acute MIs.[50] Angina was not found to be useful in predicting outcome. The investigators stated their belief that reduced exercise duration is an indicator of LV failure and owes its predictive value to this association. The exercise-test variables of duration, PVCs, and ST-segment depression ranked ahead of the clinical variables of vascular congestion, cardiomegaly, and prior MI in predictive value. This is the first study that considered standard clinical risk predictors along with the exercise test, and the exercise test proved superior to the clinical variables. The exercise test variables ranked in the following order: (1) exercise duration, (2) PVCs, and (3) ST segment depression. Patients unable to reach an exercise capacity of 4 METs had a relative risk of 15. Exertional hypotension (a maximal systolic BP of less than 130) generated an odds ratio of 5, but a drop in SBP was not predictive. Standardized regression coefficients showed that all three exercise variables had a stronger association with 1-year cardiac mortality than any of the clinical variables that constitute the Norris index. However, by this multivariate analysis, ST-segment depression was not statisically associated with 1-year mortality. The predictive ability of the multiple logistic regression model was tested using a jackknife procedure. Contingency table analysis was used to relate individual exercise variables to other data and to outcome for comparisons to other studies.

De Feyter and colleagues, from the Free University Hospital in Amsterdam, have reported the prognostic value of exercise testing and cardiac catheterization 6 to 8 weeks after MI. Their study provides data on a consecutive series of 179 survivors of acute MI who had a symptom-limited Bruce test. In this study, the following cardiac catheterization variables were also considered: number of vessels, ejection fraction, left ventricular end-diastolic volume, wall-motion abnormalities, and left anterior descending artery involvement. Fifty-eight patients with an exercise time of

10 minutes or more had a very low risk for cardiac death or reinfarction. No treadmill markers resulted in a higher risk group, whereas three-vessel disease or a left ventricular ejection fraction of 30% or less was predictive of high risk. The mortality was 22% in patients with an EF less than 30% or with three-vessel disease; 1% in patients with an EF greater than 30% or with one or two vessel disease. Clinical variables were not considered.

Jelinek and co-workers from Melbourne have presented their findings in 188 patients with an uncomplicated MI who underwent bicycle testing on the day of discharge (about day 10) and returned to work at a median of 6 weeks after MI.[51] They considered the total duration of exercise, maximal heart rate, maximal blood pressure, and ST-segment shifts. Secondary risk factors for recurrence of heart attack were found to be angina before the MI, angina on the exercise test, and radiological heart failure. There was no difference between the two groups for maximal work load, maximal heart rate, maximal systolic blood pressure, or maximal double product. The risk factors for total events were angina before MI, angina during exercise testing, and x-ray findings of CHF. No other variables were predictive including ST-segment depression, but only chi-square analysis was performed.

Madsen has reported findings from symptom-limited bicycle testing at Grostrup Hospital in Denmark.[52] The study population included 886 patients discharged between 1977 and 1980 after an MI. Nearly 50% of the patients were excluded from testing because of age, CHF, or other clinical reasons. A bicycle protocol that started at 50 watts and increased 50 watts each 6 minutes until maximal effort was used. During the 1-year follow-up time, few patients were on beta-blockers, and no one underwent CABS. Madsen considered angina, ST-segment depression, PVCs, duration of exercise, maximal heart rate, and maximal rate pressure product as possible risk markers. A wide variety of clinical markers were considered also. The most important exercise test variables were duration of exercise and PVCs. Prediction of death was not different with clinical or exercise test variables or their combination. For reinfarction, the predictive value was significantly higher for the exercise test variables than the combined set.

Gibson and colleagues applied predischarge quantitative exercise thallium scintigraphy in 140 consecutive patients with an uncomplicated MI.[53] The results were compared with submaximal treadmill testing and coronary angiography. During the follow-up time, 7 patients died and 9 suffered recurrent myocardial infarction. Included in their coronary events was clinical progression of angina pectoris. This confuses analysis, since the test responses are compared between those with and without combined events. There was no difference in clinical characteristics between those with and those without events including ejection fraction. The only variables that were different during treadmill testing were achievement of target heart rate and the occurrence of angina. The presentation of data did not permit determination of the test modalities that were able to be compared to predict death or nonfatal recurrent MI. For the cut-point values chosen, it appeared that no testing modality was significantly different for sensitivity of detecting those who were going to die. They ranged from the treadmill with the lowest sensitivity, to coronary angiography, to thallium scintigraphy, which had the greatest sensitivity for allowing prediction of a nonfatal MI. They mentioned that mortality was 4× higher in those with ST-segment depression and angina with borderline significance, PVCs were not predictive, and those with hypotension and ischemia had more complications. However, this univariate analysis is in question because sufficient data are not presented. This is a very disappointing report, since this study is one of the most complete but suffers from a lack of proper statistical analysis. The low mortality (5%) also seriously reduced the statistical power of the tests to detect differences between groups.

Norris and co-workers from Green Lane Hospital in New Zealand reported the determinants of reinfarction and sudden death in male survivors of a first MI younger than 60 years (mean 50) who underwent exercise testing and coronary angiography 4 weeks after MI.[54] Between January 1977 and June 1982, 425 men suitable were admitted to the hospital. Of these, 7% died in the hospital, leaving 395 survivors. Of these 395, 315 (80%) underwent exercise testing, and 325 (82%) underwent coronary angiography. Exercise testing was performed at 2.5 miles per hour starting at 0% grade and gradually increasing to 15%. Total cardiac mortality was best predicted by ejection fraction and by a coronary prognostic index dependent on age, history of infarct, and chest x-ray findings. Neither the severity of coronary artery lesions nor the results of exercise testing were predictive of mortality. Reinfarction could not be predicted by any clinical or angiographic variable.

Williams and co-workers from Ottawa Civic Hospital compared clinical and treadmill variables for the prediction of outcome after MI.[55] They considered the relative prognostic merits of 15 clinical and 10 predischarge exercise test variables in 226 patients. A submaximal treadmill test was performed on 205 patients (88%) to a mean work load of 6 METs an average of 12 days after MI. During the first year of observation, 3.4% of the patients developed unstable angina, 6.8% had a recurrent infarction, and 6% died. Twelve percent underwent coronary bypass surgery. Among those who did not have a treadmill test, there was a 31% death rate. The predictors of death were found to be resting ST-segment depression, a high creatine phosphokinase level, a poor exercise tolerance, and a history of prior MI.

Jenning and co-workers at Newcastle on Tyne considered 1253 patients admitted over 1 year to their critical care unit; 503 sustained an MI, but only 289 were less than 66 years of age.[56] Of these 289, 18% died in the hospital and 36% were excluded from study because of LBBB, ischemic pain, or other complications; 49 could not be tested before discharge for logistic reasons. Using univariate analysis, exertional hypotension generated a risk ratio of 8; inability to complete the protocol, a risk ratio of 8; and an excessive heart rate response, a risk ratio of 4. No survival analysis techniques were employed; only chi-square and t-tests were used.

Fioretti and co-workers from the Thorax Center in Rotterdam have evaluated the relative merits of resting ejection fraction by radionuclide ventriculography and the predischarge exercise test for predicting prognosis in hospital survivors of MI.[57] A symptom-limited bicycle test was performed with increments of 10 watts/min. The Frank leads were computer processed; 43% had abnormal ST-segment depression, and approximately 40% were taking beta-blockers. The hospital mortality was 13%, and 19 additional patients out of 214 died in the subsequent follow-up period (9%). Mortality was 33% for patients with an ejection fraction less that 20%, 19% for patients with an ejection fraction between the 20 and 39, and 3% for patients with an ejection fraction greater than 40%. Mortality was high (23%) in 47 patients excluded from performing exercise tests because of heart failure or other limitations. The patients could be stratified further into intermediate-risk groups according to an increase in systolic blood pressure during exercise. Maximal work load, angina, ST-segment changes, and PVCs were less predictive. After discharge, 14% of the patients had clinical signs or symptoms of heart failure, and 38% had angina; 17 were treated with bypass surgery or angioplasty. They concluded that symptom-limited exercise testing is the method of choice, since it provides more information for patient management. This study was later expanded to 405 patients, and similar results were obtained. Discriminant function analysis demonstrated that the combination of clinical and exercise variables gave better predictive accuracy than either used alone.

Krone and co-workers reported the experience of the Multicenter Post MI Research Group using low level exercise testing after MI.[58] Fourteen hundred and seventeen patients met their criteria, and 866 consented. Of those who consented to be in the study, 77% performed the treadmill test. The protocol was done to 5 METs with V_2, V_5, and aV_F monitored on an average of 15 days after MI. The grade was 0% for 3 minutes, 5% for the next 3 minutes, and 10% for the final 3 minutes. After 1 minute at 1 mile per hour the speed was increased to 1.7 mph for the final 8 minutes. Of those who exceeded a systolic blood pressure of 110 during testing there was a 3% mortality versus 18% for those unable to do so. In those who had an absence of couplets, there was a 4% mortality, whereas it was 13% in those with couplets. In patients with a normal exercise blood pressure and no pulmonary congestion on the chest x-ray film, there was a 1% mortality versus 13% in those with either abnormality. Most of the results are presented in univariate form, with Fisher's exact test evaluation. Further analysis of selected clinical and demographic variables using stepwise logistic regression demonstrated that exercise results significantly improved the prediction model for cardiac death.

In this same study population, Dwyer and co-workers reported the experience with nonfatal events in the year after acute MI.[59] Radionuclide ventriculography and Holter monitoring were done on all subjects, and treadmill tests were performed in 76%. Thirty-two percent were readmitted (7% for bypass surgery) with a death rate of 14%. The relative risk of death in the first year after readmission was 2.6 times greater than for patients who did not have a readmission. Only an ejection fraction less than 40% and post-MI angina were predictive of readmission. Reinfarction was best predicted by predischarge angina, which carried a risk ratio of 2.5. Failure to perform the exercise test was significantly associated as well with reinfarction, but none of the treadmill variables was discriminating. They concluded that urgent referral to cardiac catheterization and CABS because of an abnormal exercise test after MI does not seem warranted.

Handler from Guy's Hospital in London has reported his findings using submaximal predischarge exercise testing.[60] Three hundred thirty-nine consecutive patients 66 years of age or less were considered. Abnormal ST-segment depression generated a risk ratio of 6, which was not significant, and elevation a risk ratio of 10, which was significant. Combined elevation and depression had a risk ratio of 13, which was statistically significant. An abnormal blood pressure response and ST-segment elevation were also predictive of heart failure. Killip classes 3 and 4 were predictive of congestive heart failure and death.

From the University of California, San Diego, Specialized Centers of Research (SCOR) comes a report prepared by Madsen[61] that attempts to answer two important questions: Can an "ischemic" exercise test response and the exercise capacity be predicted from historical and clinical data available during hospitalization? Can the patients at low or high risk of death or new MI be identified by the exercise test? To answer these questions, they analyzed data from 1469 patients discharged after an acute MI from four hospitals. Of these patients, 466, or 32%, underwent a treadmill test at discharge. The exercise test was an optional part of the SCOR multicenter study protocol. The main reasons for not performing an exercise test were advanced age, poor general condition, severe cardiac dysfunction, or complicating diseases. The 466 patients who underwent exercise testing had a lower frequency of clinical risk factors than patients who did not undergo exercise testing. Various treadmill protocols were used, but MET levels were calculated. Limiting conditions of exercise tests were angina in 16%, marked ST-segment changes in 7%, fatigue in 44%, shortness of breath in 17%, claudication in 4%, and severe arrhythmias in 2%. If no symptoms developed, the patients continued exercise until they approached 75% of maximal age adjusted heart rate. In the 9% of patients without limiting symptoms where the exercise test was stopped at a low heart rate the test was considered indeterminate. Patients taking beta-blockers were included if a heart rate greater than 100 beats/min were achieved above 6 METs. Medications taken during the testing time included digoxin in 26% and beta-blockers in 53%. Patients with bundle branch block or left ventricular hypertrophy or those receiving digoxin therapy had test results considered indeterminate. Thus 92 patients with indeterminate test results were excluded, leaving 374 patients. Four historical variables from hospitalization were chosen as predicting an ischemic exercise test response by discriminate analysis. These included previous angina, ST-segment depression at rest, beta-blocking agents on discharge, and age; however, prediction was poor. When there was an attempt to predict who would have an exercise capacity of 4 METs or less, univariate analysis revealed several factors historically that were different. These included age, previous MI, angina, hypertension, heart failure,

resting ST-segment changes, and ejection fraction. However, multivariate analysis found only age and ST-segment changes at rest to be significant. In the 295 patients followed 1 year with satisfactory exercise tests, among exercise test variables tested univariately, only exercise capacity in METs and the occurrence of exercise-induced ST-segment depresssion were important for predicting death or a new MI within 1 year. A discriminate analysis using all exercise test variables selected only the exercise capacity in METs. The total correct classification was 75%. In the low-risk group of patients (72% of patients with an exercise capacity greater than 4 METs), fewer than 2% died or had a new MI within 1 year. In the high-risk group of patients (29% of patients with an exercise capacity less than or equal to 4 METs), 18% had a cardiac end point. They concluded that an ischemic exercise test response could not be reliably predicted from historical or clinical variables from the hospitalization. Patients likely to have good exercise capacity would be identified by use of age and ST-segment changes at rest. Good exercise capacity is the most important exercise test variable for identifying those with a very low risk of death and new MI within a year. A group of patients at relatively high risk can be identified by a poor exercise capacity.

Jespersen and colleagues from two Danish Hospitals have reported a series of 126 consecutive patients selected because they could exercise and had no evidence of prior MI, unstable angina pectoris, or severe heart failure and were less than 71 years of age.[62] The nine patients with ST-segment depression and subsequent cardiac events did not differ in any of their clinical or exercise test features from the patients without ST-segment depression. One patient who had ST-segment depression underwent CABS because of angina refractory to medical management. During the year of follow-up study, there were nine major cardiac events, six being fatal, in the 46 patients who developed ST-segment depression. Only three cardiac events (all deaths) occurred in 80 patients without exercise-induced ST-segment depression. The subgroup with exercise-induced ST-segment depression had annual death rates and reinfarction of 13% and 17% respectively, and the annual rate of cardiac death was 4% in the subgroup without ST-segment depression. The estimates of cardiac event–free probability showed a significantly worse prognosis for patients with ST-segment depression. Exercise-induced angina pectoris was not predictive for further cardiac events. There was no significant difference for rate pressure product, estimated VO_2, or arrhythmias in those with cardiac events.

Summary of prognostic indicators from exercise tests

The inconsistencies found in these studies make it difficult to develop an algorithm for intervention in post-MI patients. One of the best means of selecting a high-risk group is to consider an individual too sick to undergo exercise testing. Possible biases because of this clinical selection process as well as the characteristics associated with being admitted to the academic centers from which these reports come must be considered. Following will be specific summaries grouped by each of the exercise test risk markers. Only studies reporting statistically significant results are cited. From the previous summaries of each study where the definitions for an abnormal responses were given, it is apparent that often several different responses under each heading are being considered together by summarizing across studies (that is, the thresholds for abnormal PVCs, exercise capacity, or systolic blood pressure response differ). In addition, not all the exercise predictors were considered by the various investigators; such studies are indicated in Table 9-2 with an *NR* for "not reported" in the appropriate test response column.

The five exercise test variables suggested to have prognostic importance are ST-segment depression (and sometimes elevation), exercise test–induced angina, poor exercise capacity (or excessive heart rate response to a low work load), a blunted systolic BP response (or exertional hypotension), and PVCs. Because they involve the same populations and institutions and usually obtained the same results, the following studies are grouped together: Théroux and Waters (Montreal Heart Institute); Sami, Davidson, and DeBusk (Stanford); Hunt and Srinivasan (Royal Melbourne Hospital), Krone and Dwyer (Multicenter Post MI Group), and Fioretti (1984 and 1985, Thorax Center). Thus the results from a total of 28 centers are considered.

EXERCISE-INDUCED ST-SEGMENT SHIFTS

Nine out of the 28 centers found ST-segment depression to be significantly predictive of subsequent death; an additional 6 centers reported a positive but insignificant association. Nine centers reported a null effect, with 4 of the 28 failing to report data on ST-segment depression.

ST elevation

Sullivan and co-workers evaluated the prognostic importance of exercise-induced ST-segment elevation in 64 patients who underwent submaximal exercise testing a mean of 11 days after an acute infarct. The follow-up period was 1 year. The presence of exercise-induced ST-segment elevation was the only exercise test variable that was predictive of cardiac death. De Feyter and co-workers found that ST-segment depression indicated multivessel coronary disease (MVD), whereas ST-segment elevation indicated advanced left ventricular wall motion abnormalities and a low ejection fraction. Both shifts indicated that both MVD and advanced left ventricular wall motion abnormalities existed. In Waters' study, ST-segment elevation generated the same univariate risk as depression did, and so they were considered together. However, location of the ST shift was not specified. Saunamaki and Andersen considered ST-segment depression and elevation separately but did not specify its location. In their study, the ST responses were found to have little prognostic value. Handler found ST-segment elevation to generate a risk ratio of 10, which was significant. Combined elevation and depression had a risk ratio of 13, which was significant. Elevation was more common in anterior MIs. ST-segment elevation also predicted heart failure. These results are too inconsistently reported to make a conclusion, and clearly ST-segment elevation has a different meaning in Q-wave and non–Q wave MIs though this is rarely considered.

Exercise-induced arrhythmias

Only five out of 28 centers reported exercise test–induced PVCs to indicate a significant increase in risk. Four centers did not include results regarding PVCs; nine centers reported null or negative associations of PVCs with mortality.

Exercise capacity

Nine centers out of 28 reported that a low exercise capacity or an excessive heart rate response to exercise indicated a high-risk group. Five additional centers reported nonsignificant positive associations, Stanford reported a positive association in only one of three studies, whereas 10 of the 28 centers failed to report sufficent data on this variable to assess its effect.

Exercise-induced angina

Only five of 28 centers reported exercise test–induced angina to indicate a significantly increased risk group. Eight centers failed to report angina data. Seven of the remaining 11 reported nonsignificant positive associations.

Systolic blood pressure response to exercise

Nine of 28 centers found that inadequate or abnormal systolic blood pressure response to exercise significantly identified a high–risk group; 11 of the centers failed to report data, and four of the remaining six reported a nonsignificant positive association.

Comparison of exercise data to clinical data

An important question to be resolved is: Does the exercise test give more predictive information than the standard clinical risk predictors? Attempts to establish risk have included scores based on clinical features of the MI and historical information such as the Norris and Peel indices. There are reasons other than prognostication for performing exercise testing, but given the need to cost-account, all possible justification for performing a procedure is needed.

Kentala and associates assessed clinical parameters including a careful history of prior activity level. The prognostic power of clinical and ECG variables recorded soon after MI and in connection with the exercise test were analyzed by stepwise multiple discriminant analysis. They found that both clinical and exercise variables were important. Patients dying within 2 years had a low exercise systolic BP. With longer follow-up time, the exercise BP had a weaker influence. At the 4- and 6-year points, an abnormal resting terminal P-wave was the best predictor of poor prognosis. This probably identified a group with mild heart failure. For patients who suddenly died after 2 years, the T-wave changes after exercise, which possibly indicated subendocardial injury, were common. Patients with a high level of physical activity before their MI were less likely to die suddenly. Of the many factors considered, an abnormal apical impulse, T-wave inversion after exercise, prior CPR, sedentary life-style before infarction, and occurrence of PVCs during exercise were of discriminatory value in relation to sudden death.

Granath and co-workers found that analysis of clinical data in the critical care unit failed to produce any differences between survivors and those who died, though there were more deaths among those patients who had a previous MI. Saunamaki and Andersen demonstrated that exercise testing variables including PVCs and a poor SBP-HR change in response to exercise still were able to be predictive of risk within the strata of CHF, prior MI, and anterior MI. The exercise variables outperformed these important clinical parameters. Weld found the exercise test variables of duration, PVCs, and ST-segment depression to be ranked in that order ahead of the clinical variables of x-ray vascular congestion, prior MI, and x-ray cardiomegaly in predictive value.

De Feyter were unable to identify from treadmill markers a higher risk group, whereas three-vessel disease or a left ventricular ejection fraction of 30% or less did. Madsen and Gilpin found that in those who underwent testing, clinical variables were better able to be predictive of outcome

than those in the nontested group. The most important exercise test variables were exercise duration and PVCs; however, they improved prediction of reinfarction but not death. Although exercise test variables were selected by discriminant analysis, the correct total classification of deaths and survivors was not improved. The total correct prediction was 71% for clinical data were used alone, 67% for exercise data alone, and 71% for both combined.

DeBusk and colleagues found that prior MI or angina, or recurrence of pain in the critical care unit identified the 10% of patients with the highest rate of reinfarction and death within 6 months (18%). Clinical contradictions to exercise testing identified another 40% with an intermediate risk (6.4%). In those who underwent treadmill testing, ST-segment depression, and low peak work load were selected before any clinical variables or ambulatory ECG data in the logistic regression analysis. Gibson and co-workers found no difference in univariate comparison of clinical variables between those with or without events; even the ejection fraction was similar.

Norris found that total cardiac mortality was best predicted by EF and by an index dependent on age, history of MI, and chest x-ray findings. Neither the severity of coronary lesions nor the results of exercise testing predicted mortality. Reinfarction could not be predicted by any clinical exercise test or angiographic variable. William and colleagues considered the relative prognostic merits of 15 clinical and 10 predischarge exercise test variables in 226 patients. The predictors of death were found to be resting ST-segment depression, a high creatine phosphokinase, a poor exercise tolerance, and a history of prior MI.

Jennings and colleagues found that the Norris index score (age, prior MI, x-ray abnormalities) of less than 3 was associated with a 12% mortality and a score of more than 12 with a mortality of 85%. Fioretti and co-workers evaluated the relative merits of resting EF by radionuclide ventriculography and the predischarge exercise test. Mortality was 33% for patients with an EF less that 20%, 19% for patients with an EF between 20 and 39, and 3% for patients with an EF greater than 40%. Mortality was high (23%) in 47 patients excluded from performing exercise tests because of heart failure or other limitations.

Krone and co-workers found that among those not able to take a treadmill test there was a 14% mortality compared to 5% in those who were able to take it. In patients with a normal exercise blood pressure and no pulmonary congestion on the chest x-ray film, there was a 1% mortality versus 13% in those with either abnormality. In this same population, Dwyer and co-workers reported the experience with nonfatal events in the year after MI. Thirty-two percent were readmitted (7% for CABS) with a death rate of 14% and a risk ratio of 2.6. Only an EF less than 40% and postinfarction angina were predictive of readmission. Reinfarction was best predicted by predischarge angina. Failure to perform the exercise test was significantly associated with these events, but none of the treadmill variables was discriminating.

Waters and colleagues found that predictors by the Cox regression model were different in the first and the second year of follow-up study. During the first year, ST-segment shift in either direction, a flat blood pressure response, or angina within the 48 hours after admission were predictors ("markers of ischemia"). During the second year, a history of prior MI, the QRS score, or PVCs were independent risk predictors ("markers of left ventricular dysfunction"). This is illogical and disagrees with the findings of other investigators.

In summary, the results are mixed regarding whether the exercise test gives information that can predict death and reinfarction better than the clinical features. Remember that clinical judgment to exclude patients from testing identifies the highest risk group and that the threshold for doing so must be quite variable.

Clinical design features

The column headings used in Table 9-2, and separately listed in the accompanying box, are the important features of the study design that could affect the findings. Following is a discussion of these features.

Exercise protocol. Bicycle protocols, especially a supine protocol like Velasco used, can give different responses from those of a treadmill. Most protocols were continuous, but some were not progressive in work load increments. The standard Bruce protocol starts at a relatively high work load (4 or 5 METs). Heart rate responses at submaximal levels can be affected by the protocol as well as by beta-blockade, fitness, and anxiety.

End points of exercise test. If stopped at a certain amount of ST-segment shift, MET level, or heart rate, then the end-point response cannot be considered as a continuous variable nor can a higher value, which might be more discriminating, be reached.

ECG leads monitored. Use of different electrode placements make comparisons between studies difficult. Because of the visual location and effects of Q waves, 12-lead recordings are needed in post-MI patients.

Time after myocardial infarction when exercise test was performed. "Stunned" myocardium and deconditioning affect predischarge testing more than they affect hemodynamic responses later. ST-seg-

---

CHARACTERISTICS THAT CAN DIFFER AS TO METHODOLOGY BETWEEN STUDIES

Patients excluded
Entrance criteria
Age range, gender
Infarct mix (that is, non–Q wave, inferior/anterior/lateral Q-wave)
Patients with prior MI and those with or without complications
Prior coronary artery bypass surgery
History of congestive heart failure and angina
Myocardial infarction size
Follow-up thoroughness and length
Percentage of patients undergoing CABS or PTCA during follow-up study and whether they are
    censored
Cardiac events (CABS should not be used as an end point)
Mortality during follow-up study (Are they a high-risk or a low-risk group?)
Reinfarction rate
Exercise protocol
Time after myocardial infarction when test was performed
End points of test
Leads monitored and how ST-segment elevation is considered
Medications taken after discharge from hospital and at time of exercise test
Test responses considered and their cut points (PVCs, ST, SBP, exercise capacity, angina)
Statistical methods (multivariate survival analysis techniques are required; if univariate techniques
    are used, they should include Kaplan-Meier survival curves)

ment responses appear more labile early after MI. The responses differ at various times after MI as well, with a spontaneous improvement in hemodynamics occurring by 2 months. The contrast in the spontaneous improvement in both ejection fraction and functional capacity but their failure to correlate with each other makes them difficult to interpret. The studies that included exercise testing at multiple times found the same responses to have a different predictive value at the specific times the tests were performed. There is a spontaneous improvement during the first year after MI in the blunted blood pressure response to exercise that occurs particularly in large anterior MIs.

MI mix (that is, Q-wave location). Each MI location has a different prognosis and different "normal" response to exercise. Exercise predictors may be different in each type.

Inclusion of non–Q wave MIs. After much controversy regarding the risk of having a "subendocardial" MI, a study from the Mayo Clinic appears to clarify the stituation.[63] From 1960 to 1979, 1221 residents of Rochester, Minnesota, had an MI as the first manifestation of coronary heart disease; 784 had a transmural (Q-wave), and 353 had a non–Q wave MI. The 30-day mortality was 18% among transmural and 9% in subendocardial MIs. No significant difference was found in the rates of reinfarction, CABS, or mortality over the next 5 years. Congestive heart failure was more common among patients with transmural MIs, and angina was more common among patient with non–Q wave MIs. This review and other data support the concept that ST-segment depression and exercise effectively stratify patients after a non–Q wave MI.

Thoroughness and length of follow-up observation. Those lost to follow-up study most likely have a higher percentage of deaths. Also, follow-up variations affect analysis if censored data cannot be handled adequately with the statistical program. Mortality changes over time, and predictors change.

Percentage of patients undergoing CABS (or PTCA) during follow-up. CABS could alter mortality and affect outcome prediction. Also, patients with ischemic predictors would be selected to have this procedure more frequently. These patients should be censored at the time of intervention, but such censoring is not random.

Cardiac events considered as end points. The only clear-cut end points that should be considered from an epidemiological point of view are death and reinfarction. Separation or distinction of sudden death makes little sense and may confuse the analysis, particularly if those with sudden death are compared to all others (including non-

sudden cardiac death). Noncardiac deaths are often difficult to distinguish and lead to biased results but may play a confusing role, particularly in older populations. However, only 50% to 70% of the deaths in the usual age group studied are attributable to cardiovascular causes. CABS is not a valid end point and should be considered as a censored outcome. It is clearly related to certain exercise test results that physicians feel motivated to "fix" with that procedure. "Instability" or progression of symptoms (CHF or angina) are unclear end points that cannot be used for epidemiological purposes. Unfortunately it is difficult to predict infarction or reinfarction. We assume it is caused by ischemia and should be predicted by ischemic responses, but this does not appear to be the case. The end points of infarct-free survival are both infarction and death.

Mortality during follow-up study. If there is a low mortality, more patients are needed to find a statistical difference between those with or without certain variables. Some studies have compensated for this by using unclear end points and by combining end points.

Prior MI patients included or not. Prior MI is an important predictive variable that is dependent on the number and severity of the prior MIs. Patients with prior large MIs are biased toward being admitted with non–Q wave MIs, since another transmural MI increases their likelihood of dying before hospitalization. Few studies have tried to account for the number or severity of prior MIs.

Exclusion criteria. Clearly, clinical judgment applied to the post-MI population to exclude patients from exercise testing allows identification of the highest risk group. Although this process involves consideration of complicating illnesses and age, cardiac dysfunction and ischemia are considered as well.

Age range and sex. Women are believed to have a higher MI mortality and certainly are known to respond differently from men to exercise testing. Because of this, they should be considered separately, but the studies do not contain a sufficent number for valid analysis. Death rates are directly related to age.

Medications taken after discharge from hospital and at time of test. Digoxin causes ST-segment depression but is usually taken for congestive heart failure thus implicating an ischemic cause for a potential death because of left ventricular dysfunction. Digoxin administration after MI may actually be an independent risk predictor and may act by predisposing to ventricular dysrhythmias. Beta-blockers affect blood pressure and heart rate response and improve survival.

STATISTICAL CRITIQUE OF THE PROGNOSTIC STUDIES

There are several general problems that are apparent across many of the studies. The purpose of a specific study is not always clear; there is confusion evident between the desire to develop a prediction algorithm that will be of practical clinical use in patient treatment and the desire to demonstrate an association of exercise testing responses to subsequent cardiac events in any form. Development of a prediction algorithm requires an approach to validation that is quite different from the testing of the statistical significance of an effect, as is done in many of the studies. Although effect-size estimation is probably the most clinically relevant procedure, most of the studies report only significance test results, perhaps with some means or frequency differences cited. None of the studies reported effect-size estimates with confidence intervals, even though this is the well-established method of reporting estimation results.

If investigators (and journal editors) insist on using hypothesis testing in studies that should be estimation problems, they should also be conscientious about reporting power computations for any negative results. Lack of this computation makes it difficult to judge whether a nonsignificant test is a likely result of a study design with low power to detect significant differences rather than an accurate reflection of no association between the population parameters.

Finally, many of the studies reviewed failed to provide enough details about the data to allow independent evaluation of the investigators' conclusions. Such details are especially necessary to compare results across different studies. Recomputation of effects may be required to compare studies that have reported results in different formats. The number of "?" appearing in the exercise test risk markers column of Table 9-2 illustrates how often data reported were insufficient to compute even the direction of the associations in the study (whether the association is "significant").

Common areas of difficulty include selection biases, a relatively rare outcome of interest, use of multiple end points, and unequal follow-up times. Many of the studies fail to be specific enough about the target population of interest. Selection biases in the patients studied may be too severe for the results to be considered representative of the general population. However, if the limited target population is carefully specified, other investigators can use the additional information gained from those patients in designing further research even if the results are not generally applicable. Evaluation of possible biases requires information on patients who were eligible for the study but declined to participate, or who dropped out of the study after their initial entry. A few of the investigators have reported on such nonparticipants or follow-up losses, but many do not report more than the number of individuals involved.

The most desirable end point for analyses in these studies is death because it is the most well-defined end point, even though some noncardiac deaths may be included in the results. However, this is a relatively rare outcome requiring that large numbers of patients be tested and followed. Failure to include enough patients in a study can lead to reduced precision of estimates or low power to detect differences because of low effective sample size; effective sample size is limited by the number of deaths in the study group. One approach to attempt to deal with small numbers of deaths is the use of multiple end points, often combined. However, this practice may obscure underlying relationships for several reasons. End points other than death, such as angina, cannot be well enough defined to avoid extensive misclassification errors. A potentially more serious issue when end points are combined is independent of the precision of the end-point measurement. Different end points may be related to different mechanisms and thus may have different associations with the test markers. Such differences will confound any attempt to measure associations using combined end points. Perhaps the worst pitfall is the use of an end point to assess associations that may be influenced by the exercise test result; studies that have included CABS as an end point have fallen prey to this trap.

Finally the problem of unequal time periods in follow-up observation of patients cannot be ignored. This problem can be circumvented in the design of a study by use of a limited period for entry into the study, with a follow-up time that will allow the study to be completed with sufficient events. This approach requires that the follow-up time be limited enough to minimize loss-to-follow-up problems. Adjustments for unequal follow-up time can also be made in the analysis phase of the study, but these were not used in most of the studies.

Only one fourth of the research centers reported any use of multivariate techniques. Computer programs for such analyses were certainly widely available after 1980; only five of the 28 centers have reports limited to before 1981, when access to such analysis tools may have been more difficult. None of the studies reported multivariate estimates of effect, even though the effect estimate is at least as sensitive to error from exclusive univariate analysis as significance tests. It is true that multivariate techniques often have stricter assumptions than some of the univariate techniques available and should not be used without initial screening with univariate analysis. Even if univariate estimates are given for comparison to other studies, the multivariate results should be reported so that the extent of adjustment necessary for interrelationships can be assessed.

The other major analysis issue is the problem of unequal follow-up time. Unequal follow-up time that is not controlled in the design of a study must be handled in the analysis of the data. Unequal follow-up time of patients can be treated as censored data. A typical approach in biomedical research for analysis of censored time-to-response data is to use survival analysis techniques. This approach was used in several of the more recent studies. However, a fundamental assumption of most survival techniques is that the censoring is random with respect to the outcome of interest. This assumption cannot be evaluated without there being a report on those patients who were lost to follow-up observation either because of dropping out of the study or because of lack of complete follow-up time attributable to late entry into the study. Information on those who have dropped out could be gathered by death-certificate searches or other techniques; reports on such persons are often missing from the studies reviewed. Including patients who had censored observations because of short follow-up time must be considered carefully, since the risk of subsequent cardiac events is known to change with time. Multivariate approaches to survival analysis are available using proportional hazard regression models or other hazard functions. However, these models may be relatively insensitive to modeling of interactions among the variables. In addition, the results may not be readily interpretable in terms useful to clinicians.

Other approaches to the problem of censored data are possible. One solution often used in epidemiological research is computations in the form of events per person-time, or person-time incidence. Another approach that avoids the inclusion of short-term follow-up patients is to stop entry into the study early enough so that all patients available can be followed for a fixed time. A limited, fixed time of follow-up study can also help reduce the number of dropouts, since the likelihood of losing a patient from the study increases with time. One approach to be avoided that was used in several of the studies is to count merely events in various subgroups without regard to differences in follow-up time. Data reported in such a way is essentially meaningless.

Survival analysis is appropriate when outcome measurements represent the time to occurrence of some event (that is, death or reinfarction). If differences in important covariates or prognostic variables exist at entry between the groups to be compared, the investigator must be concerned with the analysis of the survival experience as influenced by that difference. To adjust for these differences in prognostic variables, stratified analysis or a covariance type of survival analysis could be done. If there are many covariates, the number of strata can quickly become large, with few subjects in each. Moreover, if a covariate is continuous, it must be divided into intervals and each interval assigned to a score or rank before it can be used in a stratified analysis. Cox proposed a regression model that allows for analysis of censored survival data adjusting for continuous as well as discrete covariates, thus avoiding these two problems. This model, also called the "proportional hazards model," rests on the assumption that the hazard rate, or "force of mortality," can be expressed as a product of two terms. Available statistical packages allow for incomplete data; that is, there are cases for which the response is not observed but the data (time in study) are included in the analysis. This case could occur in the study of survival where an individual may remain alive at the close of the observation period or may drop out before the end. The Cox survival analysis allows for covariates that can be selected in a stepwise fashion. The covariates or prognostic factors usually represent either inherited differences among the study subjects or constitute a set of one or more indicator variables representing different groups. The covariates may also describe changes in a patient's prognostic status as a function of time. The Cox proportional hazards regression model rests on the presumption that death rates may be modeled as log-linear functions of the covariates. A regression coefficient that relates the effect of each covariate to the survival function is estimated.

The Cox model is currently favored; however few investigators have compared the various techniques in one data set. Madsen and co-workers compared two software versions of the Cox multivariate analysis, stepwise discriminant analysis, and recursive partitioning in a post-MI population.[64] They concluded that all four techniques gave equally precise prognostic evaluations but that recursive partitioning was easier to use and the Cox models were more accurate. Gilpin and co-workers at UCSD evaluated several multivariate statistical methods in two different hospital populations to predict 30-day mortality and survival after MI.[65] The methods evaluated were linear discriminant analysis, logistic regression, recursive partitioning, and nearest neighbor. Variables used were identified as predictive univariately from the base hospital and were obtained during the first 24 hours. Linear discriminant analysis available in BMDP is based on the assumption of normality among the predictor variables, whereas logistic regression is based on the assumption that the log of the classification function is a linear function of the fitted coefficents. Recursive partitioning makes no assumption regarding normality and can detect interactions among variables and handles missing data. The nearest neighbor procedure is based on the concept that in the multidimensional space defined by the variables a patient would likely have the same outcome as another patient in that space. It cannot detect interaction or assign importance. Linear discriminant analysis, logistic regression, or recursive partitioning all performed similarily within a given population though each used the information contained in the prognostic variables differently. Application between different populations of prediction schemes based on linear discriminant analysis and logistic regression was shown to be feasible, but prior validation is essential.

Temporal changes in risk

It is well documented that changes in the risk of subsequent cardiac events occurs within the first year after MI. Such underlying changes in the hazard function indicate that there may be temporal changes in the effects of any related risk markers. Evaluation of this effect requires time-dependent modeling or conditional analysis with respect to time. Waters and co-workers are the only investigators to have addressed this problem. One expected effect of not considering the temporal changes in risk is that estimates of effect size may be biased toward the null over intervals that span several risk periods.

Metanalysis considerations

Metanalysis is a statistical approach to develop a consensus from an existing body of research. It is a quantitative approach to reviewing research using a variety of statistical techniques for sorting, classifying, and summarizing information from the findings of many studies. It is also the application of research methodology to the characteristics and findings of studies. This includes problem selection, hypothesis formulation, the definition and measurement of constructs and variables, sampling, and data analysis.

The application of metanalysis to a body of research involves three stages. First, a complete literature search analogous to the collection of data in an experimental study is conducted. Second, the important characteristics and findings of relevant studies are classified. Third, statistical techniques are applied to the compiled data. This last stage can involve descriptive, correlational, and inferential statistical analysis. The statistical techniques applied here are sign testing, correlations, and weighted regression analysis. Sign testing is a statistical test that evaluates the proportions of findings and determines if they are related by more than chance.

Although scientific truth relies on reproducibility, clinical studies often do not agree because of the effect of confounding variables that at times can be accounted for by statistical techniques. When metanalysis was applied, it became apparent that an electronic spreadsheet facilitated the process. After word processing, electronic spread sheets are the most common software used in microcomputers. The first of these was VisiCalc (1979) and its introduction was the greatest impetus for the use of personal computers in the office. These programs create a matrix of cells indexed by column and row headings. The cells can be adjusted for size and data presentation. Once data are entered, they can be moved, deleted, copied, sorted, and subjected to mathematical manipulation. However useful these programs have been in business, there has been little application in medicine.

To identify the studies previously presented, Med-line was searched using the keywords of exercise testing and myocardial infarction. Studies were included if they attempted to evaluate the relationship between exercise test variables and cardiac events during a follow-up period and were published before 1988. The review data were entered into the spreadsheet, and tables were directly printed from the program. The spreadsheet program allowed for very flexible data entry. Column and row headings were specified without excessive care for priority, appearance, or order, since data ranges could be easily moved, ordered alphabetically or numerically, copied, or deleted. Graphic capabilities made it possible to present the data in various graphic formats (pies, bars, and x-y plots) and to visualize the relationships between data in columns or rows, or both. Facile identification and separation of subgroups was possible; the latter being the second step in the application of metanalysis.

Initial analysis consisted in searching and sorting findings within the spreadsheet. Studies were categorized as early, or predischarge, testing (arbritarily set at less than 3 weeks after MI) and late, postdischarge, testing (3 weeks or greater) and placed in Table 9-3. The studies were then subgrouped to see if differences were attributable to maximal or submaximal end points for exercise testing and placed in Table 9-4. Other exploratory

Table 9-3   Results of studies grouped by whether testing was done before 3 weeks after myocardial infarction or at 3 weeks or later

Investigator		End point	Exercise test risk markers				
			SBP	PVCs	ExCap	Angina	ST
Early or predischarge (13 institutional studies)							
7	MHI	sub	+*	+	+	NR	8×*
9	Starling	sub	5×	2×	NR	4×	4×
10	Weld	sub	5×*	2×*	19×*	2×	2×
12	Velasco	sub	3×	2×	NR	3×	4×*
14	Jelinek	max	−	NR	+	2×*	1
15	Madsen	max	+*	+*	+*	?	1
16	Gibson	sub	NR	NR	NR	1	1
18	Williams	sub	2×	−	2×*	2×	1
19	Jennings	sub	8×*	1	8×*	?	1
20	Fioretti	max	+*	+	+*	1	−
21	MCPMIgrp	sub	8×*	2×	3×*	3×*	1
22	Handler	sub	5×*	1	8×*	1	2×
23	SCOR	sub	1	2×	9×*	2×	3×
No. significant out of 13			7	2	8	3	2
No. reporting positively			10	8	10	7	7
No. reporting analysis			12	12	10	12	13
Late or postdischarge (11 institutional studies)							
1	Ericsson	sub	NR	4×	?	?	NR
2	Kentala	max	+	+	NR	NR	+*
3	Granath	sub	NR	2×*	2×	2×	NR
4	Smith	sub	NR	−	NR	NR	6×*
5	Hunt	sub	NR	1	NR	4×*	3×*
6	Stanford	max	NR	NR	+*	1	8×*
8	Koppes	max	?	?	?	?	?
11	Saunamaki	max	3×*	2×*	NR	NR	1
13	De Feyter	max	NR	3×	+	2×	1
17	Norris	max	NR	NR	?	?	1
24	Jespersen	max	1	1	1	1	3×*
No. significant out of 11			1	2	1	1	5
No. reporting positively			2	5	3	3	5
No. reporting analysis			4	9	7	8	9

*Statistically significant.

subgroupings included examining American studies versus studies from other countries and selection of the "best" studies. Subset analysis by whether women or patients with prior or non−Q wave MIs were included was limited by the small number of studies that used these features as exclusion criteria as well as by the suprising number of studies that did not make this information available. The same could be said for analysis of the data regarding cardiac medications. Therefore the percentages of these clinical features were correlated and regressed against the risk ratios found for the exercise risk markers.

Because of the varied statistical treatments used by the studies analyzed as well as the lack of complete reporting by some investigators, exer-

cise responses were associated with relative risk by both quantified univariate or multivariate analysis or by unquantified multivariate analysis. Risk ratios from the former were used in regression and correlation analysis whether the reported value was statistically significant. All values were plotted in x-y graphs. For plotting purposes, if the risk ratios were not available, arbitrary values of positive or negative 1.6 and 1.3 were used for significant and nonsignificant multivariate ratios respectively.

Initial data analysis consisted in the construction of a correlation matrix consisting of Pearson product moment correlations for the risk ratios of the five exercise test responses with each of the following clinical variables: percent tested, per-

Table 9-4 Results of studies grouped by whether the end point was maximal or submaximal

	Investigators	Exercise test risk markers				
		SBP	PVCs	ExCap	Angina	ST
Submaximal testing (14 institutional studies)						
1	Ericsson	NR	4×	?	?	NR
3	Granath	NR	2×*	2×	2×	NR
4	Smith	NR	−	NR	NR	6×*
5	Hunt	NR	1	NR	4×*	3×*
7	MHI	+*	+	+	NR	8×*
9	Starling	5×	2×	NR	4×	4×
10	Weld	5×*	2×*	19×*	2×	2×
12	Velasco	3×	2×	NR	3×*	4×*
16	Gibson	NR	NR	NR	+	+
18	Williams	2×	−	2×*	2×	1
19	Jennings	8×*	1	8×*	?	1
21	MCPMIgrp	8×*	2×	3×*	3×*	1
22	Handler	5×*	1	8×*	1	2×
23	SCOR	1	2×	9×*	2×	3×
No. significant out of 14		5	2	6	3	4
No. reporting positively		8	8	8	8	9
No. reporting analysis		9	13	9	10	12
Maximal testing (10 institutional studies)						
2	Kentala	+	+	NR	NR	+*
6	Stanford	NR	NR	+*	1	8×*
8	Koppes	?	?	?	?	?
11	Saunamaki	3×*	2×*	NR	NR	1
13	De Feyter	NR	3×	+	2×	1
14	Jelinek	−	NR	+	2×*	1
15	Madsen	+*	+*	+*	?	1
17	Norris	NR	NR	?	?	1
20	Fioretti	+*	+	+*	1	−
24	Jespersen	1	1	1	1	3×*
No. significant out of 10		3	2	3	1	3
No. reporting positively		4	5	5	2	3
No. reporting analysis		7	7	8	8	10

*Statistically significant.

cent females, percent of prior MI, percent with each Q-wave location, percent on digoxin, percent on a beta-blocking agent, percent subsequent mortality if tested, and percent mortality if not tested. Subsequently, if the correlation was greater than 0.30 between a ratio of an exercise test response risk and one of the above, they were selected for regression analysis. Regression was performed on each pair selected. To adjust for differences in sample size between studies (that is, the results of a study with only 60 subjects should not have the same effect on decision analysis as a study with 120 patients), regression analysis was weighted by the number of patients exercise tested in each study. Resulting f values were tested for confidence levels. Regression equations

associated with a p value equal or less than 0.10 are reported. The correlations are listed on Table 9-5.

As part of metanalysis, sign testing was applied to the findings in table 9-2. Since it is not possible to ascertain the directions of the nonsignificant associations listed as "?" in Table 9-2, metanalysis conclusions must be tentative. Some researchers probably did not evaluate markers that are not reported (NR), but others are likely to have failed to report null or negative findings. The most generous evaluation would be to omit studies that did not report results for a particular marker; the most conservative approach would be to include these studies and to assume that any unreported results were not positive associations. Results are pre-

Table 9-5 Matrix of correlation of the prevalence of variables with risk ratios in the post-MI studies described in Table 9-2

| | % Ex tested | % women | % prior MI | % SE MI | % AMI | % IP MI | % on DIG | % on BB | Mortality | | Exercise test risk markers | | | |
									If ET done	If not done	SBP	PVC	ExCap	Angina
% women	.23													
% prior MI	.01	.37												
% SE MI	.51	.22	.04											
% Ant MI	-.39	-.15	.44	-.57										
% IP MI	-.32	-.45	.05	-.67	.07									
% Dig	.15	.04	.29	.25	-.06	-.21								
% BB	-.17	.22	.31	.35	.24	-.17	.10							
Mort if ET	.09	-.15		-.12	.08	.14	.39	-.26						
Mort no ET	.60*	.21	-.01	.39	.14	-.61	.33	.21	.38					
BP	-.13	.14	.42	-.08	.60	.18	-.03	.21	-.15	.31	-.10			
PVC	.20	-.21	.38	-.53	.28	.09	.16	-.33	-.08	-.99	.20	.23		
ExCap	.04	.25	.28	-.65	.41	.46	.50	.00	-.15	-.45	.43	.48	.01	
Angina	-.40	-.34	.14	-.39	.26	.19	.40	.34	.15	-.73*	-.40	-.09	.13	
ST	-.28	-.49*	.04	-.37	.20	.64*	-.35	-.33	-.18	-.68*				.42

Ex tested, % of study population that underwent exercise test, % of women included in the study, % *MI*, Percentage of the types of MIs included: *Prior*, prior MI; *AMI*, anterior Q-wave MI; *IP*, inferior or posterior MI; *SE*, subendocardial or non–Q wave MI; % *on*, percentage of patients receiving digoxin (*Dig*) or a beta-blocker (*BB*) at the time of treadmill testing. *mortality if ET done*, death rate in patients who underwent exercise testing; *if not done*; mortality in those who were excluded from exercise testing; *BP*, abnormal systolic BP response; *PVC*, abnormal PVCs; *ExCap*, abnormally low exercise capacity; *angina*, angina induced by test; *ST*, abnormal ST-segment response (usually only depression).

sented for both stituations with upper and lower bounds on the overall published results on exercise test markers as predictors of death.

If there were not a true underlying association of a risk marker with death, we would expect that 50% of studies would report positive association based on chance. "Statistical significance" is not considered here; only the directions of the *observed* associations. With only studies with any reported effect being used as the denominator, the generous estimates of the percentages of positive associations reported for SBP (12 centers reporting positive associations/18 centers presenting any results for systolic BP), PVCs (14/23), ExCap (14/18), angina (12/20), and ST (15/19) are 72%, 61%, 78%, 60%, and 63% respectively. Only the *systolic blood pressure* and *exercise capacity* proportions are significantly different from chance by a sign test. The conservative estimates using all 28 studies as the denominator are 46%, 50%, 50%, 43%, and 54% respectively. None of these are different from chance. In consideration of the probable publishing bias against negative findings, the true situations are likely to be closer to the conservative computations than to the generous ones.

Subgrouping by timing and target. Subgrouping by early, predischarge, testing (arbitrarily set at less than 3 weeks after MI) and late, or postdischarge, testing (3 weeks or greater) yielded the findings in Table 9-3. Notice that all the predictors except for ST shifts were reported positively more than 50% of the time during predischarge testing and not during postdischarge testing. To see if these differences were attributable to maximal or submaximal end points for exercise testing, Table 9-4 was constructed. Although during submaximal testing the exercise predictors were more likely to be associated with positivity than maximal testing, the finding was not as strong.

Subgrouping the studies by whether or not they were performed early or late, as was done in Table 9-3, shows that the highest rate of positive predictors and the highest risk ratios occur with early testing. With only studies of early exercise testing with any reported effect being used as the denominator, the generous estimates of the percentages of positive associations reported for BP (10 centers reporting positive associations/12 centers presenting any results for SBP), PVCs (8/12), ExCap (10/10), angina (7/12), and ST (7/13) are 83%, 67%, 100%, 58%, and 54% respectively. Only the SBP and ExCap were significant, but none of the exercise test responses was significant for testing done after discharge (50%, 56%, 43%, 38%, and 56% respectively). In Table 9-4, the studies are divided into those that used maximal and those that used submaximal end points for ex-

ercise testing. With only studies of submaximal exercise testing with any reported effect being used as the denominator, the generous estimates of the percentages of positive associations reported for BP (8 centers reporting positive associations/9 centers presenting any results for SBP), PVCs (8/13), ExCap (8/9), angina (8/10), and ST (9/12) are 89%, 63%, 89%, 80%, and 75% respectively. All exercise responses except for PVCs were significantly associated with a poor outcome with submaximal testing, and none of the exercise test responses with maximal testing were significant (57%, 71%, 63%, 25%, and 30% respectively). Other exploratory subgroupings including American studies versus studies from other countries and selection of the "best" studies failed to produce test performance differences.

Correlation of prevalence of variables with risk ratios. Under the criteria described for inclusion for regression analysis, 24 pairs of variables qualified for additional analysis. Of these, the following pair's weighted regression displayed $p = 0.10$ and >0.05: (1) percent mortality in those not tested was negatively related to ST ($p = 0.06$) and to angina ($p = 0.10$) risk ratios; (2) ST risk ratio was negatively related to the percent taking digoxin ($p = 0.10$). Additionally, ST risk ratio was negatively related to percent females in the studies and positively to the percent with inferior or posterior MIs, both with high confidence levels: $p = 0.03$ and 0.01 respectively. Lastly, the relationship between %Tested and %Mortality in those tested was examined: as the proportion of patients tested increased, the mortality increases in those not tested.

Since metanalysis is an attempt to consider information from a pool of data (but at the study level, without actually pooling data), problems arise in comparing results from studies with different protocols. Differences in types of exercise tests, ECG leads used, and others increase the difficulties of summarizing the research by metanalysis, particularly since effect sizes cannot be calculated from the data reported in many of the studies. Even though all the published studies are considered, there is probably a serious publishing bias both by authors and editors toward excluding negative results. This occurs at two levels: completely negative studies may not get submitted or published, and complete data on all risk markers evaluated may not be reported. Often not even the direction of a possible effect can be computed for a particular exercise test result.

SUMMARY

The benefits of performing an exercise test in post MI patients are listed in the box. Submitting pa-

---

**BENEFITS OF EXERCISE TESTING
AFTER MYOCARDIAL INFARCTION**

Predischarge submaximal test

Setting safe exercise levels (exercise
  prescription)
Optimizing discharge
Altering medical therapy
Sorting for intensity of follow-up observation
First step in rehabilitation—assurance,
  encouragement
Reassuring spouse
Recognizing exercise induced ischemia
  and dysrhythmias

Maximal test for return to normal activities

Determining limitations
Prognostication
Reassuring employers
Determining level of disability
Sorting for invasive studies
Deciding on medications
Exercise prescription
Continued rehabilitation

---

tients to exercise testing can expedite and optimize their discharge from the hospital. The patient's response to exercise, his or her work capacity, and limiting factors at the time of discharge can be assessed by the exercise test. An exercise test before discharge is important for giving a patient guidelines for exercise at home, reassuring each of his or her physical status, and determining the risk of complications. It provides a safe basis for advising the patient to resume or increase his or her activity level and return to work. The test can demonstrate to the patient, relatives, or employer the effect of the myocardial infarction on the capacity for physical performance. Psychologically, it can cause an improvement in the patient's self-confidence by making the patient less anxious about daily physical activities. The test has been helpful in reassuring spouses of post-MI patients of their physical capabilities. The psychological effect of performing well on the exercise test is impressive. Many patients increase their activity and actually rehabilitate themselves after being encouraged and reassured by their response to this test.

The angiographic studies correlating results with post MI exercise testing involved populations that were very selected, in particular containing a higher prevalence of patients with angina, since they are more likely to undergo angiography. In some studies, an abnormal test result was considered to be angina or ST-segment depression, and the results for each response could not be separated. Few of these studies considered the other exercise test responses that have been associated with a poor prognosis. Review of the studies demonstrated a limited sensitivity and specificity for identification of patients with multivessel disease (MVD). Certainly the sensitivity for detecting those with left main and three-vessel disease is higher. The poor specificity could lead to more angiography than is necessary. This leads to unnecessary procedures, since there is always the tendency to "do something," despite the absence of data that survival is improved.

One consistent finding in the review of the post MI exercise test studies that included a follow-up study for cardiac end points is that patients who met whatever criteria set forth for exercise testing were at a lower risk than patients not tested. This finding supports the clinical judgment of the skilled clinician. In the complete data set from the review, only an abnormal systolic blood pressure response or a low exercise capacity were significantly associated with a poor outcome. These responses are so powerful because they can be associated with deaths from either ischemia or congestive heart failure. When the studies were subgrouped by whether testing was done early or late, a high proportion of early test results indicated a poor outcome. This may mean that the risk predictors from exercise testing can identify only the patients that die early after MI, that is, before later testing can be done. Submaximal testing resulted in the highest proportion of positive associations and the highest risk ratios. This means that the higher work loads are associated with a better prognosis despite the other responses.

Regression analysis of risk ratios of the test responses and the prevalence of clinical features lead to other interesting hypotheses. Surprisingly, the highest correlations for the exercise test risk markers were obtained with the mortality in the patients excluded from testing. The negative correlations indicate that the higher the mortality in those excluded, the less able the exercise test responses are to identify a high-risk group. Mortality in those excluded correlates directly with the percent exercise tested; that is, the greater the percentage tested out of an MI population, the higher the risk for death in those excluded. However, neither the percentage tested nor the mortality in those tested correlated well with the exercise test results. Therefore the more skilled the clinician is at selecting a high-risk group and excluding them from exercise testing, the poorer the exercise test functions for identifying high-risk patients because of the characteristics of the population who remain to be tested. One hypothesis from these results is that the exercise test is most useful for risk stratification in a setting where good clinicians are not available.

Other significant weighted regressions included the relationships between the risk ratios for ST-segment shifts and percentage women and percentage of patients receiving digoxin. There were negative correlations, and so an abnormal ST-segment response generated a higher risk in studies that included a lower percentage of women or a

lower percentage of patients receiving digoxin.

Who should undergo coronary angiography after MI for consideration of CABS to improve survival? By working backward through known associations and relationships, one can derive the clinical description of the high-risk patient who potentially could have improved survival with CABS. The randomized trials of CABS have demonstrated that patients with three-vessel or left main disease with an ejection fraction of 30% to 50% have improved survival with surgery as compared to medical therapy. Athough coronary heart

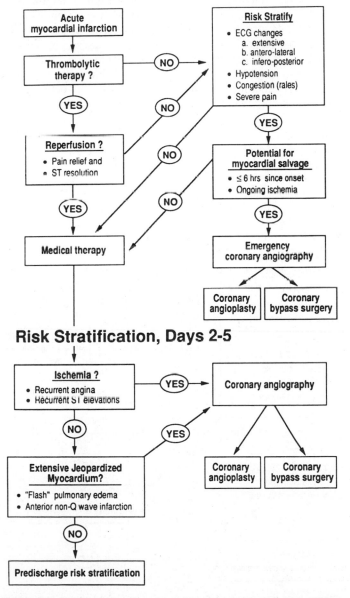

Figure 9-1 (From Krone RJ: *Am Intern Med* 116:223-237, 1992.)

disease can cause myocardial fibrosis and decreased ventricular function without overt MIs by signs or symptoms, this is unusual. Studies have shown that 15% to 25% of MIs are silent, but in these cases the diagnosis was made by the electrocardiogram. The clinical picture, either by history or by ECG, that would result in an ejection fraction from 30% to 50% would include patients with large anterior MIs, a history or ECG pattern of multiple MIs, transmural MIs followed by subendocardial MIs, or a history of transient congestive heart failure with an MI. In addition, physical findings of ventricular dyskinesia or cardiomegaly on palpation would support this. Thus clinical and electrocardiographic features predict those with decreased ventricular function. Noninvasive testing (that is, radionuclide ventriculography and echocardiography) could also be utilized. Although its sensitivity is decreased in one- or two-vessel disease, the exercise ECG is approximately 90% sensitive for three-vessel or left main disease. Angina is also very common in this group of patients. Therefore the following profile

identifies the high-risk patient after an MI who should undergo coronary angiography: the patient with a history or ECG findings of a large anterior MI or multiple MIs or abnormal precordial movements or a history of transient congestive heart failure, or any combination, and signs and symptoms of severe myocardial ischemia on the exercise test. Severe ischemia is characterized by the occurrence of ST-segment depression or angina, or both, at a double product less than 20,000 and less than 5 METs of exercise capacity. If there are no contraindications to CABS in these patients, they should be considered for coronary angiography. Post-MI patients who should be considered for reasons other than improved survival are those whose angina is not controlled satisfactorily with medications and those in whom either the diagnosis of MI or the cause of chest pain after MI is uncertain. This "logical" algorithm requires validation.

The failure of exercise-induced ST-segment depression to be consistently associated with increased risk in patients after myocardial infarction

Risk Stratification: Predischarge

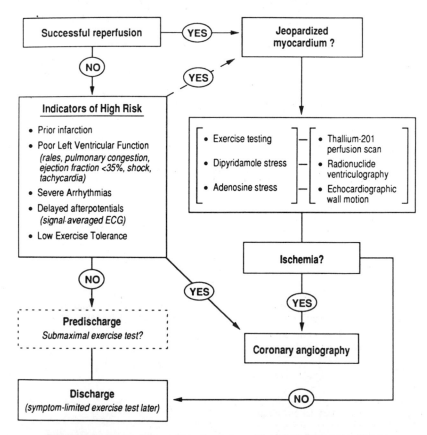

Figure 9-2 (From Krone RJ: *Am Intern Med* 116:223-237, 1992.)

was hard to explain until recently. This failure could be a result of population differences and the resting ECG. To test this we studied 198 males who survived a myocardial infarction, underwent a submaximal predischarge treadmill test, and were followed for cardiac events for 2 years.[66] Abnormal ST-segment depression was associated with twice the risk for death, and the risk increased to 11 times in patients without diagnostic Q-waves, similar to the results by Krone in patients with an initial non–Q wave myocardial infarction.[67] These results indicate that the difference in the prognostic value of the post–myocardial infarction exercise-induced ST depression between studies may be attributable to variations in the prevalence of the patterns of the rest ECG among study populations. Angiographic studies, however, have demonstrated that exercise-induced ST-segment depression is associated with severe coronary artery disease whether Q waves are present. The conflicting results from follow-up observation and angiographic studies most probably relates to the fact that early mortality is strongly associated with left ventricular damage whereas later mortality is associated with ischemia and severe coronary artery disease. Krone has nicely summarized the use of noninvasive testing in risk stratification after MI in Figure 9-1, and Figure 9-2 illustrates his recommendations.[68] These are a summary of previous recommendations and are very pertinent to clinical practice.

It is important to note that risk stratification is very effective and that routine coronary angiography is not indicated after myocardial infarction whether thrombolysis has been utilized. Also, mild degrees of ischemia (that is, occasional angina pectoris, 1 mm exercise-induced ST-segment depression) are not ominous after a myocardial infarction.

REFERENCES

1. May GS, Eberlein KA, Furberg CD, et al: Secondary prevention after myocardial infarction: a review of long-term trials, *Prog Cardiovasc Dis* 24:331-352, 1982.
2. Torkelson LO: Rehabilitation of the patient with acute myocardial infarciton, *J Chronic Disability* 17:685-704, 1964.
3. Ibsen H, Kjoller E, Styperek J, Pedersen A: Routine exercise ECG three weeks after acute myocardial infarction, *Acta Med Scand* 198:463-469, 1975.
4. Niederberger M: Values and limitations of exercise testing after myocardial infarction (monograph), Vienna, 1977, Verlag Brüder Hollinek, pp 3-45.
5. Markiewicz W, Houston N, DeBusk RF: Exercise testing soon after myocardial infarction, *Circulation* 56:26-31, 1977.
6. Sivarajan ES, Bruce RA, Lindskog BD, et al: Treadmill test responses to an early exercise program after myocardial infarction: a randomized study, *Circulation* 65:1420-1428, 1982.
7. Taylor CD, Bandura A, Ewart CK, et al: Exercise testing to enhance wives' confidence in their husbands' cardiac capability soon after clinically uncomplicated acute myocardial infarction, *Am J Cardiol* 55:635-638, 1985.
8. Ewart CK, Taylor CB, Reese LB, DeBusk RF: Effects of early postmyocardial infarction exercise testing on self-perception and subsequent physical activity, *Am J Cardiol* 51:1076-1080, 1983.
9. Handler CE, Sowton E: A comparison of the Naughton and modified Bruce treadmill exercise protocols in their ability to detect ischaemic abnormalities six weeks after myocardial infarction, *Eur Heart J* 5:752-755, 1984.
10. Starling MR, Crawford MH, ORourke RA: Superiority of selected treadmill exercise protocols predischarge and six weeks postinfarction for detecting ischemic abnormalities, *Am Heart J* 104:1054-1059, 1982.
11. Starling MR, Crawford MH, Kennedy GT, O'Rourke RA: Exercise testing early after myocardial infarction: predictive value of subsequent unstable angina and death, *Am J Cardiol* 46:909-914, 1980.
12. Handler CE, Sowton E: Diurnal variation in symptom-limited exercise test responses six weeks after myocardial infarction, *Eur Heart J* 6:444-450, 1985.
13. Starling MR, Crawford MH, Kennedy GT, O'Rourke RA: Treadmill exercise tests predischarge and six weeks post–myocardial infarction to detect abnormalities of known prognostic value, *Ann Intern Med* 94:721-727, 1981.
14. Wohl AJ, Lewis HR, Campbell W, et al: Cardiovascular function during early recovery from acute myocardial infarction, *Circulation* 56:931-937, 1977.
15. Haskell WL, Savin W, Oldridge N, DeBusk R: Factors influencing estimated oxygen uptake during exercise testing soon after myocardial infarction, *Am J Cardiol* 50:299-304, 1982.
16. Castellanet MJ, Greenberg PS, Ellestad MH: Comparison of S-T segment changes on exercise testing with angiographic findings in patients with prior myocardial infarction, *Am J Cardiol* 42:29-35, 1978.
17. Ahnve S, Savvides M, Abouantoun S, et al: Can ischemia be recognized when Q waves are present on the resting electrocardiogram? *Am Heart J* 110:1016-1020, 1986.
18. Miranda C, Herbert W, Dubach P, et al: Post MI exercise testing: non Q wave vs Q wave, *Circulation* 84:2357-2365, 1991.
19. Weiner DA: Prognostic value of exercise testing early after myocardial infarction, *J Cardiac Rehabil* 3:114-122, 1983.
20. Paine TD, Dye LE, Roitman DI, et al: Relation of graded exercise testing findings after myocardial infarction to extent of coronary artery disease and left ventricular dysfunction, *Am J Cardiol* 42:716-723, 1978.
21. Dillahunt PH, Miller AB: Early treadmill testing after myocardial infarction, *Chest* 76:150-155, 1979.
22. Sammel NL, Wilson RL, Norris RM, et al: Angiocardiography and exercise testing at one month after a first myocardial infarction, *Aust NZ J Med* 10:182-187, 1980.
23. Fuller CM, Raizner AE, Verani MS, et al: Early postmyocardial infarction treadmill stress testing: an accurate predictor of multivessel coronary disease and subsequent cardiac events, *Ann Intern Med* 94:734-739, 1981.
24. Boschat J, Rigaud M, Bardet J, et al: Treadmill exercise testing and coronary cineangiography following first myocardial infarction, *J Cardiac Rehabil* 1:206-211, 1981.
25. Schwartz KM, Turner JD, Sheffield LT, et al: Limited exercise testing soon after myocardial infarction: correlation with early coronary and left ventricular angiography, *Ann Intern Med* 94:727-734, 1981.
26. Starling MR, Crawford MH, Richards KL, O'Rourke RA: Predictive value of early postmyocardial infarction

modified treadmill exercise testing in multivessel coronary artery disease detection, *Am Heart J* 102:169-175, 1981.

27. de Feyter PJ, van den Brand M, Serruys PW, Wijns W: Early angiography after myocardial infarction: What have we learned? *Am Heart J* 109:194-199, 1985.

28. Akhras F, Upward J, Keates J, Jackson G: Early exercise testing and elective coronary artery bypass surgery after uncomplicated myocardial infarction: effect on morbidity and mortality, *Br Heart J* 52:413-417, 1984.

29. Morris DD, Rozanski A, Berman DS, et al: Noninvasive prediction of the angiographic extent of coronary artery disease after myocardial infarction: comparison of clinical bicycle exercise, electrocardiographic and ventriculographic parameters, *Circulation* 70:192-201, 1984.

30. van der Wall EE, van Eenige MJ, Visser FC, et al: Thallium-201 exercise testing in patients 6-8 weeks after myocardial infarction: limited value for the detection of multivessel disease, *Eur Heart J* 6:29-36, 1985.

31. Veenbrink WG, Van der Werf T, Westerhof PW, et al: Is there an indication for coronary angiography in patients under 60 years of age with no or minimal angina pectoris after a first myocardial infarction? *Br Heart J* 53:30-35, 1985.

32. Sia STB, MacDonald PS, Horowitz JD, et al: Usefulness of early exercise testing after non-Q-wave myocardial infarction in predicting prognosis, *Am J Cardiol* 57:738-744, 1986.

33. Laupacis A, LaBelle R, Goeree R, Cairns J: The cost-effectiveness of routine post myocardial infarction exercise stress testing, *Can J Cardiol* 6:157-163, 1990.

34. Ericsson M, Granath A, Ohlsen P, et al: Arrhythmias and symptoms during treadmill testing three weeks after myocardial infarction in 100 patients, *Br Heart J* 35:787-790, 1973.

35. Kentala E: Physical fitness and feasibility of physical rehabilitation after myocardial infarction in men of working age, *Ann Clin Res* 4(suppl 9):1-84, 1972.

36. Granath A, Södermark T, Winge T, et al: Early work load tests for evaluation of long-term prognosis of acute myocardial infarction, *Br Heart J* 39:758-765, 1977.

37. Smith JW, Dennis CA, Gassmann A, et al: Exercise testing three weeks after myocardial infarction, *Chest* 75:12-16, 1979.

38. Hunt D, Hamer A, Duffield A, et al: Predictors of reinfarction and sudden death in a high-risk group of acute myocardial infarction survivors, *Lancet* 1:233-236, 1979.

39. Srinivasan M, Young A, Baker G, et al: The value of postcardiac infarction exercise stress testing: identification of a group at high risk, *Med J Aust* 2:466-467, 1981.

40. Sami M, Kraemer H, DeBusk RF: The prognostic significance of serial exercise testing after myocardial infarction, *Circulation* 60:1238-1246, 1979.

41. Davidson DM, DeBusk RF: Prognostic value of a single exercise test 3 weeks after uncomplicated myocardial infarction, *Circulation* 61:236-241, 1980.

42. DeBusk RF, Dennis CA: "Submaximal" predischarge exercise testing after acute myocardial infarction: Who needs it? *Am J Cardiol* 55:499-500, 1985.

43. Théroux P, Marpole DGF, Bourassa MG: Exercise stress testing in the post–myocardial infarction patient, *Am J Cardiol* 52:664-667, 1983.

44. Waters DA, Bosch X, Bouchard A, et al: Comparison of clinical variables and variables derived from a limited predischarge exercise test as predictors of early and late mortality after myocardial infarction, *J Am Coll Cardiol* 5:1-8, 1985.

45. Koppes GM, Kruyer W, Beckmann CH, Jones FG: Response to exercise early after uncomplicated acute myo-

cardial infarction in patients receiving no medication: long-term follow-up, *Am J Cardiol* 46:764-769, 1980.

46. Starling MR, Kennedy GT, Crawford MH, ORourke RA: Comparative predictive value of ST-segment depression or angina during early and repeat postinfarction exercise tests, *Chest* 86:845-849, 1984.

47. Saunamaki KI, Andersen JD: Early exercise test in the assessment of long-term prognosis after acute myocardial infarction, *Acta Med Scand* 209:185-191, 1981.

48. Saunamaki KI, Anderson JD: Early exercise test vs clinical variables in the long-term prognostic management after myocardial infarction, *Acta Med Scand* 212:47-52, 1982.

49. Velasco J, Tormo V, Ferrer LM, et al: Early exercise test for evaluation of long-term prognosis after uncomplicated myocardial infarction, *Eur Heart J* 2:401-407, 1981.

50. Weld FM: Exercise testing after myocardial infarction, *J Cardiac Rehabil* 5:20-27, 1985.

51. Jelinek VM, Ziffer RW, McDonald IG, et al: Early exercise testing and mobilization after myocardial infarction, *Med J Aust* 2:589-593, 1977.

52. Madsen EB, Gilpin E: Prognostic value of exercise test variables after myocardial infarction, *J Cardiac Rehabil* 3:481-488, 1983.

53. Gibson RS, Watson DD, Craddock GB, et al: Prediction of cardiac events after uncomplicated myocardial infarction: a prospective study comparing predischarge exercise thallium-201 scintigraphy and coronary angiography, *Circulation* 68:321-336, 1983.

54. Norris RM, Barnaby PF, Brandt PWT, et al: Prognosis after recovery from first acute myocardial infarction: determinants of reinfarction and sudden death, *Am J Cardiol* 53:408-413, 1984.

55. Williams WL, Nair RC, Higginson LA, et al: Comparison of clinical and treadmill variables for the prediction of outcome after myocardial infarction, *J Am Coll Cardiol* 4:477-486, 1984.

56. Jennings K, Reid DS, Hawkins T, Julian DJ: Role of exercise testing early after myocardial infarction in identifying candidates for coronary surgery, *Br Med J* 288:185-187, 1984.

57. Fioretti P, Deckers JW, Brower RW, et al: Predischarge stress test after myocardial infarction in the old age: results and prognostic value, *Eur Heart J* 5:101-104, 1984.

58. Krone RJ, Gillespie JA, Weld FM, et al: Low-level exercise testing after myocardial infarction: usefulness in enhancing clinical risk stratification, *Circulation* 71:80-89, 1985.

59. Dwyer EM, McMaster P, Greenberg H: Nonfatal cardiac events and recurrent infarction in the year after acute myocardial infarction, *J Am Coll Cardiol* 4:695-702, 1984.

60. Handler CE: Exercise testing to identify high risk patients after myocardial infarction, *J R Coll Phys London* 18:124-127, 1984.

61. Madsen EB, Gilpin E: How much prognostic information do exercise test data add to clinical data after acute myocardial infarction, *Int J Cardiol* 4:15-27, 1983.

62. Jespersen CM, Kassis E, Edeling CJ, Madsen JK: The prognostic value of maximal exercise testing soon after first MI, *Eur Heart J* 6:769-772, 1985.

63. Connolly DC, Elveback LR: Coronary heart disease in residents of Rochester, Minnesota. VI. Hospital and posthospital course of patients with transmural and subendocardial myocardial infarction, *Mayo Clin Proc* 60:375-381, 1985.

64. Madsen EB, Gilpin E, Henning H: Short-term prognosis in acute myocardial infarction: evaluation of different prediction methods, *Am Heart J* 107:1241-1251, 1984.

65. Gilpin E, Olshen R, Henning H, Ross J: Risk prediction after myocardial infarction: comparison of three multi-variate methodologies, *Cardiology* 70:73-84, 1983.

66. Klein J, Froelicher VF, Detrano R, et al: Does the rest electrocardiogram after myocardial infarction determine the predictive value of exercise-induced ST depression? A 2 year follow-up study in a veteran population, *J Am Coll Cardiol* 14:305-311, 1989.

67. Krone RJ, Dwyer EM Jr, Greenberg H, et al: Risk stratification in patients with first non–Q wave infarction: limited value of the early low level exercise test after uncomplicated infarcts: the Multicenter Post-Infarction Research Group, *J Am Coll Cardiol* 14:31-37, 1989.

68. Krone RJ: The role of risk stratification in the early management of a myocardial infarction, *Ann Intern Med* 116:223-237, 1992.

10 Special Application

Screening Apparently Healthy Individuals

DEFINITION

Screening can be defined as the presumptive identification of unrecognized disease by the utilization of procedures that can be applied rapidly. The relative value of techniques for identifying individuals who have asymptomatic coronary heart disease (CHD) should be assessed in order to direct preventive efforts toward those with such disease.

CRITERIA

Eight criteria have been proposed for the selection of a screening procedure: (1) the procedure is acceptable and appropriate; (2) the quantity and quality of life can be favorably altered; (3) the results of intervention outweigh any adverse effects; (4) the target disease has an asymptomatic period during which its outcome can be altered; (5) acceptable treatments are available; (6) the prevalence and seriousness of the disease justify the costs of intervention; (7) the procedure is relatively easy and inexpensive; and, (8) sufficient resources are available. In addition, *seven guides* have been recommended for deciding whether a community screening program does more harm than good: (1) has the program's effectiveness been demonstrated in a randomized trial and, if so, (2) are efficacious treatments available; (3) does the current burden of suffering warrant screening; (4) is there a good screening test; (5) does the program reach those who could benefit from it; (6) can the health care system cope with the screening program; and (7) will those who had a positive screening comply with subsequent advice and interventions?

The process of primary prevention of coronary heart disease could be facilitated by targeting asymptomatic individuals with early disease. Thus it is advisable to evaluate screening methods for detection of coronary artery disease before death or disability occurs. Risk-factor screening and resting techniques including the ECG have limited sensitivity, and so exercise testing, which brings out abnormalities not present at rest, could increase sensitivity. Various techniques have been recommended to improve the sensitivity and specificity of exercise testing; these are new computerized and noncomputerized electrocardiographic criteria, other exercise test responses, cardiac radionuclide procedures, systolic time intervals, cardiokymography, cardiac fluoroscopy, digital radiographic imaging, echocardiography, and the computerized application of bayesian statistics using risk factors and risk markers. These techniques may improve attempts to screen for latent coronary heart disease. Limited data indicate that angiographically documented asymptomatic coronary disease may have a relatively good prognosis compared with symptomatic disease and rarely should lead to coronary artery bypass surgery. Individuals identified by screening should be prime targets for behavior modification with the hope of avoiding the usual course of this disease. Because of the high probability of restenosis (and making asymptomatic disease symptomatic), percutaneous transluminal coronary angioplasty (PTCA) should rarely be applied.

Screening has also been recommended for evaluating asymptomatic individuals in whom sudden incapacitation could compromise public safety. Such individuals include pilots, firemen, and policemen. Others who possibly should be screened are railroad engineers, air traffic controllers, and drivers of large commercial vehicles. This has not met with enthusiasm from the targeted groups because of the high false-positive rate inherent with low prevalence populations. Because a high-level exercise program designed to develop athletic performance does present a risk to sedentary, middle-aged men, it is prudent to evaluate such individuals with screening before such an exercise program is begun.

SENSITIVITY AND SPECIFICITY

For evaluation of the value of any screening test, sensitivity, specificity, predictive value, and relative risk must be demonstrated. Sensitivity is the percentage of times a test gives an abnormal response when those with disease are tested. Specificity is the percentage of times a test gives a normal response when those without disease are tested—a definition quite different from the conventional use of the word "specific." These two values are inversely related and are determined by the discriminant values or cut points chosen for the test that separate abnormals from normals. The predictive value of an abnormal test is the percentage of individuals with an abnormal test who have disease. The relative risk of an abnormal test response is the relative chance of having disease if the test is abnormal compared to having disease if the test is normal. The values for these last two terms are dependent on the prevalance of disease in the population being tested.

A basic step in applying any testing procedure for the separation of those without disease from those with a disease is to determine a test value that best separates the two groups. One problem is that there is usually a considerable overlap of measurement values of a test in the groups with and without disease. Consider two bell-shaped normal distribution curves, one representing a normal population and the other representing a population with disease, with a certain amount of overlap of the two curves (see Figure 7-1). Along the vertical axis is the number of patients and along the horizontal axis could be the value for such measurements as Q-wave size, exercise-induced ST-segment depression, or creatine phosphokinase. The optimal test would be able to achieve the most clear-cut separation of these two bell-shaped curves and minimize the overlap. Unfortunately, most tests have a considerable overlap of the range of measurements for the normal population and for those with heart disease. Therefore problems arise when a certain value is used to separate these two groups (that is, Q-wave amplitude or width, 0.1 mV of ST-segment depression, a 10 mm Hg drop in systolic blood pressure, less than 5 METs of exercise capacity, three premature ventricular beats). If the value is set far to the right (that is, 0.2 mV of ST-segment depression) to identify nearly all the normal subjects as being free of disease, the test will have a high specificity. However, a substantial number of those with disease will be called normal. If a value is chosen far to the left (that is, 0.05 mV of ST-segment depression) that identifies nearly all those with disease as being abnormal, giving the test a high sensitivity, then many normal subjects are identified as abnormal. If a cut-point value is chosen that equally mislabels the normal subjects and those with disease, the test will have its highest predictive accuracy. However, there may be reasons for wanting to adjust a test to have a relatively higher sensitivity or relatively higher specificity than possible when predictive accuracy is optimal. For instance, sensitivity should be highest in the emergency room, and the specificity should be the highest when one is doing insurance examinations. Remember that sensitivity and specificity are inversely related; that is, when sensitivity is the highest, specificity is the lowest and vice versa. Any test has a range of inversely related sensitivities and specificities that can be chosen by selection of a certain discriminant or diagnostic value. Attempts have been made to use a series of tests to improve diagnostic power, but test interaction is complex. Usually the highest sensitivity and the lowest specificity of the tests represent their combined performance.

THE RESTING ECG AS A SCREENING TECHNIQUE

As part of the Copenhagen City Heart Study, nearly 20,000 men and women, 20 years of age or older, had a resting 12-lead ECG performed.[1] The Minnesota code was used to classify the electrocardiograms. The prevalence of all electrocardiographic findings, except for axis deviation, high-amplitude R-waves, minor Q-wave abnormalities, and prolonged or short PR interval, was very low below 40 years of age in men and 50 in women. Rates for Q-wave abnormalities, left axis deviation, ST-segment depression, premature beats, and atrial fibrillation increased with age and were higher for men than for women. A strong association between total mortality and major ST-segment depression and T-wave abnormalities, Q-wave patterns, and left bundle branch block existed. During a period from 1976 to 1980, 489 subjects died, but there were only a few deaths in those under 50 years of age. Because of this death pattern and because the prevalence of ECG abnormalities was low in the young, relative risk was only significant in those 50 or older. Over 50% of the deaths were attributable to noncardiovascular specific deaths. The relative risk of ST-segment depression was as high as five times. Some Q-wave abnormalities carried a relative risk of about three times.

Rose and colleagues performed electrocardiograms (limb leads only) on 8403 male civil servants 40 to 64 years of age and coded them using the Minnesota code.[2] Coronary heart disease mortalities were established over the ensuing 5 years (657 men died). Q-waves, left axis deviation, ST-segment depression, T-wave changes, ventricular conduction defects, and atrial fibrillation were related to mortality. However, there was little significance to increased R-wave amplitude, QT interval, premature beats, or heart rate extremes. Among the 6% of men with patterns suggestive of ischemia, the subsequent coronary heart disease mortality was little more than 1% per year and even lower in those who were asymptomatic when screened. However, a five-times risk ratio was found.

As part of the Busselton City (in Australia) Study 2119 unselected subjects had a 12-lead ECG performed and coded according to the Minnesota code.[3] In addition, all subjects completed the Rose chest pain questionnaire. Subjects were between 40 and 79 years of age and included both men and women. Between 1967 and 1979, the mortality in this group was determined, and the mortality from cardiovascular disease was found to be significantly higher in those with an initial ECG that showed Q-wave and QS patterns, left axis deviation, ST-segment depression and T-wave abnormalities, atrial fibrillation, or premature ventricular beats. In subjects free of angina and other ECG abnormalities, ventricular extra systoles were associated with a significantly higher mortality from cardiovascular disease compared with controls. Q-wave patterns had the highest risk ratio (3.7×), whereas the other abnormalities had about a 2× risk ratio.

As part of the Manitoba Study, a cohort of 3983 men with a mean age of 30 years at entry were followed with annual examinations including ECG since 1948.[4] During the 30-year observation period, 70 cases of sudden death occurred in men without previous clinical manifestations of heart disease. The prevalence of ECG abnormalities before sudden death was 71%. The frequencies of these abnormalities was 31% for major ST-segment and T-wave abnormalities, 16% for ventricular extra beats, 13% for left ventricular hypertrophy, 7% for left bundle branch block. LBBB had a 14× risk for sudden death, whereas ST-segment and T-wave abnormalities, increased R-wave, and premature beats had relative risks as high as 5. It must be remembered that this was a serial ECG study with ECGs obtained usually each year and specificity was not determined.

In 2000 Framingham Study participants, the 12-lead ECG failed to correctly classify over half of the persons with clinically definite heart dis-ease.[5] The sensitivity was about 50% and specificity 90%. The utility of the ECG for assessment of prior infarction can be evaluated by comparion of results with postmortem findings or by comparison of results with survivors of a previously documented infarction. Levine and Phillips found that only 20% of old infarcts found at autopsy were correctly identified by the antemortem ECG.[6] ECG abnormalities may not persist in patients with a previously documented myocardial infarction. In the Framingham Study, 18% of the infarction patients had no ECG abnormalities on subsequent examination. Other studies have reported a 10% to 15% loss of diagnostic Q-waves in the year after MI. However, the ECG has a much stronger prognostic value in survivors of a coronary heart disease event than in apparently healthy populations.

The independent contributions of baseline major and minor ECG abnormalities to subsequent 11.5-year risk of death were explored among 9643 white men and 7990 white women 40 to 64 years of age without definite prior coronary heart disease in the Chicago Heart Association Detection Project in Industry by Liao and co-workers.[7] At baseline age, prevalence rates of major ECG abnormalities were higher in women than in men, with age-adjusted rates of 12.9% and 9.6% ($p < 0.01$) respectively. Minor ECG abnormalities were more common in men than in women (7.3% versus 4.5%, $p < 0.01$). Both major and minor ECG abnormalities were associated with an increased risk of death from coronary heart disease, all cardiovascular diseases, and all causes. The strength of these associations was greater in men than in women. When baseline age, diastolic pressure, serum cholesterol, cigarettes smoked per day, diabetes, and use of antihypertensive medication were taken into account, major abnormalities continued to be significantly related to each cause of death in both genders with much larger adjusted absolute excess risk and relative risk for men than for women. In multivariate analyses, minor ECG abnormalities contributed independently to risk of death in men but not clearly so in women.

Angiographic findings in asymptomatic men with resting ECG abnormalities

Cardiac catheterization was used to evaluate 298 asymptomatic, apparently healthy aircrew men with ECG abnormalities.[8] These men were identified from annual ECGs and exercise tests used to screen them for latent heart disease. Data from 27 additional symptomatic aircrew men who underwent cardiac catheterization because of mild angina pectoris were also included. The men were grouped according to the major reason for cardiac catheterization. The order of groups by increasing prevalence of significant coronary artery disease (CAD) was as follows: abnormal treadmill in a labile lead (4%), supraventricular tachycardia (14%), right bundle branch block (20%), left bundle branch block (24%), abnormal exercise-induced ST-segment depression (31%), ventricular irritability (38%), probable infarct (56%), and angina (70%). Approximately 60% of the men were completely free of angiographic coronary disease. The ECG abnormalities studied had a poorer predictive value for coronary artery disease in asymptomatic apparently healthy men than they do in a hospital or clinical population. A hypothesis based on the USAFSAM data is that a first tier of serial screening with the resting ECG could identify a subpopulation that could be more effectively screened with a next tier of testing, that is, exercise testing.

EXERCISE TESTING AS A SCREENING PROCEDURE
Economic factors

Hartley and colleagues reported an exercise testing program designed to examine large numbers of people effectively, conveniently, and inexpensively.[9] This study was designed to evaluate the possible future application of exercise testing as a routine screening tool. A bicycle ergometer was used, and multilead testing was performed. More than 1800 subjects were examined in 3 years. As many as 55 tests per day were performed at a cost of $60 to $70 each. Abnormalities uncovered were similar to those observed in other studies. The program was considered successful for rendering services conveniently, at low cost, and with accuracy.

Type of test

Maximal or near-maximal exercise tests are superior screening techniques compared with submaximal exercise tests. One shortcoming of submaximal testing is its relatively low sensitivity. Other shortcomings, specifically of a step test like the double Master's test, are that it cannot be used to evaluate exercise capacity and that the ECG is not monitored during exercise. There is a physiological fallacy in adjusting the number of steps as determined by Master according to body weight.

The advantages of a progressive, continuous exercise test with ECG and blood pressure monitoring during the test have been discussed elsewhere. Numerous studies using such a test to screen asymptomatic individuals have been reported without subsequent follow-up data. Nevertheless, these studies have demonstrated that maximal testing is a more sensitive method than submaximal tests and

that abnormal responses correlate directly with other risk factors.

FOLLOW-UP STUDIES THAT HAVE UTILIZED EXERCISE TESTING

The following discusses the follow-up studies that utilized maximal or near-maximal exercise testing to screen asymptomatic individuals for latent coronary heart disease. The populations in these studies were tested and followed for the coronary heart disease end points of angina, acute myocardial infarction, and death. Later distinction will be made as to the results of these studies by the end points utilized, and they will be divided into two groups: angina included as an end point (Table 10-1) and distinct end points (Table 10-2). Table 10-3 lists the end points in all the studies for comparison. There has been controversy over whether, in the absence of conventional risk factors, exercise testing provides additional prognostic information in normal men. Another concern is whether the knowledge of having an abnormal exercise test makes an individual more likely to report angina.

Bruce and colleagues studied 221 clinically normal men in Seattle who were 35 to 82 years of age.[10] A CB_5 bipolar lead was used, and 0.1 mV or more of ST-segment depression was the criterion for an abnormal response. The patients were monitored in the sitting position after exercise. Ten percent of them had abnormal ST-segment responses to the symptom-limited maximal treadmill test.

Aronow and Cassidy tested 100 normal men in Los Angeles, 38 to 64 years of age, and followed them for 5 years.[11] Risk-factor analysis was not performed, but all subjects were normotensive. A V_5 lead was used, and 0.1 mV or more of ST-segment depression was the criterion for an abnormal response. The patients were monitored in the supine position after exercise.

Cumming and colleagues reported their 3-year follow-up data for coronary heart disease end points in 510 asymptomatic men 40 to 65 years of age.[12] Maximal or near-maximal effort was performed and a CM_5 lead was monitored. The criterion for abnormal was 0.2 mV or more of ST-segment depression, and the patients were monitored in the supine position after exercise. Twelve percent had an initial abnormal response to a bicycle exercise test. Subjects with an abnormal response had a higher prevalence of hypertension and hypercholesterolemia.

At USAFSAM, 1390 asymptomatic men 20 to 54 years of age who did not have any of the known causes for false-positive treadmill tests were screened for latent coronary heart disease by max-

Table 10-1 Screening studies that included angina as an end point

	Number	Years followed	Incidence of CHD (%)	Sens. (%)	Spec. (%)	Predictive value + (%)	Risk ratio
Bruce	221	5	2.3	60	91	14	14×
Aronow	100	5	9.0	67	92	46	14×
Cumming	510	3	4.7	58	90	25	10×
Froelicher	1390	6	3.3	61	92	20	14×
Allen	356	5	9.6	41	79	17	2.4×
Manca	947	5	5.0	67	84	18	10×
	508(w)	5	1.6	88	73	5	15×
MacIntyre	578	8	6.9	16	97	26	4×
McHenry	916	13	7.1	14	98	39	6×
		AVERAGES*		48	90	26	9×

CHD, Coronary heart disease; *Sens.*, sensitivity; *Spec.*, specificity; *w*, women.
*Averages do not include women.

Table 10-2 Four screening studies with distinct end points only (not angina)

	Number	Years followed	Incidence of CHD (%)	Sens. (%)	Spec. (%)	Predictive value + (%)	Risk ratio
Seattle Heart Watch	2365	6	2.0	30	91	5	3.5×
MRFIT (SI)	6217	6-8	1.7	17	88	2.2	1.4×
(UC)	6205		1.9	34	88	5.2	3.7×
LRC (Gordon)	3630	8	2.2	28	96	12	6×
(Ekelund)	3806	7	1.8	29	95	7	5×
			AVERAGES	27	91	6	4×

LRC, Lipid Research Clinics Coronary Primary Prevention Trial; *MRFIT*, Multiple Risk Factor Intervention Trial; *SI*, special intervention group; *UC*, usual care group.

imal treadmill testing and were followed for a mean of 6.3 years.[13] A CC$_5$ lead was mainly used, but additional leads were obtained in the supine position after exercise. The criterion for abnormal was 0.1 mV or more of horizontal or downsloping ST-segment depression.

In Italy, Manca and colleagues studied 947 men and 508 women who were referred for exercise testing because of atypical chest pain.[14] Those with typical symptoms of angina pectoris, valvular disease, hypertension, bundle branch block, dysrhythmias, Wolff-Parkinson-White syndrome, left ventricular hypertrophy with strain, significant resting repolarization abnormalities, and previous myocardial infarction were excluded. No patient received drugs such as digitalis, beta-blockers, antidysrhythmics, or diuretics in the 2 weeks preceding exercise testing. Exercise was carried out after routine hyperventilation, using a supine bicycle, until at least 85% of the predicted maximal heart rate was reached. The conventional 12 electrocardiographic leads were recorded during and after the exercise test. The criterion for an abnormal response was 0.1 mV or more of horizontal

or downsloping ST-segment depression. Eighteen percent of the men and 28% of the women had an abnormal electrocardiographic response. The end points for coronary disease were myocardial infarction or sudden death, and there was a mean follow-up time of 5.2 years. The overall incidence of coronary disease was 5% in the men and 1.6% in the women. The sensitivity was 67% in the men versus 88% in the women. The specificity of the test in the men was 84% versus 73% in the women. The predictive value of a positive test was 18% in men but only 5% in women. Men with positive test results had a relative risk of 10 for developing clinical manifestations of coronary heart disease; the relative risk for women with positive test results was 15. This study clearly shows how predictive value is influenced by the prevalence of coronary heart disease in the population under study and that the specificity of the exercise test is lower in women.

Allen and colleagues reported a 5-year follow-up study of 888 asymptomatic men and women without known coronary heart disease who had initially undergone maximal treadmill test-

Table 10-3 Events used as end points for follow-up studies

	Number	Events	Total deaths	Cardiovascular deaths	MI	CABS	AP
Aronow	100	9	3	3	4	1	1
Bruce	221	5	NR	1	1		3
Cumming	510	26	5	3	8		13
McHenry	916	65	8	8	26		30
MacIntyre	548	38	NR	10	16	6	6
Allen	888	48	NR	?	?	NR	?
Froelicher	1390	65	47	25	82	35	11
Seattle Heart Watch	2365	65	47	25	82	35	11
MRFIT (SI)	6427	265	115	NR	NR	NR	NR
(UC)	6438	260	124	NR	NR	NR	NR
LRC	3630	NR	151	75	NR	NR	NR

AP, Angina pectoris; *CABS*, coronary bypass surgery; *MI*, myocardial infarction; *MRFIT*, Multiple Risk Factor Intervention Trial; *NR*, not reported; *SI*, special intervention group, *UC*, usual care group; *?*, used as end point.

ing.[15] When tested, none of the subjects was receiving medications that would affect the electrocardiogram. None had pathological Q-waves or other abnormalities. None had clinical evidence of pulmonary disease or vascular disease. No subject who was included developed serious dysrhythmias, conduction abnormalities, or chest pain in conjunction with the exercise test. Maximal treadmill testing was performed using the Ellestad protocol, and leads CM_5, V_1, and a bipolar vertical lead were recorded. Subjects were exercised until they reached 100% of predicted maximal heart rate, fatigue, or pronounced dyspnea. Flat ST-segment depression of 0.1 mV or greater and downsloping of the ST-segment were considered a positive response. Subjects with major ST-segment changes at rest were excluded. If there were minor changes in the ST-segment before exercise, an additional 0.15 mV of depression at 80 msec from the J-point were required to indicate an abnormal exercise test. R-wave amplitude was measured for an average of six beats during a control period and immediately after exercise, and an increase or no change in the R-wave immediately after exercise compared with control was defined as an abnormal response. A decrease in R-wave amplitude was defined as a normal response. The original population included 1077 subjects, and 888 (82.5%) were contacted for follow-up study. Of the 113 subjects who initially had abnormal exercise tests, 105 were located (92.9%). There was a 1.1% incidence of coronary heart disease per year. End points for coronary heart disease were angina pectoris, myocardial infarction, or sudden cardiac death.

Only 2 of 221 men 40 years of age or less developed heart-disease end points, and neither of the two had ST-segment abnormalities, abnormal R-wave response, or exercise duration of 5 minutes or less. Hence, in this study, abnormal results did not correlate with subsequent coronary heart disease in asymptomatic men 40 years of age or younger. These results contrast with those of the USAFSAM study of 563 men 30 to 39 years of age in whom a 1.4% incidence of coronary disease was found. The exercise ECG was found to have a 50% sensitivity, 95% specificity, 13% predictive value, and risk ratio of 17, and thus it still had value in this age range.

Allen and colleagues concluded that the exercise test was of value only in men older than 40 years of age. For these men, subsequent coronary heart disease within 5 years was predicted by an abnormal ST-segment response, an increase or no change in R-wave, and an exercise duration of 5 minutes or less. The ST-segment, R-wave, and exercise duration criteria had sensitivities of 41%, 47%, and 26% respectively. With the test results interpreted as abnormal when either ST-segment or R-wave criteria were present, sensitivity was 65%. Adding exercise duration of 5 minutes or less as a third alternative criterion for a positive test did not change sensitivity. When all three criteria were present, a sensitivity of 29% with a specificity of 100% was achieved. In men older than 40 years of age, the ST-segment criteria had the above-mentioned sensitivity of 41%, specificity of 79%, predictive value of 17%, and risk ratio of 2.4. With the exception of predictive value, these values are strikingly lower than those found in earlier studies, including results previously presented by this group.

Of the 311 women whom Allen and colleagues followed, 10 developed coronary heart disease end points. The authors found that ST-segment depression and R-wave response did not correlate with subsequent development of coronary heart disease. Exercise duration of 3 minutes or less, however, proved to be a significant predictor of coronary heart disease. Four of 13 women with a low exercise time developed coronary heart disease. When used as a criterion for abnormal, exercise duration of 3 minutes or less in asymptomatic women had a sensitivity of 40%, specificity of 97%, predictive value of 31%, and risk ratio of 15. Limited follow-up study of 80% of the original population and the low incidence of coronary disease end points in women and in men younger than 40 years of age are limitations of this study.

Bruce and colleagues recently reported a 6-year follow-up study of 2365 clinically healthy men (mean age 45 years) who were exercise tested as part of the Seattle Heart Watch.[16] They underwent symptom-limited maximal treadmill testing using neither ST-segment depression nor target heart rates as end points of maximal exercise. The Bruce protocol was used, and the electrocardiogram was monitored with a bipolar CB_5 lead. Conventional risk factors were assessed at the time of the initial examination in a subset of the population. Follow-up data were obtained by questionnaire, with morbidity defined as hospital admission. Forty-seven men (2%) experienced coronary heart disease morbidity or mortality. Univariate analysis of the individual conventional risk factors (positive family history, hypertension, smoking, hypercholesterolemia) did not show a statistically significant increase in the 5-year probability of primary coronary heart disease events. Only when the sum of risk factors in an individual were assessed did conventional risk factors become statistically significant in relation to the event rate. Four variables from treadmill testing were predictive: (1) exercise duration less than 6 minutes (which requires 6 or 7 METS, or multiples of resting oxygen requirement), (2) 0.1 mV of ST-segment depression during recovery, (3) greater than 10% heart rate impairment (defined as the percent reduction of age-adjusted maximal heart rate), and (4) chest pain during maximal exertion. The ST-segment criteria had a sensitivity of 30%, specificity of 89%, predictive value of 5.3%, and risk ratio of 3.3. Angina and exercise duration each had sensitivities of about 6%. Heart rate impairment had a sensitivity of 19% and was comparable to ST-segment depression for the other parameters.

Table 10-4 summarizes the performance of the exercise test predictors. The presence of two or more of the exercise test predictors identified men in all age groups who were at increased risk. Furthermore, it was found that in the presence of one or more conventional risk factors and as the prevalence of exertional risk predictors rose from none to any three, the relative risk rose from 1 to 30. The group that had one or more conventional risk factors and two or more exertional risk predictors was found to have the highest 5-year probability of primary coronary heart disease. In the absence of conventional risk factors, however, exercise testing in this study failed to provide additional prognostic information in normal men.

MacIntyre and colleagues performed maximal exercise tests on 548 fit, healthy middle-aged former aviators at the Naval Aerospace Medical Laboratory.[17] To be included, subjects had to have no clinical evidence of heart or lung disease as determined by history, physical examination, chest x-ray findings, and a completely normal resting electrocardiogram. Leads X, Y, Z, and V_5 were analyzed only after exercise for 0.1 mV or more of horizontal depression 80 msec after QRS end. Criteria for coronary disease after an 8-year follow-up study were sudden death, myocardial infarction, coronary artery bypass surgery, or angina. The predictive value of the test was not significantly greater in those with the cardinal risk factors. An abnormal exercise electrocardiogram generated a higher risk ratio than the risk factors.

McHenry and co-workers reported the results of an 8- to 15-year follow-up study of 916 apparently healthy men between 27 and 55 years of age (mean 37 years) who underwent serial medical and exercise test evaluations.[18] In 1968, the Indiana University School of Medicine entered into an agreement with the Indiana State Police Department to provide employees with periodic medical evaluations including treadmill tests. This report covers their experience with the first male employees who underwent initial medical evaluations between July 1968 and June 1975 and includes a follow-up examination for all subjects through June 1983. A CC_5 lead was monitored and 1 mm or more horizontal or downsloping ST-segment depression during or after exercise was considered abnormal. A modified Balke protocol was used for all treadmill tests and most were symptom limited. Serial evaluations were planned at 2- to 5-year intervals; however, about 15% of subjects elected not to return after their initial evaluation. During the initial evaluation, there were 23 subjects with an abnormal ST-segment response. During follow-up period there were 9 coronary events in this group: 8 cases of angina and 1 of sudden death. With serial testing, an additional 38 subjects experienced conversion to abnormal ST-segment response. During follow-up period there were 12 coronary events in this group, 10 cases of angina, 1 MI, and 1 "other." There were 833 subjects with normal

Table 10-4   Performance of exercise test variables and risk factors in detecting asymptomatic coronary artery disease

First author	Abnormal response	Sensitivity (%)	Specificity (%)	Predictive (%)	Risk ratio
Allen	ST ↓	41	79	17	2
	RWA	47	78	19	3
	TM time <5 min	27	96	43	6
	ST ↓ + RWA	40	86	27	5
	ST ↓ + TM time <5 min	24	99	71	11
	RWA + TM time <5 min	33	99	82	12
	ST ↓ + RWA + TM time <5 min	29	100	100	17
Bruce	ST ↓	30	91	5	3.5
	Angina on TM	6	99	15	8
	TM time <6 min	6	99	19	10
	HRI	19	93	7	4
	≥1 RF + ≥2 ExRP	19		46	18
Uhl	≥0.3mV ST	36	79	38	2
	Onset ST ↓ in stage I	33	64	23	1
	TM time <10 min	46	92	67	4
	Persistent ST ↓ (6 min)	28	87	43	6
	RWA	28	87	42	2
	≥1 RF + ≥2 ExRP	55	86	84	4
	≥1 RF + ≥3 ExRP to detect multivessel disease	37	98	89	4.5

ExRP, Exercise risk predictor; *HRI*, heart rate impairment; *RF*, risk factor; *RWA*, R-wave amplitude abnormality; *ST ↓*, ST-segment depression; *TM*, treadmill test.

ST-segment responses to exercise with all tests. In this group, there were 44 coronary events; 25 MI, 7 sudden deaths, and 12 diagnosed as having angina. They concluded that an abnormal ST-segment response to exercise, predicted angina pectoris but not other coronary events.

McHenry and co-workers did not present sensitivity-specificity calculations, but the data they reported enabled the calculations shown in table 10-1. The suprisingly low sensitivity from initial testing is probably attributable to the long follow-up period. An abnormal test result indicates obstructive coronary disease, which was most likely not present initially in most subjects who developed end points but developed later during the 12 years. An analysis of the treadmill test performance at 5 years, a time similar to that of prior studies reporting a higher sensitivity, would be most informative, but it is probable that the treadmill test is much less sensitive in asymptomatic men than previously demonstrated. They found that serial testing did not improve the predictive value of the test and that angina was the main cardiac event predicted. Sudden death was actually more common in the individuals with normal test results. The USAFSAM study also had angina as its most common end point, and both studies support the concept that the knowledge of an abnormal exercise test makes an individual more likely to report angina.

The Multiple Risk Factor Intervention Trial (MRFIT), a coronary heart disease (CAD) primary prevention trial, examined the effect of a special intervention (SI) program to reduce cholesterol, high blood pressure, and cigarette smoking in men 35 to 57 years old.[19] Half of the 12,866 participants were randomly assigned to usual care (UC) in the community. During a 6- to 8-year follow-up period the CAD mortality was 7% lower in the SI than in the UC group, a nonsignificant difference. A prior subgroup hypothesis proposed that men with an abnormal exercise ECG would particularly benefit from intervention. Measured by computer an abnormal ST integral of -16 μV-sec, was observed in 12.5% of the men at baseline level and was associated with a $3\times$ risk of CAD death within the UC group. In the subgroup with a normal ECG, there was no significant SI-UC difference in the CAD mortality. In contrast, there was a 57% lower death rate among men in the SI group with an abnormal test compared with men in the UC group. The relative risks (SI/UC) in these two strata were significantly different. These findings indicate that men with elevated risk factors who have an abnormal exercise ECG may benefit from risk factor reduction. This study certainly is the largest and probably the most reliable for demonstrating the predictive accuracy of exercise testing in an asymptomatic population, since only cardiac deaths were considered the end point as opposed to angina in most of the other studies.

Rautaharju and co-workers presented the prognostic value of the exercise electrocardiogram in the 6438 usual care men of MRFIT in relation to fatal and nonfatal coronary heart disease events, rest electrocardiographic abnormalities, and coronary heart disease risk factors.[20] An abnormal response to exercise, defined as an ST-depression integral of -16 µV-sec or more, was observed in 12.2% of the men. There was a nearly fourfold increase in 7-year coronary mortality among men with an abnormal response to exercise compared with men with a normal ST-segment in exercise (risk ratio 3.8, 95% confidence limits 2.5 to 5.5). The risk ratio for coronary death, adjusted for age, diastolic blood pressure, serum cholesterol, and smoking status at baseline value, was 3.5, and the corresponding adjusted risk ratio for death from all causes was 1.6. A similar trend toward excess coronary events was seen for angina pectoris (risk ratio of 1.6). The trend was not significant for nonfatal myocardial infarction. Multivariate analyses indicated that the ST-depression integral was a strong independent predictor of future coronary death ($p < 0.001$). Men with an abnormal electrocardiogram at rest (mainly high-amplitude R-waves) and an abnormal ST response to exercise had an over sixfold relative risk for coronary death compared with men with an abnormal electrocardiogram at rest and a normal ST response to exercise.

Gordon and colleagues presented one of many interesting analyses of the Lipid Research Clinics Mortality Follow-Up Study.[21] More than 3600 white men, from 30 to 79 years of age and without a history of myocardial infarction, underwent submaximal treadmill tests as part of their baseline elevation. The exercise test was conducted according to a common protocol and coded centrally; depression of the ST-segment by at least 1 mm (visual coding) or 10 µV-sec (ST-segment integral, computer coding) signified a positive test result. Concurrent measurements of age, blood pressure, history of cigarette smoking, and plasma levels of lipids, lipoproteins, and glucose, as well as other coronary risk factors, were obtained. Cumulative mortality from cardiovascular disease was 11.9%

(22/185) over an 8.1-year mean follow-up period among men with a positive exercise test result versus 1.2% (36/2993) over an 8.6-year mean follow-up period among men with a negative test result. Three fourths (43) of these deaths were attributable to coronary heart disease. The relative risk for cardiovascular mortality associated with a positive exercise test was 9.3 before and 4.6 after age adjustment. Cardiovascular mortalities were especially elevated (relative risk 15.6 before and 5.1 after age adjustment) among the 82 men whose exercise tests were adjudged "strongly" positive based on degree and timing of the ischemic electrocardiographic response. A positive exercise test was also moderately associated with noncardiovascular mortality; the relative risk for all-cause mortality was 7.2 before and 3.4 after age adjustment. The relative risk for cardiovascular mortality associated with an abnormal exercise test was not appreciably altered by covariance adjustment for known coronary risk factors other than age. An abnormal exercise test result was a stronger predictor of cardiovascular death than were high levels of low-density lipoprotein cholesterol, low levels of high-density lipoprotein cholesterol, smoking, hyperglycemia, or hypertension. Its influence on risk of cardiovascular death was equivalent to that of a 17.4-year increment in age.

Ekelund and colleagues attempted to predict coronary heart disease morbidity and mortality in hypercholesterolemic men from an exercise test performed as part of the Lipid Research Clinics Coronary Primary Prevention Trial.[22] For study of whether the test was more predictive for hypercholesterolemic men (that is, thus increasing the pretest probability for disease), data from 3806 asymptomatic hypercholesterolemic men were analyzed. All the men had performed a submaximal treadmill test at baseline level before they were assigned to the cholestyramine or placebo treatment group. A test was abnormal if the ST-segment was displaced by ≥ 1 mm (visual code) or there was ≥ 10 µV-sec change in the ST-segment integral (computer code), or both. The prevalence of an abnormal test was 8.3%. During the 7- to 10-year (mean 7.4) follow-up period, the mortality from coronary heart disease was 6.7% (21 of 315) in men with an abnormal test and 1.3% (46 of 3460) in men with a negative test (placebo and cholestyramine groups combined). The age-adjusted mortality ratio for an abnormal test, compared with a negative test, was 6.7 in the placebo group and 4.8 in the cholestyramine group. Cox's proportional hazards model demonstrated that the risk of death from coronary heart disease associated with an abnormal test was 5.7 times higher in the placebo group and 4.9 times higher in the cholestyramine group after adjustment for age, lipids, and other risk factors. An abnormal test was not significantly associated with nonfatal myocardial infarction.

Josephson and co-workers analyzed the results of serial exercise tests performed at two to four intervals in 726 men and women volunteers, 22 to 84 years of age (mean, 55.1 years) from the Baltimore Longitudinal Study of Aging.[23] All subjects were free of cardiovascular disease at entry by history, physical examination, and resting 12-lead electrocardiogram. Over a mean overall follow-up time of 7.4 years, coronary events occurred in 34 of 178 (19.1%) of those with an abnormal ST response to exercise versus 30 of 548 (5.5%) in those with a normal response ($p = 0.001$). Angina pectoris was the most common presenting coronary event regardless of ST-segment exercise response. Among individuals with an abnormal ST-segment response, the incidence of events was virtually identical for those with an initially abnormal response (group 1) and for those who converted from a normal to an abnormal response (group 2), 19.8% versus 18.5%. After adjustment for standard coronary risk factors by proportional hazards regression analysis, the risk of a coronary event relative to subjects with persistently normal ST-segment responses (group 3) remained nearly identical in the two groups, 2.72 in group 1 ($p < 0.003$) and 2.80 in group 2 ($p < 0.002$). Thus, in asymptomatic individuals, conversion from a normal to an abnormal exercise ST-segment response is associated with a prognosis similar to an initially abnormal response and is not a more specific marker for future coronary events.

Gordon and co-workers analyzed smoking, physical activity, and other predictors of endurance and heart rate response to exercise in asymptomatic hypercholesterolemic men.[24] The association of known coronary risk factors with progressive submaximal treadmill exercise test performance was studied in 6238 asymptomatic white 34- to 60-year-old hypercholesterolemic men screened between 1973 and 1976 for the Lipid Research Clinics Coronary Primary Prevention Trial. Both cigarette smoking and habitual physical inactivity were associated with a doubling of the rate of symptom-related discontinuation of the exercise test; the tests of sedentary smokers were discontinued at four times the rate observed for active nonsmokers. Smaller increases in heart rate were observed during exercise testing in physically active men and in smokers than that in their sedentary and nonsmoking counterparts. Thus smoking, like habitual physical activity, reduced the heart rate required to sustain a given external work load. However, the heart rates of smokers tended

to remain elevated after exercise, whereas those of physically active men returned more rapidly toward resting levels. Age, Quetelet index, and low plasma levels of high-density-lipoprotein cholesterol were also strong predictors of decreased exercise capacity, whereas resting heart rate and blood pressure levels were significant predictors of heart rate response. Comparison of these results with those previously reported for ischemic electrocardiographic changes in this cohort indicates that coronary risk factors may selectively influence specific aspects of exercise test performance.

Relevance to the silent ischemia issue

The use of the exercise ECG for predicting prognosis in asymptomatic individuals has again become of interest because of the poor predictive power of the ST-segment response being reported in recent studies and the citation of these studies in regard to silent ischemia. The Seattle Heart Watch study was the first study that reported quite different results from previous studies. These results were different from Bruce's earlier findings. The explanation became apparent from considering the end points used. The earlier studies all considered angina pectoris as one of the cardiac events or end points. In the Seattle Heart Watch, the angina end point had to be associated with a hospital admission diagnosis of angina, making it a more definite cardiac end point. The other recent studies considered only distinct end points such as death or MI and not angina.

When the studies are separated by those that used angina as an end point (Table 10-1), the average sensitivity was 50%, predictive value was 26%, and risk ratio was 9 times. This means that 26% or one out of four with ST-segment depression would have a cardiac event including angina during approximately 5 years of follow-up observation. However, when the studies that used only distinct end points were considered (Table 10-2), much poorer results were obtained. The sensitivity was 27% and the predictive value was 6%. Only 6%, or 1 out of 17, with ST-segment depression would have a distinct end point during follow-up study. Rather than 1 cardiac event out of 4 with ST-segment depression, it turns out to be 1 out of 17. This means that 16 out of 17 abnormal responses are false positives. This finding must be considered, since these studies are being cited as showing the dangers of silent ischemia. Silent ischemia induced by exercise testing in apparently healthy men is not so predictive of a poor outcome as once believed. Also, the use of the exercise test for screening is even more misleading than previously appreciated because of the higher false-positive rate. The earlier better results can be explained by the cardiac concerns caused by an abnormal exercise test. Individuals with abnormal tests would be more likely to report chest pain, and doctors would be more likely to diagnose it as angina given the exercise test results. In the only study of its kind, Hedblad obtained similar results when using ambulatory Holter monitoring.[25] Table 10-5 demonstrates his findings in the asymptomatic and symptomatic subjects he studied.

The nonselective utilization of exercise testing for screening apparently healthy individuals should be discouraged because of the poor predictive value of only 1 mm of ST-segment depression. Unfortunately, this "abnormal" response leads to psychological and vocational disability as well as unnecessary medical expenses and risks. When this response is no longer equated with disease, then perhaps the test could be used in such individuals for setting exercise prescriptions and for motivational purposes. Only combinations of other abnormal responses and 2 mm ST-segment depression should be considered as predictive of increased risk for exercise related cardiovascular events.

Exercise testing and coronary angiography in asymptomatic populations

Froelicher and colleagues performed cardiac catheterization on 111 asymptomatic men with an abnormal ST-segment depression in response to a treadmill test. Only one third of the subjects had at least one lesion equal to or greater than 50% luminal narrowing of a major coronary artery. Table 10-4 summarizes the influence of the resting ECG on the prediction value. Resting mild ST-segment depression that appears on serial ECGs and persists increases the predictive value of an abnormal exercise test. Borer and colleagues reported angiographic findings in 11 asymptomatic individuals with hyperlipidemia and an abnormal exercise

test. Only 37% were found to have coronary artery occlusions.[26]

Barnard and colleagues used near-maximal treadmill testing to screen randomly selected Los Angeles firefighters.[27] Ten percent had abnormal exercise-induced ST-segment depression despite few risk factors for coronary disease. Six men with an abnormal exercise test result elected to undergo cardiac catheterization. One had severe three-vessel disease, and another had a 50% obstruction of the left circumflex coronary artery. The other four men had normal studies.

Uhl and colleagues have reported their findings in 255 asymptomatic men who underwent coronary angiography for an abnormal ST-segment response to exercise testing over a 7-year period at the USAFSAM.[28] None of the clinical or ECG variables were able to detect those with significant diseases. The three exercise test responses with high likelihood ratio were (1) at least 0.3 mV of depression, (2) persistence of ST-segment depression 6 minutes after exercise, and (3) an estimated oxygen uptake of less than 9 METs. However, because of their low sensitivity and predictive value, it was necessary to combine them with risk factors. A combination of any risk factor and two exercise responses was highly predictive (89%) but insensitive (39%) for any coronary disease. However, this combination had a sensitivity of 55% and a predictive value of 84% for two- or three-vessel diseases.

Erikssen and colleagues reported angiographic findings in 105 men 40 to 59 years of age of a working population with one or more of the following criteria: (1) a questionnaire for angina pectoris positive on interview or either (2) typical angina or (3) ST-segment depression as responses to a near-maximal bicycle test.[29] The exercise test had a predictive value of 84% if a slowly ascending ST-segment was included. The higher predictive value in this study may be attributable to the older age of their population and inclusion of men with angina. Of the 36 who were found to have normal coronary arteries, a 7-year follow-up study revealed that 3 died of sudden death, 4 received a diagnosis of cardiomyopathy, and 1 had developed aortic valve disease.[30] They had a relative decline in their physical performance over the follow-up period. Thallium studies were normal, but the radionuclide ventriculogram revealed a subnormal increase in ejection fraction during exercise in half of them.

Kemp and colleagues evaluated 7-year survival in patients having normal or near-normal coronary arteriograms using data from the Coronary Artery Surgery Study (CASS) registry of 21,487 consecutive coronary arteriograms taken in 15 clinical

Table 10-5   The Holter study of Hedblad reporting results of screening in both asymptomatic and symptomatic populations

History of CAD	ST depression on Holter	Number	MI/deaths	Risk ratio
yes	no	34	2(5.9%)	2.6×
	yes	19	7(39%)	16×
no	no	262	6(2.3%)	1×
	yes	79	8(10.8%)	4.4×

From Hedblad B: *Eur Heart J* 10:149-158, 1989.
CAD, Coronary heart disease = previous myocardial infarction, *MI,* or positive Rose questionnaire result.

sites.[31] Of these, 4051 arteriograms were normal or near normal, and the patients had normal left ventricular function as judged by absence of a history of congestive heart failure, no reported segmental wall-motion abnormality, and an ejection fraction of at least 50%; 3136 arteriograms were entirely normal, and the remaining 915 revealed mild disease with less than 50% stenosis in one or more segments. Of the total number, 843 patients had exercise tests, and of these, 195 had abnormal ST-segment depression. The 7-year survival rate was 96% for the patients with a normal arteriogram and 92% for those whose study revealed mild disease. They noted that the ECG response to exercise was a nonpredictive variable. This is in contrast to the 7-year follow-up study of only 36 apparently healthy middle-aged men with a positive exercise test and normal coronary arteriograms reported by Erikssen. Erikssen concluded that patients with an abnormal exercise test result could not be assured of a good prognosis on the basis of a normal coronary arteriogram. The CASS data do not support this conclusion. There were 195 subjects with abnormal ST-segment depression, and Kemp and co-workers were unable to show any predictive value of even considerable amounts of depression. If exercise-induced ST-segment depression is attributable to ischemia in patients with normal coronaries, it is not related to a disease process that has a strong effect on mortality over 7 years of follow-up study. In general, these angiographic studies confirm the low predictive value of an abnormal exercise test response also found in the epidemiological studies of populations with a low prevalence of CHD.

Labile ST shifts. McHenry performed serial exercise tests on 900 presumably healthy men and identified 14 men with labile ST-T changes with standing or hyperventilation and abnormal ST-segment depression at exercise.[32] At a 7-year follow-up time, none had manifested a coronary event, whereas in 24 men with exercise-induced ST changes but no labile ST-T wave phenomena before exercise, 10 (42%) had a coronary event.[33]

Exercise-induced dysrhythmias. Few studies in asymptomatic subjects have evaluated exercise-induced ventricular premature beats for detecting coronary disease. In the USAFSAM study of 1390 men, only 39 men (2.1%) of the population developed "ominous" dysrhythmias. The risk ratio of developing coronary disease over 6 years of follow-up observation with these dysrhythmias was 3:1, however, the predictive value was only 10%, and sensitivity only 6.7%. Thus dysrhythmias induced by exercise testing have not been helpful in detecting latent coronary disease in apparently healthy men.

Busby and co-workers studied 1160 subjects 21 to 96 years of age who underwent maximal exercise treadmill testing an average of 2.4 times.[34] Eighty (6.9% developed frequent [$\geq$10% of beats in any 1 minute] or repetitive [$\geq$3 beats in a row] ventricular ectopic beats on at least one test. These 80 individuals were significantly older than the group without such arrhythmia (63.8 $\pm$ 12.5 versus 50.0 $\pm$ 16.1 years, $p < 0.001$). A striking age-related increase in the prevalence of frequent or repetitive exercise-induced ventricular ectopic beats was seen in men ($p < 0.0001$) but not in women. The prevalence of electrocardiographic abnormalities at rest, exercise-induced ST-segment depression and thallium perfusion defects, duration of treadmill exercise, maximal heart rate, systolic blood pressure, and rate-pressure product did not differ between these 80 study subjects with frequent exercise-induced ventricular ectopic beats and a control group matched for age and sex. Furthermore, the incidence of cardiac events (angina pectoris, nonfatal myocardial infarction, cardiac syncope, or cardiac death) (10% versus 12.5%) as well as noncardiac mortality (each 7.5%) was found to be similar for the study and control groups, respectively, over a mean follow-up period of 5.6 years. No study subjects required antiarrhythmic drugs over this interval. Thus frequent or repetitive exercise-induced ventricular ectopic beats in these predominantly older, asymptomatic individuals without apparent heart disease do not predict increased cardiac morbidity or mortality and therefore do not require specific therapy.

Techniques to improve screening

Numerous techniques have been recommended to improve the sensitivity and specificity of exercise testing. Various computerized criteria for ischemia have been proposed, as well as new standard visual ST criteria. In addition, there are ancillary techniques that could possibly improve the discriminating power of the exercise test. These methods are listed in the box on the next page.

Electrocardiographic criteria. Hollenberg has applied his computerized treadmill score in an asymptomatic United States Army population with success.[35] Okin and co-workers compared the ST/HR index and the rate-recovery loop with standard electrocardiographic criteria for prediction of CHD events in 3168 asymptomatic men and women in the Framingham Offspring Study who underwent treadmill testing. These individuals were free of clinical and ECG evidence of heart disease.[36] After a mean follow-up period of 4.3 years, there were 65 new CHD events: four sudden deaths, 24 new myocardial infarctions, and 37 new cases of angina pectoris. When a Cox pro-

---

ANCILLARY TECHNIQUES DISCUSSED THAT HAVE BEEN USED TO SCREEN FOR ASYMPTOMATIC CORONARY HEART DISEASE

Thallium perfusion imaging
Radionuclide ventriculography during bicycle exercise and post treadmill exercise
Cardiac fluoroscopy for coronary artery calcification (enhanced with digital subtraction angiography)
Cardiokymography
Total cholesterol/high-density-lipoprotein ratio, conventional risk factors
ECG-gated chest x-ray film before and after exercise
Computerized multifactorial risk prediction using bayesian statistics
Systolic time intervals during and after exercise
Digital subtraction angiography with intravenous injection of contrast to visualize the coronary arteries
Echocardiography (or Doppler imaging) during and after exercise (even after treadmill)

---

portional hazards model with adjustment for age and sex was used, an abnormal exercise electrocardiogram by standard criteria (≥ 0.1 mV of horizontal or downsloping ST-segment depression) was not predictive of new CHD events ($\chi^2 = 0.40$; $p = 0.52$). In contrast, stratification according to the presence or absence of an abnormal ST/HR index (≥ 1.6 μV/beat/min) and an abnormal (counterclockwise) rate-recovery loop was associated with CHD event risk ($\chi^2 = 9.45$; $p < 0.01$) and separated subjects into three groups with varying risks of coronary events: *high risk,* when both tests were abnormal (relative risk 3.6; 95% confidence interval, 2.4 to 5.4); *intermediate risk,* when either the ST/HR index or the rate-recovery loop was abnormal (relative risk, 1.9; 95% confidence interval, 1.3 to 2.8); *low risk,* when both tests showed negative results. After multivariate adjustment for age, sex, smoking, total cholesterol level, fasting glucose level, diastolic blood pressure, and electrocardiographic evidence of left ventricular hypertrophy, the combined ST/HR index and rate-recovery loop criteria remained predictive of coronary events ($\chi^2 = 5.45$; $p = 0.02$). This study is hard to explain, since in all previous similar studies simple ST criteria were associated with cardiovascular events. The results obtained still did not justify screening asymptomatic individuals because of the high false-positive rate. Angina was included as an end point, and this is a problem as previously noted.

Thallium exercise testing. Caralis and colleagues used thallium exercise testing and coronary angiography to evaluate asymptomatic individuals with abnormal ST-segment responses to exercise testing.[37] Of 3496 consecutive treadmill exercise tests performed primarily on asymptomatic individuals, 22 developed 0.2 mV or more of asymp-

tomatic horizontal ST-segment depression. These individuals had physical examinations, routine laboratory studies, chest x-ray films, and resting electrocardiograms, all of which were normal. Fifteen of these 22 patients agreed to be evaluated further with thallium and coronary angiography. These 15 included 14 men and one woman; the mean age was 52. Thallium was administered intravenously for separate rest and exercise myocardial studies. Myocardial imaging began 10 minutes after administration, and imaging in each of the views required 8 to 12 minutes. The rest and subsequent exercise studies were performed 1 week apart, and all the resting studies were normal. The thallium was injected at peak bicycle exercise, and patients were encouraged to keep a constant level of exercise for an additional 1 minute. Rest and exercise studies were examined together and considered positive for ischemia only if a new perfusion defect involved more than 15% of the left ventricular circumference. Of the 15 asymptomatic individuals with horizontal ST-segment depression on exercise testing, 5 had normal scans with exercise, whereas 10 individuals developed new defects. The angiographic criterion for abnormal was based on 70% luminal narrowing. Four of the 5 individuals with normal exercise thallium images had normal coronary angiograms, and 1 had an abnormal angiogram. Of the 10 with abnormal exercise scans, 9 had significant narrowing of two or more major coronary arteries and 1 patient had essentially normal coronary vessels. Hence, once subjects were selected on the basis of an abnormal exercise test, the thallium exercise scans classified 13 of 15 patients properly.

Nolewajka and colleagues performed thallium treadmill tests on 58 asymptomatic men as part of a screening study.[38] The risk for coronary heart disease was determined by use of the Framingham risk equation, based on age, cholesterol, systolic blood pressure, cigarette-smoking history, left ventricular hypertrophy on the electrocardiogram, and glucose intolerance. The risk calculation was greater in those with abnormal exercise studies compared with those who had normal studies. Five of the subjects had electrocardiographic left ventricular hypertrophy, 6 had abnormal exercise-induced ST-segment depression, and 6 had abnormal thallium scans (5 consistent with ischemia, 1 with scar). Three of the subjects with abnormal thallium studies underwent coronary angiography, and all had normal coronary arteries. Surprisingly, 2 of these had left bundle branch block (1 with exercise only, the other at rest). The disappointment of these results was compounded by profound psychological stress to the individuals who were told they had "abnormal" results.

Uhl and colleagues performed thallium exercise tests on 119 aircrewmen before undergoing coronary angiography because of abnormal treadmill test results or serial ECG changes.[39] Of these, 41 men had significant angiographic disease (equal or greater than 50% occlusion) for a predictive value of the ECG screening procedures of 21%. The sensitivity of the computer-enhanced thallium exercise test was 95%, as compared with 68% for analog Polaroid interpretation, and its specificity was 90%. There were mixed results in the 10 men who had minimal angiographic disease (less than 50% occlusion); 10 had abnormal scans, and 5 had normal scans. The high sensitivity and specificity of the computer-enhanced thallium exercise test in this population of apparently healthy men is a strong support for its use as a second-line screening procedure. If both an abnormal exercise electrocardiogram and an abnormal perfusion scintigram had been required before angiography was performed, 136 of those free of coronary disease would not have needed to undergo angiography.

To examine whether thallium scintigraphy improved the predictive value of exercise-induced ST-segment depression, Fleg and co-workers performed maximal treadmill tests and thallium scans on 407 asymptomatic volunteers 40 to 96 years of age (mean = 60) from the Baltimore Longitudinal Study on Aging.[40] The prevalence of exercise-induced silent ischemia, defined by concordant ST-segment depression and a thallium perfusion defect, increased more than sevenfold from 2% in the fifth and sixth decades to 15% in the ninth decade. Over a mean follow-up period of 4.6 years, cardiac events developed in 9.8% of subjects and consisted of 20 cases of new angina pectoris, 13 myocardial infarctions, and seven deaths. Events occurred in 7% of individuals with both negative thallium scan and ECG, 8% of those with either test positive, and 48% of those in whom both tests were positive ($p < 0.001$). By proportional hazards analysis, age, hypertension, exercise duration, and a concordant positive ECG and thallium scan result were independent predictors of coronary events. Furthermore, those with positive ECG and thallium scan had a 3.6-fold relative risk for subsequent coronary events, independent of conventional risk factors. Radionuclide left ventricular angiography during exercise has not been reported in any substantial number of asymptomatic subjects, but its low specificity makes its use impractical.

Cardiokymography. The cardiokymograph is an electronic device that produces a representation of regional left ventricular wall motion noninvasively. It generates an electromagnetic field, and motion within the field causes a change in the frequency of an oscillator. A change in frequency is converted into a change in voltage proportional to the motion. The cardiokymograph produces a recording similar to the apexcardiogram and the kinetocardiogram. The advantage of the cardiokymograph is that it records absolute cardiac motion without chest motion, thus eliminating the distortion problem inherent in both the apexcardiogram and the kinetocardiogram. There is considerable tissue penetration, and so the cardiokymograph responds to deeper cardiac motion as well as precordial surface movement. Cardiokymographic recordings have been shown to be predictive of ventriculographic wall-motion abnormalities.

Silverberg and colleagues reported their use of the cardiokymograph after exercise in 157 patients, including 27 apparently healthy volunteers and 130 patients with suspected coronary heart disease who underwent coronary angiography.[41] The subjects performed a progressive symptom-limited maximal treadmill test. The cardiokymograph was recorded within 2 minutes of termination of exercise, and every minute thereafter for 10 minutes. Two sets of empiric criteria for an abnormal cardiokymographic pattern were defined in relation to known effects of ischemia on regional wall motion. The first abnormality was defined as paradoxical systolic outward motion. The second abnormality was defined as development of total absence of inward motion, a resultant holosystolic outward motion, or systolic outward motion occurring for less than the entire period of ejection but not preceded by inward motion. For detecting coronary heart disease in atypical chest pain patients, the cardiokymogram had a higher sensitivity, specificity, and predictive value than the electrocardiogram did. However, no statistical difference existed between the electrocardiogram and the cardiokymogram in asymptomatic patients. Exercise-induced cardiokymographic abnormalities persisted longer during recovery than the electrocardiographic changes did.

Alexander and co-workers utilized cardiokymography as part of a serial testing evaluation of 287 asymptomatic subjects. Type II cardiokymographic abnormalities occurred in 10 subjects, five of whom had coronary disease. The resultant sensitivity of 63% and specificity of 74% and predictive value of 50% was more effective than horizontal ST-segment depression (25%, 89%, and 50% respectively) and was the second best single screening tool (thallium scintigraphy was best).

A multicenter study has demonstrated the diagnostic accuracy of cardiokymography recorded 2 to 3 minutes after exercise in 617 patients undergoing cardiac catheterization.[42] Of these patients, 29% had prior MI. There were 12 participating centers using a standardized protocol. Adequate cardiokymographic (CKG) tracings, which were obtained in 82% of patients, were dependent on the skill of the operator and on certain patient characteristics. Of the 327 patients without prior MI who had technically adequate CKG and ECG tracings, 166 (51%) had coronary disease. Both the sensitivity and specificity of CKG (71% and 88% respectively) were significantly greater than the values for the exercise ECG (61% and 76% respectively). Coronary artery disease and multivessel disease were present in 98% and 68% respectively of the 70 patients with both abnormal CKG and ECG results and in 15% and 5% respectively of the 132 patients with both studies normal. The CKG was most helpful in those patients in whom the posttest probability of coronary disease was between 21% and 72% after the exercise ECG. In these patients, an abnormal concordantly positive CKG result increased the probability of coronary disease to between 67% and 100%, whereas a normal response decreased it to between 12% and 15%. In the subgroup of 102 patients undergoing concomitant exercise thallium testing, the sensitivity and specificity for the thallium scintigraphy (81% and 80% respectively) were similar to the values for CKG (72% and 84% respectively).

To determine which subgroup of patients derive the most benefit from testing, they categorized the chest pain complaints of the 327 patients without prior MI undergoing testing for the purpose of diagnosis into four symptom groups: (1) *Typical angina*. A history of typical angina pectoris in men was very predictive of both coronary artery disease (85%) and multivessel disease (51%). An abnormal exercise ECG increased the probability of coronary disease to 94%. In these patients, an abnor-

mal CKG only slightly increased the probability of coronary disease (to 95%), whereas a normal CKG was still associated with a high probability. (2) *Atypical angina*. 51% of these men and 33% of these women had coronary artery disease. An abnormal exercise ECG increased the probability of coronary disease to 90% in men and to 86% in women, whereas a negative result was associated with a probability of 27% in men and 25% in women. A normal exercise ECG in patients with atypical angina was still associated with a 37% probability of coronary disease in men and a 20% probability in women. In these patients, when the CKG was normal, the probability of coronary disease (15% in men and 12% in women) and of multivessel disease (5% in men and 3% in women) was very low. (3) *Nonischemic chest pain*. Of 43 patients, 24% had coronary disease and 7% had multivessel disease. An abnormal ST-segment response resulted in a 45% probability of coronary disease, whereas a negative ECG result was associated with a 17% probability. In the 14 patients with an abnormal exercise ECG, a positive CKG response increased the probability of coronary disease to 80%. In the 30 patients with negative ECG, a negative CKG response, which was present in 26 patients, lowered the probability to 8%, and none had multivessel disease. (4) *Asymptomatic*. There were too few individuals for analysis.

This study confirms that the CKG performed during exercise testing improves the diagnostic accuracy of the ECG response and is a cost-effective indicator of myocardial ischemia. Unfortunately, this device is no longer available commercially. The seismocardiograph is a similar device now available but not yet validated. The technical skills and need for breath holding after exercise were impediments in the widespread acceptance of this procedure, but failure to obtain reimbursement is the more likely explanation.

Coronary artery calcification on fluoroscopic examination. Langou and colleagues reported the use of cardiac fluoroscopy as a prescreening tool in asymptomatic men before exercise tests.[43] In one study, 129 healthy men (average age 49) were evaluated with cardiac fluoroscopy to detect coronary artery calcification, followed by a submaximal exercise test. Of the 108 subjects who completed the exercise test, 37, or 34%, had at least one fluoroscopically detected calcified coronary artery. Of this group of subjects with positive fluoroscopic findings, 13 (35%) had an abnormal ST-segment response to the exercise test. Of the 68 subjects with normal fluoroscopy, only 3 (4%) had an abnormal exercise response. Consequently those with calcification of at least one coronary artery had a ninefold increased risk of having an abnormal exercise electrocardiographic test. Of the 16 subjects with an abnormal exercise test, 81% had calcification of at least one coronary artery. The location of the calcific deposit conferred greater risk for exercise-induced ischemic changes than multivessel involvement did. Forty-seven percent of men with calcification in the left anterior descending coronary artery had an abnormal exercise electrocardiogram versus 33% and 16% of persons with left circumflex and right coronary artery calcifications respectively.

In a second study, the 13 men who had both coronary artery calcification and an abnormal exercise test had coronary angiography. They had a mean age of 44, none had any symptoms or signs of coronary disease, and all had a normal resting electrocardiogram. Coronary artery calcification was first detected by fluoroscopy in a single artery in 10 men, in two arteries in 2 men, and in three arteries in 1 man. On angiography, coronary artery disease was considered clinically significant if there was greater than 50% luminal narrowing in any major coronary branch. Coronary arteriography revealed 12 men with clinically significant coronary artery disease: single-vessel disease in 4, double in 5, and triple in 3 men. One man had only a minor lesion. In a 3-year follow-up study in these 13 patients, 3 had developed typical angina and 1 had developed a Q-wave MI. The results of this study indicate that the combination of coronary artery calcification and an abnormal exercise test may be highly predictive of coronary heart disease.

To evaluate variability in the reported accuracy of fluoroscopically detected coronary calcific deposits for predicting angiographic disease, Gianrossi and colleagues applied metanalysis to 13 consecutively published reports comparing the results of cardiac fluoroscopy with coronary angiography.[44] Population characteristics and technical and methodological factors were analyzed. Sensitivity and specificity for predicting serious coronary disease compare quite well with those from the literature on the exercise ECG and thallium scintigram. Sensitivity for any disease averaged 58% and specificity 82%, and for severe disease sensitivity averaged 87% and specificity 59%. Sensitivity increases and specificity decreases more significantly with patient age, and sensitivity is paradoxically lower in laboratories testing patients with more severe disease, as well as when 70% rather than 50% diameter narrowing is used to define angiographic disease. Work-up and test review bias were also significantly related to reported accuracy.

Detrano has used digitally enhanced fluoroscopy to visualize coronary artery calcifications. Initial results indicate that it may have its greatest predictive accuracy in younger individuals. This investigator is in the process of performing a large National Institutes of Health–sponsored trial to test the hypothesis that this technique is the most cost-effective screening tool available.[45]

Lipid screening. Total cholesterol to high-density lipoprotein cholesterol (TC-HDL) ratios have been shown to be directly correlated with coronary heart disease risk. In a study by Williams and colleagues on 2568 asymptomatic men, a TC-HDL ratio of 4 correlated with a very low coronary heart disease conventional risk factor rating, and a TC-HDL ratio of 8 was correlated with a very high risk for coronary heart disease.

Uhl and colleagues measured fasting total cholesterol and high-density lipoproteins in 572 asymptomatic aircrewmen.[46] Of these, 132 had an abnormal treadmill test and underwent coronary angiography. Coronary disease defined as a lesion of 50% or greater diameter narrowing was found in 16, with the rest having minimal ($n = 14$) or no coronary artery disease ($n = 102$). The 14 men with minimal coronary artery disease had TC-HDL ratios that differed from the normals ($p < 0.001$). Two of the 16 with angiographic coronary artery disease had TC-HDL ratios of less than 6, whereas four of the 102 angiographic normal subjects had a ratio of greater than 6. Only 42 of 440 (9.5%) with a normal treadmill test had a TC-HDL ratio greater than 6; 87% of those with coronary heart disease had TC-HDL ratios greater than 6. This ratio generated a risk of 172. A limitation of this study is that true sensitivity cannot be determined because only those with an abnormal treadmill test underwent coronary angiography.

At the USAFSAM, 255 totally asymptomatic men underwent cardiac catheterization because of at least 0.1 mV of ST-segment depression. Sixty-five men had at least 50% coronary artery narrowing. Thus the predictive value of ST-segment changes was only 24%. Five risk factors were studied (smoking, hypertension, hypercholesterolemia, a family history tendency, and glucose intolerance), and univariate analysis did not increase the predictive value. However, 41 men had no abnormal risk factors, and their odds ratio was over 3:1 with hypercholesterolemia alone or the presence of three risk factors. The presence of at least one risk factor and two or more exercise variables identified as predictive (including 0.3 mV of ST-segment depression early, persistent ST-segment depression after exercise, or exercise duration under 10 minutes) identified over half the cases of two- or three-vessel disease with a predictive value of 84%.

Computer probability estimates. Diamond and

Forrester have reviewed the literature to estimate pretest likelihood of disease by age, sex, symptoms, and the Framingham risk equation (based on blood pressure, smoking, glucose intolerance, resting electrocardiogram, and cholesterol).[47] In addition, they have considered the sensitivity and specificity of four diagnostic tests (the exercise test, cardiokymography, thallium, and cardiac fluoroscopy) and applied Bayes' theorem. This information has been assimilated in a computer program written in BASIC that can be used to determine probabilities of coronary disease for a given individual after entry of any of the above data. (CADENZA is the acronym for this program).

Essentially, they derived a system of decision analysis that prescreens patients before they undergo more expensive tests. This enhances the predictive value of these noninvasive tests by selection of a subgroup with a greater pretest likelihood of disease (perhaps with a 15% to 40% prevalence) so that the posttest probability of an abnormal test will be raised to 60% or even to 80%.

The biggest weakness of this approach is that the sensitivities and specificities of the secondary tests is not certain, and it is uncertain how they interact because of similar inadequacies. In addition, a step approach that uses risk markers to identify a high-risk group excludes the majority of individuals who will eventually get coronary disease. This approach concentrates the preventive effect on the small, high-risk group while ignoring the majority of individuals in the moderate-risk range who will contribute larger numbers but at a lesser rate to disease end points.

Hlatky and co-workers attempted to validate two available methods of probability calculation by comparing their diagnostic accuracy with that of cardiologists.[48] Ninety-one cardiologists evaluated the clinical summaries of eight randomly selected patients. For each patient, the cardiologist assessed the probability of coronary heart disease after reviewing the clinical history, physical examination, and laboratory data, including an exercise test. The probability of coronary disease was also obtained for each patient using identical information from (1) a published table of data based on age, sex, symptoms, and degree of ST-segment change during exercise and (2) CADENZA using the age, sex, risk factors, rest electrocardiogram, and multiple exercise measurements. With the coronary angiogram as the standard, average diagnostic accuracy was best for the computer program.

Prognosis in asymptomatic patients with angiographic coronary artery disease

Hammermeister and colleagues reported the effects of coronary artery bypass surgery on asymptomatic or mildly symptomatic angina patients who were studied as part of the Seattle Heart Watch.[49] The report was based on 227 medically treated and 392 surgically treated patients who were nonrandomly assigned to medical or surgical therapy. Cox's analysis was used to correct for the differences in baseline characteristics. Patients with three-vessel disease who underwent surgery had significantly improved survival, but surgically treated patients with one-vessel disease and two-vessel disease did not. The results of this study indicate that surgery may be indicated in the asymptomatic or mildly symptomatic patient with three-vessel disease, moderate impairment of left ventricular function (ejection fraction 31% to 50%), good distal vessels, and no other major medical illness. Asymptomatic patients with normal left ventricular function (ejection fraction greater than 51%) had an excellent prognosis regardless of the treatment.

Hickman and colleagues at USAFSAM followed for 5 years 90 men 45 to 54 years of age with asymptomatic angiographic coronary disease without previous MI.[50] Sixteen patients developed angina, 4 had myocardial infarctions, and 2 died suddenly. The events were not significantly different in those with one-, two-, or three-vessel disease. They concluded that in asymptomatic patients with angiographic coronary disease, the 5-year prognosis was good even in those with high-risk lesions. Conventional risk factors predicted risk more than the angiographic severity of disease did. Angina, an indistinct end point, was the most common initial event.

Kent and co-workers have reported 147 asymptomatic or mildly symptomatic patients with coronary heart disease who were followed prospectively for an average of 2 years.[51] None had significant one-vessel, 31% had two-vessel, and 41% had three-vessel coronary disease. The ejection fraction was 55% or greater in 70% of the patients. Thirty-five percent of the patients had a normal electrocardiogram, whereas 30% had evidence of a previous myocardial infarction. During the follow-up period there were eight deaths. There was an annual mortality of 3% for the entire group, 1.5% for patients with one- and two-vessel disease, and 6% for those with three-vessel disease. In those with three-vessel disease, exercise testing enabled better identification of high-risk and low-risk groups. Despite a history of mild symptoms, 25% of the patients with three-vessel disease exhibited poor exercise tolerance; of these, 40% either died (for an annual mortality of 9%) or had progressive symptoms requiring an operation. In those with good exercise capacity, only 22% died or had progressive symptoms, giving an annual mortality of 4%. The prognosis is excellent in patients with no or mild symptoms with one- or two-vessel disease. In those with three-vessel disease and good exercise capacity, there was an annual mortality of 4%, versus 9% in those with three-vessel disease and poor exercise capacity.

Multiple testing procedures to detect coronary artery disease

A program of serial testing to detect latent coronary heart disease was evaluated by the U.S. Army. Screening was considered necessary before a mandatory exercise program was initial for all personnel older than 40 years. The screening tests were applied in a sequential manner in an attempt to eliminate low-risk patients from further testing and to enhance the pretest likelihood of disease in the remaining subset. An initial history, physical examination, and rest electrocardiogram were performed on 285 men and 2 women over 40 years of age (mean age 44). A fasting biochemical profile was obtained, and a risk-factor index based on the Framingham data base was calculated. All subjects underwent maximal exercise testing. All were encouraged to exercise to exhaustion and the average METs was 10 (range 7 to 18). Pre- and postexercise CKGs were performed. A risk factor index over 5.0 was considered abnormal. An abnormal ST-segment response occurred in 4 men, and an "abnormal nondiagnostic" response, defined as upsloping ST-segment changes, occurred in 15 men. Six men had frequent exercise-induced PVC's. These 26 men underwent cardiac fluoroscopy and thallium scintigraphy. Seven men had abnormal thallium scintigraphic findings, 6 underwent cardiac catheterization, and 1 died of a MI. One man with a low-risk index and normal treadmill test, cardiokymogram, and fluoroscopic findings had a MI after 6 months of follow-up study. No patient had coronary calcification. An abnormal ST-segment response was insensitive and not highly predictive of coronary disease. Cardiokymography had a 63% sensitivity, a 74% specificity, and a predictive value of 50% and was the most accurate individual test. Risk-factor analysis was not predictive, and only when there were two or more risk factors and an abnormal cardiokymogram was screening accuracy improved.

Zoltick and co-workers reported preliminary results with application of the United States Army Cardiovascular Screening Program.[52] A two-tier staged approach was initiated for a cardiovascular screening program for all active duty army personnel over 40 years of age. Criteria for primary cardiovascular screen failure include any one of the following abnormalities: (1) Framingham risk index ≥5%; (2) abnormal cardiovascular history or examination; (3) abnormal electrocardiogram; and (4) fasting blood glucose ≥115 mg/dl. Failure of the primary screen requires the taking of a secondary screening test, which includes an internal medicine or cardiology consultation and a maximum treadmill test or further sequential follow-up study. During the follow-up period, recommendations are made for risk-factor modification and exercise programs. Between June 1981 and August 1983, 42,752 individuals were screened. Of these, 23,428 (55%) cleared the primary screen, 7279 (17%) cleared the secondary screen, and 1040 (2.4%) did not pass the secondary screen. We hope that the long-term results of this important study will be published soon.

Secondary prevention and testing

Hypothetically, if a method of secondary prevention were proved and available today, the following three-step approach to screening for asymptomatic coronary heart disease in men over 35 years of age appears reasonable. First, chest pain history, risk factor analysis, and a resting electrocardiogram should be obtained. If any data collected place the individual at risk, the second step should be a maximal exercise test. If this test is interpreted as abnormal based on ST-segment shifts and perhaps other abnormal responses, the third step should be utilization of thallium exercise scintigraphy, cardiac fluoroscopy, or cardiokymography. The lack of data on the diagnostic value of these tools in asymptomatic individuals prevents strict recommendations at this time. Good clinical judgment must be exercised to avoid producing "cardiac cripples" by mislabeling healthy people. The severity of the abnormal response must be considered. Most often it is appropriate to follow an asymptomatic individual with only abnormal ST-segment depression.

Exercise testing for exercise programs

There are multiple reasons for doing an exercise test before initiating an exercise program. The optimal exercise prescription, based on a percentage of an individual's maximal heart rate or oxygen consumption (50% to 80%) or one that exceeds the gas-exchange anaerobic threshold, can be written only after an exercise test is performed. The best way to assess the risk of an adverse reaction during exercise is to observe the individual during exercise. The level of exercise training then can be set at a level below that at which adverse responses or symptoms occur. Some individuals motivated by popular misconceptions about the benefits of exercise may disregard their natural "warning systems" and push themselves into dangerous levels of ischemia.

An individual with a good exercise capacity and only 0.1 mV of ST-segment depression at maximal exercise has a relatively low risk of cardiovascular events in the next several years compared to an individual with pronounced ST-segment depression at a low heart rate or systolic blood pressure or both. Most individuals with an abnormal test can be put safely into an exercise program if the level of intensity of the exercise at which the response occurs is considered. Such patients can be followed with risk factor modification rather than being excluded from exercise or their livelihood.

Siscovick and co-workers determined whether the exercise electrocardiogram predicted acute cardiac events during moderate or strenuous physical activity among 3617 asymptomatic, hypercholesterolemic men (age range, 35 to 59 years) who were followed up in the Coronary Primary Prevention Trial.[53] Submaximal exercise test results were obtained at entry and at annual follow-up visits in years 2 through 7. ST-segment depression or elevation (≥ 1 mm or 10 μV-sec) was considered to be an abnormal result. The circumstances that surrounded each nonfatal myocardial infarction and coronary heart disease death were determined through a record review. The cumulative incidence of activity-related acute cardiac events was 2% during a mean follow-up period of 7.4 years. The risk was increased 2.6-fold in the presence of clinically silent, exercise-induced ST-segment changes at entry (95% confidence interval [CI], 1.3 to 5.2) after adjustment for 11 other potential risk factors. Of 62 men who experienced an activity related event, 11 had an abnormal test result at entry (sensitivity, 18%; 95% CI, 8 to 27). The specificity of the entry exercise test was 92% (95% CI, 91 to 93). The sensitivity and specificity were similar when the length of follow-up time was restricted to 1 year after testing. For a newly abnormal test result on a follow-up visit, the sensitivity was 24% (95% CI, 12 to 36), and the specificity was 85% (95% CI, 84 to 86); for any abnormal test result during the study (mean number of tests per subject, 6.2) the sensitivity was 37% (95% CI, 25 to 49) and the specificity was 79% (95% CI, 77 to 80). Their findings indicated that the presence of clinically silent, exercise-induced, ischemic ST-segment changes on a submaximal test was associated with an increased risk of activity-related acute cardiac events. However, this test was not sensitive when used to predict the occurrence of activity-related events among asymptomatic, hypercholesterolemic men. For this reason, the utility of the submaximal exercise test to assess the safety of physical activity among asymp-

tomatic men at risk of coronary heart disease is likely to be limited.

Exercise testing is indicated before entering an exercise program for individuals with a strong family history of coronary disease (that is, family members less than 60 years of age with a coronary event), the presence of increased risk factors (particularly serum cholesterol), or any symptoms suggestive of myocardial ischemia currently or in the past. In addition, there is clearly a group of patients who self-select for exercise testing. They may request the test even though they deny having any symptoms.

High-risk selection. A problem with using exercise testing only in those patients with identified abnormal risk factors is that a large number of patients with coronary artery disease would be excluded. Thus this approach increases the pretest probability of coronary artery disease and improves the predictive value of an abnormal response but leaves a large number of patients with potential coronary artery disease without the potential benefits of this screening technique. It has been hypothesized that this approach concentrates the preventive influence on the small, high-risk group but excludes the majority of individuals in the moderate-risk range.

Further testing. A major problem with performing an exercise test in apparently healthy people is the difficulty associated with a "positive" response. Thallium planar imaging test appears to have relatively high sensitivity (80%) and specificity (90%), but it requires experienced readers and a good laboratory.[54] It is, however, superior to SPECT or radionuclide ventriculography, which in some studies has had a specificity as low as 60%. In some patients, a clearly abnormal secondary study may ultimately require coronary arteriography to assess coronary anatomy. It is necessary to see if there is an overlap in calling false positives; that is, the exercise electrocardiogram and thallium could be abnormal in women because of attenuation by breast tissue causing cold spots, and the X phenomena causing ST-segment depression.[55] Also, thallium may be falsely positive for unknown reasons in mitral valve prolapse as the exercise electrocardiogram is. Remember that a low specificity must be avoided in screening.

Exercise testing for special screening purposes: pilots

Unfortunately, politics and economic factors are two of the strongest factors influencing the use of exercise testing in subjects with flying responsibilities.[56] The pool of available pilots is obviously an important national resource. If there are many pilots available, society is more likely to be more strict with regulations regarding flying standards. Clearly, physicians must be concerned with public safety. Allowing an individual with an increased health risk to take responsiblity for many other peoples' lives could result in a tragedy. The presence of a back-up pilot and the effect of modern technology on flying do not lessen the stresses of this occupation. There are numerous situations of very high stress, such as takeoffs and landings, where it might not be possible for another person in the cockpit to take over control of the aircraft and thus a disaster might not be averted if the key pilot were to have a cardiac event. In general, pilots are a highly motivated, intelligent group of men who feel a high level of reponsibility for the performance of their work. Flying is their livelihood, however, and most of them love it so dearly that they may conceal medical information that could endanger their flying status. In addition, the stress of work often leaves them unable to maintain a healthy life-style. The stress of altering one's circadian cycle and trying to navigate in and out of today's busy airports, leaves many of them overweight, deconditioned, and smoking heavily. Whenever possible, health professionals should recommend that these men and women have the full benefits of modern preventive medicine, including the periodic assessment of physical work capacity, response to stress, and risk factors for coronary atherosclerosis.

SUMMARY

Recent studies greatly change our understanding of the application of exercise testing as a screening tool. These studies were additional follow-up studies and one angiographic study from the CASS population where 195 individuals with abnormal exercise-induced ST-segment depression and normal coronary angiograms were followed for 7 years. No increased incidence of cardiac events was found, and so the concerns raised by Erikssen's findings in 36 subjects that they were still at increased risk have not been substantiated. The new follow-up studies (MRFIT, Seattle Heart Watch, Lipid Research Clinics, and Indiana State Police) have shown quite different results compared to prior studies, mainly because distinct cardiac end points and not angina were required. The first 10 prospective studies of exercise testing in asymptomatic individuals included angina as a cardiac disease end point. This led to a bias for individuals with abnormal tests to report angina subsequently or to be misdiagnosed as having angina. When only distinct end points (death or myo-

cardial infarction) were used, as in the MRFIT, Lipid Research Clinics, Indiana State Police, or the Seattle Heart Watch studies, the results were very discouraging. The test could identify only one third of the patients with distinct events, and 95% of abnormal responders were false positives; that is, they did not die or have a myocardial infarction. The predictive value of the abnormal maximal exercise electrocardiogram ranged from 5% to 46% in the studies reviewed. However, in the studies using appropriate end points (other than angina pectoris) only 5% of the abnormal responders developed coronary heart disease over the follow-up period. Thus more than 90% of the abnormal responders were false positives. Some of these individuals have coronary disease that has yet to manifest itself, but angiographic studies have supported this high-false positive rate when the exercise test was used in asymptomatic populations. Moreover, the CASS study indicates that such individuals have a good prognosis. In a second Lipid Research Clinics study, only patients with elevated cholesterols were considered, and yet only a 6% positive prediction value was found. These results in a population first screened for a risk factor to increase the pretest prevalence of disease argue strongly against the routine use of exercise testing as a screening tool. The iatrogenic problems resulting from screening must be considered.

Some individuals who eventually develop coronary disease will change on retesting from a normal to an abnormal response. However, McHenry and Fleg have reported that a change from a negative to a positive test is no more predictive than an initially abnormal test is. One individual has even been reported who changed from a normal to an abnormal test but was free of angiographically significant disease.[57] Fleg has also demonstrated that thallium scintigraphy should be the first choice in the evaluation of asymptomatic individuals with an abnormal exercise test.

Exercise testing may prove to have value in asymptomatic populations other than for screening. Bruce and colleagues examined the motivational effects of maximal exercise testing for modifying risk factors and health habits.[58] A questionnaire was sent to nearly 3000 men 35 to 65 years of age who had undergone symptom-limited treadmill testing at least 1 year earlier. Individuals were asked if the treadmill test motivated them to stop smoking (if already a smoker), increase daily exercise, purposely lose weight, reduce the amount of dietary fat, or take medication for hypertension. There was a 69% response to this questionnaire, and 63% of the responders indicated that they had modified one or more risk factors and health habits and that they attributed this change to the exercise test. In fact, a greater percentage of patients with decreased exercise capacity, compared with normal subjects, reported a modification of risk factors or health habits.

Given the current approaches competing for health care resources, it is best to screen only those who request it, those with multiple abnormal risk factors, those with worrisome medical histories, or a family history of premature cardiovascular disease. It is difficult to choose a chronological age after which exercise testing is necessary as a screening technique before one begins an exercise program, since physiological age is important. In general, if the exercise is more strenuous than vigorous walking, most individuals over 50 years of age will benefit from such screening. The potential problems resulting from screening must be considered, and the results of testing must be applied using the predictive model and bayesian statistics. Test results must be thought of as probability statements and not as absolutes. The recent data from treadmill screening studies convincingly demonstrate the inappropriateness of including exercise testing as part of routine health maintenance in apparently healthy individuals. If it is used to classify asymptomatic individuals as having or not having coronary artery disease, it is very ineffective and causes more harm (psychological, work and insurance status, cost for more tests, and so on) than good by misclassifying many normals as having disease.

REFERENCES

1. Oster E, Schnohr H, Jensen G, et al: Electrocardiographic findings and their association with mortality in the Copenhagen City Heart Study, *Eur Heart J* 2:317-328, 1981.
2. Rose G, Baxter PJ, Reid DD, McCartney P: Prevalence and prognosis of electrocardiogram findings in middle-aged men, *Br Heart J* 15:636-643, 1978.
3. Cullen K, Stenhouse NS, Wearne KL, Cumpston GN: Electrocardiograms and 13 year cardiovascular mortality in Busselton study, *Br Heart J* 47:209-212, 1982.
4. Rabkin SW, Mathewson FAL, Tate RB: The electrocardiogram in apparently healthy men and the risk of sudden death, *Br Heart J* 47:546-552, 1982.
5. Dawber TR, Kannnel WB, Love DE, Streeper RB: The Framingham Study, *Circulation* 5:559-566, 1952.
6. Levine HD, Phillips E: The electrocardiogram and MI, *N Engl J Med* 245:833-842, 1951.
7. Liao Y, Liu K, Dyer A, et al: Major and minor electrocardiographic abnormalities and risk of death from coronary heart disease, cardiovascular diseases and all causes in men and women, *J Am Coll Cardiol* 12:1494-1500, 1988.
8. Froelicher VF, Thompson AJ, Wolthuis R, et al: Angiographic findings in asymptomatic aircrewmen with electrocardiographic abnormalities, *Am J Cardiol* 39:32-39, 1977.
9. Hartley LH, Herd JA, Day WC, et al: An exercise testing program for large populations, *JAMA* 241:269-275, 1979.
10. Bruce RA, McDonough JR: Stress testing in screening for cardiovascular disease, *Bull NY Acad Med* 45:1288-1295, 1969.
11. Aronow WS, Cassidy J: Five year follow-up of double Master's test, maximal treadmill stress test, and resting and postexercise apexcardiogram in asymptomatic persons, *Circulation* 52:616-622, 1975.
12. Cumming GR, Samm J, Borysyk L, et al: Electrocardiographic changes during exercise in asymptomatic men: 3-year follow-up, *Can Med Assoc J* 112:578-585, 1975.
13. Froelicher VF, Thomas M, Pillow C, et al: An epidemiological study of asymptomatic men screened with exercise testing for latent coronary heart disease, *Am J Cardiol* 34:770-779, 1975.
14. Manca C, Barilli AL, Dei Cas L, et al: Multivariate analysis of exercise ST depression and coronary risk factors in asymptomatic men, *Eur Heart J* 3:2-8, 1982.
15. Allen WH, Aronow WS, Goodman P, Stinson P: Five-year follow-up of maximal treadmill stress test in asymptomatic men and women, *Circulation* 62:522-531, 1980.
16. Bruce RA, Fisher LD, Hossack KF: Validation of exercise-enhanced risk assessment of coronary heart disease events: longitudinal changes in incidence in Seattle community practice, *J Am Coll Cardiol* 5:875-881, 1985.
17. MacIntyre NR, Kunkler JR, Mitchell RE, et al: Eight-year follow-up of exercise electrocardiograms in healthy, middle-aged aviators, *Aviat Space Environ Med* 52:256-259, 1981.
18. McHenry PL, O'Donnell J, Morris SN, Jordan JJ: The abnormal exercise electrocardiogram in apparently healthy men: a predictor of angina pectoris as an initial coronary event during long-term follow-up, *Circulation* 70:547-551, 1984.
19. Multiple Risk Factor Intervention Research Group: Exercise electrocardiogram and coronary heart disease mortality in the multiple risk factor intervention trial, *Am J Cardiol* 55:16-24, 1985.
20. Rautaharju PM, Prineas RJ, Eifler WJ, et al: Prognostic value of exercise electrocardiogram in men at high risk of future coronary heart disease: multiple risk factor intervention trial experience, *J Am Coll Cardiol* 8:1-10, 1986.
21. Gordon DL, Ekelund LG, Karon JM, et al: Predictive value of the exercise tolerance test for mortality in North American men: the Lipid Research Clinics Mortality Follow-Up Study, *Circulation* 74:252-261, 1986.
22. Ekelund LG, Suchindran CM, McMahon RP, et al: Coronary heart disease mortality and mortality in hypercholesterolemic men predicted from an exercise test: the Lipid Research Clinics Coronary Primary Prevention Trial, *J Am Coll Cardiol* 14:556-563, 1989.
23. Josephson RA, Shefrin E, Lakatta EG, et al: Can serial exercise testing improve the prediction of coronary events in asymptomatic individuals? *Circulation* 81:20-24, 1990.
24. Gordon DJ, Leon AS, Ekelund LG, et al: Smoking, physical activity, and other predictors of endurance and heart rate response to exercise in asymptomatic hypercholesterolemic men, *Am J Epidemiol* 125:587-600, 1987.
25. Hedblad B, Juul-Möller S, Svensson K, et al: Increased mortality in men with ST segment depression during 24 h ambulatory long-term ECG recording, *Eur Heart J* 10:149-158, 1989.
26. Borer JS, Brensike JF, Redwood DR, et al: Limitations of the electrocardiographic response to exercise in predicting coronary artery disease, *N Eng J Med* 193:367-375, 1975.
27. Barnard RJ, Gardner GW, Diaco NV, Kattus AA: Near-maximal ECG stress testing and coronary artery disease risk factor analysis in Los Angeles City fire fighters, *J Occupational Med* 18:818-827, 1975.
28. Uhl GS, Hopkirk AC, Hickman JR, et al: Predictive im-

plications of clinical and exercise variables in detecting significant coronary artery disease in asymptomatic men, *J Cardiac Rehabil* 4:245-252, 1984.

29. Erikssen J, Enge I, Forfang K, Storstein O: False positive diagnostic tests and coronary angiographic findings in 105 presumably healthy males, *Circulation* 54:371-376, 1976.

30. Erikssen J, Dale J, Rottwelt K, Myhre E: False suspicion of coronary heart disease: a 7 year follow-up study of 36 apparently healthy middle-aged men, *Circulation* 68:490-497, 1983.

31. Kemp HG, Kronmal RA, Vlietstra RE, Frye RL: Seven year survival of patients with normal and near normal coronary arteriograms: a CASS registry study, *J Am Coll Cardiol* 7:479-483, 1986.

32. McHenry PL. Exercise-induced ventricular arrhythmias: prevalence, mechanisms, and prognostic implications, Philadelphia, 1992, Lippincott.

33. McHenry P, Morris S, Kavalier M: Comparative study of exercise-induced ventricular arrhythmias in normal subjects and patients with documented coronary artery disease, *Am J Cardiol* 37:609-616, 1976.

34. Busby MJ, Shefrin EA, Fleg JL: Prevalence and long-term significance of exercise-induced frequent or repetitive ventricular ectopic beats in apparently healthy volunteers, *J Am Coll Cardiol* 14:1659-1665, 1989.

35. Hollenberg M, Zoltick JM, Go M, et al: Comparison of a quantitative treadmill exercise score with standard electrocardiographic criteria in screening asymptomatic young men for coronary artery disease, *N Engl J Med* 313(10):600-606, 1985.

36. Okin PM, Anderson KM, Levy D, Kligfield P: Heart rate adjustment of exercise-induced ST segment depression: improved risk stratification in the Framingham Offspring Study, *Circulation* 83:866-874, 1991.

37. Caralis DG, Bailey I, Kennedy HL, Pitt B: Thallium-201 myocardial imaging in evaluation of asymptomatic individuals with ischemic ST segment depression on exercise electrocardiogram, *Br Heart J* 42:562-571, 1979.

38. Nolewajka AJ, Kostuk WJ, Howard J, et al: [201]Thallium stress myocardial imaging: an evaluation of fifty-eight asymptomatic males, *Clin Cardiol* 4:134-142, 1981.

39. Uhl GS, Kay TN, Hickman JR: Computer-enhanced thallium-scintigrams in asymptomatic men with abnormal exercise tests, *Am J Cardiol* 48:1037-1046, 1981.

40. Fleg JL, Gerstenblith G, Zonderman AB, et al: Prevalence and prognostic significance of exercise-induced silent myocardial ischemia detected by thallium scintigraphy and electrocardiography in asymptomatic volunteers, *Circulation* 81:428-436, 1990.

41. Silverberg RA, Diamond GA, Vas R, et al: Noninvasive diagnosis of coronary artery disease: the cardiokymographic stress test, *Circulation* 61:579-589, 1980.

42. Weiner DA: Accuracy of cardiokymography during exercise testing: results of a multicenter study, *J Am Coll Cardiol* 6:502-509, 1985.

43. Langou RA, Huang EK, Kelley MJ, et al: Predictive accuracy of coronary artery calcification and abnormal exercise test for coronary artery disease in asymptomatic man, *Circulation* 62:1196-1202, 1981.

44. Gianrossi R, Detrano R, Colombo A, Froelicher VF: Cardiac fluoroscopy for the diagnosis of coronary artery disease: a meta-analytic review, *Am Heart J* 120:1179-1188, 1990.

45. Detrano R, Froelicher V: Diagnosis and treatment: a logical approach to screening for coronary artery disease, *Ann Intern Med* 106:846-852, 1987.

46. Uhl GS, Troxler RG, Hickman JR, Clark D: Angiographic correlation of coronary artery disease with high density lipoprotein cholesterol in asymptomatic men, *Am J Cardiol* 48:903-911, 1981.

47. Diamond GA, Forrester JS: Analysis of probability as an aid in the clinical diagnosis of coronary artery disease, *N Engl J Med* 300:1350-1359, 1979.

48. Hlatky M, Bovinick E, Brundage B: Diagnostic accuracy of cardiologists compared with probability calculations using Bayes' rule, *Am J Cardiol* 49:192-197, 1982.

49. Hammermeister KE, DeRouen TA, Dodge HT: Effect of coronary surgery on survival in asymptomatic and minimally symptomatic patients, *Circulation* 62:98-104, 1980.

50. Hickman JR, Uhl GS, Cook RL, et al: A natural history study of asymptomatic coronary disease, *Am J Cardiol* 45:422-430, 1980.

51. Kent KM, Rosing DR, Ewels CJ, et al: Prognosis of asymptomatic or mildly symptomatic patients with coronary artery disease, *Am J Cardiol* 49:1823-1831, 1982.

52. Zoltick JM, McAllister HA, Bedynek JL: The United States Army Cardiovascular Screening Program, *J Cardiac Rehabil* 4:530-535, 1984.

53. Siscovick DS, Ekelund LG, Johnson JL, et al: Sensitivity of exercise electrocardiography for acute cardiac events during moderate and strenuous physical activity, *Arch Intern Med* 151:325-330, 1991.

54. Fagan LF, Shaw L, Kong BA, et al: Prognostic value of exercise thallium scintigraphy in patients with good exercise tolerance and a normal or abnormal exercise electrocardiogram and suspected or confirmed coronary artery disease, *Am J Cardiol* 69:607-611, 1992.

55. Gavrielides S, Kaski JC, Galassi AR, et al: Recovery-phase patterns of ST segment depression in the heart rate domain cannot distinguish between anginal patients with coronary artery disease and patients with syndrome X, *Am Heart J* 122(6):1593-1598, 1991.

56. Bruce RA, Fisher LD: Clinical medicine: exercise-enhanced risk factors for coronary heart disease vs. age as criteria for mandatory retirement of healthy pilots, *Aviation Space and Environmental Medicine* 58:792-798, 1987.

57. Thompson AJ, Froelicher VF: Kugel's artery as a major collateral channel in severe coronary disease, *Aviation Space and Environmental Medicine* 45:1276-1280, 1974.

58. Bruce RA, DeRouen TA, Hossack KF: Pilot study examining the motivational effects of maximal exercise testng to modify risk factors and health habits, *Cardiology* 66:111, 1980.

11 Miscellaneous Other Applications

EVALUATION OF TREATMENTS

The exercise test can be used to evaluate the effects of both medical and surgical treatment. The effects of various medications including nitrates, digitalis, and antihypertensive agents have been evaluated by exercise testing. Although exercise testing has been used to evaluate patients before and after coronary artery bypass surgery and coronary angioplasty, a definitive comparison has not been possible. One problem with using treadmill time or work load rather than measuring maximal oxygen uptake in serial studies is that people learn to perform treadmill walking more efficiently. Thus treadmill time or work load can increase during serial studies without any improvement in cardiovascular function. Thus it is important to include the measurement of ventilatory oxygen uptake when the effects of medical or surgical treatment are being evaluated by treadmill testing.

Evaluation of antianginal agents

Reproducibility. Since studies using standard exercise testing are required by the Food and Drug Administration before approval of antianginal agents, it is important to know the reproducibility of exercise variables in patients with angina. To evaluate reproducibility, Sullivan and co-workers at UCSD studied 14 angina patients with 3 consecutive days of treadmill testing.[1] A random effects analysis of variance (ANOVA) model was used to measure reliability and to determine any trends in the test results. The intraclass correlation coefficient (ICC), a generalization of the Pearson product-moment correlation coefficient for bivariate data, served as the measure of reliability. The results are summarized in Table 11-1. Prior studies evaluating the changes of work performance in patients with angina pectoris concentrated on improvements in total exercise time. Smokler and

Lasvik, using moderately severe angina as an end point, observed coefficients of variation (standard deviation divided by the mean times 100) of approximately 5% for total treadmill time.[2] Similar results were obtained by Sullivan, who found a coefficient of variation of 6% for peak time. However, when the intraclass coefficient (ICC) was determined to test for reproducibility, a rather low value of 0.70 was obtained. The addition of a given amount to each observation of a parameter would increase the mean without affecting the standard deviation and thus lower the coefficient of variation. The ICC, like the Pearson product-moment correlation coefficient, is not affected by the addition or multiplication of a given number to the observations. An example of this is observed at peak exercise where there is a lower coefficient of variation (6%) than at the onset of angina (11%) but reproducibility, as defined by the ICC, was the same (0.70). During sequential exercise testing, many investigators have noted an increase in total treadmill time in normals, angina patients, and CHF patients. In the study by Sullivan and colleagues, we observed better reproducibility for oxygen uptake when compared to time at each analysis point.

The ability to reproducibly determine angina during exercise testing is critical to the evaluation of therapeutic interventions. Previous investigations have included a baseline exercise test in which the patient becomes familiar with the exercise testing equipment and staff. Studies by Redwood and others have stressed the importance of a properly designed exercise test protocol when evaluating patients with stable angina pectoris.[3] In the study by Sullivan and colleagues the baseline test familiarized the patient with the equipment and staff and evaluated their exercise capacity. From this, an individualized protocol was designed to al-

Table 11-1 Standard deviation of change of two measurements (SD), intraclass correlation (ICC), coefficient of variation (CV) at peak exercise, onset of angina, and gas-exchange anaerobic threshold (ATge)

Variable	Peak exercise			Onset of angina			ATgc		
	SD	ICC	CV (%)	SD	ICC	CV (%)	SD	ICC	CV (%)
Time (sec)	58	0.70	6 ± 6	65	0.70	11 ± 6	65	0.70	15 ± 9
VO_2 (L/min)	0.150	0.88	6 ± 4	0.152	0.85	6 ± 4	0.113	0.83	7 ± 4
Double product ($\times 10^3$)	2.6	0.90	9 ± 5	2.0	0.75	8 ± 5	2.2	0.75	8 ± 6
Heart rate (beats/min)	7	0.94	4 ± 2	6	0.89	4 ± 2	8	0.83	4 ± 4
ST60 X (mV)	0.06	0.80	34 ± 25	0.03	0.79	31 ± 25	0.03	0.78	45 ± 29
ST60 GD (mV)	0.05	0.83	23 ± 21	0.04	0.65	25 ± 16	0.05	0.65	53 ± 34

X, Lead X; *GD*, lead with greatest depression.

low the patient sufficient time on the treadmill before stopping because of angina. Redwood has suggested that exercise capacity at the onset of angina can be optimally evaluated using a progressive exercise test that elicits chest pain within 3 to 6 minutes. Also, increments in work should not exceed 20 watts, or approximately 2 METs for a 75 kg man. In our study, the onset of angina occurred at a mean of approximately 6 minutes. In the individualized protocols the increments in work did not exceed 2 METs and in most cases were approximately 1 MET. The advantage of the individualized protocol over one protocol for all patients is that it provides a gradual increase in work and is specific for each patient's exercise capacity.

The criterion for stopping the exercise test was the patient's subjective angina corresponding to that level of pain at which they would normally stop to take a sublingual dose of nitroglycerin. The use of the Borg pain scale produced a wide range of numerical end points. It would appear that there is individual variation in the amount of tolerable angina before an activity is stopped. The reproducibility of the double product, a noninvasive estimate of myocardial oxygen demand, was excellent at peak exercise (0.90) but somewhat low at the onset of angina and the gas-exchange anaerobic threshold (ATge) (0.75 for both). The poorer reproducibility at the onset of angina and the ATge may be explained by the fact that blood pressure was measured every 2 minutes. The observed improvement in the ICC for the heart rate when compared to double product at the onset of angina (0.89) and the ATge (0.83) and a slight increase at peak exercise (0.94) supports this contention. Thus, when systolic blood pressure is difficult to obtain, heart rate may be used as a reproducible noninvasive estimate of myocardial oxygen demand.

Previous studies involving patients with angina have reported high coefficients of variation for the amount of ST-segment displacement. However, here again the failure of the coefficient of variation to depict a reproducible variable is evident. When one is considering the ICC for lead X, the reproducibility is good (0.80) at peak exercise, the onset of angina, and ATge, though the coefficients of variation range from 31% to 45%. Although not nearly as reproducible at the onset of angina or ATge (0.65), the ECG lead with the greatest ST-segment displacement is reproducible at peak exercise (0.83).

Conclusions from the study of Sulivan and colleagues include these points: (1) measured oxygen uptake should be used instead of total exercise time because it is a more reproducible measure of aerobic exercise capacity, (2) the ventilatory threshold is a reproducible submaximal exercise variable at which to evaluate myocardial ischemia and myocardial oxygen demand, (3) a pretrial exercise test allows the patient to become familiar with the exercise testing staff, the equipment, and the nature of his or her anginal end points, (4) the treadmill protocol should be designed for the patient's exercise capacity with 2 MET or less increments per stage, (5) computerized techniques for ECG analysis provide reproducible measurement of ST-segment displacement, and (6) statistical methods based on the estimate of the measurement error associated with a particular variable can be used by the clinician or investigator to better plan and evaluate an intervention.

Variable anginal threshold. Waters and colleagues investigated the frequency and mechanism of variable-threshold angina by performing seven treadmill tests in each of 28 patients with stable-effort angina and exercise-induced ST-segment depression. Each patient had tests at 8 A.M. on 4 days within a 2-week period and on one of these days had three additional tests at 9 A.M., 11 A.M., and 4 P.M. Time to 0.1 mV of ST-segment depression increased from 277 + 172 seconds on day 1 to 319 ± 186 seconds on day 2, 352 ± 213 seconds on day 3, and 356 ± 207 seconds on day 4 ($p <$ 0.05). Rate-pressure product at 0.1 mV of ST-segment depression remained constant. Similarly, time to 0.1 mV of ST-segment depression increased from 333 ± 197 seconds at 8 A.M. to 371 ± 201 seconds at 9 A.M. and 401 ± 207 seconds at 11 A.M. and decreased to 371 ± 189 seconds at 4 P.M. ($p < 0.01$). Again, rate-pressure product at 0.1 mV of ST-segment depression remained constant. The standard deviation for time to 0.1 mV of ST-segment depression was 22% ± 11%. The standard deviation for rate-pressure product at 0.1 mV of ST-segment depression was significantly less at 8.4% ± 2.8%. In 78 (40%) of the 196 tests, time to 0.1 mV of ST-segment depression was less than 80% or greater than 120% of the patient's mean; in contrast, rate-pressure product at 0.1 mV of ST-segment depression was less than 80% or greater than 120% of the patient's mean in only three tests (1.5%). They found considerable variability in exercise tolerance in patients with effort angina, even when rate-pressure product at the onset of ischemia remained fixed. They concluded that a history of variable threshold angina does not necessarily imply variations in coronary tone.

Evaluation of long-acting nitrates. It has been difficult to demonstrate the efficacy of long-acting nitrate preparations in the treatment of angina pectoris. There are available more objective measurements during exercise testing that could make this possible, but they rarely have been applied. A key question that we have tried to answer is, Can gas-exchange variables and computerized ST-segment analysis accurately and reproducibly detect beneficial changes during exercise in angina patients treated acutely with sublingually placed nitrates or after treatment with long-acting nitrate preparations? Do these beneficial changes persist after chronic administration of the long-acting agents for 2 weeks?[4]

The use of organic nitrates in the treatment of angina dates back to the nineteenth century when the English physician Brunton discovered the vasodepressor activity of amyl nitrate, by inhalation, and noted the immediate but transient relief of angina. Subsequent findings by Murrell, in 1879, established the use of sublingually placed nitroglycerin for the treatment of angina as well as its use as a prophylactic agent before exertion.

Symptoms of effort angina are produced by a transient imbalance between the supply and demand of myocardial oxygen. The deficiency in myocardial oxygen is a result of increased myocardial demand in the face of restricted myocardial blood flow. Effort angina pectoris must be distinguished from spontaneous angina pectoris, in which coronary spasm plays an important role. Typical effort angina is highly predictive of obstructive coronary artery disease. It has been noted, however, that only one third of all patients examined at necropsy with significant coronary atherosclerosis have a history of angina pectoris. It is not clear why some patients with obstructive coronary artery disease have pain whereas others having the same degree of obstruction do not manifest this symptom. The chest pain associated with angina is usually relieved promptly by sublingually administered nitroglycerin.

Why is there controversy and disparate results with clinical studies of the use of the long acting nitrates? Some of the explanations for this include the following: (1) acute (single-dose) effects can be demonstrated for the long-acting preparations, but when the agents are given chronically, tolerance can develop; (2) there is a definite placebo effect involved in the treatment of angina; (3) nitrate blood levels are dificult to measure, but some modes of delivery clearly do not result in effective blood levels; (4) large increases of nitrates in the blood may be more effective than those at a chronic level; (5) treadmill time or work load is not a reproducible measurement; and (6) more objective measurements using expired gases and computerized ST-segment analysis rarely have been used.

Most studies evaluating antianginal agents have relied on changes in treadmill time for assessment of drug efficacy. VO_2 max has been rarely performed in patients with angina. End points in anginal patients are often very subjective, and the grading of angina to arrive at a consistent end point has not resolved even this problem. Therefore researchers have looked at submaximal end points as measures of change. These have included ST-segment depression, anginal threshold, the heart rate and blood pressure response to exercise, and more recently anaerobic threshold. Anginal patients should be able to walk longer on the treadmill because they become anaerobic later because of improved cardiac performance during exercise after use of an antianginal medication. This improvement has not been demonstrated as yet but offers the opportunity for more objective and safer evaluation of antianginal agents. An additional methodology is to assess ST-segment changes using computer methodology and to see if this objective estimate of myocardial ischemia is altered by antianginal agents.

Measurements should be made at the following points:

1. Supine and sitting heart rate and blood pressure. Rationale: the action of nitrates may be attributable to dropping BP. Previous studies have found a relationship of change in VO_2 to drop in BP. If this is demonstrated, a nitrate effect could be documented or titrated in the office by changes in resting BP.
2. Standard workload. We have used 3.0 mph at a 5% grade as a "standard" submaximal work load that most anginal patients can achieve.
3. Submaximal heart rate and double product. These parameters are chosen specifically for each individual using his baseline testing. The heart rate and the double product where definite abnormal ST-segment depression is first seen is the value used for subsequent comparisons.
4. Ventilatory anaerobic threshold—submaximal point chosen by gas-analysis techniques.
5. Onset of angina—patient's first perception of usual angina.
6. Maximal exercise—last 30 seconds of treadmill exercise.

With these considerations, we designed several studies to evaluate the effects of long-acting nitrates on treadmill test variables. The following describes the methodology we have used: After the baseline test, the patients underwent exercise testing at the same time of day separated by 1 week. The baseline test was given to evaluate their current clinical condition and allow them to become familiar with the procedure. All testing was done in the fasting state, with no food eaten for at least 3 hours. Individualized protocols were designed to provide small increments in work to allow the patients sufficient time on the treadmill before reaching a symptom-limited end point. These protocols conformed to guidelines for testing patients with stable angina pectoris outlined by Redwood and co-workers. Each patient's subjective perception of angina was evaluated using the Borg scale. The patients were taught the proper hand signals to indicate the severity of pain. The points of analysis were the onset of angina and peak angina, corresponding to that level of pain at which the patient would normally stop exercise to take a sublingual nitroglycerin pill. The following measurements were derived from the gas-exchange data: minute ventilation (VE, liters/min at BTPS); oxygen uptake (VO_2, ml/kg/min, liters/min); carbon dioxide production (VCO_2, liters/min); respiratory exchange ratio (RER, VCO_2/VO_2); and the ventilatory equivalent for oxygen (VE/VO_2).

Evaluation Of pentaerythritol tetranitrate. We evaluated the efficacy of oral sustained-release pentaerythritol tetranitrate (PETN) in 11 patients with stable angina pectoris using a double-blind, randomized-study design. Treadmill testing with the direct measurement of expired gas–exchange variables was determined at 1, 6, and 10 hours after administration of PETN or matching placebo. Changes in resting standing and supine heart rates (mean increases 4 and 5 beats/min respectively) and supine systolic blood pressure (mean decrease 9 mm Hg) were observed 1 hour after PETN administration. There were no significant changes in any of the resting hemodynamic variables measured at 6 and 10 hours. One and 6 hours after PETN, ventilation and the ventilatory oxygen consumption were increased at peak exercise. Total treadmill time did not differ between PETN and placebo at any time period investigated.

The response to drug differs according to its administration between when given only on the day of the test versus when given for days (chronic administration as in clinical practice) preceding the first day of exercise testing. Parker has demonstrated partial tolerance to the hemodynamic effects of isosorbide dinitrate within 48 hours of initiating therapy.[5] Thadani and co-workers demonstrated that acute resting hemodynamic and exercise variables in angina patients are attenuated during chronic therapy.[6] Resting hemodynamic changes that persisted for 8 hours during acute therapy were demonstrable for only 4 hours during chronic therapy. Similarly, significant increases in exercise capacity were observed for 8 hours after acute and only 2 hours during chronic therapy.

Evaluation of transdermal nitroglycerin (TDN). Transdermally administered nitroglycerin systems are advertised to offer 24-hour relief from angina pectoris. The basis for this extended therapeutic effect was inferred from studies documenting constant plasma nitroglycerin levels 24 hours after transdermal application and from preliminary studies in patients with angina pectoris. However, recent controlled studies have produced conflicting results as to the efficacy of TDN systems in patients with angina. Thompson observed significant increases in treadmill time at 2 and 26 hours after application of individually titrated patches.[7] In contrast, other investigators have been unable to document significant changes in exercise capacity 24 hours after application of TDN, though increases in exercise time were observed at intervals up to 8 hours.

We studied 16 patients with stable angina pectoris in a double-blind crossover manner utilizing treadmill exercise testing with direct measurement of ventilatory oxygen uptake, 1 and 24 hours after application of a 20 cm^2 TDN system and identical placebo.[8] Testing was performed after a 3-day lead-in period on either an active patch or a placebo. Points of analysis were peak angina and the submaximal work load occuring at 4 minutes of exercise. No statistically significant differences were observed between TDN and placebo in any of the resting hemodynamic or peak angina variables at 1 or 24 hours. A significant increase in the double product at the submaximal work load was observed 1 hour after TDN relative to placebo. However, no significant differences were observed in any of the other measured variables at the submaximal work load, 1 or 24 hours after TDN.

A chronically administered, once daily application of 20 cm² TDN was ineffective in altering the exercise capacity in our patients with angina pectoris. A combination of factors would appear responsible for this. In investigations demonstrating an increase in exercise capacity with TDN, a titration period was initiated before the study to determine the maximally tolerated dosage. This was not done in the present study. In addition, the timing of the initial test, 1 hour after application of the transdermal system, may have been too early to detect significant changes in exercise capacity because of inadequate blood nitroglycerin levels.

The development of tolerance is another explanation. Twenty-four hours after transdermal application blood nitroglycerin concentrations have been observed to be similiar to concentrations obtained at 2 and 8 hours. However, changes in exercise capacity recorded at 2 and 8 hours after transdermal application did not persist up to 24 hours. Although blood nitroglycerin levels at any time period after transdermal application are lower than those observed during oral nitrate therapy, the lack of effect observed at 24 hours in the present study may in part be attributable to a nitrate tolerance acquired during the 3-day lead-in period. Tolerance to organic nitrates when given chronically occurs within 48 hours after initiating therapy. There were no positive effects of TDN at a submaximal work load where reductions in myocardial oxygen supply and demand were hypothesized to occur.

Correlation of changes in resting systolic blood pressure (SBP) with exercise capacity.

Although the effectiveness of nitrates for the long-term prophylaxis of exertional angina is controversial, investigations utilizing large doses have demonstrated persistent physiological effects. During a titration period, the observation of a 10 mm Hg decrease in resting SBP or a 10 beat/min increase in resting heart rate, or both parameters, has been utilized in studies attempting to demonstrate an increase in exercise capacity after nitrate administration. These criteria have served a dual purpose of documenting physiological changes in variables known to affect myocardial oxygen demand and to identify subjects nonresponsive to nitrates before inclusion in a study. If after nitrate administration changes in blood pressure or heart rate are correlated with changes in exercise capacity, the utilization of these variables by the clinician could identify patients expected to improve exercise tolerance during nitrate therapy.

To determine if these practical criteria could predict improved exercise capacity in patients with angina pectoris treated with nitrates we included both nitrate-responsive and nitrate-nonresponsive subjects. Nineteen patients with stable angina pectoris were studied in a double-blind placebo-controlled manner. Significant increases in resting heart rate and peak oxygen uptake and decreases in resting SBP were observed 1 hour after nitrate relative to placebo. Changes in peak oxygen uptake and total treadmill time during nitrate administration relative to placebo correlated to changes in resting supine systolic and diastolic blood pressure ($r = -0.54$ to -0.62) but not to changes in resting heart rate. The multiple regression correlation coefficient utilizing the changes in supine systolic and diastolic blood pressure during nitrate administration relative to placebo as independent variables was $r = 0.66$ when compared to changes in peak oxygen uptake. These results indicate that during administration of nitrates a decrease in resting systolic and diastolic blood pressure may be essential to ensure increases in exercise capacity. On the other hand, a lack of blood pressure response to nitrates is indicative of no improvement in exercise tolerance. Thus in the clinical setting these parameters should be utilized as the basis for nitrate titration.

Improvement in oxygen uptake and treadmill time was noted in 10/11 patients with a greater than 5 mm Hg drop in supine SBP. Whereas in five of the remaining seven patients without a greater than 5 mm Hg drop in supine SBP there was no improvement in exercise capacity. Multiple regression analysis utilizing changes in resting supine systolic and diastolic blood pressure during nitrate administration relative to placebo as independent variables resulted in significant correlations with changes in oxygen uptake and total treadmill time. This is the first statistical proof for the previously intuitive concept of equating changes in resting SBP with improvement in exercise capacity in angina pectoris patients receiving nitrates. Patients who had the greatest drop in systolic and diastolic blood pressure had the greatest increase in peak oxygen uptake and total treadmill time. On the other hand, those patients in which administration of nitrates did not affect resting blood pressure did not improve their exercise capacity. There was a correlation between the drop in resting SBP and the increase in VO_2 max.

Studies demonstrating the positive effects of nitrates on exercise capacity have utilized a titration criterion of a 10 mm Hg fall in resting SBP or a 10 beat/min increase in heart rate. The increased heart rate criteria is based on the baroreceptor-mediated rise in heart rate caused by decreased arterial pressure. Reichek has emphasized the importance of individual nitrate titration to achieve an optimal physiologic response. Standard doses of nitrates produced variability in the hemodynamic and exercise response. These results indicate that clinicians should document changes in resting systolic and diastolic blood pressure in anginal patients receiving nitrate therapy. It would appear that the greater the drop in systolic and diastolic blood pressure the greater the benefit. The magnitude of this change in blood pressure may be limited by symptoms of headaches, hypotension, or possible nitrate tolerance during chronic administration. On the other hand, a lack of blood pressure response after nitrate administration indicates little or no therapeutic effect and warrants a reevaluation of therapy.

Safety of placebo in studying antianginal agents. Because the safety of withholding standard therapy and enrolling patients with stable angina in placebo-controlled trials was not known, Glasser and co-workers identified all events leading to dropout from trials of 12 antianginal drugs submitted in support of new drug applications to the U.S. Food and Drug Administration.[9] Persons who dropped out of the trials were classified according to cause from adverse cardiovascular events or other causes without knowledge of drug assignment. There were 3161 subjects who entered any randomized, double-blind phase of placebo-controlled protocols; 197 (6.2%) withdrew because of cardiovascular events. There was no difference in risk of adverse events between drug and placebo groups. A prospectively defined subgroup analysis showed that groups who received calcium antagonists were at an increased risk of dropout compared with placebo groups, primarily because of a disproportionate number of adverse events in studies of one drug. In conclusion, there were few adverse experiences associated with short-term placebo use. Withholding active treatment for treatment of angina does not increase the risk of serious cardiac events.

Evaluation of percutaneous transluminal coronary angioplasty (PTCA)

Berger and co-workers reported follow-up data in 183 patients who had undergone PTCA at least 1 year earlier.[10] The duration of follow-up ranged from 1 to 5 years. Subjective clinical information was obtained in all patients and exercise testing in 91. PTCA was initially successful in 141 patients (79%). Of the 42 patients in whom PTCA was unsuccessful, 26 underwent CABG, whereas 16 were maintained on medical therapy. When compared to the medical patients at the time of follow-up, successful PTCA patients experienced less angina (13% versus 47%), used less nitroglycerin (25% versus 73%), were hospitalized less often for chest pain (8% versus 31%), and subjectively felt their condition had improved (96% versus 20%). During exercise testing, the prevalence of angina was less (9% versus 43%), and exercise duration was greater (8.2 minutes versus 5.8 minutes) among PTCA patients. However, there were no significant differences in ST-segment depression (26% PTCA patients versus 55% medical patients). No pre-PTCA exercise testing is reported. There were no significant differences in the incidence of subsequent myocardial infarction, mortality, or the need for CABS. For these variables no differences were seen between the CABG and PTCA groups.

Vandormael and colleagues reported the safety and short-term benefit of multilesion PTCA in 135 patients, 66 of whom had a minimum of 6 months of follow-up time.[11] Primary success, defined as successful dilatation of the most critical lesion or all lesions attempted, occurred in 87% of the 135 patients. Complete revascularization was achieved in 46% of the 117 patients with a primary success. Of the 66 patients eligible for 6-month follow-up study, 80% had an uncomplicated course and required no further procedures. Clinical improvement by at least one angina functional class was observed in 90% of the patients. Cardiac events, including a second revascularization procedure, were significantly more common in patients who had incomplete versus complete revascularization. All patients who had a primary success demonstrated clinical improvement with a reduction in symptoms or improved exercise tolerance. Exercise-induced angina occurred in 11 (12%) and an abnormal exercise ECG in 30 (32%) of the 95 patients with post-PTCA exercise test data. Exercise-induced angina occurred in 1 (2%) of 46 patients with complete revascularization versus 10 (20%) of 49 patients with incomplete revascularization; an abnormal exercise electrocardiogram occurred in 9 versus 21 patients respectively. Of 57 patients who had paired exercise test data before and after angioplasty, exercise-induced angina occurred in 56% of patients before the procedure compared with only 11% of patients after angioplasty. Exercise-induced ST-segment depression of more than

0.1 mV occurred in 75% of patients before PTCA versus 32% of the procedure. After patients were stratified according to completeness of revascularization, the number of patients with exercise-induced angina was reduced to zero when complete revascularization was obtained; the difference was less pronounced in the patients who had incomplete revascularization. The incidence of exercise-induced ST-segment depression of more than 0.1 mV was significantly reduced in patients who had complete and incomplete revascularization compared with that before angioplasty.

Rosing and colleagues reported that exercise testing after successful PTCA exhibited improved ECG and symptomatic responses, as well as improved myocardial perfusion and global and regional left ventricular function (by radionuclide ventriculography, RNV).[12] Sixty-six patients were studied before and after successful PTCA. Surprisingly, only 33% had abnormal ST-segment depression, whereas 68% had angina during initial TM testing. Follow-up studies an average of 8 months after the successful procedure showed 7% to have ST-segment depression or angina during treadmill studies, and there were no abnormal studies with thallium scintigraphy. RNV demonstrated similar ejection fractions at rest before and after PTCA but there was an improvement of 9% ($p < 0.001$) in the exercise ejection fraction at follow-up testing. However, 52% of patients with paired data still had an abnormal RNV study result after successful PTCA.

Ernst and co-workers in the Netherlands described the results of functional and anatomic follow-up study of 25 patients who underwent PTCA.[13] All patients had subjective and objective evidence of coronary artery disease mainly because of proximal discrete one-vessel disease. Patients were studied before PTCA, within 14 days after, and at 4 to 8 months later. History, exercise ECG, thallium scintigraphy, and technetium ejection fraction were performed at rest in maximal exercise. The mean stenosis of a dilated vessel decreased significantly from 83% to 38%. The functional status of the patients improved as reflected by a decrease in anginal complaints and an increase in negative ECGs, exercise level, and ejection fraction response. The ejection fraction response to exercise was the most reliable way to discover a possible restenosis in the late follow-up period.

Prediction of restenosis with the exercise test. To demonstrate whether a treadmill test could be predictive of restenosis in 289 patients 6 months after a successful emergency angioplasty of the infarct-related artery for acute myocardial infarction Honan and co-workers performed the following

study.[14] After excluding those with interim interventions, medical events, or medical contraindications to follow-up testing, both a treadmill test and a cardiac catheterization were completed in 144 patients, 88% of those eligible for this assessment. Of six follow-up clinical and treadmill variables examined by multivariable logistic regression analysis, only exercise ST-segment deviation was independently correlated with restenosis at follow-up testing. The clinical diagnosis of angina at follow-up testing, though marginally related to restenosis when considered by itself ($p = 0.04$), did not add significant information once ST-segment deviation was known. The sensitivity of ST deviation of 0.10 mV or greater for detection of restenosis was only 24% (13 of 55 patients), and the specificity was 88% (75 of 85 patients). The sensitivity of exercise-induced ST-segment deviation for detection of restenosis was not affected by extent or severity of wall-motion abnormalities at follow-up testing, by the timing of thrombolytic therapy or of angioplasty, or by the presence of collateral blood flow at the time of acute angiography. A second multivariable analysis evaluating the association of the same variables with the number of vessels with significant coronary disease at the sixth-month catheterization found an association with both exercise ST deviation and exercise duration. Angina symptoms and exercise treadmill test results in this population had limited value for prediction of anatomic restenosis 6 months after emergency angioplasty for acute myocardial infarction.

Bengtson and co-workers studied 303 consecutive patients with successful PTCA and without a recent myocardial infarction.[15] Among the 228 patients without interval cardiac events, early repeat revascularization, or contraindications to treadmill testing, 209 (92%) underwent follow-up angiography, and 200 also had a follow-up treadmill test and formed the study population. Restenosis ($\geq 75\%$ luminal diameter stenosis) occurred in 50 patients (25%). Five variables were individually associated with a higher risk of restenosis: recurrent angina, exercise-induced angina, a positive treadmill test result, more exercise ST-segment deviation, and a lower maximum exercise heart rate. However, only exercise-induced angina, recurrent angina, and a positive treadmill test were independent predictors of restenosis. Using these three variables, patient subsets could be identified with restenosis rates ranging from 11% to 83%. The exercise treadmill test added independent information to symptom status about the risk of restenosis after elective PTCA. Nevertheless, 20% of patients with restenosis had neither recurrent angina nor exercise-induced ischemia at follow-up study.

Wijns and colleagues at the Thoraxcenter evaluated exercise testing and thallium scintigraphy in being predictive of recurrence of angina pectoris and restenosis after a primary successful PTCA.[16] In 89 patients, a symptom-limited exercise ECG and thallium scintigraphy were performed 4 weeks after they had undergone successful PTCA. No information is given on pre-PTCA testing. Patients were followed for 6 months or until recurrence of angina. They all underwent a repeat coronary angiography at 6 months or earlier if symptoms recurred. PTCA was considered successful if the patients had no symptoms and if the stenosis was reduced to less than 50% of the luminal diameter. Restenosis was defined as an increase of the stenosis of more than 50% luminal diameter. The ability of the thallium scintigram (presence of a reversible defect) to be predictive of recurrence of angina was 66% versus 38% for the exercise ECG (ST-segment depression or angina at peak work load). Restenosis was predicted in 74% of patients by thallium but only in 50% of patients by the exercise ECG. Thallium was highly predictive, but the ECG was not. Restenosis had occurred to some extent already at 4 weeks after the PTCA in most patients in whom it was going to occur.

Evaluation of CABS patients. Hultgren and co-workers analyzed the 5-year effect of medical versus surgical treatment on symptoms and exercise performance in patients with stable angina who entered the Veterans Administration Cooperative Study from 1972 to 1974.[17] Exercise testing revealed comparable changes to symptoms and physical performance. At 1 year, surgical patients had fewer tests stopped by angina compared with medical patients (28% versus 64%) and a higher estimated oxygen consumption (26 versus 21 ml/kg/minute) and treadmill duration (7.3 versus 4.9 minutes). Other measures of exercise performance were comparably improved. At 5 years, exercise performance of surgical patients remained superior to that of medical patients, but the treatment difference was smaller. The beneficial effect of surgical treatment in patients with stable angina was maintained, with only a modest increase in symptoms and a slight decrease in exercise performance at 5 years compared with 1 year. Benefits of surgery were still substantially superior to medical treatment at 5 years.

Ryan and the CASS group reported the results of exercise testing performed in 81% of the 780 patients randomized at entry.[18] The cumulative survival at the end of a 7-year follow-up study was 90% for those assigned to surgical treatment and 88% for those assigned to medical therapy. The survival rates did not differ significantly from either those of the entire randomized cohort or those of the 149 patients who did not have a qualifying exercise test at the entry point. No differences in important baseline characteristics existed between those who were exercised and those not exercised at entry. Stratification of patients according to the degree of ST-segment depression and final exercise stage achieved during a Bruce treadmill test (final stage) failed to show any significant differences in 7-year survival rates between medically and surgically assigned patients. Additionally no differences in survival were noted within either the medical or surgical groups regardless of the degree of ST-segment depression or the final stage achieved. The presence of exercise-induced angina, however, identified patients who had a survival advantage if assigned to surgical therapy, with a 7-year survival rate of 94% compared with 87% of medically assigned patients. This advantage was observed primarily in the subset of patients with three-vessel coronary artery disease and impaired left ventricular function. These survival rates are incredibly low and indicate that the population is highly selected toward a low-risk group.

Gohlke and co-workers evaluated exercise responses in patients with different angiographically defined degrees of revascularization with serial exercise tests in 435 patients 1 to 6 years after CABS.[19] All patients had undergone postoperative angiography 2 to 12 months after CABS to determine the degree of revascularization achieved. Revascularization was complete in 182, sufficient in 176, and incomplete in 57 patients. Twenty patients had all grafts occluded. Exercise capacity, angina threshold, maximal double product, prevalence of ≥ 0.1 mV of exercise-induced ST-segment depression, and the prevalence of the combination of ST-segment depression plus angina pectoris were determined in serial supine bicycle tests. Patients with complete, sufficient, and incomplete revascularization showed improvement of all exercise parameters for 6, 4, and 1 year after CABS respectively. In those with the best result, the prevalence of ST-segment depression preoperatively was 76% and was 20%, 22%, 20%, 27%, 34%, and 33% in successive years. The prevalence also decreased in patients whose grafts became occluded. Patients with all grafts occluded had improvement of only some exercise parameters. Exercise capacity was improved by 50% in patients with complete and sufficient revascularization at 1 year and still by 30% at 5 years. Surprisingly, it was also improved in patients with incomplete revascularization or with all grafts occluded.

To determine whether preoperative exercise testing adds important independent prognostic information in patients undergoing CABS, Weiner and the CASS group analyzed 35 variables in 1241 enrolled patients. All patients underwent a treadmill test before CABS and were followed for 7 years. Survival in this surgical cohort was 90.6%. Multivariate stepwise discriminant analysis identified the left ventricular score and the final exercise stage achieved as the two most important independent predictors of postoperative survival. In a subgroup of 416 patients with three-vessel coronary disease and preserved left ventricular function, the probability of postoperative survival at 7 years ranged from 95% for those patients able to exercise to 10 METs to 83% for those whose exercise capacity was less than 5 METs. Exercise capacity was found to be an important independent predictor of postoperative survival.

Comparison of PTCA and CABS

Coronary artery bypass grafting (CABG) is an accepted procedure in the management of angina pectoris refractory to medical treatment. It has also been documented to improve survival in selected patients.[20-22] Percutaneous transluminal coronary angioplasty (PTCA) has become a widely used alternative to CABG.[23] Gruentzig and associates[24] initially advocated the use of PTCA only for patients with a discrete stenosis of a single coronary artery, but the application of coronary angioplasty to narrowings in more than one coronary artery has recently increased, and encouraging results have been reported. The usefulness of exercise testing before and after interventions or treatments to document results is obvious. Since PTCA is now routinely applied in multivessel disease, such a comparison can indeed be very helpful in the clinical choice of revascularization procedures. Dubach performed a retrospective assessment of veterans being treated at Long Beach Veterans Affairs Medical Center.[25] All patients identified as having undergone exercise testing before and after PTCA and CABG were considered for selection according to medication status and timing of exercise tests. Twenty-eight patients formed the CABG group, and 38 patients formed the PTCA group. Since the timing of the tests was according to usual clinical practices, the exercise tests were performed an average of 2.5 weeks after PTCA and 5 months after CABG. The medication status was comparable, but there were significantly more patients with multivessel disease in the CABG group than in the PTCA group ($p < 0.001$). CABG was found to be significantly more effective in decreasing signs ($p < 0.001$) and symptoms ($p = 0.04$) of ischemia than PTCA, but there were no significant differences in estimated aerobic capacity (1.8 METs versus 2.2 METs).

This section compares the exercise responses in patients who have had clinically successful revascularizations. The medical publications were reviewed for studies reporting exercise testing both before and after revascularization with CABG or PTCA. Twenty-seven reports were found, and their results summarized in Table 11-2. Medication status, percentage with multivessel disease, and methods of exercise capacity measurement differed between studies. However, the results could be tabulated to permit comparison. As shown in Table 11-2, more than twice as many patients had multivessel disease in the CABG studies as in the PTCA studies. Hemodynamic improvements and lessening of ischemia during exercise testing were comparable in both groups. Remember, however, that in assessing therapeutic approaches, there are multiple considerations including efficacy, cost, convenience, and safety. Only CABG has been shown to improve survival in only certain anatomic subsets of patients.

Efficacy of an intervention can be assessed noninvasively by exercise testing, since signs and symptoms of ischemia can be demonstrated and exercise capacity can be measured. Table 11-1 summarizes the important points of the most complete studies that compared the pre- and post-exercise test variables in patients who underwent either PTCA or CABG. As can be appreciated, there is great variability in the results reported, especially in the reduction of angina pectoris and in the normalization of the ST-segment. This variability is attributable to the problems inherent in such comparisons, including differences in medications, percentage of patients with multivessel disease, the interval between intervention and testing, and the experience of the individuals performing the revascularization procedures. With regard to medications, digoxin can cause ST-segment depression not attributable to ischemia or alter the amount of ST-segment depression relative to the double product. Also, beta-blockers can alter the ST-segment response relative to double product and ameliorate angina with or without altering the ST-segment response.

Despite the much lower percentage of patients with multivessel disease included in the PTCA groups (28% versus 80% in CABG group), the average reduction in angina pectoris and in ST-segment depression in the pooled studies are similar: 49% in angina and 40% in ST-segment depression after PTCA and 50% and 35% after CABG respectively (Table 11-2). Meier and co-workers have provided the only data comparing the exercise test results in patients who have undergone PTCA to those who have undergone CABG. However, their CABG group was composed of patients in whom PTCA failed.[26] Thus the patients

Table 11-2 Review of the studies that included exercise testing both before and after either PTCA or CABG

Number	Medication	Multi-vessel disease (%)	Exercise capacity Before	Change (%)	Mean maximal heart rate (bpm) Before	After	Maximal double product Before	After	Angina pectoris during ET Before	After	Abnormal ST-segment response (%) Before	After
PTCA (percutaneous transluminal coronary angioplasty)												
Rod	14 BB and Dig NR	0%	6.2 METs	10%	138	149	27	30	71%	7%	(1.0 mm, 0.2 mm)	
Suzuki	14 Off BB, Dig, Nit	0%	14 min	14%	122	145	20	25	57%	21%	36%	7%
Rousing	45 Off BB, Dig, Nit	6%	7.6 min	38%					67%	7%	33%	7%
Kent	32 Off BB, Nit	14%	7 ± 2 min	143%					28%	1%	—	—
Scholl	36 Off Dig, Nit	17%	7.5 min	37%			21	31	NA	8%	56%	20%
Meier	132 NA	41%	74 watts	86%					97%	23%	72%	21%
Gruenzig	133 NA	42%	47% APN	67%					100%	33%	79%	10%
Vandormael	57 Off medications	84%	6.2 min	35%					56%	11%	75%	32%
Dubach	38 Usual medications	50%	6.8 METs	27%	126	142	21	25	71%	39%	76%	47%
TOTAL	501 Average	28%		51%	128	145	22	28	68%	19%	61%	21%
CABG (coronary artery bypass graft)												
Guiney	40 Off Dig, BB	85%	NA	61%					95%	8%	95%	38%
Gohlke	467 NA	87%	62 watts	47%			19	24	54%	5%	79%	28%
Hultgren	190 NA	48%	5.0 min	40%	130	142	21	24	71%	28%	38%	25%
Bartel	123 Dig and BB NR	80%	NA	NA	130	142			100%	32%	67%	36%
Kloster	38 NA	84%	388 kpm/min	63%	107	119			100%	17%	71%	56%
Lapin	46 NA	64%	NA	16%			21	24	85%	20%	73%	26%
Frick	45 BB and Nit NR	100%	569 kpm/min	26%	124	135	21	24	40%	Decrease	(2.8 mm, 1.5 mm)	
Meier	28 NA	41%	68 watts	79%					89%	29%	82%	14%
Dubach	28 Used medications	93%	6.0 METs	37%	122	134	12	14	50%	7%	61%	29%
TOTAL	1005 Average	80%		41%	123	134	19	22	67%	17%	69%	34%

APN, Age-predicted exercise capacity; *BB*, beta-blocker; *bpm*, beats per minute; *Dig*, digoxin; *ET*, exercise test; *kpm/min*, kilogram-meters/minute; *maximal double product*, systolic blood pressure × heart rate at maximal × 10^3; *METs*, 3.5 cc (or ml) of O_2/kg/min; *NA*, no: available; *Nit*, nitrates; *NR*, not restricted.
From Dubach P et al: Exercise test responses, *J Cardiovasc Rehabil* 10:120-125, 1990.

were not primarily assigned to CABG. Those patients who underwent PTCA had a higher work capacity 1, 2, and 3 years after revascularization compared with the CABG group. It is difficult to generalize their results or contrast them with other studies.

Ideally one should obtain exercise test variables immediately after CABG or PTCA respectively to have comparable situations. It has been demonstrated that within 5 to 6 months after PTCA 30% to 35% of the dilated vessels restenose.[27] After CABG, about 10% to 15% of the grafts are occluded in the first 6 months. But whereas patients after PTCA will be able to perform a symptom-limited exercise test within days after the procedure,[28] patients after CABG will be able to do so only weeks or months after the operation, during which time the highest rate of early graft occlusions is reported.[29] An interesting report suggested, however, that although testing within a day after PTCA seems safe but a reported 5% incidence of acute occlusion in patients with intimal dissection makes it prudent to wait in patients with this angiographic finding at PTCA.[30]

The evaluation of success of a therapeutic procedure is related to the technical and clinical goals set for that procedure, and this evaluation may be different for PTCA and CABG. In a patient with stable angina pectoris, for example, the goal is the elimination of exertional pain. In an elderly patient with associated noncardiac disease in whom coronary artery bypass surgery would be too hazardous, the goal may be to reduce the severity of angina pectoris to acceptable levels. When PTCA is used for treating unstable angina, baseline exercise test data are usually not available. This review suggests that CABG and PTCA result in a similar decrease in the signs and symptoms of exercise-induced ischemia. However, the severity of coronary disease was milder in those who underwent PTCA.

The ACME (Angioplasty Compared to Medical Treatment) trial was a randomized comparison of patients with single-vessel coronary artery disease treated with medical management or PTCA. The patients in the PTCA group increased their exercise-test total time and angina-free time relative to the medically treated group.[31]

EVALUATION OF PATIENTS FOR SURGERY

Carliner and colleagues performed a prospective study of preoperative exercise testing in 200 patients older that 40 years scheduled for elective major noncardiac surgery under general anesthesia.[32] The exercise test showed ST-segment depression in 32 patients (16%). The patients were followed with serial pre- and postoperative ECGs

and determinations of creatine kinase and CK-MB. Six patients (3%) had primary postoperative end points: 3 (1.5%) died, and 3 (1.5%) had myocardial infarctions. Secondary end points of suspected postoperative myocardial ischemia or injury diagnosed by ECG or elevation in CK-MB levels occurred in 27 patients (14%). End point events were more common in patients 70 years of age or older. End-point events were also more common in patients with an abnormal (positive or equivocal) exercise test reponse than in those with a negative response (27% versus 14%); however, preoperative exercise results were not statistically significant independent predictors of cardiac risk. Using multivariate analysis, the only statistically significant independent predictor of risk was the preoperative ECG. End-point events were more common in patients with an abnormal ECG than in those with a normal ECG (23% versus 7%). Because the results of exercise testing do not appear to add substantially to the risk separation provided by the ECG at rest, exercise testing is not recommended as a routine preoperative method for assessment of perioperative risk in older patients who are being evaluated before major elective noncardiac surgery under general anesthesia.[33]

Other studies have considered exercise testing specifically to evaluate patients before vascular surgery.[34-37] This is a very controversial area currently, but non–exercise stress methodologies seem to be favored. Difficulty in evaluating comparative evaluation tactics arises because of the low perioperative event rate (1% to 4%). It largely seems to be related to anesthetic approaches, and "prophylactic" coronary surgery or dilatation procedures are rarely indicated. It is interesting that most events occur within 3 days after operation rather than during the operation itself.

Evaluation of patients with high blood pressure

Franz investigated the blood pressure response during and after exercise in 552 males to determine if an exercise test is suitable for differentiating normotensive subjects and hypertensive subjects.[38] Patients suffering from mild hypertension showed significantly higher blood pressures at 100 watts and after exercise than age-matched normotensives and significantly lower values than stable hypertensives. In addition, the systolic pressure response to bicycle exercise was significantly influenced by age. Using the upper limits of blood pressure during and after exercise, 50% of the patients with borderline hypertension could be classified as hypertensives. Their blood pressure response at 100 watts did not significantly differ from the patients with mild hypertension. In contrast, in the 50% who acted negatively to exercise testing, the systolic blood pressure response at 100 watts was significantly lower than that of those demonstrating a positive reaction. They had exactly the same diastolic pressure value as the normotensives. This study indicates that the assessment of blood pressure during exercise may be useful in distinguishing between normotensive and hypertensive patients and in making estimates of blood pressure response to daily stress more accurate. However, this has not been reproduced by other investigators.

EVALUATION OF EXERCISE CAPACITY

The exercise test can be used to evaluate the exercise capacity of asymptomatic individuals or of patients with various forms of heart disease. Patients who exaggerate their symptoms or who mainly have a psychological impairment often can be identified. Exercise testing can more accurately measure the degree of cardiac impairment than a physician's assessment of exercise capacity can. As previously described, maximal oxygen uptake, either directly measured or estimated, is the best noninvasive measurement of functional capacity. Being unable to complete the first stage of the Bruce test (a maximal oxygen consumption below 18 cc (or ml) of O_2/kg/min or 5 METs) has been found to have a poor prognosis in several studies despite either medical or surgical treatment. The determination of a patient's exercise capacity affords an objective measurement of the degree of cardiopulmonary impairment and can be useful in patient management. Exercise testing can also be used to evaluate the effects of training, whether it be part of an athletic program, a fitness program, or a rehabilitation program. A maximal oxygen uptake of 40 cc of O_2/kg/min (11 METs) is the lowest level of fitness, and measurements of up to 80 cc of O_2/kg/min (20 METs) can be obtained in Olympic-class long distance runners. Following a trainee's progress in an exercise program with serial exercise testing can optimize the training program, and it is often a good way to encourage adherence.

EVALUATION OF DYSRHYTHMIAS

An exercise test can be used to evaluate patients with dysrhythmias or to induce dysrhythmias in patients with the appropriate symptoms. The dysrhythmias that can be evaluated include premature ventricular contractions (PVCs), sick sinus syndrome, and various degrees of heart block. Ambulatory monitoring or isometric exercise often allows detection of a higher prevalence of dysrhythmias, including more serious dysrhythmias than

dynamic exercise testing does. The findings in each of these tests, however, may have different significances. Some antiarrhythmic agents (such as flecainide) have a proarrhythmic proclivity that is brought out only by exercise.

Lown believes that maximal exercise testing is useful for detection of arrhythmias and assessment of antiarrhythmic drug efficacy. Because few reports document the safety in patients with malignant ventricular arrhythmias, Lown and colleagues reviewed the complications of symptom-limited exercise in 263 patients with such arrhythmias who underwent a total of 1377 maximal treadmill tests.[39] Seventy-four percent of the population studied had a history of ventricular fibrillation or hemodynamically compromising ventricular tachycardia, and the remainder had experienced ventricular tachycardia in the setting of either recent MI or poor left ventricular function. A complication was defined as the occurrence of arrhythmia during exercise testing—ventricular fibrillation, ventricular tachycardia, or bradycardia—that mandated immediate medical treatment. Complications were noted in 24 patients (9.1%) during 32 tests (2.3%), whereas 239 patients (90.9%) were free of complications during 1345 tests (97.7%). There were no deaths, MIs, or lasting morbid events. Clinical descriptors associated with complications included male sex, presence of coronary artery disease, and a history of exertional arrhythmia. Clinical variables previously considered to confer increased risk during exercise, such as poor left ventricular function, high-grade ventricular arrhythmias before or during exercise, exertional hypotension, and ST-segment depression, were not predictive of complications. Occurrence of a complication was also unaffected by the use of antiarrhythmic drugs at the time of exercise. Complication frequency in their study group was compared with that in a reference population of 3444 cardiac patients without histories of symptomatic arrhythmia who underwent 8221 exercise tests. Of these, four subjects (0.12%) developed ventricular fibrillation (0.05% of tests) without fatality or lasting morbidity. They concluded that maximal exercise testing can be conducted safely in patients with malignant arrhythmias, and clinical variables previously considered to confer risk during exercise are not predictive of complications.

Lown and colleagues also compared the provocation of PVCs in a standard exercise test with provocation of PVCs in an abbreviated form of testing (minitesting) that seemed to approximate more closely the demands of daily activities. The miniprotocol was as follows: the treadmill was kept at 12% elevation, and the speed began at 1.7

mph and was increased every 15 seconds to the following levels: 2.5, 3.4, 4.2, 5.5, 6.0 mph. It was then kept at 6.5 mph until the test was completed. The study involved 52 patients with known or suspected history of ventricular arrhythmia—42 men and 10 women, average age 49 years. Hemodynamic and ST-segment changes were similar during both forms of testing. Thirty-seven patients (71%) undergoing a standard exercise test exhibited PVCs, whereas 32 (62%) did so during the minitesting. Of 13 patients with repetitive PVCs, standard exercise testing as well as minitesting provoked the same degree of PVCs in 10. In two patients, the yield of these complex forms of PVCs was higher with minitesting and in one patient with standard exercise testing. This abbreviated protocol may be useful for patients undergoing serial exercise studies to provide assessment of drug efficacy for the suppression of PVCs.

Woelfel and colleagues studied 14 patients with exercise-induced ventricular tachycardia (VT) with serial treadmill testing.[40] Those with reproducible VT were treated with a beta-blocking agent and later with verapamil. In 11 patients (79%), VT of similar rate, morphologic characteristics, and duration was reproduced on two consecutive treadmill tests performed 1 to 14 days apart. Beta-blockade prevented recurrent VT during acute testing in 10 of 11 patients and during chronic therapy in 9. Eight patients had a consistent relation between a critical sinus rate and the onset of VT. In these patients, successful therapy correlated with preventing achievement of the critical sinus rate during maximal exercise. They also found verapamil to be effective in this group.

Sami and co-workers performed a retrospective study to examine the prognostic significance of exercise-induced ventricular arrhythmia in patients with stable coronary artery disease (CAD) who were included in the multicenter patient registry of the Coronary Artery Surgery Study.[41] The population included 1486 patients selected from 1975 to 1979 and followed an average of 4.3 years. All underwent a standard Bruce exercise test and had CAD by cardiac catheterization at entry. Patients were classified depending on whether they had minimal or significant CAD. They were further subclassified depending on whether they had exercise-induced ventricular arrhythmia (EIA). Patients with minimal CAD and EIA (16 patients) and 229 patients without had similar clinical and angiographic characteristics except for the average ejection fraction (EF), which was 50% for those with and 64% for those without PVCs. A hundred thirty patients with significant CAD and EIAs had a higher prevalence of previous MI, a lower mean EF, and a higher proportion with at least two cor-

onary arteries significantly narrowed than those without EIAs and significant CAD (1111 patients). The 5-year event-free survival was not influenced by the presence of EIA; it was 76% and 88% in those with minimal CAD or with EIAs respectively and 71% and 76% in both groups with significant CAD respectively. Using a stepwise Cox regression analysis of selected clinical and angiographic risk factors, they found that the only independent significant risk factors for cardiac events were the number of coronary arteries diseased and the EF.

Califf and co-workers at Duke studied the prognostic information provided by ventricular arrhythmias associated with treadmill testing in 1293 consecutive nonsurgically treated patients undergoing an exercise test within 6 weeks of cardiac catheterization.[42] The 236 patients with simple ventricular arrhythmias (at least one PVC but without paired complexes or ventricular tachycardia) had a higher prevalence of significant CAD (57% versus 44%), three-vessel disease (31% versus 17%), and abnormal left ventricular function (43% versus 24%) than patients without ventricular arrhythmias had. Patients with paired complexes or ventricular tachycardia had an even higher prevalence of significant coronary artery disease (75%), three-vessel disease (39%), and abnormal left ventricular function (54%).

In the 620 patients with significant CAD, patients with paired complexes or ventricular tachycardia had a lower 3-year survival rate (75%) than patients with simple ventricular arrhythmias (83%) and patients with no ventricular arrhythmias (90%) had. Ventricular arrhythmias were found to add independent prognostic information to the noninvasive evaluation, including history, physical examination, chest x-ray examination, ECG, and other exercise test variables ($p = 0.03$). Ventricular arrhythmias made no independent contribution once the cardiac catheterization data were known. In patients without significant coronary artery disease, no relation between ventricular arrhythmias and survival was found.

Weiner and co-workers investigated the determinants and prognostic significance of ventricular arrhythmias during exercise testing.[43] Eighty-six patients with such arrhythmias were identified from a consecutive series of 446 patients who underwent treadmill testing and cardiac catheterization. The prevalence of these arrhythmias was 19% in the total group but increased to 30% in the 120 patients with three-vessel or left main CAD. Patients with exercise-induced arrhythmias were more likely to have three-vessel or left main CAD, a lower resting EF, 0.2 mV of ST-segment depression, and more severe segmental wall-motion abnormalities than patients without this finding. Re-

Table 11-3 Prognostic value of exercise-induced ventricular arrhythmias

			Mortality	
Study	Number	Follow-up (years)	With EIVA (%)	Without EIVA (%)
Nair	280	3.9	No difference	
Weiner	446	5.3	14 (any)	10
			20 (complex)	
Califf	1293	3	17 (simple)	10
			25 (complex)	
Sami	1486	4.3	29 (any)	24

peat exercise testing in 22 patients with exercise-induced arrhythmias after CABS revealed that persistence of these arrhythmias was associated with either severe wall motion abnormalities preoperatively or residual ST-segment depression during the postoperative exercise testing. At a mean follow-up period of 5.3 years, the presence of exercise-induced ventricular arrhythmias was not associated with increased cardiac mortality in the medically treated patients. These last four studies are summarized in Table 11-3.

EVALUATION OF PATIENTS WITH ATRIAL FIBRILLATION

The reported prevalence of atrial fibrillation (AF) has varied widely, but it is directly related to age. Kannel and co-workers, in a 22-year analysis from the Framingham Study, described the onset of chronic AF in 49 of 2325 males and 49 of 2866 females.[44] This represents an overall 2% chance of developing AF in 20 years. They noted a direct relationship between the incidence of AF and age ranging from approximately 0.2% cases at 25 to 34 to greater than 3% at 55 to 64 years of age. Only 30 men and 18 women had no history of concomitant cardiovascular disease, and the other 50 cases were preceded more frequently than controls by congestive heart failure and rheumatic heart disease whereas males had, in addition, stroke and hypertension as precursors. Stroke was an antecedent predictor of AF, suggestive of transient or intermittent AF being a possible cause of cerebral emboli. There was an increased mortality associated with the onset of AF: within 6 years, 60% of males and 45% of females died. In a 30-year follow-up study of 43 individuals with AF but without cardiovascular disease, Framingham researchers found them to have an increased risk for strokes. In a similar population study from Mayo Clinic, individuals with "lone AF" were found to have a good prognosis. Rose and co-workers

screened 18,403 male civil servants and found the prevalence of AF to be 0.2% in those 40 to 49 years of age, 0.4% in those 50 to 59, and 1% in those 60 to 64. Those with AF had a mortality more than three times that of age-matched peers. Campbell and colleagues studied 2254 subjects over 65 years of age and found the prevalence of AF to be 2%. They also noted a higher prevalence (5%) in subjects over 75 years of age. Thus studies document that AF is an important clinical problem that will increase in prevalence as the population grows older. One problem managing patients with chronic AF has been how to obtain the optimal medical control of their cardiovascular response to exercise.

Response to exercise in patients with atrial fibrillation (AF)

Submaximal exercise testing. Several authors have noted that patients in AF have an inordinately fast ventricular response during the first stage of an exercise test. Aberg and co-workers noted that the largest increment in ventricular rate occurred during the first stage of exercise and was greater than 45% of the total increase in heart rate.[45] Likewise, Hornsten and Bruce have noted an increase in ventricular response from 83 to 152 beats/min during stage I and a maximal response of 176 at least two stages later.[46] In fact, most studies evaluating pharmacological efficacy in heart rate control have used only a submaximal exercise level to evaluate heart rate decrease. Most studies used only a submaximal level to evaluate and have focused on heart rate control rather than exercise capacity.

In calculating the percent change in heart rate at submaximal stages (that is, 3.0 mph/0% grade and anaerobic threshold) in a study we did at the Long Beach VAMC, we took the HR at that level, subtracted resting HR, and then divided by the difference between maximal HR and resting HR. Our findings are consistent with a rapid increase in HR during the lowest work loads, with smaller incremental changes approaching maximal. This contrasts with the linear relationship between HR and work load in subjects in normal sinus rhythm.

David and colleagues used timolol to control resting and submaximal exercise heart rate (bicycle exercise for 1 minute at 300 kilogram-meters or kpm/minute followed by 2 minutes at 450 kpm/min).[47] They found digoxin to be ineffective both at regular and high doses and that timolol alone reduced heart rate more effectively than digoxin at high or low dose. A study by Yehalom compared practolol to placebo in 28 patients. Each patient underwent submaximal bicycle exercise at 200 to 300 kpm/min and noted a significant decrease in resting and exercise HR, which fell in slow and fast HR groups with the addition of practolol. Klein and co-workers described the use of verapamil in 23 patients treated with digoxin for chronic AF and noted a decrease in heart rate at rest and during submaximal bicycle exercise. The "slow" heart rate group demonstrated little response to verapamil. Redfors studied 11 subjects in AF who were prescribed increasing amounts of digoxin. A nonlinear increase in heart rate occurred at low dose but became more linear at higher doses of digoxin. Digoxin had the least effect on heart rate at maximum work loads.

Maximal exercise testing. Hornsten and Bruce compared 25 men and 40 women in chronic AF to a similar population matched by age, sex, and cardiac functional status but in sinus rhythm. Maximal treadmill tests were performed with use of the Bruce protocol. They noted significantly decreased heart rates at rest (83 versus 76), at submaximal (152 versus 124), and maximal work loads (176 versus 150), and in recovery for the patients in AF compared to those in sinus rhythm. The mean exercise time for men in AF was 371 seconds (predicted VO_2 of 18 cc/kg/min) as compared to 377 seconds for men in sinus rhythm; for women in AF, 283 seconds (predicted VO_2 of 25 cc/kg/min) versus 272 seconds for those in sinus rhythm. All the patients had rheumatic heart disease, which explains the mean functional aerobic impairment (FAI) of 35%.

Aberg and co-workers performed two bicycle tests on 24 patients in chronic AF all of whom had valvular heart disease. The first test was performed with the patient receiving a "maintenance" lower dose and the second receiving a high dose of digoxin. During exercise, the heart rate was lower on higher doses of digoxin ranging from 5 to 25 beats/min. There was a higher work load at a heart rate of 110 in subjects on the higher dose, but there was no significant change in maximum work; mean maximum heart rate was 157 with an estimated VO_2 of 12 cc/kg/min from a bicycle mean work load of 283 kpm/min. The functional aerobic impairment of 60% was secondary to the intrinsic heart disease. Aberg and co-workers also studied 195 patients with a mean age of 47 years in chronic AF who had advanced valvular heart disease and all were using digitalis. Each test involved "steady-state" bicycle ergometry with progressively increasing work loads at 100 kpm/min. The work load at a heart rate of 110 was reduced as was the mean maximum work load when they were compared to normals, and the FAI was 60%. Mean maximum work load was 275 kpm/min, which is equivalent to an estimated VO_2 of 12 cc/kg/min. The largest percentage increase in heart

rate occurred from rest to load I (approximately 45%) with less of an increase in the other two loads. Aberg and co-workers performed a third study involving 15 patients with advanced valvular heart disease to look at reproducibility of heart rates on two consecutive bicycle tests. The initial mean maximum heart rate was 138 beats/min at a work load of 337 kpm/min (est VO_2 of 13 cc/kg/min) and a functional aerobic impairment (FAI) of 55%. They noted that patients with a high work capacity had less of a heart rate change between tests than those with a low work capacity.

Davidson and Hagan studied seven men and four women with a mean age of 55 years who were in chronic AF; 10 had rheumatic valvular disease. Maximal treadmill tests were performed before and after each digoxin dosage change. Two patients were receiving propranolol. Heart rate response at stage I fell from a mean of 163 beats/min to 146 beats/min at optimal digoxin dose. There was no significant change in heart rate response at maximal exertion—176 to 166 beats/min—but at 2 minutes into recovery a mean heart rate of 98 fell to 86 beats/min at optimal dosaging. Duration of exercise increased from 3.6 to 5.2 minutes. Khalsa and co-workers studied 11 patients with maximal bicycle exercise before direct-current cardioversion. Nine were NYHA class II or worse and most had enlarged hearts on chest x-ray film. They reached a mean maximal heart rate of 142 and a mean work load of 98 watts.

Lang and colleagues studied 20 patients in chronic AF on digoxin therapy with an optimal verapamil dose followed by a double-blind crossover analysis. Bicycle testing was performed with 3-minute stages up to maximal effort. The heart rate was significantly lowered at rest and during all work loads, but the SBP was lowered only at maximum effort. Maximum exercise duration was increased from 219 to 292 seconds. Again the maximal capacity was low, since they included patients with NYHA class II or III.

Molajo and co-workers described the use of corwin, a new beta-adrenergic receptor (partial) agonist in 10 patients in chronic AF taking digoxin.[48] Two were NYHA class III and the rest were I and II. Eight of 10 subjects had rheumatic mitral valve disease, and one had ischemic heart disease. The study was a 2-week-per-phase, double-blind, crossover study with a 1-week washout interim period. A maximum symptom-limited Bruce protocol was used. Heart rate (HR) response was significantly reduced while they received corwin: The rest HR fell from 80 to 73, 3-minute exercise HR from 132 to 105, and peak exercise from 162 to 120. Mean maximum exercise time increased from 215 seconds to 257 seconds while they received corwin. Functional aerobic impairment was 55% and is consistent with the intrinsic heart disease and the NYHA class II or worse in 7 of their patients.

In a multicenter study, DiBianco and colleagues evaluated the effects of nadolol on the heart rate response to maximal treadmill exercise in 20 patients with AF of greater than 2.5 months of duration.[49] The study involved a randomized, double-blind, crossover comparison of nadolol and placebo. The treadmill protocol used was a modified maximal Bruce protocol that began with a 3-minute stage at 1.7 mph and 0% grade. Digoxin was continued at a stable dose in 17 of 20 patients. The heart rate reduction was significant at rest (92 to 73), at 3 minutes of submaximal exertion (153 to 111), and at maximum effort (175 to 126). There was a decrease in exercise time from 466 ± 143 seconds while they received a placebo (estimated VO_2 25 cc/kg/min) to 380 ± 143 seconds (estimated VO_2 21 cc/kg/min) while they received nadolol. The authors focused mainly on heart rate control rather than on the exercise capacity. The FAI of 40% is consistent with intrinsic heart disease no doubt present in their patients with cardiomyopathy or rheumatic heart disease.

Atwood studied 34 consecutive male volunteers ranging in age from 49 to 87 years with chronic AF (duration greater than 6 months).[50] Acutely ill patients, those with angina, those receiving beta-blockers or calcium antagonists, and those with severe lung disease or thyroid dysfunction were excluded. All but one patient were taking digoxin. None of the patients was in congestive heart failure at the time of the study, and all were of functional class I or II. All patients had normal left ventricular function by echocardiography except for those with the diagnosis of cardiomyopathy. Patients were exercised on a treadmill using individualized protocols designed such that this maximal exercise test lasted between 10 to 12 minutes. Respiratory gas-exchange variables were determined continuously throughout the exercise test. The number of QRS complexes multiplied by 10 in a 6-second rhythm strip at the end of each minute was used to determine heart rate. Analysis of hemodynamic and pulmonary gas-exchange variables were performed at a submaximal work load reached by all tested (3.0 mph/0% grade), the gas-exchange anaerobic threshold (ATge), and maximal exertion. Our patients in chronic atrial fibrillation had decreased values of absolute VO_2 at ATge but had a mean percent of maximal oxygen uptake at ATge comparable to that in a population in normal sinus rhythm. VO_2 related to age and heart rate at maximal effort related to age demonstrated a wide scatter because of the small number of patients and the diversity of heart diseases included.

Table 11-4 summarizes the results of the nine studies of maximal testing for comparison with our findings. Our study was the first to provide measured oxygen uptake. FAI is calculated by the formula: estimated VO_2 (from work load performed; that is, treadmill time) minus predicted VO_2 (from age) divided by predicted VO_2 max. We obtained a higher aerobic capacity probably by excluding patients in congestive heart failure and including more patients with "lone" AF, fewer patients with valvular heart disease, and a majority of patients with normal left ventricular function by echocardiogram. Using the equation of Max HR equals 206 minus 0.6 times Age (206 − 0.6 × 60), we found that a mean maximal HR of 176 for our population is exactly as expected for this age group in normals. Consistent with other studies, the mean submaximal heart rate in our study was inordinately high, and the heart rate exhibited the greatest percent increment at that time.

Effect of drugs on exercise performance in patients with chronic atrial fibrillation. In patients with chronic AF, the primary goal of therapy is to control the rapid heart rate response at rest and during exercise. Digoxin has been the drug of choice to control resting heart rate. However, digoxin has limited effectiveness in controlling heart rates during exercise or other stresses. The concomitant use of beta-adrenergic receptor or calcium-channel blocking agents with digoxin has been recommended as a better means of controlling heart rate.

A concern with beta-adrenergic receptor blockade therapy is the possible reduction in cardiac output resulting not only from reduction in maximal heart rate, but also from the depression of myocardial function. If a significant reduction in cardiac output occurs, maximal oxygen uptake would be decreased causing a reduction in exercise capacity. Studies in normal subjects have provided conflicting results as to the effect of beta-blocking agents on maximal oxygen uptake and other ventilatory variables associated with aerobic capacity. Similarly, in studies of patients with AF, the effect of beta-blockade on maximal exercise capacity has been inconclusive, and none of the studies have included measurements of ventilatory parameters. To investigate the effect of maximum dose (600 mg) celiprolol, a $beta_1$-selective adrenergic receptor blocker, on hemodynamic and respiratory gas-exchange variables in patients with chronic AF during maximal exercise testing, Atwood and our group performed the following study.

Nine male patients (mean age 65 years) with chronic AF, eight treated with digoxin, underwent

Table 11-4   Results of maximal exercise testing in patients with atrial fibrillation

Investigator	Hornsten	Aberg	Aberg	Aberg	Khalsa	Davidson	Lang	Molajo	DiBianco	Atwood
Year	1968	1972	1972	1977	1979	1979	1983	1984	1984	1986
Number of patients	65	179	24	15	11	11	20	10	20	34
Mean age	50	47	45	45	56	55	59	52	60	66
Exercise protocol	Bruce	Bike	Bike	Bike	Bike	Bruce	Bike	Bruce	Modified Bruce	Modified B-W
Mean Max HR	176	134	157	138	142	176	169	162	175	171
est METs	5	3.5	3.5	4	5.7	6.5	4.5	5	7	8
est VO_2	18	12	12	13	20	23	15	18	25	27
FAI	35%	60%	60%	55%	30%	50%	50%	55%	10%	11%
Measured VO_2	—	—	—	—	—	—	—	—	—	21

B-W, Balke-Ware protocol; *est,* estimated; *FAI,* functional aerobic impairment; *HR,* heart rate; *Max,* maximal; *MET,* 3.5 cc of O_2/kg/min; VO_2, ventilatory oxygen consumption in cc of O_2/kg/min.

a randomized, double-blind maximal-dose celiprolol/placebo study using exercise testing with measured ventilatory parameters to assess the effect of beta-blockade on exercise capacity.[51] We observed a significant decrease in heart rate and systolic blood pressure at the submaximal work load of 3 mph/0% grade during celiprolol administration, which is similar to previous data obtained in normal subjects and patients in atrial fibrillation. The fact that celiprolol did not alter gas-exchange variables such as minute ventilation, oxygen uptake, and respiratory exchange ratio is consistent with studies in normal subjects.

A significant decrease in heart rate and systolic blood pressure occurred at the ATge during celiprolol therapy, which is similar to data acquired in normal subjects and patients with coronary artery disease taking beta-blockers. The observed reduction in oxygen uptake at the ATge during celiprolol usage is consistent with the study by Peterson and co-workers but not with studies by Sklar and Hughson and MacFarlane. The discrepancies with these studies appear attributable to (1) medication and dosage level used (celiprolol at maximum dose versus propranolol at moderate dose); (2) chronicity of administration (for 1 week versus one oral dose); (3) population differences (young normal subjects versus older patients with heart disease); (4) pharmacokinetics and testing times (2 hours after receiving celiprolol, which reaches its peak level 2 to 4 hours later versus in the Sklar study 4 hours after propranolol, which peaks at 1 to 2 hours); (5) differences in testing protocols.

In subjects in normal sinus rhythm, the effect of beta-adrenergic receptor blockade on maximal oxygen uptake has been controversial. Authors have noted either a decrease in oxygen uptake with

beta-adrenergic receptor blockade or no change at all. Wilmore and co-workers list several possible causes for such variable findings—some of which include the type of beta-blocker (selective or nonselective with or without intrinsic sympathomimetic activity), method of medication administration (intravenous or oral), timing of test with respect to peak medication effect, length of time on medication (hours, days, weeks), dosage level (high versus low), exercise protocol (using treadmill or cycle ergometry), subject motivation and age, and even the statistical analysis used.

Few studies in patients with atrial fibrillation have addressed the effect of beta-adrenergic receptor blockade on maximal exertion. Di Bianco and co-workers in a multicenter trial involving 20 subjects in AF looked at the exercise heart rate response to AF while the subjects were receiving placebo and digoxin versus nadolol and digoxin. They noted not only a reduction in heart rate and systolic pressure, but also a significant reduction in exercise time from placebo of 466 seconds to 380 seconds while nadolol was taken. This implied a reduced exercise capacity, but the authors focused on the reduced heart rate response and the safety of nadolol. In another study with 10 patients, Molajo and co-workers noted a reduction of maximal heart rate but also noted a significant increase in exercise time from 215 seconds during the placebo and digoxin phase to 257 seconds after administration of digoxin and corwin, a beta-adrenergic receptor antagonist with partial beta-agonist activity and some positive inotropic properties. However, the improved exercise time was 40 seconds in the same stage II of the Bruce protocol. In addition, the population tested had mild-to-moderate congestive heart failure, and the Bruce protocol with its rigorous first stages explains why this population had such a very low total treadmill time.

From a clinical standpoint, the addition of a beta-blocker for heart rate control in patients with chronic AF makes sense when the only goal is to reduce myocardial oxygen demand through reduction of heart rate such as that in patients with angina pectoris. However, in adding beta-blocker therapy there is the risk of compromising VO_2 because of the negative chronotropic and inotropic effects associated with these agents. A maximum dose of beta-blockade exerted negative chronotropic and inotropic effects, consequently leading to decreased exercise capacity, but perhaps a lower dose would have normalized the heart rate without a change in the VO_2 oxygen uptake.

Treatment with diltiazem. Since a calcium antagonist may offer chronotropic control but less negative inotropic effect, it could be more advantageous in the treatment of atrial fibrillation. Therefore we tested these patients after stabilizing them with diltiazem.[52] They exhibited an improvement in treadmill time and no decrease in VO_2 max with good heart rate control. This leads us to believe that diltiazem is the agent of choice for these patients.

Clinically the decrease in the ATge and the reduction in oxygen uptake at higher work loads becomes important in patients who desire an active life-style. Since the patient perceives an equivalent amount of work as being harder during beta-adrenergic receptor blockade, their motivation to engage in previous activities may be affected. Results from the present study indicate that the use of beta-adrenergic receptor blockers in patients with AF is a double-edged sword. The effective control of submaximal exercise heart rates must be weighed against the impairment in oxygen delivery at moderate to heavy work loads. The key to therapy in patients with AF would appear to be normalizing the heart rate response to exercise without affecting the ATge or maximal oxygen uptake, and this can be done with a calcium antagonist.

Evaluation of valvular heart disease

Exercise testing has been utilized in the evaluation of patients with valvular heart disease. It has been used to qualify the amount of disability caused by their disease, to reproduce any exercise-induced set of symptoms, and to evaluate their response to medical and surgical intervention. The exercise electrocardiogram (ECG) has been used as a means to identify concurrent coronary artery disease (CAD), but there is a high prevalence of false-positive responses (ST-segment depression not attributable to ischemia) because of the frequent baseline ECG abnormalities and left ventricular (LV)

hypertrophy. Some physicians have used the exercise test to help decide when surgery is indicated. Exercise testing has been utilized most in patients with aortic stenosis, and so this section will emphasize evaluation of this valvular abnormality.[53,54]

Aortic stenosis. Effort syncope in patients with aortic stenosis (AS) is an important and well-appreciated symptom. Most guidelines regarding exercise testing list moderate to severe AS as a contraindication for exercise testing because of concern with syncope and cardiac arrest.

Physiological mechanisms of effort syncope. From the time that syncope in AS was first described, with reduced systolic pressure during syncope, an absence of pulses and apical impulse, and the disappearance of murmurs, various mechanisms have been hypothesized for effort syncope in AS. Carotid artery hyperreactivity and inadequate cardiac output leading to "cerebral anemia" and syncope have been proposed. An inability to increase cardiac output during exercise because of LV failure or arrhythmias could be the cause.

The most plausible explanation for syncope during exercise in patients with AS is that of LV stretch baroreceptor stimulation or mechanoreceptor stimulation with concomitant arterial hypotension, reduced venous return, and bradycardia. Elevation of left arterial and LV pressure in dogs can cause a decrease in venous return and a fall in systemic vascular resistance that is most prominent during extrasystoles. The abrupt elevation of LV systolic pressure without a corresponding rise in aortic pressure could allow LV baroreceptors to produce "a violent depressor reflex." This could lead to bradycardia, peripheral vasodilatation, and hypotension, which would reduce coronary arterial flow and result in LV dysfunction and arrhythmias.

The forearm vascular response in normal subjects to leg exercise is vasoconstriction. In the patients with AS, forearm vasodilatation and increased forearm blood flow occurs. Forearm vasodilatation can revert to vasoconstriction during exercise after aortic valve replacement. Activation of LV baroreceptors could result in reflex vasodilatation with arterial hypotension and reduce coronary artery perfusion. This reflex plays a role in inhibition of the sympathetic drive. Reflex withdrawal of the adrenergic vasoconstrictor tone in the muscles as well as the skin in response to an elevation of LV pressures can occur.

Exercise testing in subjects with aortic stenosis. Although studies have delineated possible mechanisms for effort syncope in AS, a review of the literature (Table 11-5) demonstrates rare complications from exercise testing when such testing is performed with appropriate caution and monitoring. While predominantly used in pediatric cardi-

Table 11-5 Review of studies that reported exercise testing in patients with aortic stenosis

Parameter	Halloran	Chandramouli	Aronow	Whitmer	James	Barton	Niemala	Kveselis*	Linderholm†	Nylander
Number	31	44	19	23	65	11	14	12	20	91
Age (years)	(8-17)‡	(5-19)	(35-56)	11	12	12 (6-20)	46 ± 5	13 ± 3	58 ± 14	65 (52-78)
Mode	Bike	Treadmill	Treadmill	Bike	Bike	Treadmill	Bike	Bike	Bike	Bike
Mean value area (cm^2)	1.22 ± 0.74	NA	NA	NA	NA	NA	1.0 ± 0.6	0.60 ± 0.16	NA	(0.48-1.63)
Mean valve gradient (mm Hg)	50	(10-112)	(53-80)	86 (30-235)	(<30->70)	38 (14-80)	NA	59 ± 18	57 ± 23	(18-64)
Maximal heart rate (beats/min)	(160-200)	NA	NA	NA	(183-194)	182	150 ± 17	180 ± 17	NA	NA
Exercise capacity	NA	NA	NA			NA	520 kpm/min	800 kpm/min	500 kpm/min	NA
Angina (%)	0	0	0	(0-29)	6	9	0	0	35	29
>1.0 mm ST-segment depression (%)	48	27	37	(71-100)	(38-89)	54	NA	100	x̄ = 1.33 ± 0.8	NA
Abnormal blood pressure response (%)	NA	NA	NA	NA	(0-32)	63	NA	58	NA	NA

Modified from Atwood JE, Kawanishi S, Myers JA, et al: *Chest* 93:1085, 1988.
NA, Not available; *kpm/min*, kilogram-meters/minute.
*Selected subgroup with >1.0 mm ST-segment depression.
†Selected subgroup without CAD.
‡Parentheses denote range.

ology for assessment of congenital AS and the need for surgical therapy, exercise testing has more recently been performed with appropriate caution and monitoring. Although predominantly used in pediatric cardiology to assess congenital AS and the need for surgical therapy, exercise testing has more recently been performed in adults to resolve problems when there is a disparity between history and clinical findings. Since Doppler echocardiography has been available, asymptomatic AS in the elderly has also become a challenging therapeutic decision.

Exercise testing in children with valvular stenosis has been used to distinguish who would benefit from surgery. However, this was before Doppler echocardiography was available. In children with congenital AS who were tested by bicycle exercise, those with gradients of 60 mm Hg or greater had 2 mm or more ST-segment depression. An exercise profile consisting of ST-segment depression of 2 mm or more, a decreased SBP response of 2 SD below normal and a decreased total work capacity of 2 SD below normal has been proposed. Two or more of these abnormal exercise responses occurred predominantly among those with a resting gradient of greater than 70 mm Hg.

In adults with AS, Scandinavian cardiologists have reported no complications in over 600 tests. In a series of 50,000 exercise tests performed in Sweden, only two deaths were reported—one of the two deaths reported was in a patient with AS. A "coronary insufficiency index score" expressed in degree of ST-segment depression relative to predicted exercise capacity was predictive of CAD even in patients who had LVH and were receiving digitalis.

Exercise testing is a relatively safe test in both the pediatric and adult patient when appropriately performed. Attention should be focused on the minute-by-minute response of the blood pressure, the patient's symptoms, the heart rate for slowing, and premature ventricular and atrial arrhythmias. In the presence of an abnormal BP response, a patient with AS should undergo at least a 2-minute cooldown walk at a lower stage of exertion to avoid the acute LV volume overload that may occur when placed supine. As in the elderly, detrained, and CAD patient, when one is testing patients with AS, low-level protocols should be used.

Exercise plays an important role in the objective assessment of symptoms, hemodynamic response, and functional capacity. Whether ST-segment depression indicates significant CAD remains unclear. By performing exercise testing preoperatively and postoperatively, one can quantify the benefits of surgery and baseline impairment. Exercise testing offers the opportunity to evaluate objectively any disparities between history and clinical findings, for example, in the elderly "asymptomatic subject" with physical or Doppler findings of severe AS. Often the echocardiographic studies are inadequate in such patients, particularly when they are smokers. When Doppler echocardiography reveals a significant gradient in the asymptomatic patient with normal exercise capacity, he could be followed closely until symptoms develop. In patients with an inadequate SBP response to exercise or a fall in SBP from the resting value when symptoms occur, surgery appears to be indicated.

EVALUATION FOR AN INDIVIDUALIZED EXERCISE PROGRAM

The exercise test can be used to evaluate the safety of participating in an exercise program and can help formulate an exercise prescription. Because of the wide scatter of maximal heart rate when plotted against age, it is much better to determine what an individual's maximal rate is, in order to assign a target for training, rather than give a predicted value. In certain individuals, it would be advantageous to evaluate objectively their response to exercise in a monitored situation before one embarks on an exercise program. In adult fitness or cardiac rehabilitation programs, an exercise test can be used to progress an individual safely to a higher level of performance. Also, the improvement in exercise performance secondary to training demonstrated by an exercise test can be an effective incentive and encouragement to people in such programs. If the goal of an exercise program is maximum physiological benefit as opposed to optimal health, training at or above the anaerobic threshold determined by gas exchange or lactate levels is indicated.

SUMMARY

The results from studies determining the risk of exercise-induced premature ventricular contractions and more serious ventricular dysrhythmias are mixed, but the prognosis appears to relate more to the "company they keep" than to the arrhythmias themselves. Some investigators contend that exercise testing is a better means of evaluating arrhythmic patients than other testing modalities. Certainly, exercise-induced arrhythmias are best studied with exercise. The studies evaluating antianginal agents have been greatly hampered by the increase in treadmill time that occurs merely by performing serial tests. For this reason, expired-gas analysis is frequently being added to protocols evaluating therapeutic agents. The studies of coronary artery bypass surgery and percutaneous transluminal coronary angioplasty are confounded by differences in medications before and after intervention and by the low rate of abnormal preintervention studies in the patients undergoing percutaneous transluminal coronary angioplasty who have mostly single-vessel disease. Standard exercise testing does not appear to be very helpful in the prediction of restenosis. From one study, we must conclude that exercise testing has little value in the evaluation of patients before noncardiac surgery. Further work in this area is needed but nonexercise stress modalities are playing an important role. Other applications of exercise testing include its use for evaluating patients with unstable angina, valvular heart disease, and intermittent claudication.

REFERENCES

1. Sullivan M, Genter F, Savvides M, et al: The reproducibility of hemodynamic, electrocardiographic, and gas exchange data during treadmill exercise in patients with stable angina pectoris, *Chest* 86:375-382, 1984.
2. Sklar J, Johnston GD, Overlie P, et al: The effects of a cardioselective (metoprolol) and a nonselective (propranolol) beta-adrenergic blocker on the response to dynamic exercise in normal men, *Circulation* 65:894-899, 1982.
3. Redwood DR, Rosing DR, Goldstein RE, et al: Importance of the design of an exercise protocol in the evaluation of patients with angina pectoris, *Circulation* 43:618-628, 1971.
4. Abrams J: The mystery of nitrate resistance, *Am J Cardiol* 68:1393-1396, 1991.
5. Parker JO, VanKoughnett KA, Fung HL: Transdermal isosorbide dinitrate in angina pectoris: effect of acute and sustained therapy, *Am J Cardiol* 54:8-13, 1984.
6. Thadani U, Manyari D, Parker JO, Fung HL: Tolerance to the circulatory effects of oral isosorbide dinitrate: rate of development and cross-tolerance to glyceryl trinitrate, *Circulation* 61:526-535, 1980.
7. Thompson RH: The clinical use of transdermal delivery devices with nitroglycerin, *Angiology* 34:23-31, 1983.
8. Sullivan MA, Savvides M, Abouantoun S, et al: Failure of transdermal nitroglycerin to improve exercise capacity in patients with angina pectoris, *J Am Coll Cardiol* 5:1220-1223, 1985.
9. Glasser SP, Clark PI, Lipicky RJ, et al: Exposing patients with chronic, stable, exertional angina to placebo periods in drug trials, *JAMA* 265:1550-1554, 1991.
10. Berger E, Williams DO, Reinert S, Most AS: Sustained efficacy of percutaneous transluminal coronary angioplasty, *Am Heart J* 111:233-236, 1986.
11. Vandormael MG, Chaitman BR, Ischinger T, et al: Immediate and short-term benefit of multilesion coronary angioplasty: influence of degree of revascularization, *J Am Coll Cardiol* 6:983-991, 1985.
12. Rosing DR, Van Raden MJ, Mincemoyer RM, et al: Exercise, electrocardiographic and functional responses after percutaneous transluminal coronary angioplasty, *Am J Cardiol* 53:36C-41C, 1984.
13. Ernst S, Hillebrand FA, Klein B, et al: The value of exercise tests in the follow-up of patients who underwent

transluminal coronary angioplasty, *Int J Cardiol* 7:267-279, 1985.
14. Honan MB, Bengtson JR, Pryor DB, et al: Exercise treadmill testing is a poor predictor of anatomic restenosis after angioplasty for acute myocardial infarction, *Circulation* 80:1585-1594, 1989.
15. Bengtson JR, Mark DB, Honan MB, et al: Detection of restenosis after elective percutaneous transluminal coronary angioplasty using the exercise treadmill test, *Am J Cardiol* 65:28-34, 1990.
16. Wijns W, Serruys PW, Simoons ML, et al: Predictive value of early maximal exercise test and thallium scintigraphy after successful percutaneous transluminal coronary angioplasty, *Br Heart J* 53:194-200, 1985.
17. Hultgren HN, Peduzzik P, Ketre K, Takoro T: The 5 year effect of bypass surgery on relief of angina and exercise performance, *Circulation* 72:V79-V83, 1985.
18. Ryan TJ, Weiner DA, McCabe CH, et al: Exercise testing in the Coronary Artery Surgery Study randomized population, *Circulation* 72:V31-38, 1985.
19. Gohlke H, Gohlke-Barwolf C, Samek L, et al: Serial exercise testing up to 6 years after coronary bypass surgery: behavior of exercise parameters in groups with different degrees of revascularization determined by postoperative angiography, *Am J Cardiol* 51:1301-1306, 1983.
20. Read RC, Murphy ML, Hultgren HN, Takaro T: Survival of men treated for chronic stable angina pectoris: a cooperative randomized study, *J Thorac Cardiovasc Surg* 75:1-16, 1978.
21. European Coronary Surgery Study Group: Long-term results of prospective randomized study of coronary artery bypass surgery in stable angina pectoris, *Lancet* 2:1173-1180, 1982.
22. CASS principal investigators and their associates: Coronary Artery Surgery Study (CASS): a randomized trial of coronary artery bypass surgery—survival data, *Circulation* 68:939-950, 1983.
23. Kent KM: Coronary angioplasty: a decade of experience, *N Engl J Med* 316:1148-1150, 1987.
24. Grüntzig AR, Senning A, Siegenthaler WE: Nonoperative dilatation of coronary-artery stenosis: percutaneous transluminal coronary angioplasty, *N Engl J Med* 301:61-68, 1979.
25. Dubach P, Froelicher V, Atwood JE, et al: A comparison of the exercise test responses pre/post revascularization: Does coronary artery bypass surgery produce better results than percutaneous transluminal coronary angioplasty? *J Cardiovasc Rehabil* 10:120-125, 1990.
26. Meier B, Gruentzig AR, Siegenthaler WE, Schlumpf M: Long-term exercise performance after percutaneous transluminal coronary angioplasty and coronary artery bypass grafting, *Circulation* 68:796-802, 1983.
27. King SB, Talley JD: Coronary arteriography and percutaneous transluminal coronary angioplasty: changing patterns of use and results, *Circulation* 79(suppl I):I-19-I-23, 1989.
28. Deligonul U, Vandormael MG, Younis LT, Chaitman BR: Prognostic significance of silent myocardial ischemia detected by early treadmill exercise after coronary angioplasty, *Am J Cardiol* 64:1-5, 1989.
29. Grondin CM, Campeau L, Thornton JC, et al: Coronary artery bypass grafting with saphenous vein, *Circulation* 79(suppl I):I-24-I-29, 1989.
30. Sionis D, Vrolix M, Glazier J, et al: Early exercise testing after successful PTCA: a word of caution, *Am Heart J* 123:530-532, 1992.
31. Parisi AF, Folland ED, Hartigan P, on behalf of the Veterans Affairs ACME Investigators: A comparison of angioplasty with medical therapy in the treatment of single-

vessel coronary artery disease, *N Engl J Med* 326:10-16, 1992.

32. Carliner NH, Fisher ML, Plotnick GD, et al: Routine preoperative exercise testing in patients undergoing major noncardiac surgery, *Am J Cardiol* 56:51-58, 1985.

33. Goldberger AL, O'Konski M: Utility of the routine elecrocardiogram before surgery and on general hospital admission, *Ann Intern Med* 105:552-557, 1986.

34. Cutler BS, Wheeler HB, Parakos JA, Cardullo PA: Assessment of operative risk with electrocardiographic exercise testing in patients with peripheral vascular disease, *Am J Surg* 137:484-490, 1979.

35. Cutler BS, Wheeler HB, Paraskos JA, Cardullo PA: Applicability and interpretation of electrocardiographic stress testing in patients with peripheral vascular disease, *Am J Surg* 141:501-506, 1981.

36. McPhail N, Calvin JE, Shariatmadar A, et al: The use of preoperative exercise testing to predict cardiac complications after arterial reconstruction, *J Vasc Surg* 7:60-68, 1988.

37. McPhail NV, Ruddy TD, Calvin JE, et al: A comparison of dipyridamole-thallium imaging and exercise testing in the prediction of postoperative cardiac complications in patients requiring arterial reconstruction, *J Vasc Surg* 10:51-56, 1989.

38. Franz IW: Ergometry in the assessment of arterial hypertension, *Cardiology* 72:147-159, 1985.

39. Young DZ, Lampert S, Graboys TB, Lown B: Safety of maximal exercise testing in patients at high risk for ventricular arrhythmia, *Circulation* 70:184-191, 1984.

40. Woelfel A, Foster JR, McAllister RG, et al: Efficacy of verapamil in exercise-induced ventricular tachycardia, *Am J Cardiol* 56:292-297, 1985.

41. Sami M, Chaitman B, Fisher L, et al: Significance of exercise-induced ventricular arrhythmia in stable coronary artery disease: a coronary artery surgery study project, *Am J Cardiol* 54:1182, 1984.

42. Califf RM, McKinnis RA, McNeer M, et al: Prognostic value of ventricular arrhythmias associated with treadmill exercise testing in patients studied with cardiac catheterization for suspected ischemic heart disease, *J Am Coll Cardiol* 2:1060-1067, 1983.

43. Weiner DA, Levine SR, Klein MD, Ryan TJ: Ventricular arrhythmias during exercise testing: mechanism, response to coronary bypass surgery and prognostic significance, *Am J Cardiol* 53:1553, 1984.

44. Kannel W, Abbott R, Savage D, McNamara PM: Epidemiologic features of chronic atrial fibrillation, *N Engl J Med* 306:1018-1022, 1982.

45. Aberg H, Ström G, Werner I: On the reproducibility of exercise tests in patients with atrial fibrillation, *Upsala J Med Sci* 82:27-30, 1977.

46. Hornsten TR, Bruce RA: Effects of atrial fibrillation on exercise performance in patients with cardiac disease, *Circulation* 37:543-548, 1968.

47. Klein H, Pauzner H, Di Segni E, et al: The beneficial effects of verapamil in chronic atrial fibrillation, *Arch Intern Med* 139:747-749, 1979.

48. Molajo AO, Coupe MO, Bennett DH: Effect of corwin on resting and exercise heart rate and exercise tolerance in digitalized patients with chronic atrial fibrillation, *Br Heart J* 52:392-395, 1984.

49. DiBianco R, Morganroth J, Freitag JA, et al: Effects of nadolol on the spontaneous and exercise-provoked heart rate of patients with chronic atrial fibrillation receiving stable dosages of digoxin, *Am Heart J* 108:1121-1127, 1984.

50. Atwood JE, Myers J, Sullivan M, et al: Maximal exercise testing and gas exchange in patients with chronic atrial fibrillation, *J Am Coll Cardiol* 11:508-513, 1988.

51. Atwood JE, Sullivan M, Forbes S, et al: The effect of beta-adrenergic blockade on exercise performance in patients with chronic atrial fibrillation, *J Am Coll Cardiol* 10:314-320, 1987.

52. Atwood JE, Myers JN, Sullivan MJ, et al: Diltiazem and exercise performance in patients with chronic atrial fibrillation, *Chest* 93:20-25, 1988.

53. Areskog NH: Exercise testing in the evaluation of patients with valvular aortic stenosis, *Clin Physiol* 4:201-208, 1984.

54. Atwood JE, Kawanishi S, Myers J, Froelicher VF: Exercise and the heart: exercise testing in patients with aortic stenosis, *Chest* 93:1083-1087, 1988.

Stress Radionuclide Myocardial Perfusion Imaging

The addition of radionuclide imaging techniques to exercise electrocardiographic evaluations of patients with known or suspected coronary artery disease provides important diagnostic, pathophysiologic, and prognostic information that is frequently helpful in guiding patient management decisions. Imaging can be performed with either pharmacological or exercise stress, making possible evaluation of patients who cannot exercise. Stress radionuclide imaging tests may be considered in two broad categories, myocardial perfusion studies and ventricular function studies. This chapter is a discussion of myocardial perfusion imaging. Chapter 13 is a review of stress ventricular function examinations.

MYOCARDIAL PERFUSION IMAGING

Potassium is a metabolically important cation that is abundantly present in high concentration inside living cells as a result of energy-consuming transfer mechanisms that act across the cell membrane. Potassium is actively taken up from plasma and transferred into the intracellular milieu, an indication that radionuclides of potassium or potassium analogs might prove to be useful physiological markers of perfusion. The potassium analogs are the elements that occupy the same column in the periodic table—potassium, rubidium, and cesium, along with thallium in another column. Of these, thallium 201 has emerged as the clearly leading candidate for clinical imaging, which, though not ideal, has been convincingly shown with extensive investigation and experience to be a reliable and useful isotope for clinical imaging of patients with known or suspected coronary artery disease. Technetium 99m (metastable) has properties, particularly its shorter half-life, higher energy emissions, and greater clinical availability, which make it preferable to ^{201}Tl for imaging. Two ^{99m}Tc-labeled

myocardial perfusion compounds with very different properties, ^{99m}Tc-sestamibi and ^{99m}Tc-teboroxime, have recently been approved for clinical use and have been the subject of considerable investigation. Refinements in positron emission tomographic (PET) imaging, as well as the development of a generator capable of producing rubidium 82 without the need of a cyclotron, have led to renewed interest in PET myocardial perfusion imaging. Because positron imaging techniques are available only in a small number of centers at the present time, however, and because they are still considered to be investigational by most third-party carriers, this discussion deals only with single-photon isotope studies. The understanding and proper utilization of perfusion imaging, however, requires familiarity with the basic concepts of autoregulation of coronary blood flow in normal and diseased vessels, and so the discussion begins here with a brief review.

Autoregulation of coronary blood flow in normal and diseased vessels

The heart is an obligate aerobic organ that has little capacity to generate energy through anaerobic metabolism. The oxygen requirement of the heart, on a per-gram basis, is 5 times that of the rest of the body, whereas that of the left ventricle is 20 times the rest of the body. The demand of the myocardium for oxygen is primarily determined by four factors. Heart rate is the most important single determinant of myocardial oxygen demand. As heart rate increases, so does myocardial oxygen requirement. Two determinants of wall tension, intraventricular pressure and ventricular radius (by the Laplace relationship), contribute to myocardial oxygen demand. Of the two, pressure work is much more expensive in terms of oxygen requirement than volume work is. The fourth determinant of demand, which is approximately as significant as wall tension, is contractility. As contractility increases, so does oxygen requirement. Heart rate, pressure, volume, and contractility, all are variables that are influenced by exercise.

Myocardial oxygen supply must be autoregulated in order to meet the organ's high demands. Since oxygen extraction in the coronary circulation is nearly maximal at rest, the heart has little capability to increase its oxygen supply under conditions of increased demand by the mechanism of increasing extraction of the oxygen from the coronary blood flow that it is already receiving. Therefore, to increase its oxygen consumption, the heart must increase coronary blood flow. Autoregulation of coronary blood flow therefore becomes central to the heart's capability to respond to exercise.

Figure 12-1 illustrates the factors that control myocardial oxygen supply at rest.[1] Coronary perfusion pressure is the difference between central aortic pressure and right atrial pressure, since the coronary venous drainage empties into the right atrium through the coronary sinus. In the left ventricle, coronary flow is primarily a diastolic event. There is some flow to the epicardial vessels during systole, but this flow serves primarily a capacitance function. There is virtually no flow to the endocardium during systole. Because of its lower pressure, the right ventricle receives some of its nutrient flow during systole. For practical purposes, however, it is primarily aortic diastolic pressure that drives coronary perfusion.

In opposition to this perfusion pressure there is resistance. In the coronary system resistance exists at three primary levels, which can be thought of as R1, R2 and R3 resistance. The R1 resistance vessels are composed of the epicardial coronary arteries as well as the larger intramyocardial vessels. Primarily these are the vessels that are seen on a coronary angiogram. These vessels serve largely a capacitance function, contributing comparatively little to resistance, as illustrated in Figure 12-1. Downstream are the R2 vessels, which are the small intramyocardial arteries and precapillary arterioles. Proportionately, these vessels contribute much more resistance to flow. Since the coronary vessels must penetrate through the myocardial muscle, any force that is transmitted against the muscle from within the cavity is also transmitted against the vessels that are within the wall. This is the R3 component of resistance. Importantly, the R3 component of resistance is unevenly distributed across the myocardium, being greatest in the subendocardium and least in the subepicardium. This single factor largely accounts for the greater vulnerability of the subendocardium to ischemic injury.

The response of the normal coronary circulation to exercise is illustrated in Figure 12-2. During aerobic exercise, blood pressure normally increases, but it is primarily systolic pressure that rises. Diastolic pressure normally does not rise. Effective coronary perfusion pressure therefore goes up very little during exercise. Myocardial ox-

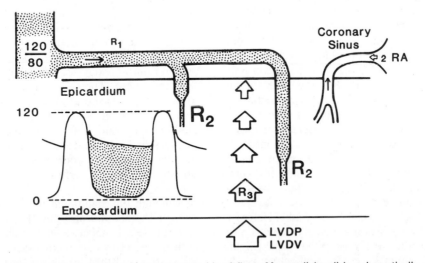

Figure 12-1   Factors that determine coronary blood flow. Myocardial wall is schematically represented from epicardial to endocardial surfaces. Coronary artery originates from the ascending aorta. Coronary venous drains through the coronary sinus to the right atrium. Left ventricular and central aortic pressure are shown, as well as three levels of resistance to perfusion: R1, R2, and R3. (From Follansbee WP: The heart in vasculitis. In LeRoy EC, editor: *Systemic vasculitis: the biologic basis,* New York, 1992, Marcel Dekker.)

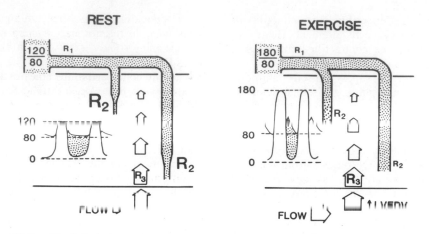

Figure 12-2   Physiological response of coronary system to exercise, *right,* in comparison to rest, *left.* The increase in coronary flow during exercise is primarily mediated by a decrease in resistance at the level of the R2 vessels. (From Follansbee WP: The heart in vasculitis. In LeRoy EC, editor: *Systemic vasculitis: the biologic basis,* New York, 1992, Marcel Dekker.)

ygen demand increases to maximum levels, which are as much as three to four times baseline levels, by virtue of the increased heart rate, systolic blood pressure, and contractility. Changes in ventricular volume vary depending on the type and position of exercise. This increased myocardial oxygen demand must be met by increased coronary blood flow. Since perfusion pressure does not effectively increase, the increased flow can be accomplished only by decreasing resistance. The R1 vessels vasodilate somewhat during exercise, but since they contribute little to resistance at rest, this exercise response has little effect on perfusion. The R2 vessels, however, have the capacity to vasodilate. They can decrease their resistance to approximately 25% of the baseline value. The R3 component of resistance should change very little during exercise in normal subjects. If perfusion pressure is kept the same and R2 resistance falls to 25% of resting levels, flow has the potential capacity to increase approximately fourfold. This magnitude of increased flow is seldom achieved during exercise except in highly conditioned athletes. Pharmacological vasodilatation of the R2 vessels with agents like dipyridamole or adenosine, however, does produce levels of flow that are of this magnitude.

The patient with coronary artery atherosclerosis has increased R1 vessel resistance to flow as a result of the obstructive plaque in the vessel (Figure 12-3, left). There is a pressure gradient across the stenosis in the vessel. Despite the presence of obstructions of up to 90%, however, resting flow through these vessels is maintained at or near resting levels. To compensate for the increase in resistance to flow in the R1 vessel, and the autoreg-

ulatory control mechanisms mediate a vasodilator response at the level of the R2 vessels. This decrease in resistance at the R2 level compensates for the increased resistance at the level of the R1 vessels, and so total resistance is kept within the normal range and resting flow is preserved. With critical obstructions, diastolic myocardial function is also frequently abnormal, causing an increase in the R3 component of resistance, which also must be overcome by R2 vessel vasodilatation.

Although flow in the distribution of the narrowed vessel is preserved at rest, the vasodilator reserve is partially or even totally expended in the process. In response to exercise, therefore, there is limited remaining vasodilating reserve available to mediate an increase in flow during exercise (Figure 12-3, right). As myocardial oxygen demand goes up during exercise, the R2 vessels dilate to their maximum. Thereafter, as demand continues to increase, myocardial oxygen supply cannot increase any further, and ischemia results. With increasing ischemia, left ventricular end-diastolic pressure and end-diastolic volume increase, and they increase the R3 component of resistance and further compromise perfusion, particularly to the subendocardium.

Although this traditional model of exercise-induced ischemia indicates that flow through an obstructed vessel increases in response to exercise until the point of maximum vasodilatation of the R2 vessels and then levels off despite increasing demand, it is probably an oversimplification. Schwartz and colleagues described a study in dogs in which they placed a snare around the circumflex coronary artery to simulate an obstruction (Figure 12-4). They observed that virtually imme-

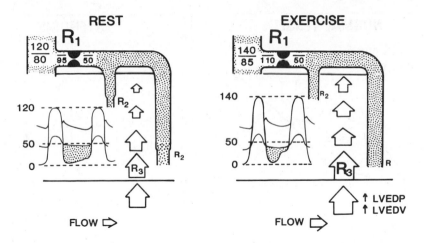

Figure 12-3   Effects of a coronary atherosclerotic obstruction on resting coronary blood flow, *left*. Resting coronary blood flow is preserved despite the presence of a pronounced obstruction in the R1 vessel, because of compensatory vasodilatation of the R2 vessels. The vasodilating reserve of the R2 vessels downstream from the atherosclerotic obstruction during exercise, *right*, is decreased because it is partially or even completely expended in protecting flow at rest. As ischemia develops, the ventricle develops both diastolic and then systolic dysfunction, which results in an increase in the R3 component of resistance, further worsening the ischemia. (From Follansbee WP: The heart in vasculitis. In LeRoy EC, editor: *Systemic vasculitis: the biologic basis,* New York, 1992, Marcel Dekker.)

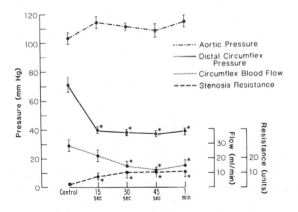

Figure 12-4   The mean hemodynamic changes occurring during the first minute of exercise in the presence of a critical circumflex stenosis, induced by a snare, are shown in a canine experiment. *Asterisks,* Significant differences from control values (*p* <0.025). Flow through the stenotic vessel decreased virtually immediately with the onset of exercise. (From Schwartz JS et al: *Am J Cardiol* 50:1409-1413, 1982.)

diately with the onset of exercise the flow through the narrowed vessel decreased. It did not increase and then plateau as would be predicted by the traditional model of exercise-induced ischemia, but instead promptly decreased. Perfusion pressure downstream from the obstruction fell greatly. The next question became, Why did the flow decrease? Two primary possibilities are suggested. One is

that as perfusion pressure beyond the obstruction falls because of the exponential increase in resistance to flow across the obstruction as flow increases, intravascular distending pressure decreases and the vessel passively collapses upon itself, resulting in worsening of the obstruction. The alternative explanation is that there is dynamic vasoconstriction at the site of the atherosclerotic plaque in response to exercise that acutely worsens the obstruction and results in a decrease in flow.

Gage and coinvestigators reported findings from an elegant study on patients in a catheterization laboratory that addressed this question.[3] Using quantitative angiographic techniques, they measured the size of the epicardial (R1) vessels at rest (Figure 12-5). The resting lumen diameter is plotted as 100%. The response of normal vessels is shown in the lefthand illustration. Group I patients were exercised. Promptly with the onset of exercise, the lumen of the R1 vessel increased by approximately 20%. At peak exercise, the patient was given nitroglycerin sublingually, and the vessels further dilated. Patients who were pretreated with intracoronary nitroglycerin before exercise (group 2) showed a prompt increase in R1 vessel diameter, with little further change during subsequent exercise. The response of the atherosclerotic vessels to the same protocol is shown in the righthand illustration of Figure 12-5. In response to exercise, there was an immediate prominent de-

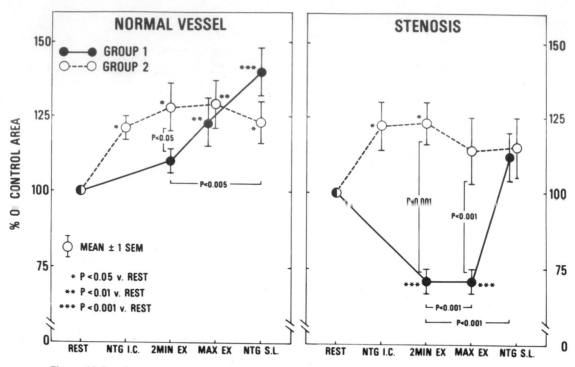

Figure 12-5 Coronary artery luminal diameter was measured in normal and abnormal vessels of patients undergoing coronary angiography, using quantitative techniques. The responses of normal and stenotic coronary arteries to dynamic exercise in patients without (group 1) and with (group 2) pretreatment with nitroglycerin are shown expressed as percent of resting luminal area. Normal vessels, *at left,* dilated during exercise to 123% of control values and dilated further to 140% with the sublingual administration of nitroglycerin at peak exercise. Intracoronary nitroglycerin induced dilatation of normal vessels to 121% of resting values. The dilatation persisted at the same level during subsequent exercise. In contrast to the response in normal vessels, in stenotic vessels, *at right,* exercise induced a narrowing of stenoses to 71% of control. This worsening stenosis reversed to 112% of control with sublingual administration of nitroglycerin at peak exercise. Intracoronary administration of nitroglycerin before exercise (group 2) produced a dilatation of stenoses to 122% of resting size, which did not change significantly during exercise. The exercise-induced narrowing of the vessel was prevented by the nitroglycerin, an indication that the worsening obstruction during exercise is attributable to arterial vasoconstriction at the site of the stenosis, which is prevented or reversed by nitroglycerin treatment. (From Gage JE et al: *Circulation* 73:865-876, 1986.)

crease in the lumen size at the site of the atherosclerotic plaque, the opposite of the normal response. With sublingual administration of nitroglycerin at peak exercise, the lumen increased to about 110% of baseline value. If the patient was pretreated with intracoronary nitroglycerin (group 2), the decrease in lumen diameter during exercise no longer occurred. These observations strongly indicate that there may be an active vasoconstricting response of the R1 vessels during exercise in the presence of atherosclerosis that results in a decrease in flow through the diseased vessel. This vasoconstricting response is prevented by nitroglycerin. The vasomotor control of the vessel is mediated at least in part by the endothelium. In the presence of endothelial damage, stimuli that

normally cause vasodilatation instead cause vasoconstriction.

The use of exercise testing with perfusion imaging is predicated on the differential flow response to increased myocardial oxygen demand of normal compared to abnormal vessels. The disparity in flow is produced by exercise, typically resulting in ischemia. At peak exercise the perfusion-imaging agent is injected. Its distribution will reflect peak regional blood flow, providing the ability to image the deficient perfusion response of the abnormal vessels. Pharmacological stress testing, by virtue of producing maximum R2 vessel vasodilatation, increases coronary flow to levels that even exceed normal peak levels achieved during exercise. The perfusion indicator will again reflect the regional variation in flow response, allowing detection of the presence of disease.

Thallium scintigraphy

The thallium analogs potassium 43, rubidium 81, and cesium 129 are single-photon emitting radiopharmaceuticals, but each has a comparatively high energy spectrum of gamma-ray emissions, which require special shielding and collimation for clinical imaging. Both potassium 43 and rubidium 81 provide relatively low target-to-background ratios of myocardial uptake, limiting their utility as myocardial perfusion tracers. Uptake of cesium 129 is too slow to make it a useful marker of ischemia. For these and other reasons, these radionuclides have not been found to be useful for clinical imaging. [201]Tl, however, has properties that have proved to be suitable in widespread clinical application.

Radiochemistry and kinetics. When ^{201}Tl is administered intravenously as a chloride salt, it is rapidly and efficiently extracted from the blood pool, entering the intracellular space including that in the myocardium. Myocardial uptake of thallium after injection at rest reaches 80% of maximum within 1 minute, though it does not peak for 24 minutes.[4] [201]Tl uptake in areas with reduced flow at rest is both decreased and delayed.[5] Okada and co-workers demonstrated that myocardial thallium uptake during stress (in this experiment done by norepinephrine infusion) peaks within 1 minute of injection.[6] Uptake in areas perfused by stenosed vessels is slower, peaking approximately 2 minutes after injection. The difference in time to peak uptake when one compares rest to stress injections reflects the pronounced increase in coronary blood flow and therefore the ^{201}Tl delivery that is associated with exercise. This increase results in greater initial ^{201}Tl concentration compared to blood-pool activity.

[201]Tl uptake is proportional to regional blood flow and is dependent on viable cell membranes. Thallium extraction by the myocardium is linearly related to flow at rest, during conditions of reduced flow,[7] and in the setting of increased flow associated with exercise.[8] Gould and colleagues demonstrated that at the superphysiologic flow rates associated with intravenous dipyridamole or adenosine infusion, however, ^{201}Tl extraction becomes less efficient.[9] Under these conditions, ^{201}Tl uptake falls off relative to peak flow, a finding confirmed by Melin and Becker.[10] [201]Tl uptake is not appreciably altered by propranolol, acetylstrophanthidin, insulin, or acidemia.[11] The effect of hypoxia on ^{201}Tl uptake has been somewhat more controversial but appears to be minimal.[12-14] Because splanchnic blood flow decreases while myocardial blood flow increases during exercise, the resulting target-to-background ratio of thallium uptake in the myocardium after exercise compared to the liver and gut is favorable for imaging. With pharmacologic stress, splanchnic uptake is proportionally much greater than that during exercise, resulting in a target-to-background ratio that is less desirable.

After intravenous injection of ^{201}Tl, blood pool activity rapidly decreases to very low levels coinciding with the rapid uptake of the radionuclide into cells. After initial ^{201}Tl uptake by the myocardium, activity decreases over time as radionuclide washes out of the myocardium down the concentration gradient back into the blood pool, from which it is ultimately excreted by the kidneys. The kinetics of ^{201}Tl washout reflect a complex interaction of multiple variables. When ^{201}Tl is injected directly into a coronary artery, blood pool activity is very low; intrinsic ^{201}Tl myocardial washout is monoexponential under these conditions with a half-time after resting injection of 84 minutes.[4] [201]Tl clearance is significantly faster after intracoronary injection compared to after intravenous injection. After intravenous injection, blood pool activity is greater as a result of the continuous diffusion of ^{201}Tl back into the blood pool from the large whole-body intracellular stores. As a result of this continuously renewed supply of ^{201}Tl to the blood pool, the myocardium continues to take up some ^{201}Tl from the blood pool while at the same time it is leaking ^{201}Tl back into the blood pool through its intrinsic washout.[15] The net effect is that washout is biexponential, reflecting the sum of these directionally opposite forces.[6]

After exercise, ^{201}Tl concentration in normal myocardium is greatly increased relative to the blood pool. The washout rate is faster when the concentration gradient becomes greater. In myocardium perfused by an obstructed coronary vessel, the initial ^{201}Tl concentration after exercise is less than in myocardium supplied by normal vessels. Washout from these hypoperfused areas is slower than that from the normal areas because the concentration gradient is less and because the intrinsic washout rate itself may also be decreased.[16] Time to peak myocardial activity is also delayed, and washout from the normal areas is increased.[17] As a result, ^{201}Tl activity in the abnormal areas increases over time compared to the normal areas, a phenomenon sometimes referred to as "wash-in."[18] Massie and colleagues showed that the rate of ^{201}Tl washout is decreased at lower peak exercise heart rates because of the decreased thallium concentration associated with the decreased peak coronary blood flow, a finding subsequently confirmed by Kaul and colleagues.[19,20] [201]Tl washout can be accelerated by high carbohydrate meal after injection.[21] It is not significantly effected by the ischemia that occurs after initial ^{201}Tl uptake.[22,23]

[201]Tl undergoes radioactive decay by electron capture. A proton in the nucleus captures an electron from an inner orbit, converting the proton into a neutron. The number of protons decreases by one, transforming the element from thallium to mercury, but the atomic mass number (the sum of the protons and neutrons in the nucleus) remains unchanged at 201. Mercury x rays (energy emissions originating from the electron shell) are emitted with energies ranging from 69 to 83 keV (94% abundant), and thallium gamma rays (energy emissions originating from the nucleus) are emitted with energies of 167 keV (10% abundant) and 135 keV (3% abundant.) The primary imaging window therefore is in the comparatively low energy range of 69 to 83 keV.

[201]Tl decays with a relatively long physical half-life of 73 hours, which is both an advantage and a disadvantage. The advantage is that it provides a sufficiently long shelf life to make production at centralized nuclear reactors with subsequent shipment to clinical sites a practical possibility. The disadvantage is that the radiation exposure associated with the longer half-life limits the amount of isotope that can be administered to patients, therefore decreasing the number of radioactive counts that can be acquired per unit time in building an image. As a result, image resolution is limited by count statistics. Dosimetry calculations performed by Atkins and colleagues have indicated that the total body radiation dose is 0.42 rad per 2 millicurie dose administered, with 0.68 rad exposure to the heart and 2.4 rad to the kidney.[24] The biological half-life is 57 hours. The lower large intestine is the critical target organ when ^{201}Tl is injected at peak exercise in normal subjects, receiving a calculated dose of 1.08 rad per 2 mCi administered dose.[25] In addition to its implications on dosimetry, the long physical half-life of ^{201}Tl limits its utility for serial studies with repeated measurements in a short time frame, which might be desirable, for example, in assessment of the effects of therapeutic interventions in acute infarction.

Planar thallium imaging. Clinical ^{201}Tl imaging can be performed using either planar or tomographic (single-photon emission computerized tomography, or SPECT) techniques. With planar imaging, an Anger scintillation camera detects the radioactive emissions and, interfaced to a computer system, builds an image. Typically, planar scintigrams are acquired in the anterior, 45-degree left anterior oblique, and 70-degree or lateral decubitus views for 8 to 10 minutes per view (Figure 12-6). If the heart is rotated, the best angle to profile the septum and separate the images of the left and right ventricle may not be the 45-degree LAO view. In that instance, the best view should be identified and acquired, with subsequent views obtained 45-degrees anterior and lateral to the best LAO projection. With these three projections, the perfusion areas of all three major coronary arteries can be examined, usually in more than one projection.

Because of the low energies of the predominant ^{201}Tl emissions, attenuation of activity as it passes through tissue is considerable (approximately 50% every 4 cm of tissue). Attenuation can cause artifactual perfusion defects that simulate hypoperfusion. The most common artifact is from breast attenuation, which typically affects the anterolateral wall on the anterior view, the upper septum and lateral wall on the 45-degree LAO view, and the anteroseptal wall on the 70-degree LAO view. The breast shadow is usually readily identifiable on the planar image, signaling the potentially artifactual nature of a perfusion defect. Diaphragmatic attenuation can cause perfusion defects in the inferior wall, particularly on the 70-degree LAO views. Repeating the steep LAO view with the patient lying on his or her right side will usually eliminate the artifactual defect. Inferior wall attenuation of activity can also occur from the overlying right ventricle, which is seen most commonly on the anterior projection.

Interpretation of ^{201}Tl images requires considerable experience as well as an understanding of the physiology and pathophysiology of coronary artery disease. DiCola and co-workers demonstrated that visual assessment of images is limited particularly in its ability to detect ^{201}Tl redistribution.[26] In an effort to improve the accuracy and reproducibility of image interpretation, computer techniques to quantify myocardial thallium uptake and washout have been widely utilized. To quantify thallium activity in the myocardium, it is essential that background activity and scatter radiation, which is being detected within the region of the myocardium but is in fact coming from surrounding structures contiguous to the heart, be eliminated. Because background radiation is not uniform in its distribution around the myocardium, simple uniform background subtraction will introduce artifacts. The most commonly utilized background correction method is a modification of the bilinear interpolative background-correction algorithm originally described by Goris and co-workers.[27] A box is placed around the myocardium, and all activity outside the box is eliminated. The background activity assigned to each pixel within the myocardial field is calculated by examination of

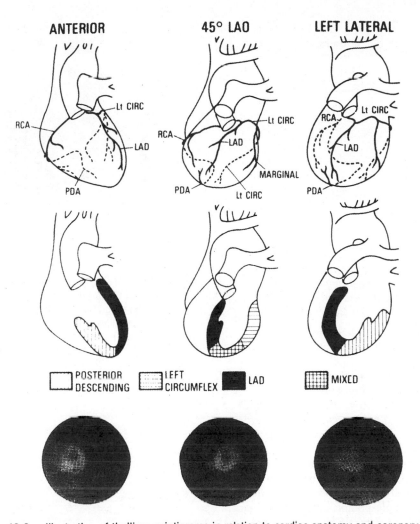

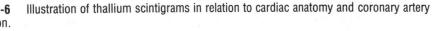

Figure 12-6   Illustration of thallium scintigrams in relation to cardiac anatomy and coronary artery distribution.

the activity at the perimeter of the box at both ends of the horizontal and vertical profiles drawn through that pixel. Watson and associates developed a weighting factor that accounts for the effect of distance on background activity (Figure 12-7).[28]

Profiles of myocardial ^{201}Tl activity can be generated from the interpolative background-corrected images by use of either horizontal slices through the myocardium,[29] or circumferential plots of peak counts per pixel in radii extending from the centroid out through the myocardium.[30,31] Perfusion defects can then be defined from the curves by one of two methods. Activity in myocardial walls can be compared to other walls in the same view. Since distribution of thallium throughout the myocardium is normally homogeneous, a decrease in activity in one wall compared

to another in the same view (usually defined as 25%, except in the inferior wall on the anterior view where it is defined as 35%) is considered to be abnormal.[29] Alternatively, the myocardial distribution can be compared to a normal reference data file, particularly when circumferential profile plots are used. Areas falling more than 2.5 standard deviations below the normal range are defined as abnormal perfusion defects. Count profiles from repeat images done 3 to 24 hours after the initial images can be compared with those from the initial images to identify ^{201}Tl redistribution, implying ischemia. The washout of ^{201}Tl activity from the various walls of the myocardium can also be quantified by comparison of the curves from the two sets of images. Maddahi and co-workers suggested that an abnormally delayed washout rate, again as compared to a normal reference file, is a

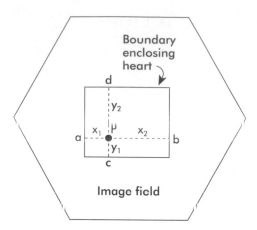

Figure 12-7 The myocardial imaging field is illustrated with a computer-defined boundary circumscribing the heart. The background activity assigned to pixel p is derived from activity at the boundary of the x (points a and b) and y (points c and d) axes through that pixel. (From Watson DD et al: *J Nucl Med* 22:577-584, 1981.)

helpful indicator of disease even in the absence of a visible perfusion defect.[32]

SPECT thallium imaging. Planar thallium imaging has theoretic intrinsic limitations because it is a two-dimensional modality. Areas of background activity overlying the heart can create an artifactual appearance of uneven myocardial uptake, which is only partially correctable by interpolative background correction. In addition, areas of normal thallium uptake within the heart can overlap areas of decreased perfusion, concealing the perfusion defect. Single-photon emission computerized tomography (SPECT) imaging affords the possibility of examining ^{201}Tl distribution in sequential tomographic slices of about 6 mm thickness, providing the potential for improved detection, localization, and quantitation of perfusion defects.

With SPECT imaging, a series of between 32 and 64 successive planar images are acquired as the camera rotates around the patient, usually in an 180-degree arc from a 45-degree RAO to a 45-degree LPO view.[33] Image data are reconstructed in the transaxial plane, utilizing a filtered back projection technique.[34] From the transaxial images, the long axis of the ventricle can be identified, from which orthogonal views can be reconstructed in the short axis, horizontal long axis, and vertical long axis planes[35] (Figure 12-8).

García and colleagues developed a method for quantitation of SPECT ^{201}Tl images that is entirely analogous to the circumferential profile method utilized in planar imaging.[36] DePasquale and co-workers further refined the technique, demonstrating that circumferential profile plots of activity in sequential short-axis slices can be represented in a

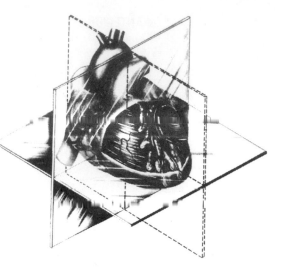

Figure 12-8 Planes of the heart. The long axis of the left ventricle is defined by the longest straight line connecting the apex of the ventricle to a central point at the base. The three planes of reconstruction of tomographic images are shown and include the horizontal and vertical long-axis projections as well as the short-axis plane, which is vertical to the long axis of the ventricle. (From Gerson MC: *Cardiac nuclear medicine,* New York, 1991, McGraw-Hill, p. 43.)

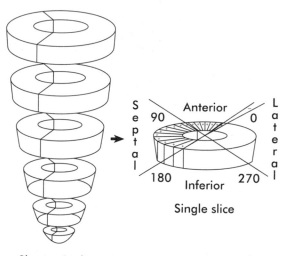

Figure 12-9 Alternating short-axis slices of the left ventricle, **A,** are displayed. The middle slice is highlighted, **B.** A septal perfusion defect extends from the apex to the base of the ventricle. The highlighted slice is divided into 40 radial sectors that subtend the anterior, septal, inferior and lateral walls. (From DePasquale EE et al: *Circulation* 77:316-327, 1988.)

polar-coordinate "bull's eye" map, providing a convenient two-dimensional representation of the three-dimensional data (Figures 12-9 and 12-10).[37] The patient profile maps can be compared to a normal reference data file, with areas falling more

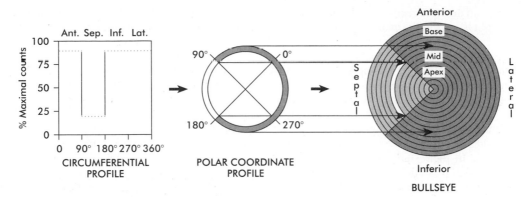

Figure 12-10   Rectangular coordinate profile plot of the maximum counts per pixel for each sector are plotted relative to the location of the sector in one slice of the tomographic image, **A.** A similar profile is generated for each slice of the image. Each profile is then converted into a polar coordinate profile, **B,** which displays the curve as a circle, representing the 40 pixels. These profiles are interpolated to produce 15 profiles per study, which are displayed as a polar coordinate map, **C.** The apex is represented at the center of the plot, and the base is at the periphery. The myocardial walls are located as shown. (From DePasquale EE et al: *Circulation* 77:316-327, 1988.)

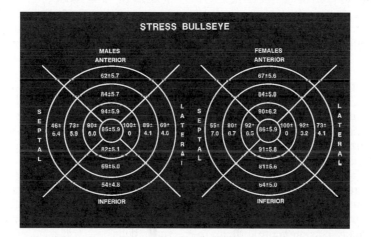

Figure 12-11   The normal distribution of ^{201}Tl activity for exercise bull's-eye plots are shown for men, *left,* and women, *right.* All regions are expressed as a percentage (± S.D.) of activity of the lateral wall near the apex. (From Eisner RL et al: *J Nucl Med* 29:1901-1909, 1988.)

than 2.5 standard deviations below the normal range being blacked out by the computer. Eisner and co-workers demonstrated that the normal reference files must be sex specific (Figure 12-11).[38]

SPECT ^{201}Tl images are subject to breast and other attenuation artifacts very similar to those that occur with planar imaging.[39] In addition, however, other potential artifacts can be introduced including those resulting from patient motion during study acquisition.[40] Apparent "upward creep" of the heart can result from patient hyperventilation early in image acquisition while the patient is still recovering from exercise, with return to a normal breathing pattern later during the acquisition. Friedman and colleagues demonstrated that this

upward creep can cause artifactual perfusion defects, particularly in the inferior and inferoseptal walls.[41] Computer methods to correct for these patient and organ motion artifacts were devised by Geckle and co-workers.[42] Other artifacts can also be introduced in tomographic imaging, including those that result from improper equipment function, such as those with unsteady center of rotation or improper head alignment, or from errors introduced during filtered-back projection and image reconstruction.

Rest thallium imaging and detection of myocardial infarction. Patients with prior or recent myocardial infarction have ^{201}Tl perfusion defects when the isotope is injected at rest. Wackers and colleagues were the first to describe resting ^{201}Tl perfusion defects in patients presenting with acute myocardial infarction.[43,44] They noted that the frequency of abnormal scintigrams was virtually 100% in patients who could be imaged within 6 hours of onset of infarction but progressively decreased to approximately 70% when imaging occurred more than 24 hours after the onset of symptoms. Tiefenbrunn and co-workers observed a somewhat higher prevalence of chronic perfusion defects after infarction. In their study of 32 patients with prior myocardial infarction, 56% of whom had transmural infarction, 94% had ^{201}Tl perfusion defects on images acquired an average of 11 months after infarction,[45] a finding similar to the previous observation of Niess and colleagues.[46]

Despite these favorable reports, the sensitivity of detection of infarction on rest thallium studies is likely to decrease as time of imaging after the infarction increases. Wackers and colleagues demonstrated that patients who were imaged serially after infarction showed a decrease in ^{201}Tl defect size over time.[44] This clinical observation is supported by the observations of disease by Bulkley and coinvestigators who noted that there is a significant subgroup of patients (38% in their study) in whom the size of the thallium perfusion defect is a significant overestimation of the histological size of the acute infarction as determined at autopsy.[47] The findings indicate that during the evolution of acute infarction the extent of myocardium that is jeopardized decreases, likely attributable both to the effects of collateral flow to the border zones of the infarction and to possible reestablishment of antegrade flow into the infarct area resulting from spontaneous thrombolysis. As a result, thallium perfusion defect size decreases, and the infarction will likely become more difficult to detect.

Resting ^{201}Tl scintigraphy is more sensitive in detecting transmural myocardial infarction than subendocardial infarction and is more sensitive in detecting anterior compared to inferior wall infarction.[48] Transmural infarctions are easier to detect, in part because the size of the infarction is typically bigger than in subendocardial infarction. Perhaps more important from an imaging standpoint, however, transmural defects are likely to be more discrete and clearly delineated from the surrounding myocardium than subendocardial defects, which typically appear as thinning of the myocardial wall. The more delineated transmural defects would be easier to see than the subendocardial defects even when there is a comparable amount of damage. Ritchie and co-workers found that SPECT ^{201}Tl imaging offers improved sensitivity for detection of prior myocardial infarction compared to planar imaging.[49]

Although ^{201}Tl perfusion defects at rest indicate probable prior myocardial infarction with irreversible damage, caution is necessary. Gerwitz and co-workers pointed out that in patients with stable but severe coronary artery disease, ^{201}Tl perfusion abnormalities that are initially present after resting injection often show redistribution when scintigrams are repeated 2 to 4 hours later. The occurrence of redistribution implies that these initial resting perfusion defects do not represent scar but rather resting ischemia.[50] In their patient sample, areas of myocardium that had resting redistribution of ^{201}Tl activity were characteristically perfused by severely diseased coronary vessels but had comparatively normal wall motion in the affected area. Somewhat in contrast to this, Stratton and co-workers noted a relationship between resting ^{201}Tl defect size using SPECT imaging and the severity of the wall-motion abnormality present in patients with prior myocardial infarction.[51] Hirsowitz and colleagues demonstrated that ^{201}Tl uptake at rest in areas of akinesis or pronounced hypokinesis indicates viable myocardium that will recover function with time.[52] Iskandrian and colleagues noted that the presence of a redistributing defect after rest ^{201}Tl injection identified patients with coronary artery disease patients with left ventricular dysfunction whose LV function would improve after coronary bypass surgery.[53] Tamaki and co-workers further supported the hypothesis that not all resting thallium perfusion defects represent irreversibly damaged myocardium with their observation that approximately 40% of myocardial segments with fixed ^{201}Tl perfusion abnormalities by SPECT imaging have evidence of increased uptake of fluorine-18 2-fluorodeoxyglucose (FDG).[54] Active glucose metabolism requires the presence of viable cells.

Although one acknowledges that thallium perfusion defect size likely decreases somewhat with time in the initial hours after infarction and that not all resting perfusion defects represent irreversibly damaged myocardium, there nevertheless has been a good correlation reported between resting ^{201}Tl defect size and size of the myocardial infarction. In the setting of acute or recent myocardial infarction, Wackers and co-workers noted a good agreement between estimation of infarct size from planar ^{201}Tl scintigrams and pathological infarct size assessed at autopsy in 23 patients.[55] Similarly, the correlation between SPECT ^{201}Tl defect size and myocardial infarction size assessed pathologically in an acute canine model has also been good.[56] Kaul and co-workers (1985),[57] Prigent and colleagues,[58] and Mahmarian and co-workers[59] have all reported a good correlation in clinical studies between myocardial infarct size and thallium defect size using SPECT ^{201}Tl imaging. Tamaki and co-workers (1982) reported a good correlation between SPECT ^{201}Tl estimate of infarct size compared to cumulative creatine phosphokinase-MB release.[60] The correlation of planar defect size with infarct size was not as good.

Okada and Boucher examined the effect of early reperfusion on resting thallium defect size in acute infarction in a canine model.[61] They noted that some dogs with acute anterior wall infarctions followed by early reperfusion had normal ^{201}Tl uptake but the washout of ^{201}Tl from the infarct area was abnormally delayed. Moore and co-workers observed that, in animals with myocardial stunning induced by repeated short periods of coronary occlusion followed by reperfusion, ^{201}Tl uptake and washout kinetics were normal.[62]

Myocardial infarction size is an important determinant of prognosis. It is therefore likely that if resting ^{201}Tl scintigraphy is a reliable indicator of the size of the infarction, it should also be a helpful clinical indicator of prognosis. Indeed multiple clinical studies have confirmed this prognostic relationship. Pérez-González and co-workers noted that 61% of patients with ^{201}Tl perfusion abnormalities involving greater than 35% of the myocardium died during a 16-month follow-up study compared to a 7% mortality in those with smaller infarctions.[63] Botvinick and co-workers noted that the ^{201}Tl defect score was a better predictor of postinfarction cardiac events than resting ejection fraction was.[64] Hakki and colleagues compared the power of thallium defect size on rest imaging, left ventricular ejection fraction assessed by radionuclide ventriculography, and frequency of ventricular ectopy on 24-hour ambulatory monitoring to determine prognosis in patients after myocardial infarction.[65] Thallium defect size was approximately equivalent to ejection fraction and ambulatory monitoring combined in predicting outcome.

In summary, rest ^{201}Tl imaging has good sensitivity for detection of myocardial infarction. The sensitivity is increased with acute infarction, transmural infarction, and probably with SPECT imaging technique. Overall, thallium defect size correlates well with the extent of myocardial infarction. However, a significant minority of subjects, particularly those with recent infarction or severe underlying anatomic disease, will have perfusion defects after rest injection that will reperfuse on redistribution scans, indicating at least a component of residual viability and therefore potential reversibility. In these clinical subsets, therefore, it is prudent to perform routine late follow-up redistribution scintigrams after rest ^{201}Tl injection. Thallium defect size on rest thallium studies is a good indicator of prognosis in patients with myocardial infarction.

Exercise thallium scintigraphy

Exercise procedure. An intravenous line is established before exercise. The patient is exercised to symptomatic maximum usually on a treadmill, utilizing a standard exercise protocol. Approximately 1 minute before peak exercise, ^{201}Tl is injected through the intravenous line, followed by a 20 ml saline flush. Because coronary blood flow decreases rapidly after exercise, it is important that the patient continue to exercise at least 30 seconds and preferably 1 minute after isotope injection to allow time for myocardial uptake while coronary blood flow is still at peak levels.

When utilizing planar scintigraphy, it is preferable to begin imaging within 5 minutes after ^{201}Tl injection because significant redistribution of activity can occur within the first 30 minutes.[66,67] With SPECT imaging, redistribution becomes apparent more slowly. In addition, it is advantageous to allow the patient more time to recover from exercise before SPECT imaging in order to avoid "upward-creep" artifacts. For this reason, it is often useful to acquire a single 45-degree LAO planar view after exercise before beginning the SPECT acquisition. This can be helpful for assessment of lung ^{201}Tl uptake, breast attenuation artifacts, and initial ^{201}Tl distribution in the perfusion areas of all three major coronary arteries. The delay in initiating the SPECT acquisition does not affect its sensitivity.

Sensitivity and specificity for detection of coronary artery disease. In an extensive analysis and review of the literature, Kotler and Diamond concluded that the sensitivity of exercise thallium scintigraphy using qualitative visual assessment for detection of coronary artery disease is 84%, and the specificity is 87%.[68] Sensitivity and specificity are enhanced when multiple observers interpret the studies together.[69] Although intraobserver variability of image interpretation is relatively low, interobserver variability is considerable, particularly when defect location is specified.[70]

Several studies have suggested that quantitative analysis of planar thallium scintigrams increases both sensitivity and specificity to approximately 90%.[32,71,72] Kaul and coinvestigators found that computer-aided analysis of thallium images is superior to visual analysis even when multiple observers are employed in the visual interpretation.[73] Abdulla and colleagues observed that computer quantitation of myocardial thallium washout rate improves the detection of segmental myocardial hypoperfusion.[74] In contrast, Niemeyer and co-workers found that quantitative analysis did not significantly add to the detection or assessment of extent of coronary artery disease when compared to visual analysis in their study of 203 patients.[75]

The finding of diffuse slow ^{201}Tl washout on quantitative scintigraphy has been proposed to be a useful indicator of extensive coronary artery disease, improving sensitivity.[76] Subsequent studies, however, have indicated that caution should be exercised in using washout analysis in clinical interpretation of studies. Kaul and co-workers demonstrated that myocardial thallium washout is influenced by other variables besides severity of coronary artery disease.[77] The peak heart rate achieved during exercise in particular will influence thallium washout rate. In a careful evaluation of 114 subjects, Becker and colleagues demonstrated that ^{201}Tl washout is strongly influenced by both exercise heart rate and exercise duration.[78] In their study, washout of ^{201}Tl from areas perfused by stenotic coronary vessels was not significantly different from normal areas in the same patients. Even in patients with a completely normal coronary angiogram, regional variabilities in thallium washout exist, probably as a result of limitations in the imaging technique.[79] For these reasons, though quantitation of ^{201}Tl washout can be a useful adjunct increasing the sensitivity of thallium scintigraphy, it also has the potential to significantly decrease specificity and should not be used as a substitute for an experienced eye in image interpretation.

Van Train and co-workers reported results of a multicenter trial that examined the sensitivity and specificity of computer quantification of planar thallium scintigrams in diagnosing coronary artery disease.[80] They found the sensitivity to be 93%, similar to the sensitivity previously reported from a single center evaluation of the same algorithm.[32] The specificity, however, was only 50%, which was substantially lower than what had been previously reported (91%). This considerable decline in specificity has been attributed to both pretest and posttest referral bias.[81] Pretest referral bias reflects a change in the prevalence of disease in the population being tested. Posttest referral bias is a result of using the noninvasive test result to identify patients who require angiography. Patients with abnormal exercise thallium scintigrams are more likely to undergo cardiac catheterization because of the study's result. For this reason, false-positive studies are preferentially overrepresented in the catheterization population. This posttest referral bias was believed to be less operative at the time of the original study when the clinical utility of the ^{201}Tl scintigraphy was less well established.

Another important consideration in assessing the specificity of exercise thallium scintigraphy is the patient sample used to define normal. Two factors are involved. First, patients without "significant" disease by coronary angiography (that is, those with less than 50% obstruction) may nevertheless have myocardial ischemia during exercise resulting from the atherosclerotic obstruction.[82,83] Coronary angiography is a poor standard for coronary artery disease, in that the appearance of the vessel as demonstrated by silhouette imaging of the vessel lumen has limited ability to predict maximum flow through the vessel. Peak coronary blood flow is less related to percentage of stenosis than it is to minimal residual luminal area, the length of stenoses present, the existence of serial lesions, the influence of collateral channels, and the level of subendocardial wall stress present during exercise. Hence some patients with "insignificant" coronary stenoses at angiography have meaningful limitations in peak coronary blood flow, which in turn can be associated with thallium perfusion defects at exercise. These apparent false-positive thallium scintigrams in fact represent false-negative coronary angiograms with respect to ischemia.

Second, patients who have sufficient clinical signs and symptoms to warrant coronary angiography might have occult cardiac disease that is unrelated to coronary atherosclerosis and thus not be true normals. This might theoretically include small vessel disease, occult myocardial or valvular disease, or abnormalities in myocardial metabolism or cellular function that are currently undescribed but contributed to the patient's original symptoms. In these patients, thallium images might not be representative of true normals, as determined from studies performed on subjects who have a very low probability of disease based upon clinical and noninvasive variables, without undergoing an invasive study.[84,85] The specificity of quantitative ^{201}Tl scintigraphy compared to a population with a low probability of disease, sometimes referred to as the normalcy rate, is substantially greater than specificity compared to angiographic normals.[80] Assessing scintigraphy compared to angiographic normals probably produces underestimates of specificity, whereas assessing it compared to clinical normals may result in overestimation of specificity.[86]

In recent years, single-photon emission computed tomography (SPECT) has been widely utilized in thallium imaging. SPECT offers potential advantages over planar imaging for identification and localization of perfusion defects, particularly by eliminating superimposition of normal areas upon abnormal areas as occurs with planar scintigraphy. The improved spatial resolution of the technique affords the possibility of improving recognition of individual vessel disease. Multiple investigators have noted that the sensitivity and specificity of SPECT ^{201}Tl imaging are comparable to those reported with planar imaging. (Table 12-1).[37,87-91] With qualitative visual analysis, the sen-

Table 12-1 Sensitivity and specificity of SPECT thallium Imaging

Author	Year	Number of subjects	Qualitative		Quantitative	
			Sens (%)	Spec (%)	Sens (%)	Spec (%)
Tamaki[87]	1984	104	80	93	91	92
DePasquale[37]	1988	210	97	68	95	71
Iskandrian[88]	1989	272	82	62		
Maddahi[89]	1989	110			95	56
Mahmarian[90]	1990	360	87	76	87	87
Van Train[91]	1990	371			94	64
TOTALS		1427	87	75	92	74

Table 12-2 Specificity of SPECT ^{201}Tl defined in angiographic normals and clinical normals

Author	Year	Angiographic normals		Low probability of disease	
		Number	Specificity (%)	Number	Specificity (%)
Iskandrian[88]	1989	58	62	131	93
Maddahi[89]	1989	18	56	28	86
Van Train[91]	1900	64	47	115	82

sitivity of SPECT ^{201}Tl imaging is estimated to be 87% and the specificity 75%. With quantitative analysis, the sensitivity is increased slightly to 92%, without apparent change in specificity (74%), though the reported specificities have ranged widely in different studies. Similar to the observations from planar scintigraphy, several studies have noted that the specificity of SPECT ^{201}Tl imaging is greater when defined in a population with a low probability of disease (normalcy rate) compared to a population with no significant disease determined by angiography (Table 12-2). Kotler and Diamond concluded from their extensive review and analysis of the literature that, overall, SPECT imaging appears to have a somewhat higher sensitivity and lower specificity than planar imaging.[68] SPECT imaging is particularly prone to artifactual attenuation defects in the inferior and posterior walls, in addition to the more common attenuation artifacts that result from the breast and diaphragm as seen in planar imaging.

Although SPECT imaging has the potential to improve the overall accuracy of thallium imaging compared to planar imaging, there are only very limited data available to substantiate this possibility. In a small study, Nohara and co-workers found that SPECT imaging provided better detection of individual vessel disease and of triple-vessel disease than planar imaging did.[92] Fintel and colleagues found that SPECT imaging using receiver-operating-characteristic analysis offers improved diagnostic performance compared to planar

imaging, at least in certain subgroups. They suggest that it is the imaging procedure of choice.[93] Overall, however, there have not been sufficient studies directly comparing planar to SPECT ^{201}Tl imaging in the same patients to permit firm conclusions about the relative accuracy of the two techniques. Additional studies are necessary.

Regardless of the technique utilized, the sensitivity of thallium imaging increases with the number of vessels involved. The sensitivity for detection of single-vessel disease is less than for multiple-vessel disease. Kotler and Diamond noted that overall sensitivity for detection of single-vessel disease by planar imaging with qualitative analysis is 78%, for double-vessel disease is 89%, and for triple-vessel disease is 92%.[68] It has not been demonstrated that quantitation of scintigrams improves detection of single-vessel disease. Maddahi and co-workers[32] and Kaul and co-workers[94] both reported no difference in detection of single-vessel disease comparing visual to quantitative analysis of planar scintigrams. However, quantitation of planar ^{201}Tl scintigrams might improve recognition of individual vessel involvement compared to visual image interpretation.[32] The results with SPECT imaging are similar. Mahmarian and co-workers found that quantitation of SPECT scintigrams did not improve the sensitivity for detection of single-vessel disease compared to visual reading.[90] Sensitivity for detection of circumflex disease is the lowest of the three major vessels using either planar[32,95] or SPECT[90,96] imaging, probably because of both its comparatively posterior location, and its smaller area of perfusion. Quantitation of planar images appears to improve detection of right coronary artery disease, whereas quantitation of SPECT images improves detection of disease in the left anterior descending and circumflex vessels.[32,37,90,93]

Because peak heart rate achieved during exercise is directly related to the peak level of coronary blood flow attained and because thallium imaging compares the relative uptake of isotope in one wall of myocardium compared to another, it is likely that sensitivity for disease detection will be related to peak heart rate. Surprisingly, however, Esquivel and colleagues found that by using careful quantitative techniques, peak heart rate did not influence the sensitivity of ^{201}Tl imaging for detection of disease in patients with symptomatic coronary artery disease.[97] However, peak heart rate might be more important in detecting disease in asymptomatic populations because such persons are likely to have less severe disease, which would require higher levels of myocardial blood flow to be detected. Furthermore, it is also likely that detection of multiple-vessel disease will also be related to heart rate, since higher levels of coronary blood flow will be necessary to allow detection of abnormalities in those vessels that have lesser severity of obstruction. Supporting this hypothesis, Stewart and co-workers noted that submaximal exercise thallium studies had only a 57% sensitivity and 46% specificity for detection of disease in non–infarct related arteries of patients with recent myocardial infarction.[98] In addition to possible effects on sensitivity, peak heart rate will help determine the severity and extent of ^{201}Tl perfusion defects, providing useful information about severity of disease. The target-to-background ratio of thallium uptake in the myocardium is also increased with increasing peak heart rates; this will result in improved image contrast. Finally, peak exercise performance itself provides information that is useful in the diagnostic and prognostic assessment of patients. For these reasons, although a sub-maximal peak heart rate during exercise may not decrease the overall sensitivity and specificity of thallium imaging for detection of coronary artery disease, higher peak heart rates are nevertheless likely to enhance the overall assessment of disease severity and distribution, as well as prognosis.

Because the predicted range of peak heart rate based on age and sex is wide, for any individual it is impossible to predict maximum heart rate with acceptable accuracy. It is therefore preferable not to stop the exercise test at any arbitrary peak heart rate, but rather to continue it to symptomatic maxi-

mum. At the conclusion of the test, one can then evaluate the peak heart rate achieved and compare it to the predicted maximum to determine the adequacy of the exercise performance for the individual. If a test is being performed to make a diagnosis of coronary artery disease or to assess its severity, it is preferable when clinically advisable to withhold a beta-blocker, diltiazem, or verapamil medication before the test. Although these medications do not directly effect thallium uptake and washout, their withdrawal will permit attainment of a higher peak heart rate during exercise. Patients should be counseled to limit their activity while they are not using the medication.

The specificity of thallium scintigraphy is decreased in the presence of left bundle branch block (LBBB). Hirzel and coinvestigators noted that all 19 of their patients with LBBB had anteroseptal perfusion defects but only 4 had left anterior descending disease at angiography.[99] In contrast to these findings, Jazmati and colleagues found a low prevalence (14%) of false-positive septal perfusion defects in their study of 93 patients with LBBB.[100] Others, however, have confirmed the high prevalence of false-positive defects in these patients.[101,102] To investigate the cause of the perfusion defects, Hirzel performed thallium imaging in 7 dogs during right ventricular pacing to simulate LBBB.[99] They noted that thallium activity in the septum was reduced to 69% of maximum during right ventricular pacing, whereas in the lateral wall it was 90%. Corresponding regional blood flow measurements showed similar decreases in septal blood flow, apparently as a result of asynchronous contraction of the septum. Some patients with LBBB have accompanying septal myocardial fibrosis. Septal perfusion defects in these instances could also be a manifestation of fibrosis as well as of the LBBB itself. The presence of an apical perfusion abnormality on SPECT studies has been reported to improve the accuracy of diagnosis of coronary disease in patients with LBBB, but the specificity of this finding has been variable.[101,103]

Exercise ^{201}Tl scintigraphy in evaluation of the postrevascularization patient. Stress thallium scintigraphy is widely used to identify the presence of recurrent ischemia in patients who have undergone prior revascularization, either by percutaneous transluminal coronary angioplasty (PTCA) or coronary artery bypass surgery (CABG).

Several researchers have investigated the utility of thallium imaging in predicting restenosis after PTCA. These were recently well summarized by DePuey.[104] Hardoff and co-workers performed atrial pacing stress studies 12 to 24 hours after PTCA in 90 patients and related the findings to late follow-up catheterization in 70 patients.[105] Of 104 dilated vessels, 38% had reversible ^{201}Tl perfusion abnormalities. These vessels were at high risk of developing late restenosis (sensitivity 77%, specificity 67%). Only 7 of 65 (11%) vessels without early redistributing ^{201}Tl defects developed late restenosis. Hence in this study stress ^{201}Tl scintigraphy very early after PTCA was predictive of late restenosis. If confirmed, these findings would have very interesting implications about the mechanisms of restenosis, an indication that the early luminal dimension after angioplasty is predictive of the late biological response.

Several studies have used exercise thallium scintigraphy 2 to 6 weeks after PTCA in an effort to predict restenosis. Miller and colleagues performed ^{201}Tl studies 4 weeks after PTCA in 50 patients who were followed for 18 months.[106] Postangioplasty gradient (greater than 20 mm Hg), reduced ^{201}Tl clearance, and transient ^{201}Tl defects were found to be additive predictors of subsequent adverse events. Breisblatt and co-workers noted that 17 of 121 PTCA patients developed chest pain within the first 4 to 6 weeks after the procedure.[107] Of these, 9 had reversible ^{201}Tl perfusion defects. All 9 developed restenosis. Of the 104 asymptomatic patients, 25% also had redistributing ^{201}Tl perfusion defects. Of these, 85% developed restenosis within 6 months, and 96% developed it by 1 year. A total of 42 patients developed restenosis within 1 year; 31 (74%) had redistributing ^{201}Tl scans at 4 to 6 weeks. Wijns and coinvestigators reported nearly identical experience in that 74% of their patients who developed restenosis within 6 months after PTCA had abnormal exercise ^{201}Tl studies at 4 weeks.[108] Somewhat in contrast to these findings, Stuckey and colleagues noted that although a redistributing ^{201}Tl perfusion abnormality was the only significant independent predictor of restenosis of the clinical, exercise, and angiographic variables that they evaluated, its sensitivity for predicting restenosis was only 39%.[109] Moreover, Manyari and co-workers noted that ^{201}Tl scans often show delayed improvement after PTCA.[110] In their study, myocardial perfusion abnormalities in the distribution of the affected artery progressively improved over time, an indication that early defects may not necessarily be assumed to be harbingers of restenosis. Their sample was highly selected, however, in that it included only patients with single-vessel disease who did not have restenosis 6 to 9 months after PTCA. Finally, Reed and coinvestigators noted that a redistributing thallium perfusion abnormality was the only independent predictor of restenosis in patients who underwent PTCA of a saphenous vein bypass graft.[111]

Taken together, these studies indicate that patients who will develop restenosis after PTCA can be identified with reasonable but certainly imperfect sensitivity and specificity by exercise ^{201}Tl scintigraphy 2 to 6 weeks after the procedure and possibly as early as within 24 hours. Exercise ^{201}Tl scintigraphy can also be utilized to identify the "culprit lesion" causing symptoms in the patient with multiple-vessel disease who could only incompletely be revascularized with PTCA.[112]

Exercise thallium scintigraphy has also been used to evaluate patency of coronary artery bypass grafts. Ritchie and colleagues reported that 54% of bypass grafts were patent in their patients with exercise-induced perfusion abnormalities, compared to 87% of grafts in the patients without exercise defects.[113] Greenberg and co-workers noted that ^{201}Tl scintigraphy had 77% sensitivity for recognizing graft occlusion, graft stenosis, or native vessel stenosis beyond graft insertion.[114] Hirzel and co-workers found a good correlation between thallium perfusion scintigrams and graft patency in their study of 54 patients.[115] They noted that the thallium findings were better predictors of graft patency than either clinical symptoms or the exercise electrocardiographic results. Forty percent of patients who were symptom free and had normal exercise electrocardiograms continued to have exercise-induced perfusion defects, indicating incomplete revascularization, whereas 53% of patients with persistent chest pain symptoms, often showing abnormal exercise electrocardiograms, had resolution of thallium perfusion defects compared to their preoperative study condition. Pfisterer and co-workers reported findings from a prospective controlled study of 55 patients who underwent exercise thallium scintigraphy preoperatively and 2 weeks and 1 year after bypass surgery.[116] The serial ^{201}Tl studies had an 80% sensitivity and 88% specificity for detection of graft occlusion, as assessed by angiography. All grafts were patent in 90% of patients who did not have new perfusion defects on follow-up evaluation.

Gibson and coinvestigators reported findings from 47 patients who underwent exercise thallium studies 4 weeks before coronary bypass surgery and again 7 weeks later.[117] Using quantitative analysis, they found that 19 of 42 (45%) persistent defects on the preoperative study showed normal perfusion postoperatively. The majority of these segments had normal or only mildly abnormal wall motion on the preoperative study. Only 21% of defects with a great reduction of thallium activity (more than 50% reduction) on the preoperative study showed improved perfusion after surgery compared to 57% of defects that had a 25% to 50% reduction in activity preoperatively (Figure 12-12).

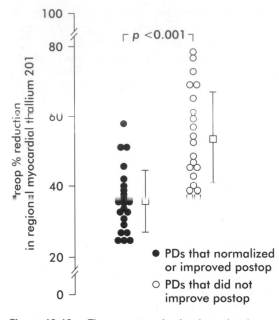

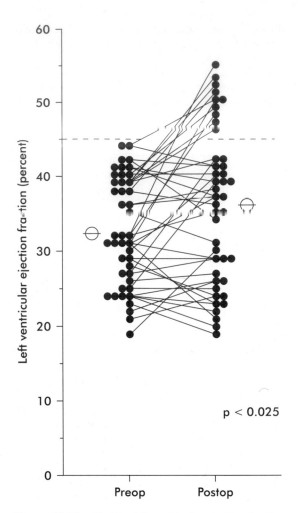

Figure 12-12 The percent reduction in regional myocardial thallium uptake is shown from 42 patients with fixed ²⁰¹Tl-perfusion defects on pre–coronary bypass examinations. Those patients who had improved or normalized ²⁰¹Tl uptake in the area of the defect postoperatively, *open circles,* had less severe perfusion defects preoperatively than those who did not improve postoperatively. (From Gibson et al: *J Am Coll Cardiol* 1:804-815, 1983.)

Figure 12-13 Resting left ventricular ejection fraction is shown before and 6 months after coronary artery bypass surgery in 43 patients with preoperative left ventricular dysfunction. *Dashed line,* Lower limit of the normal range for that laboratory. As a group, surgery resulted in only a small increase in ejection fraction. However, 15 patients (35%) had substantial increases in ejection fraction, including 10 (23%) whose ejection fraction became normalized. (From Bonow RO and Dilsizian V: *Semin Nucl Med* 21:230-241, 1991.)

Assessment of myocardial viability. Patients with chronic left ventricular dysfunction as a group have only small increases in left ventricular ejection fraction after coronary artery bypass surgery.[118] However, a subgroup of approximately 35% of these patients have substantial increases in ejection fraction, and approximately 20% will normalize their ejection fraction (Figure 12-13). This finding implies that these patients have ischemic myocardium at rest (hibernating myocardium), which is still viable and can regain function when revascularized.

Thallium perfusion abnormalities present at rest or persistent nonredistributing ²⁰¹Tl defects after exercise scintigraphy have been assumed to imply infarction and therefore nonviability of myocardium. Early pathological studies reported a strong correlation between the mass of myocardial infarction and the size of resting thallium perfusion defects.[55,119] However, some patients with large resting perfusion defects have small infarctions at autopsy.[47] In an early clinical study of 25 consecutive patients who underwent coronary bypass surgery, Rozanski and co-workers reported that 90% of segments that had reversible asynergy after revascularization had a normal thallium redistribution pattern on the preoperative exercise study.[120]

They concluded that the thallium redistribution pattern on images acquired 3 to 6 hours after exercise was a good predictor of the presence or absence of reversibility of dysfunction after revascularization.

Subsequent studies, however, have demonstrated that nonredistributing ²⁰¹Tl perfusion defects commonly represent ischemic and viable rather than infarcted tissue, which will recover if revascularized. Liu and colleagues noted that 75% of regions with persistent ²⁰¹Tl perfusion defects normalized after PTCA in their study of patients with single-vessel left anterior descending artery disease.[121] As previously discussed, multiple investigators have demonstrated that thallium perfusion defects that are present after resting injection frequently show redistribution on follow-up scans; redistribution of activity implies viable myocardium, which will regain function if revascularized.[50,53,122,123] Similar observations have been made with exercise scintigraphy. In patients with prior infarctions up to 50% of segments and in patients without infarction up to 76% of segments that have apparent fixed perfusion ^{201}Tl defects after exercise will improve after PTCA.[124] A majority of these segments with fixed ^{201}Tl perfusion defects also show active glucose metabolism by PET imaging, again an indication of viability.[54,125] Late redistribution scanning 24 hours after exercise improves the detection of reversibility of perfusion defects compared to imaging at approximately 3 to 4 hours. Occasionally, however, ^{201}Tl redistribution will be apparent in segments at 4 hours and not be present at 24 hours.[126] Although some investigators have suggested that redistribution imaging can be performed as late as 72 hours after injection, count statistics are likely to be poor.[127] Kayden and co-workers noted that thallium studies performed after separate resting injection were superior to 24-hour redistribution imaging for detection of reversibility of defects, primarily because of the poor quality of the images obtained even at 24 hours.[128]

Dilsizian and co-workers examined the role of thallium reinjection after exercise imaging for improving the detection of viable myocardium. In a study of 100 patients, 33% of 260 abnormal segments had fixed ^{201}Tl perfusion abnormalities on redistribution scintigrams obtained 3 to 4 hours after exercise.[129] In 49% of these segments, ^{201}Tl uptake improved or normalized when the images were repeated after injection of a second thallium dose. Of interest, in 5% of segments reperfusion was present on the initial redistribution images and not on the images after reinjection. In a subset of patients who underwent coronary angioplasty, 87% of segments identified as being viable on the reinjection images had normal thallium uptake and improved wall motion after PTCA. Twenty-four hour redistribution imaging adds very little additional information to that obtained from redistribution imaging done at 4 hours and again immediately after ^{201}Tl reinjection.[130] Similar to the findings of the previous study, however, 8% of segments that had reperfusion on the initial redistribution images did not have it on the repeat images taken after ^{201}Tl reinjection. Both sets of redistribution images contained virtually all the information gained by 24-hour redistribution scans, but neither early redistribution scan alone was sufficient.

Finally, Bonow and coinvestigators reported findings from a study of 16 CAD patients with chronic left ventricular dysfunction (mean ejection fraction 27%) who underwent exercise thallium scintigraphy using a reinjection protocol and a PET study with ^{18}F-fluorodeoxyglucose.[131] The combination of findings including the presence or absence of ^{201}Tl redistribution after reinjection and the severity of the perfusion defect provided concordant information to that obtained from the [18]FDG study in 88% of segments. Segments with only mild (60% to 85% of peak activity) or moderate (50% to 59% of peak activity) fixed perfusion defects after reinjection were found to be viable by [18]FDG imaging in 91% and 84% respectively. [18]FDG activity was much less in segments that had significant (less than 50% of peak) fixed ^{201}Tl defects. Further studies in larger numbers of patients will be necessary, but these initial results indicate that exercise ^{201}Tl imaging using a reinjection protocol with subsequent imaging at 4 hours, 24 hours, or at rest may provide most of the information relative to myocardial viability that is provided by [18]FDG.

Assessment of disease severity and prognosis. Equally important to its sensitivity and specificity for detecting coronary artery disease is the ability of exercise thallium scintigraphy to stratify disease severity and to assess prognosis. Several recent publications have provided excellent reviews of this topic.[68,132,133]

Exercise ^{201}Tl scintigraphy has demonstrated utility for identification of patients with left main or triple-vessel coronary artery disease. The presence of multiple perfusion defects,[134-138] increased lung uptake of thallium with exercise,[136,139,140] diffuse slow washout of ^{201}Tl activity,[76,141] and transient left ventricular dilatation during exercise[142] have all been associated with the presence of severe anatomic disease. Although thallium indicators of severe ischemia may be more common in patients with left main disease,[136] none of the parameters reliably differentiates left main disease from triple-vessel disease, a finding that is not surprising in the context of coronary pathophysiology.[76,135,136] Perfusion defects that simultaneously involve the proximal and midinterventricular septum as well as the posterolateral wall on the planar 45-degree LAO view are somewhat specific but insensitive indicators of left main disease (Figure 12-14).[134,136] Exercise ^{201}Tl scintigraphy is more sensitive than exercise electrocardiography in detecting left main or triple vessel disease;[136,138] information from the two modalities has been found to be additive in some studies[134,138,143] but not in others.[136] Nygaard and co-workers found that the combination of exercise ^{201}Tl scintigraphy and the exercise electrocardiography was no better than scintigraphy alone in identifying left main

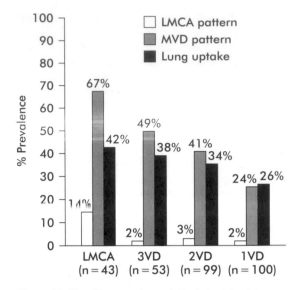

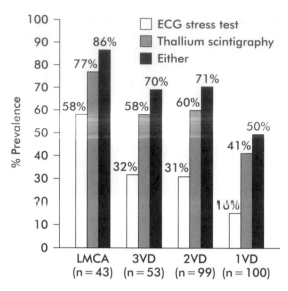

Figure 12-14   The prevalence (%) of the left main coronary artery (LMCA) scintigraphic pattern, the multivessel disease (MVD) scintigraphic pattern, and increased thallium lung uptake in patients with single (1VD), double (2VD), or triple (3VD) vessel disease or left main coronary artery disease is shown. The prevalence of the LMCA pattern and the MVD pattern were both higher in the patients with LMCA disease than in the other three groups. (From Nygaard TW et al: *Am J Cardiol* 53:462-469, 1984.)

Figure 12-15   The prevalence of high-risk thallium scintigraphic and electrocardiographic (ECG) stress test findings are shown for patients with single (1VD), double (2VD), and triple (3VD) vessel disease and with left main coronary artery disease (LMCA). (From Nygaard TW et al: *Am J Cardiol* 53:462-469, 1984.)

disease, whereas scintigraphy added significantly to the detection of severe disease compared to the exercise ECG (Figure 12-15).[136] In a later follow-up study from the same institution, however, the number of perfusion defects present, the presence or absence of ST-segment depression, and age contributed to the prediction of multiple-vessel disease (Figure 12-16).[144] Maddahi and colleagues also noted that the exercise ECG contributed significantly to the sensitivity of scintigraphy for detection of severe disease (Figure 12-17).[138] Specificity was decreased by adding the ECG variables, but the difference was not statistically significant. Overall, the cumulative findings indicate that ^{201}Tl scintigraphy is superior to exercise electrocardiography for detection of multiple-vessel coronary disease, but the exercise electrocardiogram contributes significant additional information.

Increased lung uptake of ^{201}Tl is a manifestation of left ventricular dysfunction during exercise,[145] which can be attributable either to ischemia or to underlying resting left ventricular dysfunction resulting from prior myocardial infarction or any of the other causes of myocardial damage.[139,146] When seen in the presence of normal resting ventricular function, increased lung [201]Tl

uptake indicates severe exercise-induced ischemia. The best discriminator of lung thallium uptake is the number of diseased vessels present,[147] but even patients with single-vessel left anterior descending disease can have abnormal lung ^{201}Tl uptake during exercise.[148] Hence, it is the severity of ischemia rather than the number of diseased vessels themselves that determines lung ^{201}Tl uptake. Lung ^{201}Tl uptake is also inversely related to the peak heart rate achieved during exercise and to beta-blocker therapy.[149,150] Criteria for abnormality must take these variables into account.

Quantitative analysis of ^{201}Tl scintigrams appears to increase the sensitivity for detection of left main or triple-vessel disease compared to qualitative visual analysis. In a study of 105 consecutive patients with suspected coronary artery disease, Maddahi and co-workers noted that the sensitivity of visual interpretation of ^{201}Tl scintigrams for identification of left main or triple-vessel disease was only 16%; it increased to 63% when quantitative analysis was employed (Figure 12-17).[138] It is somewhat of concern in interpreting these findings that the sensitivity of qualitative reading was so low, since an earlier study from the same laboratory reported a sensitivity for detection of triple-vessel disease using visual interpretation of 53%.[32] If the sensitivity for detection of multiple-vessel disease using qualitative analysis was underestimated in the subsequent study, it would

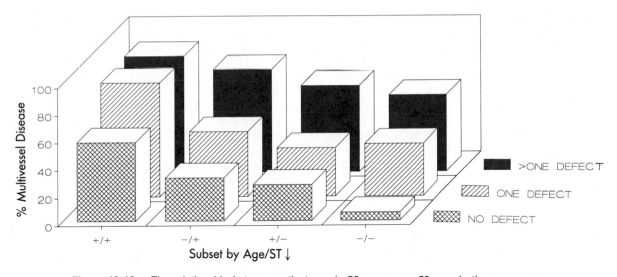

Figure 12-16   The relationship between patient age (<58 years or ≥58 years), the presence or absence of ST-segment depression on the exercise electrocardiogram, and the number of thallium-perfusion defects that are present on the scintigram are shown relative to the likelihood of multiple vessel coronary artery disease. The imaging information was the best predictor of multiple vessel disease, but both age and ST-segment depression added to its predictive power. (From Pollock SG et al: *Am J Med* 90:345-352, 1991.)

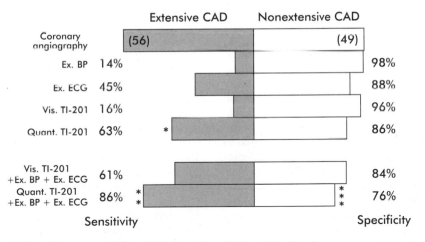

Figure 12-17   The comparative sensitivity and specificity of the blood pressure response to exercise (Ex BP), exercise electrocardiogram (Ex ECG), and exercise thallium (^{201}Tl) scintigraphy using either qualitative visual (vis) or quantitative (quant) interpretation for predicting extensive angiographic disease are shown. (From Maddahi J et al: *J Am Coll Cardiol* 7:53-60, 1986.)

have resulted in overestimation of the benefit of quantitation. However, the sensitivity of quantitative analysis was also greater in the initial study. The difference in results comparing the two studies might have been a reflection of the severity of disease in the two study populations. Iskandrian and colleagues reported that, in their experience, qualitative analysis was comparable to quantitative analysis for detection of multiple-vessel disease, and neither was specific in differentiating double-vessel disease from triple-vessel disease.[151]

Although the data are limited, SPECT ^{201}Tl imaging may improve recognition of multiple-vessel disease compared to planar imaging. Nohara and co-workers reported findings from a study that compared SPECT imaging to planar imaging in a comparatively small number of patients, approximately 40% of whom had prior myocardial infarction.[92] The sensitivity for detection of multiple-vessel disease was greater using SPECT imaging in this study, primarily because of improved recognition of circumflex vessel disease. Fintel and colleagues found that SPECT imaging provided improved recognition of circumflex and left anterior descending disease, but the benefit was primarily in patients with single-vessel disease and disease of mild severity.[93] Currently available data are insufficient to warrant conclusions about the relative sensitivity, specificity, and accuracy of SPECT imaging versus planar imaging for detection of multiple-vessel disease.

Exercise ^{201}Tl scintigraphy also has efficacy in identifying the presence of multiple-vessel disease in patients with myocardial infarction. Dunn and colleagues reported exercise ECG and ^{201}Tl scintigraphic findings from 65 patients with prior myocardial infarction.[152] Of the 40 patients with multiple-vessel disease, 85% had perfusion abnormalities in more than one area, whereas only 70% had a positive exercise ECG. On the other hand, of the 37 patients who had more than one perfusion abnormality, 92% were found to have multiple-vessel disease compared to 72% of the patients with a positive ECG. Patterson and co-workers reported similar findings in a study of 40 patients evaluated after a single transmural infarction.[153] Gibson and coinvestigators described scintigraphic findings from 42 patients with recent infarction who underwent submaximal exercise ^{201}Tl scintigraphy.[154] Of 23 clinical and laboratory variables that they considered, the presence of multiple perfusion defects was the best predictor of multi-vessel disease. The predictive accuracy of the ECG response for multiple-vessel disease was 45%, compared to 88% for scintigraphy. Abraham and colleagues found that the exercise ECG and thallium scintigrams had identical sensitivity (64%) for detection of multiple-vessel disease in their study of 103 postinfarction patients.[155] Because of the relatively lesser sensitivity for detection of disease in the right coronary artery or circumflex vessel, ^{201}Tl scintigraphy is a better predictor of multivessel disease in patients with inferior infarction (detecting additional LAD distribution ischemia) than it is in patients with anterior infarction (detecting right coronary artery or circumflex distribution ischemia.)[156]

A somewhat separate consideration from the ability of exercise ^{201}Tl scintigraphy to allow prediction of the presence of multiple-vessel disease or left main disease is its ability to help the prediction of prognosis in patients without or with prior myocardial infarction.

The patient population without prior myocardial infarction is an obviously diverse one, representing a very broad range of prognostic risk, which depends on the presence or absence of symptoms of chest discomfort, age, sex, and the presence of other coronary artery disease risk factors. The utility of ^{201}Tl scintigraphy for defining prognosis is heavily influenced by the absolute level of risk in the sample tested. Exercise thallium studies add little to the prediction of prognosis in populations who are at low risk of subsequent cardiac events based upon the history and a resting electrocardiogram. In higher risk populations ^{201}Tl imaging contributes important prognostic information.

Several studies have examined the role of exercise thallium scintigraphy in predicting prognosis of ambulatory patients with chest pain. In an early study, Brown and co-workers followed 139 consecutive patients who were managed without surgery for a mean of 3.7 years.[157] They noted that the presence of exercise-induced ^{201}Tl perfusion abnormalities was the single most important predictor of subsequent death or myocardial infarction. Other variables that were assessed did not add significantly to the information provided from scintigraphy. Iskandrian and colleagues reported similar findings from a larger study of 743 patients with known or suspected coronary disease.[158] In their study, multivariate analysis showed that the number of reperfusing ^{201}Tl defects was the most powerful predictor of subsequent cardiac events. Again no other variables added to the predictive power of the scintigraphic findings. In a follow-up study of 515 patients, Koss and co-workers noted that exercise ^{201}Tl scintigraphy was a reliable predictor of cardiac death but was not reliable in predicting nonfatal myocardial infarction.

In a study of 819 patients who were followed for 1 year, Staniloff and coinvestigators noted that the cardiac event rate at 1 year was increased tenfold in the 23% of their patients who had redistributing ^{201}Tl defects compared to the 69% of subjects who had normal or equivocal scans.[159] Of importance, the absolute risk rate in the group with unremarkable ^{201}Tl scans was extremely low (less than 1%.) The number and severity of ^{201}Tl defects added to the prognostic implication of the positive study. However, the strongest predictors of risk also occurred quite infrequently, which diminishes their utility. Ladenheim and co-workers evaluated 1689 patients who had symptoms of coronary artery disease but had no prior myocardial infarction or coronary bypass surgery.[160] They identified three variables from stepwise logistic regression analysis that were found to be independent predictors of risk. These included the number of myocardial regions with reversible ^{201}Tl defects, the maximal severity of the perfusion defects, and the peak heart rate achieved during exercise. Gill and co-workers noted in their study of

525 consecutive patients that lung thallium uptake was the single most important predictor of prognosis.[161] No other combination of variables was able to replace the information provided by lung ^{201}Tl uptake. However, this study was limited by the fact that no measurements of left ventricular function were available. The information provided from lung ^{201}Tl uptake could possibly have been provided from a measurement of resting left ventricular function, without necessitating the performance of exercise.

In 1988, Kaul and coinvestigators reported findings from two similar follow-up studies of ambulatory patients with chest pain who had undergone exercise thallium scintigraphy and coronary angiography at the University of Virginia Medical Center[162] or at the Massachusetts General Hospital[163] between 1978 and 1981. In the Virginia population, the number of diseased vessels was the most important single predictor of risk, followed by the number of segments showing ^{201}Tl redistribution. The ^{201}Tl findings were the most important predictor of nonfatal myocardial infarction. The change in heart rate with exercise and the presence of ST-segment depression during exercise also contributed independent information. Although the number of diseased vessels at angiography was the most important predictor of risk, the combined information from the exercise test and thallium scan was equally powerful in predicting prognosis as the angiographic information was. In the Massachusetts population, the lung-to-heart ratio of ^{201}Tl uptake was the single most important predictor of risk, followed by the number of diseased vessels and the change in heart rate during exercise. The findings from angiography did not add significantly to the information from the exercise ^{201}Tl study whereas the ^{201}Tl findings were marginally superior to the cardiac catheterization findings and were significantly superior to the exercise test findings. Very similar findings were described recently from a study of 432 patients in Belgium, reported by Melin and co-workers.[164] Exercise ^{201}Tl scintigraphy can also stratify risk in elderly patients with coronary artery disease.[165]

Although exercise thallium scintigraphy can provide important diagnostic and prognostic information, large subgroups of patients at low risk can be readily identified simply from the history and resting electrocardiogram. In those subgroups, ^{201}Tl scintigraphy adds little to the assessment of prognosis. In a related study to the above-cited reference, Ladenheim and coinvestigators reported follow-up findings from their study of 1659 patients.[166] In the 1451 patients who had a normal resting electrocardiogram, the clinical history provided most of the prognostic power. Neither the exercise electrocardiogram nor the ^{201}Tl study alone added to the prognostic information contained in the history. Together the two tests did add to the prognostic assessment, but the magnitude of the effect was small. In contrast, in the 208 patients who had an abnormal electrocardiogram, the history was much less useful in assessing prognosis. In that subgroup, both the exercise electrocardiogram and the ^{201}Tl study added meaningful prognostic information. The authors suggested that this is the subgroup that would benefit most from the exercise scintigraphic study.

In patients with prior myocardial infarction, exercise ^{201}Tl scintigraphy also provides useful prognostic information. The landmark study addressing this question was that of Gibson and colleagues who reported the findings from a predischarge submaximal exercise ECG, thallium scintigram, and coronary angiogram that were performed on 140 consecutive patients who had an uncomplicated myocardial infarction.[167] The cumulative probability of a subsequent cardiac event was greater in patients who were identified as being at high risk by ^{201}Tl scintigraphy, exercise testing, or angiography. Each study predicted mortality with comparable accuracy, but scintigraphy was the most sensitive in predicting recurrent infarction or progressive angina (Figure 12-18). Scintigraphy identified 94% of the high-risk patients, whereas the exercise ECG detected only 56%. Scintigraphy was also more sensitive than angiography, primarily because angiography failed to identify subsequent events in the patients who had single vessel disease, whereas 12 of 13 of these patients had abnormal scintigrams. Scintigraphy predicted low-risk status better than either exercise testing or angiography did. Abraham and co-workers noted trends toward increased cardiac events in infarct patients who had ST-segment depression during exercise, ^{201}Tl perfusion defects in areas not involved by the infarction, or multiple-vessel disease demonstrated at angiography, but none of these variables achieved statistical significance in predicting outcome.[155] The combination of the exercise ECG and ^{201}Tl findings, however, was a significant predictor of risk (relative risk 3.1).

Increased lung uptake of thallium after exercise has been associated in other studies with increased prognostic risk in postinfarction patients.[161] In infarct patients with single-vessel coronary artery disease, the presence of a redistributing ^{201}Tl perfusion abnormality is also a useful predictor of prognosis.[168] In infarction patients who were treated with thrombolytic therapy, however, predischarge submaximal exercise thallium scintigraphy may not have the same power for predicting adverse prognosis. Tilkemeier and colleagues

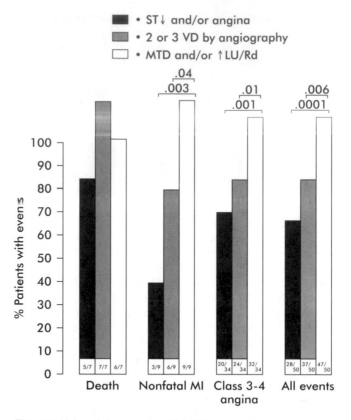

Figure 12-18 The sensitivity of the exercise ECG (ST-segment depression or angina, or both), angiogram (two- or three-vessel disease), and thallium scintigram (multiple ^{201}Tl-perfusion defects, or increased lung uptake of thallium, or both) for prediction of death, recurrent nonfatal myocardial infarction, class 3 or 4 angina, and total events are shown. (From Gibson RS et al: *Circulation* 68:321-336, 1983.)

noted that scintigraphy had only a 55% sensitivity for detection of cardiac events in the subsequent year in their 64 patients who had thrombolytic treatment, compared to 81% sensitivity in the 107 patients who did not receive thrombolytic therapy. This lower sensitivity in the intervention group could reflect the presence of more unstable plaques, which are subject to rethrombosis or progressive occlusion in this subset.

The prognostic value of exercise ^{201}Tl scintigraphy is not only in its ability to identify an adverse prognosis, but also in its ability to identify a favorable prognosis. In 1985, Wackers and colleagues reported follow-up findings from 95 patients who had chest pain but a normal quantitative exercise thallium scintigram.[170] Only 3 patients had a cardiac event (2 nonfatal MIs and 1 PTCA) over a nearly 2-year follow-up period, representing an infarction risk of 1% per year. All 3 cardiac events occurred in patients who had a high pretest probability of disease. These findings were very similar to those that were reported by Pamelia and co-workers in the same year.[171] In their 3-year follow-up study of 349 patients with chest pain and a normal ^{201}Tl study, the risk of death or myocardial infarction was 1.1% per year.[172] Wahl and colleagues also reported very similar experience in the same year. In their study, the exercise ^{201}Tl scintigram was superior to the exercise ECG in the assessment of risk, primarily because of patients who had chest pain but a nondiagnostic exercise electrocardiogram. Koss and co-workers noted that the risk of cardiac death was low in patients with chest pain who had a normal ^{201}Tl study, but noted in their study that the ^{201}Tl test had limited value in predicting risk of nonfatal myocardial infarction.[173] Nevertheless, subsequent investigators have confirmed the finding that patients who have chest pain but a normal exercise ^{201}Tl scintigram have an extremely low risk of subsequent cardiac events.[174,175]

Comparison of the sensitivity and specificity of the exercise ECG and exercise ^{201}Tl scintigraphy. In a metanalysis of 24,000 patients, Gianrossi and colleagues concluded that the sensitivity of exercise testing for diagnosis of coronary artery dis-

Table 12-3 Sensitivity of exercise ^{201}Tl scintigraphy compared to exercise electrocardiography in relation to number of diseased vessels

	Single vessel, n = 56 (%)	Double vessel, n = 40 (%)	Triple vessel, n = 40 (%)	Left main, n = 13 (%)	Total, n = 152 (%)
ST-segment depression	33 (59)*	26 (65)*	33 (77)*	11 (85)*	103 (68)*
[201]Tl imaging (qualitative)	40 (71)	31 (77)	38 (88)	11 (85)	120 (79)
[201]Tl imaging (quantitative)	46 (82)	37 (92)	42 (98)	13 (100)	138 (91)

Adapted from Kaul et al: *JAMA* 255:508-511, 1986.[179]
*$p < 0.05$ compared to quantitative thallium.

ease is 68% and the specificity is 77%.[176] They noted, however, that there is a very wide range in the reported experience that cannot be entirely accounted for from the published information. In comparison, the sensitivity of exercise ^{201}Tl scintigraphy is approximately 84%, and the specificity is 87%.[68] Exercise ^{201}Tl scintigraphy is more sensitive than exercise electrocardiography for detection of coronary artery disease at all levels of exercise and at all peak heart rates; it is particularly beneficial in patients who achieve submaximal peak heart rates during exercise.[97,177] In women, exercise scintigraphy is both more sensitive and more specific than exercise electrocardiography in the detection of coronary artery disease.[178] Exercise ^{201}Tl scintigraphy is more sensitive than exercise electrocardiography for detection of single-, double-, or triple-vessel coronary disease (Table 12-3).[179] Nygaard and co-workers noted that a high-risk test result was more prevalent using thallium scintigraphy than it was with exercise electrocardiography in patients with left main or three-vessel disease.[136]

Kotler and Diamond correctly point out, however, that it is more appropriate to compare the sensitivity and specificity of exercise electrocardiography compared to exercise ^{201}Tl scintigraphy combined with exercise electrocardiography rather than to exercise electrocardiography alone, since information from both tests is used clinically in any patients who undergo an exercise scintigraphic study.[68] They conclude that exercise scintigraphy adds to the sensitivity of exercise electrocardiography, but when the two tests are combined, specificity is decreased. Exercise scintigraphy does provide useful additional information that influences clinical decision making about the need for coronary angiography and has its greatest effect in those with an intermediate probability of disease.[180] It is primarily beneficial from a diagnostic standpoint in patients who have an abnormal resting electrocardiogram[181] or a nondiagnostic exercise electrocardiogram.[182] Physicians utilize the test more often to obtain functional information,

however, than they do simply for diagnostic information, and they consider the test to be of considerable clinical value.[183]

In asymptomatic subjects, a positive exercise ECG has a positive predictive value for diagnosing coronary artery disease of only 26%.[184] In a study of 191 healthy U.S. Air Force crewmen with positive exercise ECG results, Uhl and co-workers noted that only 21% had significant CAD at angiography.[185] Within this population, however, only 1% who had a normal thallium scan had disease at angiography, whereas 74% of those with an abnormal ^{201}Tl study had CAD at angiography. This improved diagnostic accuracy of ^{201}Tl scintigraphy in asymptomatic populations has been confirmed in other studies.[186-188] Although thallium scintigraphy is also a better indicator of prognosis in asymptomatic subjects than exercise electrocardiography is,[189] it is not cost effective to routinely use thallium scintigraphy to screen asymptomatic populations at risk.[190,191] It is preferable to perform exercise electrocardiography first in appropriate asymptomatic subjects at risk of CAD, when they have a normal baseline electrocardiogram. Thallium scintigraphy is indicated only in those who have a positive exercise ECG result. Because of the high false-positive rate associated with exercise electrocardiography in patients with an abnormal resting electrocardiogram, (particularly those with left ventricular hypertrophy, resting ST-T wave abnormality, digitalis therapy, Wolff-Parkinson-White syndrome, or bundle branch block), exercise ^{201}Tl scintigraphy is the initial screening test of choice. The appropriate asymptomatic populations in whom screening for occult CAD is appropriate is poorly defined by available data.

The prevalence of coronary artery disease in middle-aged patients with typical angina is approximately 90%, in patients with atypical chest pain is 50%, and in patients with nonanginal pain is 10%.[192] Overall, exercise ^{201}Tl scintigraphy has better sensitivity for detection of coronary artery disease in ambulatory patients with chest pain than exercise electrocardiography does.[97,192,193] Perhaps more importantly, multiple studies have shown that exercise ^{201}Tl scintigraphy has better power to stratify risk in patients with chest pain than exercise electrocardiography does.[157,160,162,163] A strongly positive ECG response to exercise (greater than 2 mm) even in patients with documented coronary artery disease is actually associated with low mortality risk with medical therapy.[194]

In postinfarction patients, development of ^{201}Tl perfusion abnormalities in more than one vascular distribution during submaximal exercise is a more sensitive and more accurate predictor of the presence of high-risk coronary anatomy than is the presence of ST-segment depression on the exercise electrocardiogram.[152,153] ST-segment depression in the postinfarction patient is a nonspecific indicator of ischemia in the absence of chest pain.[195] A normal ECG response to submaximal exercise is equally unreliable. Fully half of postinfarction patients who have a normal exercise ECG have redistributing ^{201}Tl perfusion abnormalities suggestive of ischemia, and these defects are associated with an increased risk of cardiac events over 5 years (Figure 12-19).[196] Overall, exercise ^{201}Tl scintigraphy is a better indicator of prognosis than exercise electrocardiography in postinfarction patients.[167]

In summary, exercise thallium scintigraphy appears to have better sensitivity and specificity for detection of coronary artery disease than exercise electrocardiography does and has better power to detect the presence of multiple-vessel disease or

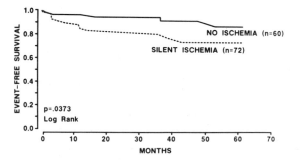

Figure 12-19 Kaplan-Meier survival curves for 132 patients who underwent a submaximal exercise test an average of 10 days after infarction and had a normal electrocardiographic response without chest pain. Despite the absence of apparent ischemia by symptoms or the electrocardiogram, 72 of the patients had redistributing thallium-perfusion abnormalities either in the area of the infarction or in a different area. Event-free survival was significantly worse in those patients who had redistributing ^{201}Tl-perfusion defects compared to those who did not. (From Gibson RS: *Curr Probl Cardiol* 13:1-72, 1988.)

increased prognostic risk in patients with or without prior infarction. Its primary benefit appears to be in subjects who have intermediate or high levels of risk based upon clinical and exercise findings.

Pharmacological stress thallium imaging. A limitation of using exercise as a modality to evaluate coronary artery disease, be it with exercise electrocardiography or exercise ^{201}Tl scintigraphy, is that many patients who have or are at risk of having coronary artery disease cannot exercise effectively. This includes patients who have peripheral vascular disease or complications of cerebrovascular disease, patients with advanced degenerative joint disease particularly when it involves the hips or knees, patients with severe obstructive pulmonary disease, many elderly patients, and many patients with diabetes mellitus, particularly those with end stage renal disease. Because of the high risk associated with known or occult coronary disease in these populations, it is desirable to be able to screen them noninvasively with regard to coronary perfusion in order to assess disease severity and prognosis. The emergence of pharmacological stress testing has provided this capability.

Pharmacological stress tests can be categorized into two groups, those that produce coronary vasodilatation as a means of assessing coronary vasodilator reserve (dipyridamole and adenosine) and those that produce ischemia by increasing myocardial oxygen demand (dobutamine).

Adenosine is a naturally occurring nucleotide that has potent cardiovascular effects that have been extensively summarized recently.[197] Although its primary cardiac effect is coronary vasodilatation,[198] it also depresses sinoatrial node and atrioventricular node function, reduces atrial contractility, attenuates the stimulatory actions of catecholamines on ventricular myocardium, decreases ventricular automaticity, and attenuates the release of norepinephrine induced by adrenergic nerve stimulation. It has vasoconstricting properties in the renal afferent arterioles and in the hepatic veins.[199] It is formed both intracellularly and extracellularly by dephosphorylation of adenosine monophosphate, and intracellularly by degradation of S-adenosylhomocysteine.[197] The primary cardiac source of adenosine appears to be the cardiomyocyte, with lesser production under normal circumstances originating in vascular endothelium.[200,201] Adenosine is a very powerful coronary vasodilator that mediates its effects through activation of purine receptors (A_1 and A_2 adenosine receptors) on vascular endothelium, resulting in a great decrease in resistance at the level of the R2 vessels. It appears to inhibit the slow inward calcium current, decreases Ca^{++} uptake, and activates adenylate cyclase. It has an extremely short biological half-life, which is measured in seconds, with primary metabolism occurring in red blood cells and coronary vascular endothelium.[197] The primary effect of dipyridamole is one of potentiating adenosine by inhibiting adenosine access to enzymatic degradation in both vascular endothelium and red blood cells.[202] Aminophylline is a direct blocker of the effects of both adenosine and dipyridamole by virtue of its effect of blocking endothelial adenosine-binding sites (Figure 12-20).

Both intravenously administered adenosine and

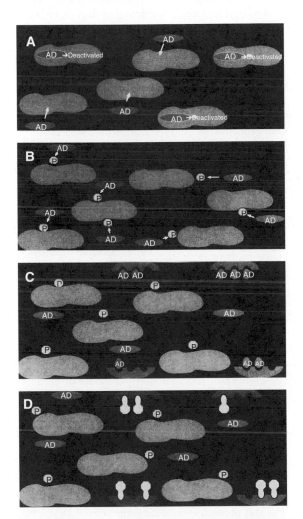

Figure 12-20   The mechanism of action of dipyridamole and adenosine are portrayed. Adenosine is metabolized primarily by the RBC membrane-bound enzyme adenosine deaminase, **A.** Dipyridamole blocks the access of adenosine to these membrane binding sites, thereby inhibiting its metabolism, **B.** Adenosine's vasodilating effect is mediated through binding to endothelial receptors, **C.** Aminophylline occupies the endothelium binding site for adenosine, directly blocking its effect, **D.** (From Botvinick EH and Dae MW: *Semin Nucl Med* 21:242-265, 1991.)

dipyridamole decrease coronary vascular resistance at the level of the R2 vessels, resulting in a considerable increase in coronary flow, which typically exceeds that attained by maximal exercise. In clinically administered doses, adenosine has a somewhat more powerful vasodilator potency than dipyridamole does, though the magnitude of effect on flow of the two agents is similar, probably because central aortic perfusion pressure decreases more with adenosine.[203] In normal coronary vessels, both endocardial and epicardial flow increase greatly with infusion of these agents. However, in the presence of a critical coronary obstruction, epicardial flow might increase only slightly in response to vasodilator infusion, whereas endocardial flow actually decreases as a result of a transmural physiological coronary steal.[204-206] The increase in flow is much greater in the distribution of normal vessels than it is in abnormal vessels because normal vessels have much greater R2 vessel vasodilator reserve. If ^{201}Tl is injected at the peak of the vasodilator effect, its myocardial distribution will reflect this disparity in flow, resulting in a regional perfusion abnormality.[207] These agents cause reduced uptake and slower clearance of ^{201}Tl in vessels with a coronary stenosis compared to a normal vascular region.[208,209]

Dipyridamole is administered by a 4-minute intravenous infusion at a dose of 0.56 mg/kg (0.14 mg/kg/min).[210,211] Its peak effect is 7 to 8 minutes after initiation of infusion, at which time ^{201}Tl is injected.[212-216] Combining dipyridamole infusion with handgrip exercise increases the peak level of coronary blood flow achieved compared to infusion alone.[217] The duration of dipyridamole effect is 30 to 60 minutes and is prolonged in hepatic failure.[202] Aminophylline can be administered by intravenous infusion beginning 3 to 4 minutes after ^{201}Tl administration, in a dose of 1 to 2 mg/kg. Prophylactic aminophylline infusion may be warranted even in the absence of early side effects in order to avoid the development of delayed side effects during imaging. Although an aminophylline dose of 75 to 100 mg is usually adequate, a dose of 250 mg can be administered by slow infusion when necessary.[202]

Adenosine is administered intravenously in a dose of 140 µg/kg/min for 4 to 6 minutes. Thallium is administered 1.5 to 2 minutes before the end of the infusion. The duration of effect of adenosine is extremely brief, approximately 1 to 2 minutes, and so aminophylline administration is rarely necessary. Because theophylline and caffeine have similar properties to aminophylline in blocking the effects of dipyridamole or adenosine, they must be withheld for 48 hours before the study.[218-220] For a dipyridamole study it is not necessary to withhold oral dipyridamole therapy, but it is necessary to withhold it for an adenosine study because the dipyridamole could prolong and potentiate the adenosine effect, possibly increasing risk of adverse reactions.

The safety and side-effect profile of intravenously administered dipyridamole is well established. There is less accumulated experience with adenosine infusion. Side effects with dipyridamole infusion are very common, primarily reflecting the vasodilating actions of the agent. The most frequent side effects are chest pain, headache, dizziness, nausea, and hypotension. ST-segment depression occurs in 8%, likely because of an intracoronary steal, which ironically may be facilitated by the presence of collateral channels.[221] The mechanism of chest pain is unclear, but it is not a specific indicator of myocardial ischemia.[222] Chest pain is a common side effect of adenosine infusion even in normal volunteers.[223]

The overall safety profile of dipyridamole infusion is quite favorable although major adverse events can rarely occur. In a recent report of Boehringer-Ingelheim's cumulative safety data representing nearly 4000 patients, the incidence of major adverse events was 0.26%.[224] Minor side effects occurred in 46%. There were 2 (0.05%) reported deaths, both attributable myocardial infarction and 2 (0.05%) other nonfatal infarctions. Three of these 4 patients had recent unstable angina. Six patients (0.15%) experienced acute bronchospasm, all reversed by aminophylline. However, severe bronchospasm leading to respiratory arrest has been reported.[225] Two recent large series reported no major side effects in studies of 800 patients.[226,227] Five studies have demonstrated that intravenous dipyridamole can be used safely in patients in the early post–myocardial infarction period.[228-232]

Side effects with adenosine infusion are also common and in many instances are similar to dipyridamole. Flushing and chest pain are the most frequent, each occurring in about 40% of patients.[199] Some degree of heart block occurs in about 6% of patients with adenosine infusion; in about 3% it is high grade. However, it resolves rapidly with discontinuation of the infusion.[199]

The reported sensitivity and specificity of intravenous dipyridamole ^{201}Tl perfusion imaging for detection of coronary artery disease are comparable to exercise ^{201}Tl imaging.[233] The sensitivity for detection of CAD, as determined from pooling results from 11 published series, is 85%, whereas the specificity is 91%.[234] Five early studies have reported comparative findings from a total of 215 patients who underwent both exercise thallium scintigraphy and dipyridamole thallium scintigraphy.[233,235-238] Combining the findings from these studies, the sensitivity of the two tests was the same at 79%.[239] The specificity of exercise scintigraphy was 92%, and that of dipyridamole scintigraphy was 95%.

Dipyridamole scintigraphy is useful in differentiating ischemic from nonischemic cardiomyopathy.[240] Increased lung uptake of ^{201}Tl after dipyridamole infusion is an indicator of the presence of CAD, though the reported findings have been mixed as to its relationship to disease severity.[241-243] Dilatation of the left ventricular cavity with dipyridamole ^{201}Tl imaging has been suggested to be a highly specific marker of triple-vessel coronary disease, reflecting diffuse subendocardial hypoperfusion.[244] Varma and colleagues demonstrated that segmental uptake and redistribution of ^{201}Tl are similar comparing exercise and dipyridamole studies in regions with and without significant coronary obstructions.[208] Quantification of ^{201}Tl washout has been noted to be predictive of the presence of CAD.[245] Of importance, however, it has been reproducibly shown, using quantitative scintigraphy, that clearance of ^{201}Tl is slower between the initial and redistribution scans with dipyridamole imaging than it is with exercise imaging.[208,246-248] Isolated washout abnormalities therefore should be used with caution in implicating CAD in the absence of perfusion defects.

There is less accumulated experience with adenosine scintigraphy, but its sensitivity and specificity appear to be quite similar to exercise scintigraphy and dipyridamole imaging. In a review of findings from 132 patients, Iskandrian noted that the sensitivity of adenosine imaging was 87% in patients with single-vessel disease, 92% in double-vessel disease, and 98% in triple-vessel disease.[199] Verani and co-workers reported a sensitivity of 83% and specificity of 81% in their study of 89 patients.[249] Most of the false-negative results were in patients with single-vessel disease. In a subsequent report summarizing their experience from over 1000 patients, they noted that the sensitivity of adenosine ^{201}Tl scintigraphy was 87% and the specificity 94%.[250] Nguyen and co-workers found that the predictive accuracy of SPECT ^{201}Tl imaging was slightly higher ($p = $ nonsignificant) with adenosine imaging compared to exercise imaging.[251] Of interest, 25 patients underwent both adenosine-perfusion imaging and adenosine echocardiography. Only 10% of the CAD patients had adenosine induced wall-motion abnormalities, whereas 80% had reversible ^{201}Tl perfusion abnormalities. Coyne and colleagues also noted similar findings comparing adenosine (sensitivity 83%, specificity 75%) to exercise (sensitivity 81%, specificity 75%) ^{201}Tl scintigraphy in their study of 100 subjects.[252] Dipyridamole and adenosine ^{201}Tl studies have not been directly compared in the same patients.

Dipyridamole ^{201}Tl scintigraphy has been found to be an effective tool for stratifying risk in various populations, similar to the experience reported using exercise scintigraphy. The presence of multiple ^{201}Tl perfusion defects, increased lung uptake after infusion, and transient left ventricular dilatation have been associated with increased prognostic risk.[243] Younis and coinvestigators evaluated 107 asymptomatic patients with coronary artery disease.[253] Using logistic regression analysis, they found that a reversible ^{201}Tl defect was the only significant predictor of subsequent cardiac events of the clinical, angiographic, and scintigraphic variables that they considered. When death or myocardial infarction were the outcome variables tested, the presence of combined fixed and redistributing perfusion defects was the only predictor of outcome. In a study of 516 consecutive patients, Hendel and colleagues noted that an abnormal dipyridamole ^{201}Tl perfusion scan was a significant independent predictor of myocardial infarction and subsequent cardiac death, increasing the risk threefold compared to those who had a negative study.[226] The presence of ^{201}Tl redistribution on the scintigram further increased the prognostic risk. The clinical presence of diabetes mellitus, prior myocardial infarction, or congestive heart failure provided additional prognostic information.

Dipyridamole ^{201}Tl scintigraphy can also be used to assess prognosis in the postinfarction patient. Leppo and co-workers performed predischarge dipyridamole ^{201}Tl studies on 51 patients with infarction.[254] Among the clinical and scintigraphic variables tested, they found that the presence of ^{201}Tl redistribution was the only significant predictor of subsequent serious cardiac events over a 19-month follow-up period. In the 26 patients who had a predischarge submaximal exercise test, the perfusion study appeared to be a better predictor of prognosis. Gimple and co-workers found that dipyridamole ^{201}Tl scintigraphy provided prognostic information similar to that provided by submaximal exercise testing, noting that ^{201}Tl redistribution outside the infarction territory was a sensitive (63%) and specific (75%) predictor of subsequent events.[255] Redistribution in the infarct zone was frequent and nonspecific in their experience. In contrast, Brown and coinvestigators performed dipyridamole scintigraphy an average of 62 hours after infarction in their study of 50 patients, without serious adverse reactions.[256] Using stepwise multivariate logistic regression analysis, they found that the presence of ^{201}Tl redistribution in the area of the prior infarction was the best and only significant predictor of subsequent ischemic events during the remainder of the patients' hospitalization. Of the 20 patients who had ^{201}Tl redistribution in the infarct zone, 45% developed further inhospital ischemic events, compared to none in the 30 patients without infarct zone ^{201}Tl redistribution. During follow-up study over the next 12 months, 3 additional patients with infarct zone redistribution developed further ischemia, whereas there were no events in the patients without redistribution. Nienaber and colleagues noted in their study of 80 consecutive postinfarction patients with chest pain that a reperfusing defect in a noninfarct territory indicated greater prognostic risk than ischemia in the infarct zone did or the presence of only a fixed perfusion abnormality.[257] Taken together, these findings indicate that a dipyridamole ^{201}Tl study can be utilized as an effective screening tool to identify postinfarction patients who do or do not require cardiac catheterization.

Boucher and colleagues demonstrated that dipyridamole ^{201}Tl scintigraphy can also be effectively utilized to identify patients at risk of cardiac events during vascular surgery.[258] They noted that the occurrence of postoperative cardiac events was not predictable from any clinical factors but did correlate with the presence of ^{201}Tl redistribution. Eagle and coinvestigators found that in patients who had no evidence of congestive heart failure, angina, prior myocardial infarction, or diabetes mellitus, risk from vascular surgery was very low; dipyridamole ^{201}Tl imaging added little to their prognostic assessment.[259] In patients with one or more of these findings, however, 50% had ^{201}Tl redistribution and nearly one half of these had postoperative ischemic events. In contrast, none of the patients in this subgroup had ischemic events in the absence of a redistributing perfusion defect. In a follow-up retrospective study of 254 patients from the same center, these investigators noted that both redistributing ^{201}Tl perfusion defects and ST-segment depression during dipyridamole infusion contribute useful prognostic information that is additive to information provided from clinical variables.[260] However, significant subgroups at high or low risk can be identified from clinical variables, and in these subgroups a scintigraphic study is probably not warranted.

Other studies have also demonstrated both the high risk that diabetic patients have associated with vascular surgery and the role of dipyridamole ^{201}Tl scintigraphy in their assessment. Lane and co-workers, for example, noted in their study of 101 diabetic patients that ^{201}Tl perfusion abnormalities were present in 80% of patients whereas operative complications occurred in only 11%.[261] However, when quantitative variables were used, the presence of multiple redistributing defects or defects in the left anterior descending distribution were helpful predictors of subsequent events. Other studies, including two very recent studies, have reaffirmed the utility of dipyridamole imaging in stratifying perioperative risk and have indicated that it adds to information available from clinical criteria and the Goldman classification.[262-264]

In contrast to these findings, Mangano and coinvestigators recently reported their experience in a prospective study of 60 consecutive patients who were candidates for dipyridamole scintigraphy and were to undergo vascular surgery.[265] Contrary to the experience of previous studies, they noted that the scintigraphic study had poor predictive power for identifying perioperative ischemic events. They stressed that in their protocol, physicians were blinded as to the results of the scintigraphic study, thus avoiding potential bias from altering management as a result of the ^{201}Tl findings. Furthermore, they performed comprehensive perioperative monitoring for ischemia to assess its relationship to postoperative complications. They found no correlation between the presence of redistributing ^{201}Tl defects and either adverse cardiac outcome or perioperative ischemia. Further studies of this issue are indicated in view of the discrepancy in these reported findings and the importance of the clinical questions involved.

Finally, dipyridamole scintigraphy has been shown to be useful in the prediction of restenosis in patients who have undergone percutaneous transluminal coronary angioplasty. Jain and coinvestigators noted that 35% of their 53 post-PTCA patients had ischemic ^{201}Tl perfusion defects with dipyridamole scintigraphy.[266] During 22 months of follow-up observation, 33% of the patients developed restenosis; 77% of these had evidence of ischemia on the post-PTCA scintigraphic study.

In summary, ^{201}Tl perfusion scintigraphy with either dipyridamole or adenosine stress has sensitivity, specificity, and prognostic utility that is comparable to that provided by exercise scintigraphy. It is a useful substitute for exercise imaging in patients who are at risk of coronary artery disease but who cannot exercise. Because vasodilator stress studies do not provide information about ischemic threshold or correlate symptoms with ischemia, exercise scintigraphy remains the procedure of choice in patients who can exercise. Although there is no reported experience as yet with adenosine ^{201}Tl perfusion imaging in stratifying prognostic risk in patients with CAD, it is very likely that it will be comparable to dipyridamole,

since dipyridamole works through its effects on adenosine metabolism, and adenosine has at least as much if not more vasodilating power.

There is much less experience with dobutamine stress ^{201}Tl scintigraphy. It has been suggested that dobutamine scintigraphy might be a useful substitute for exercise scintigraphy in patients who cannot exercise.[267,268] Dipyridamole induces greater blood flow heterogeneity than dobutamine does, an indication that dipyridamole might be superior to dobutamine for use in perfusion imaging.[269] Dobutamine, in contrast, is more effective in inducing regional myocardial dysfunction, an indication that it would be more useful as a stress modality when used with measurements of myocardial function, such as echocardiography or radionuclide ventriculography.[269] Dobutamine could be used in patients who have bronchospastic disease, in whom dipyridamole or adenosine infusion is contraindicated. Dobutamine stress perfusion imaging has been shown to be a useful screening test for stratifying risk in patients before vascular surgery.[270] More experience will be necessary in order to determine the role of stress perfusion scintigraphy using dobutamine infusion.

[99m]Technetium myocardial perfusion agents

[99m]Technetium (metastable isotope 99) has a number of advantages over ^{201}Tl as an imaging isotope. Its 150 keV energy level is better suited for conventional imaging equipment than the lower energy of ^{201}Tl is. Tissue attenuation and scatter are both less with ^{99m}Tc because of its higher energy level. The shorter half-life of ^{99m}Tc allows for administration of larger doses in clinical imaging, resulting in improved count rates and image statistics and therefore image resolution. Finally, ^{99m}Tc is more readily available than ^{201}Tl because it is generator produced. Considering these advantages, it has been hypothesized that a myocardial perfusion agent that uses a ^{99m}Tc radiolabel would provide images that are superior to those attainable with [201]Tl.

A considerable number of ^{99m}Tc-based compounds have been developed in recent years and tested as possible myocardial perfusion agents. From these, two have emerged as the leading initial candidates for clinical imaging.[271-274] Technetium-99m methoxyisobutyl isonitrile (^{99m}Tc-sestamibi) is a monovalent cation with a central Tc(I) core that is surrounded by six lipophilic ligands coordinated through the isonitrile carbon. ^{99m}Tc-teboroxime is a neutral lipophilic technetium-containing complex that is one of a group of boronic acid adducts of technetium dioxime complexes (BATOs.)

These two compounds have very different kinetics of myocardial uptake and clearance. Sestamibi has a lower fractional extraction than ^{201}Tl does, particularly at higher flow rates, whereas teboroxime has a fractional extraction that exceeds ^{201}Tl and is nearly linear even at high flow rates. However, because sestamibi has higher parenchymal cell permeability and retention efficiency than ^{201}Tl, net myocardial concentrations are similar despite its lower extraction efficiency.[275] Sestamibi is sequestered in mitochondria by the large negative transmembrane potential. As a result, the washout of sestamibi is very slow, with minimal redistribution compared to [201]Tl.[271,276] In contrast, as a neutral compound teboroxime is not trapped but instead washes out of the heart quite rapidly, with a half-life of only 20 minutes.[271] Although teboroxime can be used with exercise in clinical imaging, its rapid washout greatly limits the practicality of its application in that setting because imaging has to be completed within less than 10 minutes of injection.[277,278] Its primary utility as a stress-imaging agent therefore is in conjunction with pharmacologic stress. For that reason, this discussion focuses on sestamibi.

[99m]Tc-sestamibi. After resting injection of sestamibi, liver activity is twice that of the heart, and gallbladder activity is extremely high (Figure 12-21, *A*).[279] Liver activity falls much more quickly than myocardial activity does. Splanchnic washout can be further accelerated by a meal of whole milk. As a result, the ratio of myocardial activity to background activity becomes suitable for cardiac imaging by approximately 30 to 60 minutes after injection. After injection during exercise initial myocardial uptake is more than twice that of the liver, resulting in a target-to-background ratio of activity that is more favorable than that occurring after rest injection. Nevertheless, gallbladder activity is again quite high (Figure 12-21, *B*).

At low flow rates, myocardial uptake of sestamibi is greater than that which would be predicted by measurement of flow using microspheres. This increased uptake is probably a result of increased extraction occurring at the lower flow rates.[280] Like thallium, sestamibi underestimates flow at higher flow rates. Sestamibi washout in clinical images is small but measurable and is slightly different in normal areas compared to ischemic areas.[281] Its kinetics appear to be less sensitive to metabolic inhibitors than those of [201]Tl.[282] Uptake of sestamibi is not inhibited by myocardial stunning or by a chronic low flow state.[280,283]

Sestamibi injection can be used with exercise to evaluate coronary artery disease and exercise-induced ischemia. A first-pass radionuclide angiogram of the sestamibi bolus can be acquired, providing the possibility of measuring ventricular function and myocardial perfusion on the same study.[284-289] Because sestamibi does not get redistributed significantly, the differentiation of ischemia from infarction requires a second injection at rest to compare with exercise uptake. It may be preferable for the two studies to be performed on separate days. For pragmatic reasons, however, it is often desirable to complete the study in a single day.

Several investigators have examined the utility of performing the two studies on the same day with

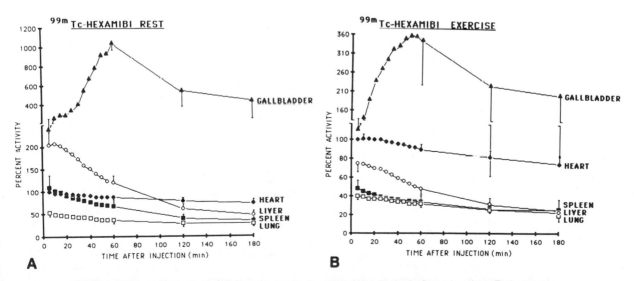

Figure 12-21   Organ time activity curves are shown at rest, **A,** and after exercise, **B,** in 5 normal volunteers each. The data are normalized to cardiac activity 5 minutes after injection. (From Wackers FJT et al: *J Nucl Med* 30:301-311, 1989.)

either the stress study first followed by the rest study, or vice versa. Borges-Neto and co-workers noted that a same-day rest/stress protocol provided image characteristics that were not significantly different from those obtained from a 2-day protocol.[290] Taillefer and colleagues concluded that performance of the rest study followed by the stress study on the same day provided the same diagnostic information as that provided by the two studies performed on separate days.[291] However, if the stress study is performed first followed by the rest study on the same day, viability of myocardium is underestimated in approximately 7% of ischemic segments.[292] In contrast to these findings, Whalley and colleagues noted that performance of the two studies on the same day, regardless of the order, resulted in a significantly higher false-negative rate than that which occurred using a 2-day protocol.[293] Further studies with larger numbers of patients will be necessary to clarify this important issue.

The sensitivity and specificity of exercise sestamibi studies for diagnosis of coronary artery disease are similar to those of exercise ^{201}Tl scintigraphy. Kahn and co-workers reported results from SPECT ^{99m}Tc-sestamibi and ^{201}Tl studies on 50 patients, 12 of whom were normal and 38 of whom had angiographic CAD.[294] The sensitivity of sestamibi in their experience, using a 2-day imaging protocol, was 95% and of ^{201}Tl was 84% (p = ns). However, the sestamibi study identified 79% of stenosed coronary arteries, whereas ^{201}Tl identified 60% ($p < 0.05$). The authors also noted that the sestamibi images were of higher quality. Taillefer and colleagues reported findings from 33 patients who were evaluated in four centers with both exercise sestamibi studies and exercise ^{201}Tl scintigraphy, again using a 2-day protocol.[295] The two studies agreed as to the findings on both a patient-by-patient comparison (88% concordance) and a segment-by-segment analysis (87% concordance). Kiat and coinvestigators reported very similar experience.[296] Sochor recently reviewed the experience of studies from Europe,[297] and Maissey and co-workers summarized published and unpublished reports, concluding that the sensitivity of exercise sestamibi is approximately 85% and is not significantly different from that of exercise ^{201}Tl scintigraphy.[298] Specificity cannot be reasonably estimated yet because there have not been sufficient studies reported. SPECT sestamibi studies appear to have improved accuracy compared to planar studies.[296,299] Quantification of sestamibi studies requires generation of new normal reference data files. Quantification of planar studies results in significant underestimation of ischemia unless a specific modified interpolative background subtraction algorithm is used.[300,301]

Although these data indicate that exercise sestamibi studies may have a sensitivity and specificity for detection of CAD which is comparable to those of ^{201}Tl, it is notable that it has not yet fulfilled expectations for improving accuracy compared to thallium.

^{99m}Tc-sestamibi studies have applicability in the evaluation of acute and prior myocardial infarction.[302] Boucher reported that resting studies have 97% sensitivity and 92% specificity for detecting infarction in their study of 118 infarct patients and 24 normals.[303] Sestamibi injection during chest pain in patients without electrocardiographic abnormalities might have utility in identifying patients with occluded vessels who are likely to evolve infarction.[304] Braat and co-workers demonstrated that sestamibi injection at the time of balloon inflation reliably demonstrates the perfusion area of the vessel, as does direct intracoronary injection during angiography.[305]

Because sestamibi does not get redistributed significantly, it offers the opportunity to assess myocardial salvage resulting from therapeutic interventions in acute infarction.[306-310] Patients can be injected with sestamibi when they present with an evolving infarction (within the limits of isotope availability), after which the therapeutic interventions can be undertaken. The patient can be imaged several hours later once he or she is stabilized, with the findings reflecting the status of myocardial perfusion that existed when the patient presented. A follow-up study can then be performed and compared to the acute-stage study to estimate the degree of myocardial salvage that resulted from the therapeutic intervention. Patients who have successful thrombolysis or successful recanalization of the infarct vessel with PTCA have greater reduction in sestamibi perfusion defect size than patients who do not recanalize.[307,308] Myocardial stunning can also be demonstrated by comparison of sestamibi defect size with ventricular function. When left ventricular ejection fraction is disproportionately reduced relative to the perfusion defect size, the possibility of reversible dysfunction caused by stunning is suggested.[311]

Compared to thallium, however, rest and exercise sestamibi studies appear to produce an underestimation of ischemia and myocardial viability. Narahara and colleagues described findings from exercise ^{201}Tl scintigrams and from rest and exercise sestamibi studies that they performed on 24 patients with coronary artery disease.[312] Although resting sestamibi defect size and ^{201}Tl redistribution defect size were very similar, exercise defects were significantly smaller in the sestamibi studies compared to those in the ^{201}Tl studies. Rocco and co-workers performed rest sestamibi studies in 26 patients with prior myocardial infarction and related the findings to wall motion assessed by equilibrium blood pool scanning.[313] Although overall there was a good correlation between perfusion defects and wall motion, they noted that 26% of territories that had absent sestamibi uptake had normal wall motion. In 8 patients who were examined before and after bypass surgery, 12 of 13 vascular territories with reduced sestamibi uptake preoperatively had improved uptake postoperatively, including all 5 segments with absent uptake initially. They concluded that the resting perfusion defects produced an underestimation of the viability of the involved myocardium. Cuocolo and coinvestigators examined 20 CAD patients who had left ventricular dysfunction.[314] Of 122 segments with fixed ^{201}Tl perfusion defects using standard exercise and redistribution scintigraphy, 47% showed enhanced uptake with ^{201}Tl reinjection. In contrast, of the same 122 segments, sestamibi scintigraphy indicated that only 18% had reversible defects. Although not all studies are in agreement,[294] these combined findings indicate that ^{201}Tl scintigraphy may be superior to sestamibi in quantifying ischemia and myocardial viability. Further study is necessary.

Sestamibi studies can also be done with dipyridamole infusion.[315] Tartagni and coinvestigators performed same-day rest and dipyridamole SPECT studies on 30 patients, who also underwent exercise ^{201}Tl scintigraphy.[316] The sensitivity (100%) and specificity (75%) of the sestamibi and ^{201}Tl studies were identical, and the identification of individual coronary artery involvement was very similar when the two techniques were compared. Kettunen and co-workers performed high-dose (0.7 mg/kg) dipyridamole infusions combined with handgrip stress in 42 patients and noted a sensitivity of 95%.[317] The sensitivity for detection of left anterior descending disease was 82%, for circumflex disease was 61%, and for right coronary artery disease was 90%. The sensitivity and specificity of the sestamibi studies were quite similar to those of ^{201}Tl performed in a subgroup of 21 patients.

Overall, therefore, sestamibi studies offer the advantages of improved image resolution, greater flexibility in imaging time, and the potential ability to assess both ventricular function and myocardial perfusion from the same test, and they have unique advantages for assessment of patients with evolving acute myocardial infarction. However, the benefit of sestamibi over thallium has not yet been demonstrated. Sestamibi has certain disadvantages compared to thallium because of its greater cost, the possible need for 2-day studies, its potential to produce an underestimation of viability compared to the reinjection thallium technique, and the substantially lesser experience with

its use compared to thallium. Its ultimate role vis-à-vis thallium imaging remains to be determined.

SUMMARY

The radionuclide imaging techniques used with either exercise stress or pharmacologic coronary artery vasodilatation provide diagnostic, pathophysiological and prognostic information that is often additive to that provided from clinical parameters and exercise electrocardiography. Myocardial perfusion imaging can be performed with thallium 201, which is still the agent of choice at the present time, or with the newer ^{99m}Tc agents sestamibi and teboroxime. Imaging can be performed using either planar or single-photon emission computerized tomography (SPECT) techniques. SPECT imaging offers the potential for improved resolution and regional localization of perfusion abnormalities, though its advantage over planar imaging has not yet been fully demonstrated. SPECT imaging appears to offer improved sensitivity, compared to planar imaging, but somewhat lower specificity. Images can be interpreted with either technique using either qualitative visual techniques, which require considerable experience and are subject to interobserver variability, or with quantitative computer techniques. Computer quantification of images improves the reproducibility of interpretation. It appears to improve detection of multiple-vessel but not single-vessel disease, possibly at the cost of somewhat lower specificity.

Thallium perfusion defects present at rest usually indicate myocardial infarction, though some resting defects will redistribute with time, representing severely ischemic but still viable myocardium. Rest thallium imaging has excellent sensitivity for detection of acute infarction; the sensitivity declines somewhat with time because the size of the defects decreases. The sensitivity is greater for transmural infarction than for subendocardial infarction. There is a significant correlation between rest thallium perfusion defect size and myocardial infarction size judged from enzymatic parameters or autopsy studies.

The sensitivity and specificity of qualitative exercise thallium scintigraphy for detection of coronary artery disease are both approximately 85%. Quantitation of images improves sensitivity to approximately 90% and increases detection of individual vessel involvement as well as the presence of multiple-vessel disease. Sensitivity increases with the number of vessels involved. The estimated specificity of the technique depends on the population used to define normal. If patients without angiographic coronary artery disease are used, the specificity of the technique is as low as 50%. However, this is probably not a representative normal population. In addition, these trials are subject to both pretest and posttest referral bias. When subjects with a low probability of coronary disease based upon clinical parameters are used to define normal, the specificity (referred to as normalcy rate) of the study increases to approximately 80% to 90%. Specificity decreases in the presence of left bundle branch block.

Exercise thallium scintigraphy has utility in the evaluation of the patient with prior revascularization therapy, whether it is with percutaneous angioplasty or coronary artery bypass surgery. The assessment of myocardial viability with thallium scintigraphy is enhanced by the use of the reinjection technique, as well as delayed imaging in selected cases at 24 hours. Using these techniques, thallium scintigraphy approaches positron emission tomography imaging with ^{18}F-fluorodeoxyglucose in the detection of viable myocardium.

Exercise thallium scintigraphy has demonstrated a capability of detecting severe anatomic coronary artery disease that is superior to that of exercise electrocardiography, but the information from the two studies is often additive. SPECT imaging appears to enhance the detection of triple-vessel or left main disease compared to planar imaging. Thallium scintigraphy also has demonstrated value in the assessment of the prognosis. Its clinical applicability in this use is dependent on the population being studied. Exercise thallium scintigraphy adds little to the prognostic assessment of populations who are at low risk of disease. Exercise ^{201}Tl scintigraphy is superior to exercise electrocardiography and is comparable to coronary angiography is the assessment of the prognosis of ambulatory patients with chest pain and in patients with recent or prior myocardial infarction. Patients with chest pain but a normal exercise thallium study have a very low incidence of cardiac events in the follow-up period.

Exercise ^{201}Tl scintigraphy is more sensitive than exercise electrocardiography in the detection of coronary artery disease at all levels of exercise and all peak heart rates and particularly adds information when the peak heart rate achieved during exercise is submaximal. It is more sensitive and more specific than exercise electrocardiography in women. ^{201}Tl scintigraphy has superior diagnostic accuracy to exercise electrocardiography in the assessment of asymptomatic subjects but is not justified for routine use in this subset. It should be reserved for use in asymptomatic subjects who are at a higher risk of coronary artery disease based upon clinical and exercise ECG parameters. Exercise ^{201}Tl scintigraphy is particularly useful in patients who have an abnormal baseline electrocardiogram.

Pharmacological stress testing with the intravenously administered coronary vasodilators dipyridamole and adenosine offers the capability for noninvasive assessment of underlying coronary disease in patients who cannot exercise. The agents have a favorable safety profile. The sensitivity and specificity for detection of coronary disease appear to be comparable to exercise imaging, and the studies have similar ability to determine prognosis. It has the disadvantage of not providing assessment of ischemic threshold or correlation of perfusion defects with clinical symptoms, nor does it provide information about functional capacity which is valuable in the assessment of prognosis and disease severity. For these reasons, exercise scintigraphy is still the preferred technique for patients who can exercise. There is insufficient experience currently available with dobutamine thallium imaging to assess its potential role.

The ^{99m}Tc perfusion agents sestamibi and teboroxime offer the advantages of ^{99m}Tc, which has energy and half-life characteristics that make it superior to ^{201}Tl for imaging. Sestamibi is different from ^{201}Tl in that it has very little redistribution with time, whereas teboroxime gets redistributed rapidly. Sestamibi can be used with exercise for assessment of coronary disease but requires separate injections at rest and during exercise, since it does not redistribute significantly. Both agents are well suited for use with pharmacological stress. The sensitivity and specificity of exercise sestamibi studies for diagnosis of coronary artery disease appears to be comparable to exercise thallium scintigraphy. It has not yet been demonstrated, however, that it is superior to ^{201}Tl, despite the superior image resolution. Sestamibi may somewhat underestimate myocardial viability compared to thallium scintigraphy. The absence of redistribution makes sestamibi particularly well suited for evaluation of patients with acute myocardial infarction.

REFERENCES

1. Follansbee WP: The heart in vasculitis. In LeRoy EC, editor: *Systemic vasculitis: the biologic basis,* New York, 1992, Marcel Dekker.
2. Schwartz JS, Tockman B, Cohn JN, et al: Exercise-induced decrease in flow through stenotic coronary arteries in the dog, *Am J Cardiol* 50:1409-1413, 1982.
3. Gage JE, Hess OM, Murakami T, et al: Vasoconstriction of stenotic coronary arteries during dynamic exercise in patients with classic angina pectoris: reversibility by nitroglycerin, *Circulation* 73:865-876, 1986.
4. Okada RD, Jacobs ML, Daggett WM, et al: Thallium-201 kinetics in nonischemic canine myocardium, *Circulation* 65:70-76, 1982.
5. Okada RD, Leppo JA, Strauss HW, et al: Mechanisms and time course for the disappearance of thallium-201 defects at rest in dogs, *Am J Cardiol* 49:699-706, 1982.

6. Okada RD: Myocardial kinetics of thallium-201 after stress in normal and perfusion-reduced canine myocardium, *Am J Cardiol* 56:969-973, 1985.

7. Chu A, Murdock RH Jr, and Cobb FR: Relation between regional distribution of thallium-201 and myocardial blood flow in normal, acutely ischemic and infarcted myocardium, *Am J Cardiol* 50:1141-1144, 1982.

8. Nielsen AP, Morris KG, Murdock R, et al: Linear relationship between the distribution of thallium-201 and blood flow in ischemic and nonischemic myocardium during rest, *Circulation* 61:797-801, 1980.

9. Gould KL, Wescott PJ, Albro PC, et al: Noninvasive assessment of coronary stenoses by myocardial perfusion imaging during pharmacologic coronary vasodilation: II, Clinical methodology and feasibility, *Am J Cardiol* 41:279-287, 1978.

10. Melin JA, Becker LC: Quantitative relationship between global left and ventricular thallium uptake and blood flow: effects of propranolol, ouabain, dipyridamole and coronary artery occlusion, *J Nucl Med* 27:641-652, 1986.

11. Hellmuth F, Weich FW, Strauss WH, et al: The extraction of thallium-201 by the myocardium, *Circulation* 56:188-192, 1977.

12. Leppo JA, Macneil PB, Moring AF, et al: Separate effects of ischemia, hypoxia, and contractility on thallium-201 kinetics in rabbit myocardium, *J Nucl Med* 27:66-74, 1986.

13. Friedman BJ, Beihn R, and Friedman JP: The effect of hypoxia on thallium kinetics in cultured chick myocardial cells, *J Nucl Med* 28.1453-1460, 1987.

14. Leppo JA: Myocardial uptake of thallium and rubidium during alterations in perfusion and oxygenation in isolated rabbit hearts, *J Nucl Med* 28:878-885, 1987.

15. Grunwald AM, Watson DD, Holzgrefe HH Jr, et al: Myocardial thallium-201 kinetics in normal and ischemic myocardium, *Circulation* 64:610-618, 1981.

16. Bergmann SR, Hack SN, Sobel BE: "Redistribution" of myocardial thallium-201 without reperfusion: implications regarding absolute quantification of perfusion, *Am J Cardiol* 49:1691 1698, 1982.

17. Beller GA, Watson DD, Ackell P, et al: Time course of thallium-201 redistribution after transient myocardial ischemia, *Circulation* 61:791-797, 1980.

18. Sklar J, Kirch D, Johnson T, et al: Slow late myocardial clearance of thallium: a characteristic phenomenon in coronary artery disease, *Circulation* 65:1504-1510, 1982.

19. Massie BM, Wisneski J, Kramer B, et al: Comparison of myocardial thallium-201 clearance after maximal and sub-maximal exercise: implications for diagnosis of coronary disease: concise communication, *J Nucl Med* 23:381-385, 1982.

20. Kaul S, Chesler DA, Pohost GM, et al: Influence of peak exercise heart rate on normal thallium-201 myocardial clearance, *J Nucl Med* 27:26-30, 1986.

21. Angello DA, Wilson RA, Palac RT: Effect of eating on thallium-201 myocardial redistribution after myocardial ischemia, *Am J Cardiol* 60:528-533, 1987.

22. Gewirtz H, Maksad AK, Most AS, et al: The effect of transient ischemia with reperfusion on thallium clearance from the myocardium, *Circulation* 61:1091-1097, 1980.

23. Okada RD, Pohost GM: Effect of decreased blood flow and ischemia on myocardial thallium clearance, *J Am Coll Cardiol* 3:744-750, 1984.

24. Atkins HL, Budinger TF, Lebowitz E, et al: Thallium-201 for medical use. Part 3: Human distribution and physical imaging properties, *J Nucl Med* 18:133-140, 1977.

25. Krahwinkel W, Herzog H, Feinendegen LE: Pharmacokinetics of thallium-201 in normal individuals after routine myocardial scintigraphy, *J Nucl Med* 29:1582-1586, 1988.

26. DiCola J, Moore M, Shearer D, et al: Limitations of visual assessment of redistribution in thallium images, *Am Heart J* 108:926-932, 1984.

27. Goris ML, Daspit SG, McLaughlin P, et al: Interpolative background subtractions, *J Nucl Med* 17:744-747, 1976.

28. Watson DD, Campbell NP, Read EK, et al: Spatial and temporal quantitation of planar thallium myocardial images, *J Nucl Med* 22:577-584, 1981.

29. Berger BC, Watson DD, Taylor GJ, et al: Quantitative thallium-201 exercise scintigraphy for detection of coronary artery disease, *J Nucl Med* 22:585-593, 1981.

30. Burow RD, Pond M, Schafer AW, et al: "Circumferential profiles": a new method for computer analysis of thallium-201 myocardial perfusion images, *J Nucl Med* 20:771-777, 1979.

31. Garcia EV, Maddahi J, Berman DS, et al: Space/time quantitation of thallium-201 myocardial scintigraphy, *J Nucl Med* 22:309-317, 1981.

32. Maddahi J, Garcia EV, Berman DS, et al: Improved noninvasive assessment of coronary artery disease by quantitative analysis of regional stress myocardial distribution and washout of thallium-201, *Circulation* 64:924-935, 1981.

33. Eisner RL, Nowak DJ, Pettigrew R, et al: Fundamentals of 180° acquisition and reconstruction in SPECT imaging, *J Nucl Med* 27:1717-1728, 1986.

34. Jaszczak RJ, Greer KL, Coleman RE: SPECT. In Rao DV, Chandra R, Graham MC, editors: *Physics of nuclear medicine: recent advances*, New York, 1984, American Institute of Physics, pp 457-482.

35. Gerson MC, Thomas SR, Van Heertum RL: Tomographic myocardial perfusion imaging. In Gerson MC, editor: *Cardiac nuclear medicine*, New York, 1991, McGraw-Hill.

36. Garcia EV, Van Train K, Maddahi J, et al: Quantification of rotational thallium-201 myocardial tomography, *J Nucl Med* 26:17-26, 1985.

37. DePasquale EF, Nody AC, DePuey EG, et al: Quantitative rotational thallium-201 tomography for identifying and localizing coronary artery disease, *Circulation* 77:316 327, 1988.

38. Eisner RL, Tamas MJ, Clininger K, et al: Normal SPECT thallium-201 bull's-eye display: gender differences, *J Nucl Med* 29:1901-1909, 1988.

39. Garver PR, Wasnich RD, Shibuya AM, et al: Appearance of breast attenuation artifacts with thallium myocardial SPECT imaging, *Clin Nucl Med* 10:694-696, 1985.

40. Friedman J, Berman DS, Van Train K, et al: Patient motion in thallium-201 myocardial SPECT imaging: an easily identified frequent source of artifactual defect, *Clin Nucl Med* 13:321-324, 1988.

41. Friedman J, Van Train K, Maddahi J, et al: "Upward creep" of the heart: a frequent source of false-positive reversible defects during thallium-201 stress-redistribution SPECT, *J Nucl Med* 30:1718-1722, 1989.

42. Geckle WJ, Frank TL, Links JM, Becker LC: Correction for patient and organ movement in SPECT: application to exercise thallium-201 cardiac imaging, *J Nucl Med* 29:441-450, 1988.

43. Wackers FJT, Schoot JB, Sokole EB, et al: Noninvasive visualization of acute myocardial infarction in man with thallium-201, *Br Heart J* 37:741-744, 1975.

44. Wackers FJT, Sokole EB, Samson G, et al: Value and limitations of thallium-201 scintigraphy in the acute phase of myocardial infarction, *N Engl J Med* 295:1-5, 1976.

45. Tiefenbrunn AJ, Biello DR, Geltman EM, et al: Gated cardiac blood pool imaging and thallium-201 myocardial scintigraphy for detection of remote myocardial infarction, *Am J Cardiol* 47:1-6, 1981.

46. Niess GS, Logic JR, Russell RO Jr, et al: Usefulness and limitations of thallium-201 myocardial scintigraphy in delineating location and size of prior myocardial infarction, *Circulation* 59:1010-1019, 1979.

47. Bulkley BH, Silverman K, Weisfeldt ML, et al: Pathologic basis of thallium-201 scintigraphic defects in patients with fatal myocardial injury, *Circulation* 60:785-792, 1979.

48. Wahl JM, Hakki A-H, Iskandrian AS, et al: Scintigraphic characterization of Q wave and non-Q-wave acute myocardial infarction, *Am Heart J* 109:769-775, 1985.

49. Ritchie JL, Williams DL, Harp G, et al: Transaxial tomography with thallium-201 for detecting remote myocardial infarction: comparison with planar imaging, *Am J Cardiol* 50:1236-1241, 1982.

50. Gewirtz H, Beller GA, Strauss HW, et al: Transient defects of resting thallium scans in patients with coronary artery disease, *Circulation* 59:707-713, 1979.

51. Stratton JR, Speck SM, Caldwell JH, et al: Relation of global and regional left ventricular function to tomographic thallium-201 myocardial perfusion in patients with prior myocardial infarction, *J Am Coll Cardiol* 12:71-77, 1988.

52. Hirsowitz GS, Lakier JB, Marks DS, et al: Sequential radionuclide angiographic assessment of left and right ventricular performance and quantitative thallium-201 scintigraphy following acute myocardial infarction, *Am Heart J* 107:934-939, 1984.

53. Iskandrian AS, Hakki A-H, Kane SA, et al: Rest and redistribution thallium-201 myocardial scintigraphy to predict improvement in left ventricular function after coronary arterial bypass grafting, *Am J Cardiol* 51:1312-1316, 1983.

54. Tamaki N, Yonekura Y, Yamashita K, et al: Relation of left ventricular perfusion and wall motion with metabolic activity in persistent defects on thallium-201 tomography in healed myocardial infarction, *Am J Cardiol* 62:202-208, 1988.

55. Wackers FJT, Becker AE, Samson G, et al: Location and size of acute transmural myocardial infarction estimated from thallium-201 scintiscans: a clinicopathologic study, *Circulation* 56:72-78, 1977.

56. Wolfe CL, Lewis SE, Corbett JR, et al: Measurement of myocardial infarction fraction using single photon emission computed tomography, *J Am Coll Cardiol* 6:145-151, 1985.

57. Kaul S, Okada RD, Pandian NG, et al: Determination of left ventricular "area at risk" with high-resolution single photon emission computerized tomography in experimental coronary occlusion, *Am Heart J* 109:1369-1374, 1985.

58. Prigent F, Maddahi J, Garcia EV, et al: Quantification of myocardial infarct size by thallium-201 single-photon emission computed tomography: experimental validation in the dig, *Circulation* 74:852-861, 1986.

59. Mahmarian JJ, Pratt CM, Borges-Neto S, et al: Quantification of infarct size by ^{201}Tl single-photon emission computed tomography during acute myocardial infarction in humans: comparison with enzymatic estimates, *Circulation* 78:831-839, 1988.

60. Tamaki S, Nakajima H, Murakami T, et al: Estimation of infarct size by myocardial emission computed tomography with thallium-201 and its relation to creatine kinase-MB release after myocardial infarction in man, *Circulation* 66:994-1001, 1982.

61. Okada RD, Boucher CA: Differentiation of viable and nonviable myocardium after acute reperfusion using serial thallium-201 imaging, *Am Heart J* 113:241-250, 1987.

62. Moore CA, Cannon J, Watson DD, et al: Thallium 201 kinetics in stunned myocardium characterized by severe postischemic systolic dysfunction, *Circulation* 81:1622-1632, 1990.

63. Pérez-González J, Botvinick EH, Dunn R, et al: The late prognostic value of scintigraphic measurement of myocardial infarction size, *Circulation* 66:960-971, 1982.

64. Botvinick EH, Pérez-González JF, Dunn R, et al: Late prognostic value of scintigraphic parameters of acute myocardial infarction size in complicated myocardial infarction without heart failure, *Am J Cardiol* 51:1045-1051, 1983.

65. Hakki AH, Nestico PF, Heo J, et al: Relative prognostic value of rest thallium-201 imaging, radionuclide ventriculography and 24-hour ambulatory electrocardiographic monitoring after acute myocardial infarction, *J Am Coll Cardiol* 10:25-32, 1987.

66. Makler PT Jr, McCarthy DM, Goldstein H, et al: Incidence of rapid resolution of defects on stress thallium scans, *Clin Nucl Med* 7:458-461, 1982.

67. Rothendler JA, Okada RD, Wilson RA, et al: Effect of a delay in commencing imaging on the ability to detect transient thallium defects, *J Nucl Med* 26:880-883, 1985.

68. Kotler TS, Diamond GA: Exercise thallium-201 scintigraphy in the diagnosis and prognosis of coronary artery disease, *Ann Intern Med* 113:684-702, 1990.

69. Okada RD, Boucher CA, Kirshenbaum HK, et al: Improved diagnostic accuracy of thallium-201 stress test using multiple observers and criteria derived from interobserver analysis of variance, *Am J Cardiol* 46:619-624, 1980.

70. Atwood JE, Jensen D, Froelicher V, et al: Agreement in human interpretation of analog thallium myocardial perfusion images, *Circulation* 64:601-609, 1981.

71. Wackers FJT, Fetterman RC, Mattera JA, et al: Quantitative planar thallium-201 stress scintigraphy: a critical evaluation of the method, *Semin Nucl Med* 15:46-66, 1985.

72. Kaul S, Boucher CA, Newell JB, et al: Determination of the quantitative thallium imaging variables that optimize detection of coronary artery disease, *J Am Coll Cardiol* 7:527-537, 1986.

73. Kaul S, Chesler DA, Okada RD, et al: Computer versus visual analysis of exercise thallium-201 images: a critical appraisal in 325 patients with chest pain, *Am Heart J* 114:1129-1137, 1987.

74. Abdulla A, Maddahi J, Garcia E, et al: Slow regional clearance of myocardial thallium-201 in the absence of perfusion defect: contribution to detection of individual coronary artery stenoses and mechanism for occurrence, *Circulation* 71:72-79, 1985.

75. Niemeyer MG, Laarman GJ, van der Wall EE, et al: Is quantitative analysis superior to visual analysis of planar thallium 201 myocardial exercise scintigraphy in the evaluation of coronary artery disease? Analysis of a prospective clinical study, *Eur J Nucl Med* 16:697-704, 1990.

76. Bateman TM, Maddahi J, Gray RJ, et al: Diffuse slow washout of myocardial thallium-201: a new scintigraphic indicator of extensive coronary artery disease, *J Am Coll Cardiol* 4:55-64, 1984.

77. Kaul S, Chelser DA, Pohost GM, et al: Influence of peak exercise heart rate on normal thallium-201 myocardial clearance, *J Nucl Med* 27:26-30, 1986.

78. Becker LC, Rogers WJ, Links JM, et al: Limitations of regional myocardial thallium clearance for identification of disease in individual coronary arteries, *J Am Coll Cardiol* 14:1491-1500, 1989.

79. Kaul S, Chesler DA, Newell JB, et al: Regional variability in the myocardial clearance of thallium-201 and its importance in determining the presence or absence of coronary artery disease, *J Am Coll Cardiol* 8:95-100, 1986.

80. Van Train KF, Berman DS, Garcia EV, et al: Quantitative analysis of stress thallium-201 myocardial scintigrams: a multicenter trial, *J Nucl Med* 1986. 27:17-25, 1986.

81. Rozanski A, Diamond GA, Berman D, et al: The declining specificity of exercise radionuclide ventriculography, *N Engl J Med* 309:518-522, 1983.

82. Brown KA, Osbakken M, Boucher CA, et al: Positive exercise thallium-201 test responses in patients with less than 50% maximal coronary stenosis: angiographic and clinical predictors, *Am J Cardiol* 55:54-57, 1985.

83. Kaul S, Newell JB, Chesler DA, et al: Quantitative thallium imaging findings in patients with normal coronary angiographic findings and in clinically normal subjects, *Am J Cardiol* 57:509-512, 1986.

84. Niemeyer MG, Laarman GJ, Lelbach S, et al: Quantitative thallium-201 myocardial exercise scintigraphy in normal subjects and patients with normal coronary arteries, *Eur J Radiol* 10:19-27, 1990.

85. Meller J, Goldsmith SJ, Rudin A, et al: Spectrum of exercise thallium-201 myocardial perfusion imaging in patients with chest pain and normal coronary angiograms, *Am J Cardiol* 43:717-723, 1979.

86. Rozanski A, Diamond GA, Forrester JS, et al: Alternative reference standards for cardiac normality: implications for diagnostic testing, *Ann Intern Med* 101:164-171, 1984.

87. Tamaki N, Yonekura Y, Mukai T, et al: Stress thallium-201 transaxial emission computed tomography: quantitative versus qualitative analysis for evaluation of coronary artery disease, *J Am Coll Cardiol* 4:1213-1221, 1984.

88. Iskandrian AS, Heo J, Kong B, et al: Effect of exercise level on the ability of thallium-201 tomographic imaging in detecting coronary artery disease: analysis of 461 patients, *J Am Coll Cardiol* 14:1477-1486, 1989.

89. Maddahi J, Van Train K, Prigent F, et al: Quantitative single photon emission computed tomography for detection and localization of coronary artery disease: optimization and prospective validation of a new technique, *J Am Coll Cardiol* 14:1689-1699, 1989.

90. Mahmarian JJ, Boyce TM, Goldberg RK, et al: Quantitative exercise thallium-201 single photon emission computed tomography for the enhanced diagnosis of ischemic heart disease, *J Am Coll Cardiol* 15:318-329, 1990.

91. Van Train KF, Maddahi J, Berman DS, et al: Quantitative analysis of tomographic stress thallium-201 myocardial scintigrams: a multicenter trial, *J Nucl Med* 31:1168-1179, 1990.

92. Nohara R, Kambara H, Suzuki Y, et al: Stress scintigraphy using single-photon emission computed tomography in the evaluation of coronary artery disease, *Am J Cardiol* 53:1250-1254, 1984.

93. Fintel DJ, Links JM, Brinker JA, et al: Improved diagnostic performance of exercise thallium-201 single photon emission computed tomography over planar imaging in the diagnosis of coronary artery disease: a receiver operating characteristic analysis, *J Am Coll Cardiol* 13:600-612, 1989.

94. Kaul S, Kiess M, Liu P, et al: Comparison of exercise electrocardiography and quantitative thallium imaging for one-vessel coronary artery disease, *Am J Cardiol* 56:257-261, 1985.

95. Massie BM, Botvinick EH, Brundage BH: Correlation of thallium-201 scintigrams with coronary anatomy: factors affecting region by region sensitivity, *Am J Cardiol* 44:616-622, 1979.

96. Korkeila P, Hietanen S, Parviainen S: Exercise thallium-201 scintigraphy in the localization of myocardial ischaemia, *Clin Physiol* 9:555-565, 1989.

97. Esquivel L, Pollock SG, Beller GA, et al: Effect of the degree of effort on the sensitivity of the exercise thallium-201 stress test in symptomatic coronary artery disease, *Am J Cardiol* 63:160-165, 1989.

98. Stewart RE, Kander N, Juni JE, et al: Submaximal exercise thallium-201 SPECT for assessment of interventional therapy in patients with acute myocardial infarction, *Am Heart J* 121:1033-1038, 1991.

99. Hirzel HO, Senn M, Nuesch K, et al: Thallium-201 scintigraphy in complete left bundle branch block, *Am J Cardiol* 53:764-769, 1984.

100. Jazmati B, Sadaniantz A, Emaus SP, et al: Exercise thallium-201 imaging in complete left bundle branch block and the prevalence of septal perfusion defects, *Am J Cardiol* 67:46-49, 1991.

101. Larcos G, Gibbons RJ, Brown ML: Diagnostic accuracy of exercise thallium-201 single-photon emission computed tomography in patients with left bundle branch block, *Am J Cardiol* 68:756-760, 1991.

102. DePuey EG, Guertler-Krawczynska E, Robbins WL: Thallium-201 SPECT in coronary artery disease patients with left bundle branch block, *J Nucl Med* 29:1479-1485, 1988.

103. Matzer L, Kiat H, Friedman JD, et al: A new approach to the assessment of tomographic thallium-201 scintigraphy in patients with left bundle branch block, *J Am Coll Cardiol* 17:1309-1317, 1991.

104. DePuey EG: Radionuclide methods to evaluate percutaneous transluminal coronary angioplasty, *Semin Nucl Med* 21:102-115, 1991.

105. Hardoff R, Shefer A, Gips S, et al: Predicting late restenosis after coronary angioplasty by very early (12-24h) thallium-201 scintigraphy: implications with regard to mechanisms of late coronary restenosis, *J Am Coll Cardiol* 15:1486-1492, 1990.

106. Miller DD, Liu P, Strauss HW, et al: Prognostic value of computer-quantitated exercise thallium imaging early after percutaneous transluminal coronary angioplasty, *J Am Coll Cardiol* 10:275-283, 1987.

107. Breisblatt WM, Weiland FL, Spaccavento LJ: Stress thallium-201 imaging after coronary angioplasty predicts restenosis and recurrent symptoms, *J Am Coll Cardiol* 12:1199-1204, 1988.

108. Wijns W, Serruys PW, Reiber JH, et al: Early detection of restenosis after successful percutaneous transluminal coronary angioplasty by exercise-redistribution thallium scintigraphy, *Am J Cardiol* 55:357-361, 1985.

109. Stuckey TD, Burwell LR, Nygaard TW, et al: Quantitative exercise thallium-201 scintigraphy for predicting angina recurrence after percutaneous transluminal coronary angioplasty, *Am J Cardiol* 63:517-521, 1989.

110. Manyari DE, Knudtson M, Kloiber R, et al: Sequential thallium-201 myocardial perfusion studies after successful percutaneous transluminal coronary artery angioplasty: delayed resolution of exercise-induced scintigraphic abnormalities, *Circulation* 77:86-95, 1988.

111. Reed DC, Beller GA, Nygaard TW, et al: The clinical efficacy and scintigraphic evaluation of post–coronary bypass patients undergoing percutaneous transluminal coronary angioplasty for recurrent angina pectoris, *Am Heart J* 117:60-71, 1989.

112. Breisblatt WM, Barness JV, Weiland F, et al: Incomplete revascularization in multivessel percutaneous transluminal coronary angioplasty: the role for stress thallium-201 imaging, *J Am Coll Cardiol* 11:1183-1190, 1988.

113. Ritchie JL, Narahara KA, Trobaugh GB, et al: Thallium-201 myocardial imaging before and after coronary revascularization: assessment of regional myocardial blood flow and graft patency, *Circulation* 56:830-836, 1977.

114. Greenberg BH, Hart R, Botvinick EH, et al: Thallium-

201 myocardial scintigraphy to evaluate patients after coronary bypass surgery, *Am J Cardiol* 42:167-176, 1978.

115. Hirzel HO, Nuesch K, Sialer G, et al: Thallium-201 exercise myocardial imaging to evaluate myocardial perfusion after coronary artery bypass surgery, *Br Heart J* 43:426-435, 1980.

116. Pfisterer M, Emmenegger H, Schmitt HE, et al: Accuracy of serial myocardial perfusion scintigraphy with thallium-201 for prediction of graft patency early and late after coronary artery bypass surgery: a controlled prospective study, *Circulation* 66:1017-1024, 1982.

117. Gibson RS, Watson DD, Taylor GJ, et al: Prospective assessment of regional myocardial perfusion before and after coronary revascularization surgery by quantitative thallium-201 scintigraphy, *J Am Coll Cardiol* 1:804-815, 1983.

118. Bonow RO, Dilsizian V: Thallium 201 for assessment of myocardial viability, *Semin Nucl Med* 21:230-241, 1991.

119. Keyes JW Jr, Brady TJ, Leonard PF, et al: Calculation of viable and infarcted myocardial mass from thallium-201 tomograms, *J Nucl Med* 22:339-343, 1981.

120. Rozanski A, Berman DS, Gray R, et al: Use of thallium-201 redistribution scintigraphy in the preoperative differentiation of reversible and nonreversible myocardial asynergy, *Circulation* 64:936-944, 1981.

121. Liu P, Kiess MC, Okada RD, et al: The persistent defect on exercise thallium imaging and its fate after myocardial revascularization: Does it represent scar or ischemia? *Am Heart J* 110:996-1001, 1985.

122. Berger BC, Watson DD, Burwell LR, et al: Redistribution of thallium at rest in patients with stable and unstable angina and the effect of coronary artery bypass surgery, *Circulation* 60:1114-1125, 1979.

123. Mori T, Minamiji K, Kurogane H, et al: Rest-injected thallium-201 imaging for assessing viability of severe asynergic regions, *J Nucl Med* 32: 1718-1724, 1991.

124. Cloninger KG, DePuey EG, Garcia EV et al: Incomplete redistribution in delayed thallium-201 single photon emission computed tomographic (SPECT) images: an overestimation of myocardial scarring, *J Am Coll Cardiol* 12:955-963, 1988.

125. Brunken R, Schwaiger M, Grover-McKay M, et al: Positron emission tomography detects tissue metabolic activity in myocardial segments with persistent thallium perfusion defects, *J Am Coll Cardiol* 10:557-567, 1987.

126. Yang LD, Berman DS, Kiat H, et al: The frequency of late reversibility in SPECT thallium-201 stress-redistribution studies, *J Am Coll Cardiol* 15:334-340, 1990.

127. Kiat H, Berman DS, Maddahi J, et al: Late reversibility of tomographic myocardial thallium-201 defects: an accurate marker of myocardial viability, *J Am Coll Cardiol* 12:1456-1463, 1988.

128. Kayden DS, Sigal S, Souffer R, et al: Thallium-201 for assessment of myocardial viability: quantitative comparison of 24-hour redistribution imaging with imaging after reinjection at rest, *J Am Coll Cardiol* 18:1480-1486, 1991.

129. Dilsizian V, Rocco TP, Freedman NMT, et al: Enhanced detection of ischemic but viable myocardium by the reinjection of thallium after stress-redistribution imaging, *N Engl J Med* 323:141-146, 1990.

130. Dilsizian V, Smeltzer WR, Freedman NMT, et al: Thallium reinjection after stress-redistribution imaging. Does 24-hour delay imaging after reinjection enhance detection of viable myocardium? *Circulation* 83:1247-1255, 1991.

131. Bonow RO, Dilsizian V, Cuocolo A, et al: Identification of viable myocardium in patients with chronic coronary artery disease and left ventricular dysfunction: comparison of thallium scintigraphy with reinjection and PET imaging with ^{18}F-fluorodeoxyglucose, *Circulation* 83:26-37, 1991.

132. Gibbons, RJ: The use of radionuclide techniques for identification of severe coronary disease, *Curr Probl Cardiol* 15:305-352, 1990.

133. Brown KA: Prognostic value of thallium-201 myocardial perfusion imaging: a diagnostic tool comes of age, *Circulation* 83:363-381, 1991.

134. Dash H, Massie BM, Botvinick EH, et al: The noninvasive identification of left main and three-vessel coronary artery disease by myocardial stress perfusion scintigraphy and treadmill exercise electrocardiography, *Circulation* 60:276-284, 1979.

135. Rehn T, Griffith LSC, Achuff SC, et al: Exercise thallium-201 myocardial imaging in left main coronary artery disease: sensitive but not specific, *Am J Cardiol* 48:217-223, 1981.

136. Nygaard TW, Gibson RS, Ryan JM, et al: Prevalence of high-risk thallium-201 scintigraphic findings in left main coronary artery stenosis: comparison with patients with multiple- and single-vessel coronary artery disease, *Am J Cardiol* 53:462-469, 1984.

137. O'Hara MJ, Lahiri A, Whittington JR, et al: Detection of high risk coronary artery disease by thallium imaging, *Br Heart J* 53:616-623, 1985.

138. Maddahi J, Abdulla A, Garcia EV, et al: Noninvasive identification of left main and triple vessel coronary artery disease: improved accuracy using quantitative analysis of regional myocardial stress distribution and washout of thallium-201, *J Am Coll Cardiol* 7:53-60, 1986.

139. Kushner FG, Okada RD, Kirshenbaum HD, et al: Lung thallium-201 uptake after stress testing in patients with coronary artery disease, *Circulation* 63:341-347, 1981.

140. Boucher CA, Zir LM, Beller GA, et al: Increased lung uptake of thallium-201 during exercise myocardial imaging: clinical, hemodynamic and angiographic implications in patients with coronary artery disease, *Am J Cardiol* 46:189-196, 1980.

141. Gewirtz H, Paladino W, Sullivan M, et al: Value and limitations of myocardial thallium washout rate in the noninvasive diagnosis of patients with triple-vessel coronary artery disease, *Am Heart J* 106:681-686, 1983.

142. Weiss AT, Berman DS, Lew AS, et al: Transient ischemic dilation of the left ventricle on stress thallium-201 scintigraphy: a marker of severe and extensive coronary artery disease, *J Am Coll Cardiol* 9:752-759, 1987.

143. McCarthy DM, Sciacca RR, Blood DK, et al: Discriminant function analysis using thallium-201 scintiscans and exercise stress test variables to predict the presence and extent of coronary artery disease, *Am J Cardiol* 49:1917-1926, 1982.

144. Pollock SG, Abbott RD, Boucher CA, et al: A model to predict multivessel coronary artery disease from the exercise thallium-201 stress test, *Am J Med* 90:345-352, 1991.

145. Boucher CA, Zir LM, Beller GA, et al: Increased lung uptake of thallium-201 during exercise myocardial imaging: clinical, hemodynamic and angiographic implications in patients with coronary artery disease, *Am J Cardiol* 46:189-196, 1980.

146. Gibson RS, Watson DD, Carabello BA, et al: Clinical implications of increased lung uptake of thallium-201 during exercise scintigraphy 2 weeks after myocardial infarction, *Am J Cardiol* 49:1586-1593, 1982.

147. Homma S, Kaul S, Boucher CA: Correlates of lung/heart ratio of thallium-201 in coronary artery disease, *J Nucl Med* 28:1531-1535, 1987.

148. Liu P, Kiess M, Okada RD, et al: Increased thallium lung uptake after exercise in isolated left anterior descending

coronary artery disease, *Am J Cardiol* 55:1469-1473, 1985.

149. Wilson RA, Okada RD, Boucher CA, et al: Radionuclide-determined changes in pulmonary blood volume and thallium lung uptake in patients with coronary artery disease, *Am J Cardiol* 51:741-748, 1983.

150. Brown KA, Boucher CA, Okada RD, et al: Quantification of pulmonary thallium activity after upright exercise in normal persons: importance of peak heart rate and propranolol usage in defining normal values, *Am J Cardiol* 53:1678-1682, 1984.

151. Iskandrian A, Hakki A, Segal BL, et al: Assessment of the myocardial perfusion pattern in patients with multivessel coronary artery disease, *Am Heart J* 106:1089-1095, 1983.

152. Dunn RF, Freedman B, Bailey IK, et al: Noninvasive prediction of multivessel disease after myocardial infarction, *Circulation* 62:726-734, 1980.

153. Patterson RE, Horowitz SF, Eng C, et al: Can noninvasive exercise test criteria identify patients with left main or 3-vessel coronary disease after a first myocardial infarction? *Am J Cardiol* 51:361-372, 1983.

154. Gibson RS, Taylor GJ, Watson DD, et al: Predicting the extent and location of coronary artery disease during the early postinfarction period by quantitative thallium-201 scintigraphy, *Am J Cardiol* 47:1010-1019, 1981.

155. Abraham RD, Freedman SB, Dunn RF, et al: Prediction of multivessel coronary artery disease and prognosis early after acute myocardial infarction by exercise electrocardiography and thallium-201 myocardial perfusion scanning, *Am J Cardiol* 58:423-427, 1986.

156. Rigo P, Bailey IK, Griffith LSC, et al: Stress thallium-201 myocardial scintigraphy for the detection of individual coronary arterial lesions in patients with and without previous myocardial infarction, *Am J Cardiol* 48:209-216, 1981.

157. Brown KA, Boucher CA, Okada RD, et al: Prognostic value of exercise thallium-201 imaging in patients presenting for evaluation of chest pain, *J Am Coll Cardiol* 1:994-1001, 1983.

158. Iskandrian AS, Hakki A, Kane-Marsch S: Prognostic implications of exercise thallium-201 scintigraphy in patients with suspected or known coronary artery disease, *Am Heart J* 110:135-143, 1985.

159. Staniloff HM, Forrester JS, Berman DS, et al: Prediction of death, myocardial infarction, and worsening chest pain using thallium scintigraphy and exercise electrocardiography, *J Nucl Med* 27:1842-1848, 1986.

160. Ladenheim ML, Pollock BH, Rozanski A, et al: Extent and severity of myocardial hypoperfusion as predictors of prognosis in patients with suspected coronary artery disease, *J Am Coll Cardiol* 7:464-471, 1986.

161. Gill JB, Ruddy TD, Newell JB, et al: Prognostic importance of thallium uptake by the lungs during exercise in coronary artery disease, *N Engl J Med* 317:1485-1489, 1987.

162. Kaul S, Lilly DR, Gascho JA, et al: Prognostic utility of the exercise thallium-201 test in ambulatory patients with chest pain: comparison with cardiac catheterization, *Circulation* 77:745-748, 1988.

163. Kaul S, Finkelstein DM, Homma S, et al: Superiority of quantitative exercise thallium-201 variables in determining long-term prognosis in ambulatory patients with chest pain: a comparison with cardiac catheterization, *J Am Coll Cardiol* 12:25-34, 1988.

164. Melin JA, Robert A, Luwaert R, et al: Additional prognostic value of exercise testing and thallium-201 scintigraphy in catheterized patients without previous myocardial infarction, *Int J Cardiol* 27:235-243, 1990.

165. Iskandrian AS, Heo J, Decoskey D, et al: Use of exercise thallium-201 imaging for risk stratification of elderly patients with coronary artery disease, *Am J Cardiol* 61:269-272, 1988.

166. Ladenheim ML, Kotler TS, Pollock BH, et al: Incremental prognostic power of clinical history, exercise electrocardiography and myocardial perfusion scintigraphy in suspected coronary artery disease, *Am J Cardiol* 59:270-277, 1987.

167. Gibson RS, Watson DD, Craddock GB, et al: Prediction of cardiac events after uncomplicated myocardial infarction: a prospective study comparing predischarge exercise thallium-201 scintigraphy and coronary angiography, *Circulation* 68:321-336, 1983.

168. Wilson WW, Gibson RS, Nygaard TW, et al: Acute myocardial infarction associated with single vessel coronary artery disease: an analysis of clinical outcome and the prognostic importance of vessel patency and residual ischemic myocardium, *J Am Coll Cardiol* 11:223-234, 1988.

169. Tilkemeier PL, Guiney TE, LaRaia PJ, et al: Prognostic value of predischarge low-level exercise thallium testing after thrombolytic treatment of acute myocardial infarction, *Am J Cardiol* 66:1203-1207, 1990.

170. Wackers FJT, Russo DJ, Russo D, et al: Prognostic significance of normal quantitative planar thallium-201 stress scintigraphy in patients with chest pain, *J Am Coll Cardiol* 6:27-30, 1985.

171. Pamelia FX, Gibson RS, Watson DD, et al: Prognosis with chest pain and normal thallium-201 exercise scintigrams, *Am J Cardiol* 55:920-926, 1985.

172. Wahl JM, Hakki A, Iskandrian AS: Prognostic implications of normal exercise thallium 201 images, *Arch Intern Med* 145:253-256, 1985.

173. Koss JH, Kobren SM, Grunwald AM, et al: Role of exercise thallium-201 myocardial perfusion scintigraphy in predicting prognosis in suspected coronary artery disease, *Am J Cardiol* 59:531-534, 1987.

174. Heo J, Thompson WO, Iskandrian AS: Prognostic implications of normal exercise thallium images, *Am J Noninvas Cardiol* 1:209-212, 1987.

175. Bairey CN, Rozanski A, Maddahi J, et al: Exercise thallium-201 scintigraphy and prognosis in typical angina pectoris and negative exercise electrocardiography, *Am J Cardiol* 64:282-287, 1989.

176. Gianrossi R, Detrano R, Mulvihill D, et al: Exercise-induced ST depression in the diagnosis of coronary artery disease: a meta-analysis, *Circulation* 80:87-98, 1989.

177. Heller GV, Ahmed I, Tilkemeier PL, et al: Comparison of chest pain, electrocardiographic changes and thallium-201 scintigraphy during varying exercise intensities in men with stable angina pectoris, *Am J Cardiol* 68:569-574, 1991.

178. Friedman TD, Greene AC, Iskandrian AS, et al: Exercise thallium-201 myocardial scintigraphy in women: correlation with coronary arteriography, *Am J Cardiol* 49:1632-1637, 1982.

179. Kaul S, Newell JB, Chesler DA, et al: Value of computer analysis of exercise thallium images in the noninvasive detection of coronary artery disease, *JAMA* 255:508-511, 1986.

180. Hlatky M, Botvinick E, Brundage B: The independent value of exercise thallium scintigraphy to physicians, *Circulation* 66:953-959, 1982.

181. Neimeyer MG, Ascoop PL, Cramer MJ, et al: Comparative value of visual and quantitative analysis of thallium-201 imaging after exercise in patients with an abnormal baseline repolarization on the electrocardiogram at rest, *Eur Heart J* 11:413-420, 1990.

182. Neimeyer MG, Cramer MJ, van der Wall EE, et al: Value of visual and quantitative analysis of thallium-201 imaging in patients with diagnostic and non-diagnostic exercise electrocardiograms, *Am J Noninvas Cardiol* 5:80-87, 1991.

183. Steinberg EP, Klag MJ, Bakal CW, et al: Exercise thallium scans: patterns of use and impact on management of patients with known or suspected coronary artery disease, *Am J Cardiol* 59:50-55, 1987.

184. Gibson RS: Comparative analysis of the diagnostic and prognostic value of exercise ECG and thallium-201 scintigraphic markers of myocardial ischemia in asymptomatic and symptomatic patients, *Cardiology Clin* 7:565-575, 1989.

185. Uhl GS, Kay TN, Hickman JR: Computer enhanced thallium scintigrams in asymptomatic men with abnormal exercise tests, *Am J Cardiol* 48:1037-1043, 1981.

186. Berman DS, Amsterdam EA, Joye JA, et al: Thallium-201 stress myocardial scintigraphy: application in asymptomatic patients with positive exercise electrocardiograms, *Am J Cardiol* 41(suppl):380, 1978.

187. Caralis DG, Bailey I, Kennedy HL, et al: Screening asymptomatic middle aged men for obstructive coronary artery disease, *Circulation* 60(suppl 2):II-149, 1979.

188. Guiney TE, Pohost GM, McKusick KA, et al: Differentiation of false- from true-positive ECG responses to exercise stress by thallium-201 perfusion imaging, *Chest* 80:4-10, 1981.

189. Fleg JL, Gerstenblith G, Becker LC, et al: Prognostic value of exercise electrocardiography and thallium scintigraphy in asymptomatic subjects, *Circulation* 68(suppl 3):III-126, 1983.

190. Detrano R, Froelicher V: A logical approach to screening for coronary artery disease, *Ann Intern Med* 106:846-852, 1987.

191. Sox HC, Littenberg B, Garber A: The role of exercise testing in screening for coronary artery disease, *Ann Intern Med* 110:456-469, 1989.

192. Gibson RS, Beller GA: Should exercise ECG testing be replaced by radioisotope methods? In Rahimtoola S, Brest A, editors: *Cardiovascular clinics: controversies in coronary artery disease,* Philadelphia, 1982, FA Davis, pp 1-31.

193. Kaul S: A look at 15 years of planar thallium-201 imaging, *Am Heart J* 118:581-601, 1989.

194. Podrid PH, Graboys TB, Lown B: Prognosis of medically treated patients with coronary-artery disease with profound ST-segment depression during exercise testing, *N Engl J Med* 305:1111-1116, 1981.

195. Gibson RS, Beller GA, Kaiser DL: Prevalence and clinical significance of painless ST segment depression during early postinfarction exercise testing, *Circulation* 75(suppl 2):II-36–II-39, 1987.

196. Gibson RS: Non-Q-wave myocardial infarction: diagnosis, prognosis, and management, *Curr Probl Cardiol* 13:1-72, 1988.

197. Belardinelli L, Linden J, Berne RM: The cardiac effects of adenosine, *Prog Cardiovasc Dis* 32:73-97, 1989.

198. Berne RM: Cardiac nucleotides in hypoxia: possible role in regulation of coronary blood flow, *Am J Physiol* 204:317-322, 1963.

199. Iskandrian AS: Single-photon emission computed tomographic thallium imaging with adenosine, dipyridamole, and exercise, *Am Heart J* 122:279-284, 1991.

200. Bardenheuer H, Whelton B, Sparks HV Jr: Adenosine release by the isolated guinea pig's heart in response to isoproterenol, acetylcholine and acidosis: the minimal role of vascular endothelium, *Circ Res* 61:594-600, 1987.

201. Deussen A, Moser G, Schrader J: Contribution of coronary endothelial cells to cardiac adenosine production, *Pflügers Arch* 406:608-614, 1986.

202. Botvinick EH, Dae MW: Dipyridamole perfusion scintigraphy, *Semin Nucl Med* 21:242-265, 1991.

203. Rossen JD, Quillen JE, Lopez AG, et al: Comparison of coronary vasodilation with intravenous dipyridamole and adenosine, *J Am Coll Cardiol* 18:485-491, 1991.

204. Beller GA, Holzgrefe HH, Watson DD: Intrinsic washout rates of thallium-201 in normal and ischemic myocardium after dipyridamole-induced vasodilation, *Circulation* 71:378-386, 1985.

205. Becker LC: Conditions for vasodilator-induced coronary steal in experimental myocardial ischemia, *Circulation* 57:1103-1110, 1978.

206. Okada RD, Leppo JA, Boucher CA, et al: Myocardial kinetics of thallium-201 after dipyridamole infusion in normal canine myocardium and in myocardium distal to a stenosis, *J Clin Invest* 69:199-201, 1982.

207. Beller GA, Holzgrefe HH, Watson DD: Effects of dipyridamole-induced vasodilation on myocardial uptake and clearance kinetics of thallium-201, *Circulation* 68:1328-1338, 1983.

208. Varma SK, Watson DD, Beller GA: Quantitative comparison of thallium-201 scintigraphy after exercise and dipyridamole in coronary artery disease, *Am J Cardiol* 64:871-877, 1989.

209. Rossen JD, Simonetti I, Marcus ML, et al: Coronary dilation with standard dose dipyridamole and dipyridamole combined with handgrip, *Circulation* 79:566-572, 1989.

210. Gould KL: Noninvasive assessment of coronary stenoses by myocardial perfusion imaging during pharmacologic coronary vasodilation. I. Physiologic basis and experimental validation, *Am J Cardiol* 41:267-278, 1978.

211. Gould KL, Westcott RJ, Albro PC, et al: Noninvasive assessment of coronary stenoses by myocardial imaging during pharmacologic coronary vasodilation. II. Clinical methodology and feasibility, *Am J Cardiol* 41:279-287, 1978.

212. Neilsen-Kudsk F, Pedersen AK: Pharmacokinetics of dipyridamole, *Acta Pharmacol Toxicol* 44:391-399, 1979.

213. Marchant E, Pichard A, Rodriguez JA, et al: Acute effect of systemic versus intracoronary dipyridamole on coronary circulation, *Am J Cardiol* 57:1401-1404, 1986.

214. Lewin MK, Labovitz AJ, Kern MJ, et al: Effect of intravenous dipyridamole on regional coronary blood flow with 1-vessel coronary artery disease: evidence against coronary steal, *Am J Cardiol* 53:718-721, 1984.

215. Okada RD, Leppo JA, Boucher CA, et al: Myocardial kinetics of thallium-201 after dipyridamole infusion in normal canine myocardium and in myocardium distal to a stenosis, *J Clin Invest* 69:199-206, 1982.

216. Mays AE Jr, Cobb FR: Relationship between regional myocardial blood flow and thallium-201 distribution in the presence of coronary artery stenosis and dipyridamole induced vasodilation, *J Clin Invest* 73:1359-1366, 1984.

217. Brown BG, Josephson MA, Petersen RB, et al: Intravenous dipyridamole combined with isometric handgrip for near maximal acute increased in coronary flow in patients with coronary artery disease, *Am J Cardiol* 48:1077-1084, 1981.

218. Smits P, Corstens FHM, Aengevaeren WRM, et al: False-negative dipyridamole-thallium-201 myocardial imaging after caffeine infusion, *J Nucl Med* 32:1538-1541, 1991.

219. Daley PJ, Mahn TH, Zielonka JS, et al: Effect of maintenance oral theophylline on dipyridamole-thallium-201 myocardial imaging using SPECT and dipyridamole-induced hemodynamic changes, *Am Heart J* 115:1185-1192, 1988.

220. Smits P, Aengevaeren WRM, Corstens FHM, et al: Caffeine reduces dipyridamole-induced myocardial ischemia, *J Nucl Med* 30:1723-1726, 1989.

221. Chambers CE, Brown KA: Dipyridamole-induced ST segment depression during thallium-201 imaging in patients with coronary artery disease: angiographic and hemodynamic determinants, *J Am Coll Cardiol* 12:37-41, 1988.

222. Pearlman JD, Boucher CA: Diagnostic value for coronary artery disease of chest pain during dipyridamole-thallium stress testing, *Am J Cardiol* 61:43-45, 1988.

223. Sylven C, Beermann B, Jonzon B, et al: Angina pectoris–like pain provoked by intravenous adenosine in healthy volunteers, *Br Med J* 293:227-230, 1986.

224. Ranhosky A, Kempthorne-Rawson J, and the Intravenous Dipyridamole Thallium Imaging Study Group: The safety of intravenous dipyridamole thallium myocardial perfusion imaging, *Circulation* 81:1205-1209, 1990.

225. Lette J, Cerino M, Laverdiere M, et al: Severe bronchospasm followed by respiratory arrest during thallium-dipyridamole imaging, *Chest* 95:1345-1347, 1989.

226. Hendel RC, Layden JJ, Leppo JA: Prognostic value of dipyridamole thallium scintigraphy for evaluation of ischemic heart disease, *J Am Coll Cardiol* 15:109-116, 1990.

227. Homma S, Gilliland Y, Guiney TE, et al: Safety of intravenous dipyridamole for stress testing with thallium imaging, *Am J Cardiol* 59:152-154, 1987.

228. Younis LT, Byers S, Shaw L, et al: Prognostic value of intravenous dipyridamole thallium scintigraphy after an acute myocardial ischemic event, *Am J Cardiol* 64:161-166, 1989.

229. Gimple LW, Hutter AM Jr, Guiney TE, et al: Prognostic utility of predischarge dipyridamole thallium imaging compared to predischarge submaximal exercise electrocardiography and maximal exercise thallium imaging after uncomplicated acute myocardial infarction, *Am J Cardiol* 64:1243-1248, 1989.

230. Brown KA, O'Meara J, Chambers CE, et al: Ability of dipyridamole-thallium-201 imaging one to four days after acute myocardial infarction to predict in-hospital and late recurrent myocardial ischemic events, *Am J Cardiol* 65:160-167, 1990.

231. Pirelli S, Inglese E, Suppa M, et al: Dipyridamole-thallium 201 scintigraphy in the early postinfarction period: safety and accuracy in predicting the extent of coronary disease and future recurrence of angina in patients suffering from their first myocardial infarction, *Eur Heart J* 9:1324-1331, 1988.

232. Bolognese L, Sarasso G, Aralda D, et al: High dose dipyridamole echocardiography early after uncomplicated acute myocardial infarction: correlation with exercise testing and coronary angiography, *J Am Coll Cardiol* 14:357-363, 1989.

233. Albro PC, Gould KL, Westcott RJ, et al: Noninvasive assessment of coronary stenoses by myocardial imaging during pharmacologic coronary vasodilation. III. Clinical trial *Am J Cardiol* 42:751-760, 1978.

234. Beller GA: Pharmacologic stress imaging, *JAMA* 265:633-638, 1991.

235. Narita M, Kurihara T, Usami M: Noninvasive detection of coronary artery disease by myocardial imaging with thallium-201: the significance of pharmacologic interventions, *Jpn Circ J* 45:127-140, 1981.

236. Wilde P, Walker P, Watt I, et al: Thallium-201 myocardial imaging: recent experience using a coronary vasodilator, *Clin Radiol* 33:43-50, 1982.

237. Timmis AD, Lutkin JE, Fenney LJ, et al: Comparison of dipyridamole and treadmill exercise for enhancing thallium-201 perfusion defects in patients with coronary artery disease, *Eur Heart J* 1:275-280, 1980.

238. Machecourt J, Denis B, Wolf JE, et al: Sensibilité et spécificité respective de la scintigraphie de myocardie réalisée après injection de thallium-201 au course de l'effort, après injection de dipyridamole et au repos: comparison chez 70 sujets coronarographiés, *Arch Mal Cœur* 74:147-156, 1981.

239. Leppo JA: Dipyridamole-thallium imaging: the lazy man's stress test, *J Nucl Med* 30:281-287, 1989.

240. Eichhorn EJ, Kosinski EJ, Lewis SM, et al: Usefulness of dipyridamole-thallium-201 perfusion scanning for distinguishing ischemic from non-ischemic cardiomyopathy, *Am J Cardiol* 62:945-951, 1988.

241. Villanueva FS, Kaul S, Smith WH, et al: Prevalence and correlates of increased lung/heart ratio of thallium-201 during dipyridamole stress imaging for suspected coronary artery disease, *Am J Cardiol* 66:1324-1328, 1990.

242. Okada RD, Dai Y, Boucher CA, et al: Significance of increased lung thallium-201 activity on serial cardiac images after dipyridamole treatment in coronary heart disease, *Am J Cardiol* 53:470-475, 1984.

243. Villaneuva FS, Watson DD, Smith WH, et al: Significance of increased lung/heart ratio on dipyridamole thallium-201 scintigraphy, *Circulation* 80(suppl II):II 210, 1989.

244. Takeishi Y, Tono-oka I, Ikeda K, et al: Dilatation of the left ventricular cavity on dipyridamole thallium-201 imaging: a new marker of triple-vessel disease, *Am Heart J* 121:466-475, 1991.

245. Okada RD, Dai Y, Boucher CA, et al: Serial thallium-201 imaging after dipyridamole for coronary disease detection: quantitative analysis using myocardial clearance, *Am Heart J* 107:475-481, 1984.

246. O'Byrne GT, Rodrigues EA, Maddahi J, et al: Comparison of myocardial washout rate of thallium-201 between rest, dipyridamole with and without aminophylline, and exercise states in normal subjects, *Am J Cardiol* 64:1022-1028, 1989.

247. Ruddy TD, Gill JB, Finkelstein DM, et al: Myocardial uptake and clearance of thallium-201 in normal subjects: comparison of dipyridamole-induced hyperemia with exercise stress, *J Am Coll Cardiol* 10:547-556, 1987.

248. O'Byrne GT, Rodrigues EA, Maddahi J, et al: Comparison of myocardial washout rate of thallium-201 between rest, dipyridamole with and without aminophylline, and exercise states in normal subjects, *Am J Cardiol* 64:1022-1028, 1989.

249. Verani MS, Mahmarian JJ, Hixson JB, et al: Diagnosis of coronary artery disease by controlled coronary vasodilation with adenosine and thallium-201 scintigraphy in patients unable to exercise, *Circulation* 82:80-87, 1990.

250. Verani MS, Mahmarian JJ: Myocardial perfusion scintigraphy during maximal coronary artery vasodilation with adenosine, *Am J Cardiol* 67:12D-17D, 1991.

251. Nguyen T, Heo J, Ogilby JD, et al: Simple photon emission computed tomography with thallium-201 during adenosine-induced coronary hyperemia: correlation with coronary arteriography, exercise thallium imaging and two-dimensional echocardiography, *J Am Coll Cardiol* 16:1375-1383, 1990.

252. Coyne EP, Belvedere DA, Vande Streek PR, et al: Thallium-201 scintigraphy after intravenous infusion of adenosine compared with exercise thallium testing in the diagnosis of coronary artery disease, *J Am Coll Cardiol* 17:1289-1994, 1991.

253. Younis LT, Byers S, Shaw L et al: Prognostic importance of silent myocardial ischemia detected by intravenous dipyridamole thallium myocardial imaging in asymptomatic patients with coronary artery disease, *J Am Coll Cardiol* 14:1635-1641, 1989.

254. Leppo JA, O'Brien J, Rothendler JA, et al: Dipyri-

damole-thallium-201 scintigraphy in the prediction of future cardiac events after acute myocardial infarction, *N Engl J Med* 310:1014-1018, 1984.

255. Gimple LW, Hutter AM, Guiney TE, et al: Prognostic utility of predischarge dipyridamole-thallium imaging compared to predischarge submaximal exercise electrocardiography and maximal exercise thallium imaging after uncomplicated acute myocardial infarction, *Am J Cardiol* 64:1243-1248, 1989.

256. Brown KA, O'Meara J, Chambers CE, et al: Ability of dipyridamole-thallium-201 imaging one to four days after acute myocardial infarction to predict in-hospital and late recurrent ischemic events, *Am J Cardiol* 65:160-167, 1990.

257. Nienaber CA, Spielmann RP, Salge D, et al: Assessment of post-infarction jeopardized myocardium by vasodilation-thallium-201 tomography: impact on risk stratification, *Eur Heart J* 11:1093-1100, 1990.

258. Boucher CA, Brewster DC, Darling RC, et al: Determination of cardiac risk by dipyridamole-thallium imaging before peripheral vascular surgery, *N Engl J Med* 312:389-394, 1985.

259. Eagle KA, Single DE, Brewster DC, et al: Dipyridamole-thallium scanning in patients undergoing vascular surgery: optimizing preoperative evaluation of cardiac risk, *JAMA* 257:2185-2189, 1987.

260. Eagle KA, Coley CM, Newell JB, et al: Combining clinical and thallium data optimizes preoperative assessment of cardiac risk before major vascular surgery, *Ann Intern Med* 110:859-866, 1989.

261. Lane SE, Lewis SM, Pippin JJ, et al: Predictive value of quantitative dipyridamole-thallium scintigraphy in assessing cardiovascular risk after vascular surgery in diabetes mellitus, *Am J Cardiol* 64:1275-1279, 1989.

262. Lette J, Waters D, Lapointe J, et al: Usefulness of the severity and extent of reversible perfusion defects during thallium-dipyridamole imaging for cardiac risk assessment before noncardiac surgery, *Am J Cardiol* 64:276-281, 1989.

263. Lette J, Waters D, Picard M: Preoperative and long-term cardiac risk assessment: predictive value of 23 clinical descriptors, 8 multivariate scoring systems and quantitative dipyridamole imaging in 360 patients, *J Am Coll Cardiol* 19(suppl):156a, 1992.

264. Younis LT, Takase B, Byers SL, et al: Enhancement of Goldman preoperative risk assessment with the use of intravenous dipyridamole thallium scintigraphy in patients referred for major nonvascular surgery, *J Am Coll Cardiol* 19(suppl):156a, 1992.

265. Mangano DT, London MJ, Tubau JF, et al: Dipyridamole thallium-201 scintigraphy as a preoperative screening test: a reexamination of its predictive potential, *Circulation* 84:493-502, 1991.

266. Jain A, Mahmarian JJ, Borges-Neto S, et al: Clinical significance of perfusion defects by thallium-201 single photon emission tomography following oral dipyridamole early after coronary angioplasty, *J Am Coll Cardiol* 11:970-976, 1988.

267. Mason JR, Palac RT, Freeman ML, et al: Thallium scintigraphy during dobutamine infusion: nonexercise-dependent screening test for coronary disease, *Am Heart J* 107:481-485, 1984.

268. Pennell DJ, Underwood SR, Swanton RH, et al: Dobutamine thallium myocaardial perfusion tomography, *J Am Coll Cardiol* 18:1471-1479, 1991.

269. Fung AY, Gallagher KP, Buda AJ: The physiologic basis of dobutamine as compared with dipyridamole stress interventions in the assessment of critical coronary stenosis, *Circulation* 76:943-951, 1987.

270. Elliott BM, Robison JG, Zellner JL, et al: Dobutamine-^{201}Tl imaging. Assessming cardiac risks associated with vascular surgery, *Circulation* 84(suppl III):III-54–III-60, 1991.

271. Beller GA, Watson DD: Physiological basis of myocardial perfusion imaging with the technetium 99m agents, *Semin Nucl Med* 21:173-181, 1991.

272. Leppo JA, DePuey EG, Johnson LL: A review of cardiac imaging with sestamibi and teboroxime, *J Nucl Med* 32:2012-2022, 1991.

273. Berman DS, Kiat H, Maddahi J: The new ^{99m}Tc myocardial perfusion imaging agents: ^{99m}Tc-sestamibi and ^{99m}Tc-teboroxime, *Circulation* 84(suppl I):I-7–I-21, 1991.

274. Maddahi J, Kiat H, Berman DS: Myocardial perfusion imaging with technetium 99m labeled agents, *Am J Cardiol* 67:27D-34D, 1991.

275. Meerdink DJ, Leppo JA: Experimental studies of the physiologic properties of technetium-99m agents: myocardial transport of perfusion imaging agents, *Am J Cardiol* 66:9E-15E, 1990.

276. Okada RD, Glover D, Gaffney T, et al: Myocardial kinetics of technetium-99m–hexakis-2-methoxy-2-methyl-propyl-isonitrile, *Circulation* 77:491-498, 1988.

277. Fleming RM, Kirkeeide RL, Taegtmeyer H, et al: Comparison of technetium-99m teboroxime tomography with automated quantitative coronary arteriography and thallium-201 tomographic imaging, *J Am Coll Cardiol* 17:1297-1302, 1991.

278. Iskandrian AS, Heo J, Nguyen T, et al: Myocardial imaging with Tc-99m teboroxime: technique and initial results, *Am Heart J* 121:889-894, 1991.

279. Wackers FJT, Berman DS, Maddahi J, et al: Technetium-99m hexakis 2-methoxyisobutyl isonitrile: human biodistribution, dosimetry, safety, and preliminary comparison to thallium-201 for myocardial perfusion imaging, *J Nucl Med* 30:301-311, 1989.

280. Beller GA, Sinusas AJ: Experimental studies of the physiologic properties of technetium-99m isonitriles, *Am J Cardiol* 66:5E-8E, 1990.

281. Taillefer R, Primeau M, Costi P, et al: Technetium-99m–sestamibi myocrdial perfusion imaging in detection of coronary artery disease: comparison between initial (1-hour) and delayed (3-hour) postexercise images, *J Nucl Med* 32:1961-1965, 1991.

282. Maublant JC, Gachon P, Moins N: Hexakis(2-methoxy isobutylisonitrile) technetium-99m and thallium-201 chloride: uptake and release in cultured myocardial cells, *J Nucl Med* 29:48-54, 1988.

283. Sinusas AJ, Watson DD, Cannon JM Jr, et al: Effect of ischemia and postischemic dysfunction on myocardial uptake of technetium-99m–labeled methoxyisobutyl isonitrile and thallium-201, *J Am Coll Cardiol* 14:1785-1793, 1989.

284. Sporn V, Balino NP, Holman BL, et al: Simultaneous measurement of ventricular function and myocardial perfusion using the technetium-99m isonitriles, *Clin Nucl Med* 13:77-81, 1988.

285. Najm YC, Timmis AD, Maisey MN, et al: The evaluation of ventricular function using gated myocardial imaging with Tc-99m MIBI, *Eur Heart J* 10:142-148, 1989.

286. Baillet GY, Mena IG, Kuperus JH, et al: Simultaneous technetium-99m MIBI angiography and myocardial perfusion imaging, *J Nucl Med* 30:38-44, 1989.

287. Jones RH, Borges-Neto S, Potts JM: Simultaneous measurement of myocardial perfusion and ventricular function during exercise from a single injection of technetium-99m sestamibi in coronary artery disease, *Am J Cardiol* 66:68E-71E, 1990.

288. Villanueva-Meyer J, Mena I, Narahara KA: Simultaneous assessment of left ventricular wall motion and myocardial perfusion with technetium-99m–methoxy isobutyl isonitrile at stress and rest in patients with angina: comparison with thallium-201 SPECT, *J Nucl Med* 31:457-463, 1990.

289. Borges-Neto S, Coleman RE, Potts JM, et al: Combined exercise radionuclide angiocardiography and single photon emission computed tomography perfusion studies for assessment of coronary artery disease, *Semin Nucl Med* 21:223-229, 1991.

290. Borges-Neto S, Coleman RE, Jones RH: Perfusion and function at rest and treadmill exercise using technetium-99m–sestamibi: comparison of one- and two-day protocols in normal volunteers, *J Nucl Med* 31:1128-1132, 1990.

291. Taillefer R, Laflamme L, Dupras G, et al: Myocardial perfusion imaging with ^{99m}Tc-methoxy-isobutyl-isonitrile (MIBI): comparison of short and long time intervals between rest and stress injections: preliminary results, *Eur J Nucl Med* 13:515-522, 1988.

292. Taillefer R, Gagnon A, Laflamme L, et al: Same day injections of ^{99m}Tc methoxyisobutyl isonitrile (hexamibi) for myocardial imaging: comparison between rest-stress and stress-rest injection sequences, *Eur J Nucl Med* 15:113-117, 1989.

293. Whalley DR, Murphy JJ, Frier M, et al: A comparison of same day and separate day injection protocols for myocardial perfusion SPECT using ^{99m}Tc-MIBI, *Nucl Med Communications* 12.99-104, 1991.

294. Kahn JK, McGhie I, Akers MS, et al: Quantitative rotational tomography with ^{201}Tl and ^{99m}Tc 2-methoxyisobutyl-isonitrile: a direct comparison in normal individuals and patients with coronary artery disease, *Circulation* 79:1282-1293, 1989.

295. Taillefer R, Dupras G, Sporn V, et al: Myocardial perfusion imaging with a new radiotracer, technetium-99m–hexamibi (methoxy isobutyl isonitrile): comparison with thallium-201 imaging, *Clin Nucl Med* 14:89-96, 1989.

296. Kiat H, Maddahi J, Roy LT, et al: Comparison of technetium 99m methoxy isobutyl isonitrile and thallium 201 for evaluation of coronary artery disease by planar and tomographic methods, *Am Heart J* 117:1-11, 1989.

297. Sochor H: Technetium-99m sestamibi in chronic coronary artery disease: the European experience, *Am J Cardiol* 66:91E–96E, 1990.

298. Maisey MN, Mistry R, Sowton E: Planar imaging techniques used with technetium-99m sestamibi to evaluate chronic myocardial ischemia, *Am J Cardiol* 66:47E-54E, 1990.

299. Maddahi J, Kiat H, Van Train KF, et al: Myocardial perfusion imaging with technetium-99m sestamibi SPECT in the evaluation of coronary artery disease, *Am J Cardiol* 66:55E-62E, 1990.

300. Sinusas AJ, Beller GA, Smith WII, et al: Quantitative planar imaging with technetium-99m methoxyisobutyl isonitrile: comparison of uptake patterns with thallium-201, *J Nucl Med* 30:1456-1463, 1989.

301. Koster K, Wackers FJT, Mattera JA, et al: Quantitative analysis of planar technetium-99m–sestamibi myocardial perfusion images using modified background subtraction, *J Nucl Med* 31:1400-1408, 1990.

302. Gibbons RJ: Technetium-99m–sestamibi in the assessment of acute myocardial infarction, *Semin Nucl Med* 21:213-222, 1991.

303. Boucher CA: Detection and location of myocardial infarction using technetium-99m sestamibi imaging at rest, *Am J Cardiol* 66:32E-35E, 1990.

304. Christian TF, Clements IP, Gibbons RJ: Noninvasive identification of myocardium at risk in patients with acute myocardial infarction and nondiagnostic electrocardiograms with technetium-99m–sestamibi, *Circulation* 83:1615-1620, 1991.

305. Braat SH, de Swart H, Janssen JH, et al: Use of technetium-99m sestamibi to determine the size of the myocardial area perfused by a coronary artery, *Am J Cardiol* 66:85E-90E, 1990.

306. Wackers FJT, Gibbons RJ, Verani MS, et al: Serial quantitative planar technetium-99m isonitrile imaging in acute myocardial infarction: efficacy for noninvasive assessment of thrombolytic therapy, *J Am Coll Cardiol* 14:861-873, 1989.

307. Wackers FJT: Thrombolytic therapy for myocardial infarction: assessment of efficacy by myocardial perfusion imaging with technetium-99m sestamibi, *Am J Cardiol* 66:36E-41E, 1990.

308. Behrenbeck T, Pellikka PA, Huber KC, et al: Primary angioplasty in myocardial infarction: assessment of improved myocardial perfusion with technetium-99m isonitrile, *J Am Coll Cardiol* 17:365-372, 1991.

309. Christian TF, Gibbons RJ, Gersh BJ: Effect of infarct location on myocardial salvage assessed by technetium-99m isonitrile, *J Am Coll Cardiol* 17:1303-1308, 1991.

310. Pfisterer M, Müller-Brand J, Spring P, et al: Assessment of the extent of jeopardized myocardium during acute coronary artery occlusion followed by reperfusion in man using technetium-99m isonitrile imaging, *Am Heart J* 122:7-12, 1991.

311. Christian TF, Behrenbeck T, Pellikka PA, et al: Mismatch of left ventricular function and infarct size demonstrated by technetium-99m isonitrile imaging after reperfusion therapy for acute myocardial infarction: identification of myocardial stunning and hyperkinesia, *J Am Coll Cardiol* 16:1632-1638, 1990.

312. Narahara KA, Villanueva-Meyer J, Thompson CJ, et al: Comparison of thallium-201 and technetium-99m hexakis 2-methoxyisobutyl isonitrile single photon emission computed tomography for estimating the extent of myocardial ischemia and infarction in coronary artery disease, *Am J Cardiol* 66:1438-1444, 1990.

313. Rocco TP, Dilsizian V, Strauss HW, et al: Technetium-99m isonitrile myocardial uptake at rest. 1. Relation to clinical markers of potential viability, *J Am Coll Cardiol* 14:1678-1684, 1989.

314. Cuocolo A, Pace L, Ricciardelli B, et al: Identification of viable myocardium in patients with chronic coronary artery disease: comparison of thallium-201 scintigraphy with reinjection and technetium-99m–methoxyisobutyl isonitrile, *J Nucl Med* 33:505-511, 1992.

315. Taillefer R: Technetium-99m sestamibi myocardial imaging: same-day rest-stress studies and dipyridamole, *Am J Cardiol* 66:80E-84E, 1990.

316. Tartagni F, Dondi M, Limonetti P, et al: Dipyridamole technetium-99m–methoxyisobutyl isonitrile tomoscintigraphic imaging for identifying diseased coronary vessels: comparison with thallium-201 stress-rest study, *J Nucl Med* 32:369-376, 1991.

317. Kettunen R, Huikuri HV, Heikkilä J, et al: Usefulness of technetium-99m-MIBI and thallium-201 in tomographic imaging combined with high-dose dipyridamole and handgrip exercise for detecting coronary artery disease, *Am J Cardiol* 68:575-579, 1991.

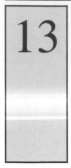

13 Exercise Radionuclide Ventricular Function Imaging

VENTRICULAR FUNCTION IMAGING
Methodology

Ventricular function can be measured both at rest and during exercise using either a first-pass or equilibrium blood pool technique. The radioactive label is ^{99m}Tc-pertechnetate. Because of its relatively short half-life, the dose of technetium that can be administered for clinical imaging provides sufficient count rate statistics to make ventricular imaging possible.

In first-pass studies, the isotope is administered as an intravenous bolus; the computer records the first transit of the bolus as it passes through the heart. The activity in the two ventricles is then temporally isolated by the computer in order that ventricular function can be quantified. Cameras with high count rate capabilities are necessary so that sufficient count statistics are achieved to provide reliable quantification of myocardial function. First-pass studies have the advantage of short study acquisition time, the ability to eliminate within limits the effects of premature beats during acquisition, and the ability to image the ventricles in the absence of significant background radioactivity. This latter factor is a particular advantage in the evaluation of right ventricular function, for which the first-pass technique is clearly the technique of choice. The disadvantages include the limited number of studies that can be performed, since each study requires a separate injection of isotope, the dependence of the technique on obtaining a tight bolus injection making a central injection preferable, and the desirability of using an imaging system with greater count rate capabilities than those achievable with the traditional Anger scintillation cameras, which are most widely utilized in clinical imaging departments.

Equilibrium blood pool studies depend on labeling the red blood cell pool with the ^{99m}Tc iso-tope, using either a direct in vivo labeling technique or a modified in vivo technique that labels the cells in a syringe, after which they are reinjected. The technique is dependent on imaging a large number of beats and summing the data from each beat to build an image with adequate count statistics. This is accomplished by gating the camera to the electrocardiogram and dividing each RR interval into segments or frames, usually between 16 and 32 frames per cycle length. An image of each frame is built by the addition of data from the successive beats and is displayed as a beating image in a continuous loop format. A major advantage of the equilibrium blood pool technique is its ability to acquire multiple images with a single radioactive injection, permitting acquisition of images from multiple viewing angles as well as during multiple stages of exercise. It can be readily performed using virtually any currently available commercial imaging system. The disadvantages include the necessity of isolating the activity of the individual cardiac chambers from surrounding activity in order to quantify function, which requires an accurate edge detection methodology, and the disruptive effect of arrhythmias on the data, unless appropriate arrhythmia rejection software are utilized.

With either technique, the ^{99m}Tc activity in the left ventricular region is determined for the complete cardiac cycle. The activity, which is directly proportional to blood volume, is represented as a ventricular time activity curve from which ejection fraction and indices of systolic and diastolic function can be derived. Both techniques have been extensively validated, demonstrating their capability to accurately quantify ventricular function.[1-7] Ejection fraction determined by the two techniques is closely correlated, though the slope of the regression is different from unity and the intercept is different from zero.[8] Equilibrium studies yield higher ejection fractions than first-pass studies do. The correlation between the two is also better with ejection fractions below 0.50, compared to those above 0.50, primarily because of the variability in quantitating small end-systolic volumes. In addition to ejection fraction and the indices of filling and ejection, regional myocardial function can be assessed by use of either visual or quantitative techniques.[9,10]

Radionuclide ventriculography can be performed during maximal exercise as well as at rest. This provides the opportunity to detect effects of exercise-induced ischemia on myocardial function. Exercise is typically performed using an upright bicycle ergometer for first-pass studies and a supine bicycle ergometer for equilibrium studies. Ejection fraction and wall motion responses to exercise are similar in the two positions, but the changes in end-systolic and end-diastolic volume are different.[11]

Exercise radionuclide ventriculography has been widely utilized in the examination of patients with known or suspected coronary artery disease. Interpretation of studies, however, requires defini-

tion of the normal response. For example, the left ventricular ejection fraction response to exercise is determined at least in part by the resting ejection fraction.[12] Normal subjects with high resting ejection fractions may not change their ejection fraction during exercise. The normal ejection fraction response to exercise is also different in women compared to men, unrelated to the levels of exercise achieved (Figure 13-1).[13,14] An apparently abnormal ejection fraction response to exercise is more common in women with chest pain and normal coronary arteries than in men.[15] Although these individuals may not represent a truly normal sample, similar findings have been noted in women with a low probability of disease based upon clinical rather than angiographic criteria.[13]

Although ejection fraction measurements are reproducible both at rest and during exercise from comparison of studies done 2 weeks apart, individual interstudy variabilities sufficient to change study interpretation are not uncommon.[16] It is imperative that conspicuous attention be paid to technique in order to obtain reproducible results. Region-of-interest selection can cause apparent abnormal ejection fraction responses to exercise

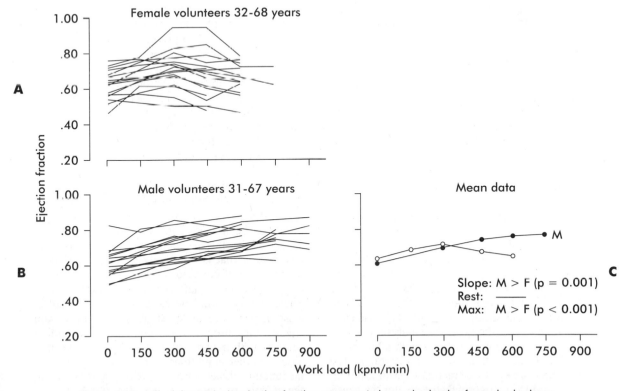

Figure 13-1   The left ventricular ejection fraction response to increasing levels of exercise is shown for female, **A,** and male, **B,** volunteers. **C,** Mean data. The normal ejection fraction response to exercise is different in women compared to men. (From Higginbotham MB et al: *Circulation* 70:357-366, 1984.)

in healthy subjects, particularly in those with high ejection fractions.[17]

Sensitivity and specificity for detection of coronary artery disease

Criteria for defining an abnormal left ventricular function response to exercise have evolved as experience with the technique has grown. In early studies, Borer and colleagues used the peak exercise ejection fraction in combination with the regional wall motion response to define an abnormal response.[18,19] Subsequent investigators, however, emphasized the change in ejection fraction during exercise compared to rest to define the normal response.[20-23] The criteria typically used was an increase of ejection fraction of ≥ 0.05 ejection fraction unit. However, the change in ejection fraction during exercise has been clearly shown to be a complex variable that is influenced by several physiological and pathophysiological factors including the resting ejection fraction,[12] the patient's age and sex,[13] and the extent and location of coronary artery disease.[24] In a study of 57 patients with angiographically normal coronary arteries, Kuo and colleagues found that the specificity of an ejection fraction increase of ≥ 0.05 unit was dependent on the level of exercise achieved.[25] In subjects who completed only one stage of exercise, it was 42%, whereas it was 75% in those who completed two levels of exercise, and 100% in those who completed at least three levels of exercise.

The ejection fraction attained at peak exercise has emerged as the preferred parameter for defining an abnormal response to exercise.[26-29] In an assessment that involved comparison of the diagnostic power of the change in ejection fraction during exercise to the peak ejection fraction attained in 736 patients, Gibbons and co-workers found that peak ejection fraction was the superior diagnostic variable.[26] This observation is logical in that peak ejection fraction reflects the effects of prior ventricular damage, which will lower the resting ejection fraction, as well as the ischemic burden that develops during exercise. Peak ejection fraction should not be considered as a discrete variable with an arbitrary cutoff point differentiating normal from abnormal but rather as a continuous variable.[26] Table 13-1 illustrates the relationship of sensitivity and specificity to peak exercise ejection fraction. Specificity in this analysis is determined from a sample of patients with a low probability of disease (that is, normalcy rate). The higher the peak ejection fraction used to differentiate normal from abnormal, the greater the sensitivity becomes for detecting coronary artery disease, while the specificity decreases. As is subsequently discussed, peak ejection fraction has also

Table 13-1 Sensitivity and specificity of peak exercise ejection fraction for diagnosis of coronary artery disease

Peak ejection fraction achieved during exercise	Sensitivity (%)	Specificity (%)
0.50	55	98
0.55	66	93
0.57	72	90
0.60	77	82
0.63	84	72
0.65	86	67

Adapted from Gibbons RJ: *Circulation* 84(suppl I):I93-I99, 1991.

been demonstrated to be the superior variable for allowing the identification of severe anatomic disease and the estimation of prognosis.[29]

The sensitivity of exercise radionuclide ventriculography for detection of coronary artery disease is greater than that of exercise electrocardiography (Table 13-2)[19,20,30-32] and is equivalent to that of exercise thallium scintigraphy (Table 13-3).[21-23,33] The increased sensitivity of exercise radionuclide ventriculography compared to exercise electrocardiography implies that mechanical manifestations of ischemia precede electrical manifestations, a finding that is confirmed by the observations of Upton and co-workers.[34] In all 10 of their normal subjects, ejection fraction increased at least 0.05 unit in the first stage of exercise. In contrast, in 11 of the patients with CAD the ejection fraction decreased during stage 1 of exercise despite the fact that none of them had either chest pain or ST-segment depression at that level of exertion.

Although the sensitivity of exercise radionuclide ventriculography has been relatively consistent in reported series and is well established, the specificity has been more controversial. Early reports suggested that the specificity approached 100%, an observation that is intuitively unrealistic, since a broad range of conditions other than coronary artery disease cause left ventricular dysfunction.[19] These overly optimistic early projections were at least in part a result of study sample bias from studies that used normal volunteers, excluding subjects with hypertension, diabetes, valvular disease, or other conditions that can affect ventricular function. Later series, however, suggested that the specificity was as low as 50%,[35] which may be somewhat of an underestimate because of posttest referral bias.[35a,35b] If specificity is defined compared to contrast angiography, there is possi-

Table 13-2   Comparison of exercise radionuclide angiography and exercise electrocardiography in the diagnosis of coronary artery disease

Source	Number of patients	Radionuclide angiography		Exercise electrocardiography	
		Sensitivity	Specificity	Sensitivity	Specificity
Borer et al[19]	84	60/63	21/21	43/63	20/21
Berger et al[20] (1979)	73	52/60	13/13	33/60	13/13
Jengo et al[30] (1979)	19	11/11	8/8	4/11	8/8
Jones et al[31] (1981)	248	151/183	43/65	103/183	56/65
TOTAL	424	274/317 (86%)	85/107 (79%)	183/317 (58%)	97/107 (91%)

Adapted from Gibbons RJ: Nuclear cardiology. In Giuliani ER, Fuster V, Gersh BJ, et al, editors: *Cardiology, fundamentals and practice,* ed 2, St. Louis, 1991, Mosby.

Table 13-3   Comparison of exercise thallium scintigraphy and exercise radionuclide ventriculography in the diagnosis of coronary artery disease

Source	Number of patients	Thallium 201		Radionuclide ventriculography	
		Sensitivity	Specificity	Sensitivity	Specificity
Johnstone et al[22] (1980)	48	30/39	9/9	35/39	9/9
Jengo et al[23] (1980)	58	39/42	15/16	41/42	16/16
Bodenheimer et al[33] (1980)	75	46/56	17/19	46/56	15/19
Caldwell et al[21] (1980)	52	35/41	11/11	38/41	6/11
TOTAL	233	150/178 (84%)	52/55 (95%)	160/178 (90%)	46/55 (84%)

From Gibbons RJ: Nuclear cardiology. In Giuliani ER, Fuster V, Gersh BJ, et al, editors: *Cardiology, fundamentals and practice,* ed 2, St. Louis, 1991, Mosby.

ble selection bias from two sources. First, patients with abnormal noninvasive tests are more likely to undergo angiography. Therefore the false-positive results will be overrepresented in catheterization comparison studies, since patients with true-negative results were unlikely to undergo angiography. Second, patients with chest pain and normal coronary angiograms may not be truly normal. Abnormalities in ventricular function during exercise in these patients could be manifestations of as-yet poorly characterized disease processes. When specificity is defined from studies of subjects who are normal defined by clinical criteria rather than by invasive testing, specificity (also referred to as normalcy rate) is approximately 80%, using peak ejection fraction as the diagnostic criterion.[28] This study, however, used a peak ejection fraction of 0.60 as the cutoff point, which results in a lower test sensitivity. Furthermore, subjects with hypertension and other disease states were again excluded. The true specificity of exercise radionuclide ventriculography therefore is likely to be somewhat greater than 50% and somewhat less than 80%.

Other radionuclide variables besides the ejection fraction response to exercise have been proposed to be helpful indicators of disease, improving the diagnostic accuracy of the test. Segmental wall-motion abnormalities present during exercise are specific for coronary disease but are insensitive.[31,28,36] Assessment of regional wall motion appears to contribute somewhat to the diagnostic accuracy of the test[26,36] but does not add independent information relative to severity of disease or prognosis.[37] Pulmonary blood volume was initially suggested to have greater sensitivity for detection of coronary artery disease than the ejection fraction response to exercise did.[38] Increased pulmonary blood volume is a manifestation of increased left ventricular filling pressure, which logically should not be as sensitive as the ejection fraction or wall-motion changes for detecting CAD because mild ischemia might be expected to impair segmental function and ejection fraction before causing elevations of filling pressure sufficient to increase pulmonary blood volume. Consistent with this speculation, subsequent studies have failed to confirm the independent diagnostic value of pulmonary blood volume.[39] The peak-systolic pressure/end-systolic volume ratio has also been suggested to be a sensitive diagnostic parameter, a theory that has a sound basis in myocardial mechanics.[40,41] However, this is a complex variable that does not appear to add significantly to the information provided by the peak exercise ejection fraction.[28]

Although peak ejection fraction appears to be the primary radionuclide variable contributing to the diagnostic assessment, the coinciding symptomatic, hemodynamic, and electrocardiographic responses to exercise contribute important additional information to the radionuclide findings. Exercise associated angina adds diagnostic information,[76] though it appears to have limited additional prognostic value.[42] The severity of exercise-induced ventricular dysfunction is independent of the presence or absence of angina during exercise.[43] The hemodynamic response to exercise has been found to provide additive information in several studies. In a multivariate discriminant analysis of data from 99 patients, DePace and colleagues noted that the change in systolic blood pressure from rest to exercise added to the radionuclide parameters for identification of severe disease.[44] In a similar study of 185 patients, Weintraub and coworkers found that peak exercise heart rate contributed additional information to peak ejection fraction and ST-segment depression.[45] In an analysis of data from 681 patients, Gibbons and colleagues noted that the peak exercise rate-pressure product was one of the four most important variables identified by logistic regression analysis for identification of patients with severe disease.[37]

Electrocardiographic findings also add significant information to the radionuclide variables for predicting disease.[45] In the above-cited study by Gibbons and colleagues, the magnitude of ST-segment depression during exercise was the most important single variable for identifying high-risk patients.[37] Currie and coinvestigators noted that two variables from the exercise radionuclide study added to clinical variables in diagnosing disease in their study of 105 men.[36] These were the presence of segmental wall motion abnormalities and the presence of considerable ST-segment depression on the exercise electrocardiogram. In an earlier study on a different sample of 736 patients, Gibbons and colleagues found that the most useful parameters for establishing a diagnosis of CAD were the peak exercise ejection fraction, peak heart rate, "ischemia score," and the presence of regional wall-motion abnormalities during exercise.[26] Hence, proper interpretation of the exercise radionuclide ventriculographic study requires consideration of these various nonimaging variables in deciding the implications of the test in the individual patient.

There are important limitations to the exercise radionuclide study that must also be considered. An adequate study requires that a patient be able to achieve a satisfactory level of stress, which can be particularly difficult in the supine position. Accurate identification of the left ventricular edge and separation from contiguous structures, particularly the left atrium, is sometimes extremely difficult to achieve, decreasing the reproducibility of the test. The importance of this variable in routine clinical imaging tends to be underestimated in the literature. Unreliable gating signals and the presence of arrhythmias during acquisition of the image significantly detract from the quality of the data. The presence of left bundle branch block can be associated with both an abnormal ejection fraction response to exercise and segmental wall-motion abnormalities in the absence of coronary artery disease.[46] Finally, although the study has utility in distinguishing ischemic from nonischemic cardiomyopathy in patients with pronounced left ventricular dysfunction at rest,[12] its sensitivity for detecting additional exercise induced ischemia in this population is reduced.[47]

Prediction of high-risk coronary anatomy

Beyond its capability to determine the presence or absence of coronary artery disease, exercise radionuclide ventriculography also provides meaningful information about disease severity and prognosis.

Since extent of anatomic coronary disease is related to prognosis and since the approach to management is at least in part dictated by the extent of anatomic disease that is present, it is desirable to have a noninvasive test capable of identifying patients with three vessel or left main coronary artery disease. The change in left ventricular ejection fraction during exercise was initially proposed to be the most useful variable from exercise radionuclide ventriculography for identification of the presence of severe anatomic disease.[48] In a recent study, Wallis and Borer found with logistic regression analysis that the change in ejection fraction during exercise was the best single predictor of "surgical" coronary anatomy whereas peak ejection fraction contributed no significant independent information.[49] Nevertheless, the change in ejection fraction during exercise is a complex variable that is clearly influenced by a variety of factors and has been only weakly correlated with the anatomic extent of disease in some studies.[50]

DePace and coinvestigators reported two of the earliest studies that were specific investigations of the utility of exercise radionuclide ventriculography for detection of anatomically extensive disease.[27,44] They noted that the peak ejection fraction achieved during exercise correlated with the anatomic extent of disease, whereas the change in ejection fraction, end-diastolic volume, or end-systolic volume did not.[27] The presence of Q-waves on the electrocardiogram, the change in systolic blood pressure during exercise, the patient's sex, and the presence of diabetes contributed to peak ejection fraction in identifying severe disease.[44] These variables were more reliable in subjects who could achieve adequate exercise end points, defined either by a peak heart rate ≥120 or by the development of chest pain or ST-segment depression.

Weintraub and coinvestigators reported results from a similar study of 185 patients.[45] Using stepwise linear discriminant analysis, they also identified peak ejection fraction, along with the magnitude of ST-segment depression and peak heart rate as being predictors of multiple-vessel disease. From these three variables they created a somewhat burdensome set of four equations that were used to predict disease severity. Patients without significant disease were correctly classified 71% of the time. Patients with three-vessel disease were correctly classified 80% of the time. Ninety percent of the patients classified as three-vessel disease had either two- or three-vessel disease.

Gibbons and colleagues examined the ability of exercise radionuclide ventriculography to discriminate severity of disease in a study of 681 patients.[37] Using logistic regression analysis, they identified seven variables that were independently predictive of the presence of three-vessel or left main coronary disease. Four of these variables—the magnitude of ST-segment depression, peak ejection fraction, peak double product, and patient sex, in that order—were the most significant, providing nearly all the information. These variables were then used to define subgroups who had low, intermediate and high probabilities of left main or three-vessel coronary artery disease (Table 13-4). Thirty-two percent of the population

was in the low-probability subgroup. Of these, only 9% had left main or three-vessel disease. Thirty-eight percent of the population was in the high-risk subgroup. Of those, 56% had left main or three-vessel disease. Based upon these four variables, the authors constructed graphical estimates of probability of severe disease for women (Figure 13-2) and for men (Figure 13-3.) Of note, at virtually any given level of peak exercise ejection fraction, peak double product, and degree of ST-segment depression, men have a greater probability of three-vessel or left main coronary artery disease than women have.

Although the radionuclide ventriculographic study provided discriminating power in identifying patients with severe anatomic disease, in a subsequent study by the same group, it was noted that in the large subset of patients who have a normal resting electrocardiogram and are not on digitalis therapy the radionuclide parameters did not add meaningful additional information to that provided from clinical findings and the exercise test.[51] In that subgroup, therefore, the addition of the imaging study may not be justified. The authors correctly point out that further investigation into this important finding is necessary. Moreover, no variable from either the exercise test or from the exercise radionuclide ventriculogram can distinguish patients with left main coronary artery disease from those who have three-vessel disease.[52]

Assessment of prognosis in patients with stable coronary artery disease

Related to the proficiency of exercise radionuclide ventriculography in identifying the presence of severe anatomic disease is its capability to distinguish subgroups of patients who have a favorable or unfavorable prognosis. A considerable number of studies have demonstrated that the exercise radionuclide study provides substantial prognostic information, though there has been some variability in reports as to the degree to which this infor-

Table 13-4   Probability of left main or three-vessel coronary artery disease in low-, intermediate-, and high-risk subgroups determined from exercise radionuclide ventriculography

Group	Number of patients in group	Patients with left main or three-vessel disease	
		Number	Percent
Low probability	216	20	9
Intermediate probability	207	51	25
High probability	258	144	56
TOTAL	681	215	32

From Gibbons RJ et al: *J Am Coll Cardiol* 11:28-34, 1988.

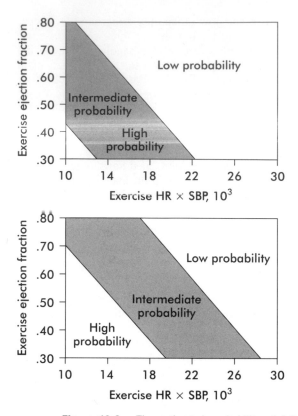

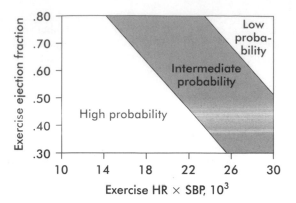

Figure 13-2 The estimated probability of left main or three-vessel coronary artery disease is shown for women with, **A,** <1 mm ST-segment depression; **B,** 1.0 mm ST-segment depression; and **C,** 2.0 mm ST-segment depression. Zones of probability are shown as predicted from the peak left ventricular ejection fraction during exercise, and the peak double product. (Exercise HR, peak heart rate achieved during exercise; SBP, systolic blood pressure.) (From Gibbons RJ et al: *J Am Coll Cardiol* 11:28-34, 1988.)

mation is independent of other clinical, exercise, and angiographic findings.

In two of the earliest studies, Bonow and co-workers at the National Institutes of Health[53] and Pryor and colleagues from Duke University[54] noted that exercise radionuclide ventriculography discriminates prognosis in patients who have coronary artery disease. In the NIH study, 117 patients with mildly symptomatic coronary artery disease and normal resting left ventricular function were assessed by coronary angiography and exercise radionuclide ventriculography. Mortality during the follow-up period was correlated with the presence of three-vessel disease as well as with the exercise ejection fraction. Of the patients who had three-vessel disease, a subgroup at high risk was identified by the presence of at least 1 mm of ST-segment depression on the exercise electrocardiogram, a decrease in ejection fraction during exercise, and a peak achieved work load of ≤120 watts. In this subset, the predicted survival at 4 years was 71%. All observed deaths occurred in

this subset, and, interestingly, all occurred in the first year.

In the Duke University study, 386 patients who had stable angina were assessed.[54] Univariate analysis identified exercise ejection fraction as the variable most closely associated with subsequent cardiac events. This was followed by resting ejection fraction, the presence of wall-motion abnormalities during exercise, and exercise time as predictors of risk. Mulitvariable analysis demonstrated that once exercise ejection fraction was known, no other radionuclide variable contributed additional prognostic information. Furthermore, the exercise ejection fraction provided most of the prognostic information that was available from coronary angiography. In a recent follow-up study from the same institution, the outcome of 1663 patients who had a clinical diagnosis of coronary artery disease and underwent exercise radionuclide ventriculography but did not have early surgical intervention was assessed.[55] Multivariable analysis revealed that clinical information provided only 5% of the

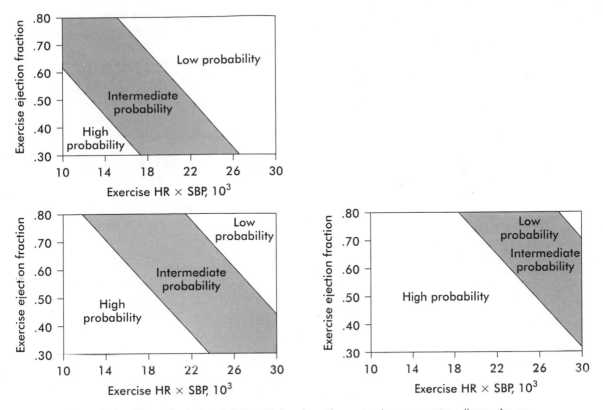

Figure 13-3   The estimated probability of left main or three-vessel coronary artery disease for men. Format and abbreviations as in Fig. 13-2. (From Gibbons RJ et al: *J Am Coll Cardiol* 11:28-34, 1988.)

prognostic power whereas radionuclide variables provided 95% of the power. Of the radionuclide variables, the exercise ejection fraction was the most important variable, providing 85% of the total information. Patients with exercise ejection fractions below 0.50 had greater mortality risk, which increased as the peak ejection fraction decreased, whereas those who had peak ejection fractions above 0.50 had a highly favorable prognosis (Figure 13-4). In a separate analysis of 571 patients from their population who had angiographically documented CAD and were treated medically, radionuclide angiographic variables were again strongly related to mortality, providing 84% of the information provided by clinical and angiographic descriptors combined.[56] The radionuclide variables were found to provide significant additional information to that provided by both clinical and catheterization findings.

In a study of 424 medically treated patients, Taliercio and colleagues from the Mayo Clinic reported somewhat different experience.[57] In their 22-month follow-up study, only three variables were found to be independently related to cardiac events in the follow-up period: the number of diseased vessels defined at angiography, the resting radionuclide ejection fraction, and age. In patients with three-vessel disease and an ejection fraction greater than 0.40, radionuclide variables were unable to differentiate subgroups with greater or lesser risk. The difference in the findings comparing this study with the NIH study[53] might be attributable to patient selection.[58] In the Mayo Clinic sample, patients with three-vessel disease had high prognostic risk even in the absence of inducible ischemia, in contrast to the patients from the NIH series. The Mayo clinic patient group was older than the NIH study population, and antianginal medications were not withheld during the exercise study. The medications might have concealed exercise-induced ischemia, thereby masking its potential power to discriminate outcome. Medications were withheld in the NIH study. Finally, 34% of the patients who were potential candidates for the Mayo Clinic study were not included because they underwent revascularization, potentially biasing outcome results of the final study population.

In a more recent study from the Mayo Clinic group, Miller and co-workers examined the prognostic information from exercise radionuclide angiography in 65 consecutive patients with one- or

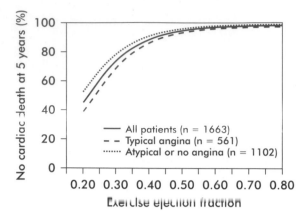

Figure 13-4 The probability of survival at 5 years is shown relative to the peak left ventricular ejection fraction achieved during exercise in 1663 patients. Patients with typical angina (*n* = 561) and atypical chest pain (*n* = 1102) are also shown separately. Mortality is strongly related to peak ejection fraction, with the inflection point being at an ejection fraction of 0.50. (From Jones RH et al: *Circulation* 84[suppl I]:I-52 to I-58, 1991.)

two-vessel disease and impaired left ventricular function (ejection fraction <0.50).[59] Univariate analysis identified severe ischemia (decrease in ejection fraction during exercise with ≥1 mm of ST-segment depression and a peak work load of ≤600 kg-m/min) on radionuclide angiography as the only variable that significantly predicted future cardiac events. In an effort to examine the possible influences of referral bias, this group also performed a population-based study, examining the outcome of 526 residents of Olmstead County who had undergone exercise radionuclide ventriculography.[60] In that sample, exercise ejection fraction, peak heart rate, age, and history of myocardial infarction were independent predictors of outcome, with exercise ejection fraction and peak heart rate being the most important.

Taken together, the cumulative findings from these studies indicate that exercise radionuclide ventriculography provides substantial prognostic information in the evaluation of patients with chronic coronary artery disease. It has yet to be fully determined in which patients this information adds meaningfully to information provided by clinical and exercise test parameters. For example, Simari and colleagues examined the outcome in 265 patients who had documented CAD, had a normal resting electrocardiogram, were not receiving digoxin therapy, and were treated with medical therapy.[61] In their study, the findings from radionuclide angiography did not add significantly to the prognostic power of exercise electrocardiography. However, this was clearly a biased sam-

ple in that 119 patients had been excluded from the trial because they underwent early revascularization with either percutaneous transluminal coronary angioplasty or bypass surgery. The group undergoing early revascularization had more severe disease. It is very likely that the findings from exercise radionuclide ventriculography contributed to the clinical decision to proceed with revascularization in these patients. The conclusions from this study have limited relevance because the exercise radionuclide study was used to identify the lower risk group, which was then treated medically. Once that subgroup was identified, the results of the radionuclide study did not further contribute to the prognostic assessment compared to the exercise test variables, but the radionuclide study was used originally to identify the subset.

Exercise radionuclide ventriculography also has prognostic utility in evaluating patients who have either mild angina or silent ischemia. Bonow and co-workers examined findings from 131 consecutive CAD patients who had preserved left ventricular function at rest with mild or no angina during medical therapy.[62] Patients who developed angina during the exercise study had more severe anatomic disease than those who did not have angina. However, exercise induced ischemia identified the group at increased prognostic risk, independent of the presence or absence of associated symptoms. Symptomatic status did not add to the prognostic information from the exercise radionuclide variables.

A subsequent study from the same group examined a related issue of prognosis in patients who had one- or two-vessel disease with left ventricular dysfunction (resting ejection fraction 0.20 to 0.40), and mild symptoms on medical therapy.[63] The ST-segment response to exercise, peak ejection fraction, and change in ejection fraction during exercise were all associated with mortality during the follow-up period. Breitenbucher and co-workers reported findings from a retrospective 5-year follow-up study of 140 patients who had unequivocal exercise-induced ischemia on a radionuclide ventriculographic examination.[64] Critical cardiac events overall were no different in the 84 patients who had silent ischemia compared to the 56 patients who had angina. Myocardial infarction or death were actually more frequent in the asymptomatic group. In part, the reason might be that more of the symptomatic patients underwent revascularization therapy.

As has been described, the specificity of exercise radionuclide ventriculography for coronary artery disease is between 50% and 80%. Miller and colleagues examined the prognostic significance of an abnormal exercise radionuclide ventriculographic study in patients who do not have anatomic coronary artery disease at angiography.[65] They followed 79 consecutive patients with these findings for a mean of 25 months. There were no mortalities and only one nonfatal myocardial infarction during the follow-up period. This subgroup therefore appears to be in a very favorable prognostic category.

Assessment of prognosis in the postinfarction patient

In the postinfarction setting, exercise radionuclide ventriculographic examination also has prognostic utility. In two early reports, Corbett and colleagues reported results of submaximal exercise ventriculographic examinations of 117 patients with recent myocardial infarction.[66,67] Patients who had anterior infarction had lower resting ejection fractions and a more abnormal left ventricular response to exercise than those with inferior infarction, though there was considerable inhomogenicity within the groups.[66] Discriminant function analysis ranked exercise changes in left ventricular ejection fraction and end-systolic volume as the most important of all clinical, exercise, and scintigraphic variables in predicting subsequent cardiac events.[67] Changes in left ventricular ejection fraction had 93% predictive power for outcome. Dewhurst and Muir noted similar findings in a report of outcome of 100 infarct patients reported in the same year.[68] In their study, exercise radionuclide ventriculography identified 88% of the 17 patients who suffered sudden death in the first 2 years after infarction. The radionuclide study was superior to either the exercise ECG response or the presence of exertional angina in identifying this high-risk subset.

Hung and coinvestigators evaluated 117 men with recent myocardial infarction with the symptom-limited treadmill exercise test, thallium scintigraphy, and radionuclide ventriculography.[69] Peak treadmill exercise level, the change in left ventricular ejection fraction during exercise, and a history of postinfarction chest pain in the coronary care unit were significantly predictive of the subsequent occurrence of cardiac death, cardiac arrest or myocardial infarction, unstable angina, congestive heart failure, or need for coronary bypass surgery. The radionuclide study contributed independent prognostic information to the treadmill test and was superior to thallium scintigraphy. These findings were not confirmed in a subsequent report by Murray and colleagues, however, who found that exercise thallium scintigraphy was the best predictor of postinfarction prognosis whereas the exercise radionuclide ventriculography study did not add to the prognostic assessment.[70] Using a Cox proportional hazards regression model,

Morris and colleagues found that resting ejection fraction and the peak exercise ejection fraction were predictors of subsequent death in their study of 106 postinfarction patients.[71] The change in ejection fraction during exercise allowed prediction of the need for subsequent coronary bypass surgery for refractory angina but did not allow prediction of other cardiac events or death. Abraham and co-workers also noted that peak exercise ejection fraction, but not the change in ejection fraction during exercise, was related to such a prognosis after infarction.[72]

It is important to note that the studies that utilized exercise radionuclide ventriculography in the assessment of a postinfarction prognosis largely predated the era of use of thrombolytic agents in the treatment of acute infarction. In a retrospective assessment of 791 consecutive patients who were referred for postinfarction exercise radionuclide ventriculographic examination over a 5-year time frame, Lavie and colleagues observed that the characteristics of the patients changed considerably, with increasing trends found in the use of thrombolytic therapy, early revascularization procedures, use of beta blockers, Q-wave infarction, inferior infarction, peak double product, exercise capacity, significant ST-segment depression during exercise, peak exercise ejection fraction, and change in ejection fraction during exercise.[73] Caution is therefore indicated in applying results from earlier prognostic trials to current postinfarction subjects. Further prospective trials will be important.

Assessment of the postrevascularization patient

There is only a limited number of studies that have examined the utility of exercise radionuclide ventriculography in the patients who have undergone previous coronary artery angioplasty or bypass surgery. It is likely that those patients who have the greatest fall in ejection fraction during exercise are the ones who are most likely to benefit from revascularization.

Kent and colleagues evaluated 59 consecutive patients who underwent coronary angioplasty.[74] They observed that left ventricular ejection fraction at rest was not different after PTCA, but peak exercise ejection fraction increased from 0.51 ± 0.03 before the procedure to 0.62 ± 0.02 ($p < 0.001$) after PTCA. Nineteen of 38 patients with a successful procedure had sustained improvement in function over 6 months of follow-up study. DePuey and co-workers examined 41 patients with exercise radionuclide ventriculography before and within 4 days after PTCA.[75] Patients who had an abnormal left ventricular response to exercise early after PTCA, defined as an increase in ejection fraction of less than 0.05 unit or the development of regional wall motion abnormalities, had more severe restenosis on follow-up angiography 4 to 12 months later. An abnormal early exercise radionuclide study was 73% accurate in predicting 50% or greater restenosis on follow up study.

Jones and colleagues examined results of exercise radionuclide ventriculographic studies of 278 patients with CAD who had low resting ejection fractions in order to assess the relationship of the radionuclide study to outcome with medical or surgical therapy.[76] Of the 172 medically treated patients, the radionuclide study identified a subgroup of 113 patients who had a 20% lower 3-year survival than the 59 patients who had a normal exercise response. Comparing all patients who had significant ischemia on the baseline study, they found that those who underwent surgical therapy had improved survival and relief of symptoms whereas those with a negative exercise study had similar outcomes with either therapy. Kronenberg and co-workers noted that the degree of postoperative improvement in exercise ejection fraction correlated with the degree of ischemia that was present on the preoperative exercise radionuclide study in their study of 36 patients,[77] a finding that was subsequently confirmed by others.[78] Improvement in regional left ventricular asynergy immediately after exercise has also been associated with improvement in function after bypass surgery.[79]

Dilsizian and colleagues used exercise radionuclide ventriculography with quantitative assessment of regional function to examine the effect of coronary bypass surgery on function of myocardial areas that could not be revascularized.[80] Twenty-four patients who had multiple-vessel disease, which included proximal circumflex or obtuse marginal disease, were studied. As a group, both global ejection fraction and the increase in ejection fraction during exercise increased postoperatively. There was no difference in the improvement comparing the 10 patients who had all vessels successfully bypassed compared with the 10 who had a circumflex vessel that either could not be bypassed or was subsequently shown to have an occluded graft. The regional ejection fraction also improved to a similar degree in the posterolateral segment in the two groups. Eight of the 10 patients with nonrevascularized circumflex coronary vessels had collaterals to that distribution from other arteries that were bypassed. The authors concluded that bypassing of other vessels might improve postoperative function in nonbypassable vessels by enhancing collateral flow. Alternatively, however, the exercise radionuclide study might be insensitive in detecting and quantifying regional myocardial dysfunction in the circumflex coronary artery distribution.

Comparative use of radionuclide ventriculography and ^{201}Tl scintigraphy

Although the information content of exercise radionuclide ventriculography is in many ways similar to that of exercise thallium scintigraphy, the latter has emerged as the more widely utilized study in the clinical evaluation of patients with known or suspected coronary artery disease. Most clinical departments currently use ^{201}Tl scintigraphy as the diagnostic procedure of choice. In part this might be because perfusion is a more direct indicator of vascular disease than function is. Changes in ventricular function might occur somewhat later than changes in perfusion, an implication that perfusion studies might be a somewhat more sensitive indicator particularly of multiple-vessel disease though this sensitivity has not been clearly established. Exercise thallium scintigraphy is unquestionably more specific than exercise ventriculography is. The advantage of the ^{99m}Tc perfusion agents compared to ^{201}Tl has not been established.

In patients with equivocal exercise electrocardiograms, exercise ^{201}Tl scintigraphy is more sensitive and more accurate than exercise radionuclide ventriculography in establishing a diagnosis of CAD.[81] Using multivariable analysis in a study of 86 patients, Borges-Neto and co-workers noted that SPECT perfusion studies, in this instance using sestamibi, provided more diagnostic information than either exercise electrocardiography or exercise radionuclide ventriculography did.[82] However, the ventricular function information did add to the information provided by the perfusion study. Dilsizian and coinvestigators noted that exercise radionuclide ventriculography was more reliable than qualitative SPECT ^{201}Tl imaging but was equally reliable to quantitative SPECT ^{201}Tl for detection of circumflex coronary artery disease.[83]

Overall, both exercise ^{201}Tl scintigraphy and exercise radionuclide ventriculography have clearly established efficacy in the establishment of a diagnosis of coronary artery disease, as well as in the assessment of its severity and prognostic implication. It is, however, relevant to note that the studies that have compared exercise ^{201}Tl scintigraphy to exercise radionuclide ventriculography are primarily older studies, which preceded the more advanced methods used with either technique today. Further comparative trials are indicated.

SUMMARY

Exercise radionuclide studies can be used for the assessment of myocardial function, using either first-pass or equilibrium blood pool techniques. Exercise radionuclide ventriculographic studies have a sensitivity for detection of coronary artery disease that is comparable to that of exercise thallium scintigraphy and are superior to exercise electrocardiography. Its specificity is somewhat less than ^{201}Tl scintigraphy. The peak left ventricular ejection fraction achieved during exercise appears to be the most useful single diagnostic variable from the study, though the change in ejection fraction during exercise has been noted in several studies to provide the most diagnostic information. The radionuclide data are additive to the clinical and exercise information in defining the diagnostic and prognostic implication of the individual patient's study.

Exercise radionuclide ventriculography has a demonstrated value in detecting severe anatomic coronary artery disease, either three-vessel disease or left main coronary disease. It also has clearly documented utility in the assessment of prognosis of the patient with coronary disease, including patients with mildly symptomatic or asymptomatic disease. The information from the exercise radionuclide study appears to be superior to angiography or exercise electrocardiography in determining prognosis, though the information from the different tests is often additive in different studies. It also has demonstrated utility in the diagnostic and prognostic evaluation of the patient with prior myocardial infarction or coronary artery revascularization, with either percutaneous transluminal coronary angioplasty or coronary artery bypass surgery.

REFERENCES

1. Burow RD, Strauss HW, Singleton R, et al: Analysis of left ventricular function from multiple gated acquisition cardiac blood pool imaging: comparison to contrast angiography, *Circulation* 56:1024-1028, 1977.
2. Wackers FJT, Berger HJ, Johnstone DE, et al: Multiple gated cardiac blood pool imaging for left ventricular ejection fraction: validation of the technique and assessment of variability, *Am J Cardiol* 43:1159-1166, 1979.
3. Marshall RC, Berger HJ, Costin JC, et al: Assessment of cardiac performance with quantitative radionuclide angiocardiography: sequential left ventricular ejection fraction, normalized left ventricular ejection rate, and regional wall motion, *Circulation* 56:820-829, 1977.
4. Berger HJ, Johnstone DE, Sands JM, et al: Response of right ventricular ejection fraction to upright bicycle exercise in coronary artery disease, *Circulation* 60:1292-1300, 1979.
5. Okada RD, Kirshenbaum HD, Kushner FG, et al: Observer variance in the qualitative evaluation of left ventricular wall motion and the quantitation of left ventricular ejection fraction using rest and exercise multigated blood pool imaging, *Circulation* 61:128-136, 1980.
6. Swain JL, Morris KG, Bruno FP, et al: Comparison of multigated radionuclide angiography with ultrasonic sonomicrometry over a wide range of ventricular function in the conscious dog, *Am J Cardiol* 46:976-982, 1980.
7. Mancini GBJ, Slutsky RA, Norris SL, et al: Radionuclide analysis of peak filling rate, filling fraction, and time to peak filling rate: response to supine bicycle exercise in nor-

mal subjects and patients with coronary disease, *Am J Cardiol* 51:43-51, 1983.
8. Kaul S, Boucher CA, Okada RD, et al: Sources of variability in the radionuclide angiographic assessment of ejection fraction: a comparison of first-pass and gated equilibrium techniques, *Am J Cardiol* 53:823-828, 1984.
9. Gibbons RJ, Morris KG, Lee K, et al: Assessment of regional left ventricular function using gated radionuclide angiography, *Am J Cardiol* 54:294-300, 1984.
10. Wasserman AG, Johnson RA, Katz RJ, et al: Detection of left ventricular wall motion abnormalities for the diagnosis of coronary artery disease: a comparision of exercise radionuclide and pacing intravenous digital ventriculography, *Am J Cardiol* 54:497-501, 1984.
11. Freeman MR, Berman DS, Staniloff H, et al: Comparision of upright and supine bicycle exercise in the detection and evaluation of extent of coronary artery disease by equilibrium radionuclide ventriculography, *Am Heart J* 102:182-188, 1981.
12. Port S, McEwan P, Cobb FR, et al: Influence of resting left ventricular function on the left ventricular response to exercise in patients with coronary artery disease, *Circulation* 63:856-863, 1981.
13. Hanley PC, Zinsmeister AR, Clements IP, et al: Gender-related differences in cardiac response to supine exercise assessed by radionuclide angiography, *J Am Coll Cardiol* 13:624-629, 1989.
14. Higginbotham MB, Morris KG, Coleman E, et al: Sex-related differences in normal cardiac response to upright exercise, *Circulation* 70:357-366, 1984.
15. Philbrick JT, Horwitz RI, Feinstein AR: Methodologic problems of exercise testing for coronary artery disease: groups, analysis and bias, *Am J Cardiol* 46:807-812, 1980.
16. Hecht HS, Josephson MA, Hopkins JM, et al: Reproducibility of equilibrium radionuclide ventriculography in patients with coronary artery disease: response of left ventricular ejection fraction and regional wall motion to supine bicycle exercise, *Am Heart J* 104:567-575, 1982.
17. Sorensen SG, Caldwell J, Ritchie J, et al: "Abnormal" responses of ejection fraction to exercise, in healthy subjects, caused by region-of-interest selection, *J Nucl Med* 22:1-7, 1981.
18. Borer JS, Bacharach SL, Green MV, et al: Real-time radionuclide cineangiography in the noninvasive evaluation of global and regional left ventricular function at rest and during exercise in patients with coronary artery disease, *N Engl J Med* 296:839-844, 1977.
19. Borer JS, Kent KM, Bacharach SL, et al: Sensitivity, specificity and predictive accuracy of radionuclide cineangiography during exercise in patients with coronary artery disease: comparison with exercise electrocardiography, *Circulation* 60:572-580, 1979.
20. Berger HJ, Reduto LA, Johnstone DE, et al: Global and regional left ventricular response to bicycle exercise in coronary artery disease: assessment by quantitative radionuclide angiocardiography, *Am J Med* 66:13-21, 1979.
21. Caldwell JH, Hamilton GW, Sorensen SG, et al: The detection of coronary artery disease with radionuclide techniques: a comparison of rest-exercise thallium imaging and ejection fraction response, *Circulation* 61:610-619, 1980.
22. Johnstone DE, Sands MJ, Berger HJ, et al: Comparison of exercise radionuclide angiocardiography and thallium-201 myocardial perfusion imaging in coronary artery disease, *Am J Cardiol* 45:1113-1119, 1980.
23. Jengo JA, Freeman R, Brizendine M, et al: Detection of coronary artery disease: Comparison of exercise stress radionuclide angiocardiography and thallium stress perfusion scanning, *Am J Cardiol* 45:535-541, 1980.
24. Leong K, Jones RH: Influence of the location of left ante-

rior descending coronary artery stenosis on left ventricular function during exercise, *Circulation* 65:109-114, 1982.

25. Kuo LC, Bolli R, Thornby J, et al: Effects of exercise tolerance, age, and gender on the specificity of radionuclide angiography: sequential ejection fraction analysis during multistage exercise, *Am Heart J* 113:1180-1189, 1987.

26. Gibbons RJ, Lee KL, Pryor D, et al: The use of radionuclide angiography in the diagnosis of coronary artery disease: a logistic regression analysis, *Circulation* 68:740-746, 1983.

27. DePace NL, Iskandrian AS, Hakki A, et al: Value of left ventricular ejection fraction during exercise in predicting the extent of coronary artery disease, *J Am Coll Cardiol* 1:1002-1010, 1983.

28. Gibbons RJ, Clements IP, Zinsmeister AR, et al: Exercise response of the systolic pressure to end systolic volume ratio in patients with coronary artery disease, *J Am Coll Cardiol* 10:33-39, 1987.

29. Gibbons RJ: Rest and exercise radionuclide angiography for diagnosis in chronic ischemic heart disease, *Circulation* 84(suppl I):I-93–I-99, 1991.

30. Jengo JA, Oren V, Conant R, et al: Effects of maximal exercise stress on left ventricular function in patients with coronary artery disease using first pass radionuclide angiocardiography: a rapid, noninvasive technique for determining ejection fraction and segmental wall motion, *Circulation* 59:60-65, 1979.

31. Jones RH, McEwan P, Newman GE, et al: Accuracy of diagnosis of coronary artery disease by radionuclide measurement of left ventricular function during rest and exercise, *Circulation* 64:586-600, 1981.

32. Gibbons RJ: Nuclear cardiology. In Guiliani ER, Fuster V, Gersh BJ, et al, editors: *Cardiology: fundamentals and practice,* ed 2, St. Louis, 1991, Mosby.

33. Bodenheimer MM, Banka VS, Fooshee CM, et al: Comparative sensitivity of the exercise electrocardiogram, thallium imaging and stress radionuclide angiography to detect the presence and severity of coronary artery disease, *Circulation* 60:1270-1278, 1979.

34. Upton MT, Rerych SK, Newman GE, et al: Detecting abnormalities in left ventricular function during exercise before angina and ST-segment depression, *Circulation* 62:341-349, 1980.

35. Gibbons RJ, Lee KL, Cobb FR, et al: Ejection fraction response to exercise in patients with chest pain and normal coronary angiograms, *Circulation* 64:952-957, 1981.

35a. Rozanski A, Diamond GA, Berman D, et al: The declining specificity of exercise radionuclide ventriculography, *N Engl J Med* 309:518-522, 1983.

35b. Rozanski A, Diamond GA, Forrester JS, et al: Alternative reference standards for cardiac normality: implications for diagnostic testing, *Ann Intern Med* 101:164-171, 1984.

36. Currie PJ, Kelly MJ, Harper RW, et al: Incremental value of clinical assessment, supine exercise electrocardiography, and biplane exercise radionuclide ventriculography in the prediction of coronary artery disease in men with chest pain, *Am J Cardiol* 52:927-935, 1983.

37. Gibbons RJ, Fyke FE, Clements IP, et al: Noninvasive identification of severe coronary artery disease using exercise radionuclide angiography, *J Am Coll Cardiol* 11:28-34, 1988.

38. Okada RD, Pohost GM, Kirshenbaum HD, et al: Radionuclide-determined change in pulmonary blood volume with exercise: improved sensitivity of multigated blood-pool scanning in detecting coronary-artery disease, *N Engl J Med* 301:569-576, 1979.

39. Hanley PC, Gibbons RJ: Value of radionuclide-determined changes in pulmonary blood volume for the detection of coronary artery disease, *Chest* 97:7-11, 1990.

40. Dehmer GJ, Lewis SE, Hillis LD, et al: Exercise-induced alterations in left ventricular volumes and the pressure-volume relationship: a sensitive indicator of left ventricular dysfunction in patients with coronary artery disease, *Circulation* 63:1008-1017, 1981.

41. Iskandrian AS, Hakki A, Bemis Ce, et al: Left ventricular end-systolic pressure-volume relation: a combined radionuclide and hemodynamic study, *Am J Cardiol* 51:1057-1061, 1983.

42. Breitenbucher A, Pfisterer M, Hoffmann A, et al: Long-term follow-up of patients with silent ischemia during exercise radionuclide angiography, *J Am Coll Cardiol* 15:999-1003, 1990.

43. Vassiliadis JV, Machac J, O'Hara M, et al: Exercise-induced myocardial dysfunction in patients with coronary artery disease with and without angina, *Am Heart J* 121:1403-1408, 1991.

44. DePace NL, Hakki A, Weinreich DJ, et al: Noninvasive assessment of coronary artery disease, *Am J Cardiol* 52:714-720, 1983.

45. Weintraub WS, Schneider RM, Seelaus PA, et al: Prospective evaluation of the severity of coronary artery disease with exercise radionuclide angiography and electrocardiography, *Am Heart J* 111:537-542, 1986.

46. Rowe DW, De Puey EG, Sonnemaker RE, et al: Left ventricular performance during exercise in patients with left bundle branch block: evaluation by gated radionuclide ventriculography, *Am Heart J* 105:66-71, 1983.

47. Port S, McEwan P, Cobb FR, et al: Influence of resting left ventricular function on the left ventricular response to exercise in patients with coronary artery disease, *Circulation* 63:856-863, 1981.

48. Campos CT, Chu HW, D'Agostino JH Jr, et al: Comparision of rest and exercise radionuclide angiography and exercise treadmill testing for diagnosis of anatomically extensive coronary artery disease, *Circulation* 67:1204-1210, 1983.

49. Wallis JB, Borer JS: Identification of "surgical" coronary anatomy by exercise radionuclide cineangiography, *Am J Cardiol* 68:1150-1157, 1991.

50. Gibbons RJ, Lee KL, Cobb FR, et al: Ejection fraction response to exercise in patients with chest pain, coronary artery disease and normal resting ventricular function, *Circulation* 66:643-648, 1982.

51. Gibbons RJ, Zinsmeister AR, Miller TD, et al: Supine exercise electrocardiography compared with exercise radionuclide angiography in noninvasive identification of severe coronary artery disease, *Ann Intern Med* 112:743-749, 1990.

52. Gibbons RJ, Fyke EF III, Brown ML, et al: Comparison of exercise performance in left main and three-vessel coronary artery disease, *Cathet Cardiovasc Diagn* 22:14-20, 1991.

53. Bonow RO, Kent KM, Rosing DR, et al: Exercise-induced ischemia in mildly symptomatic patients with coronary-artery disease and preserved left ventricular function: identification of subgroups at risk of death during medical therapy, *N Engl J Med* 311:1339-1345, 1984.

54. Pryor DB, Harrell FE Jr, Lee KL, et al: Prognostic indicators from radionuclide angiography in medically treated patients with coronary artery disease, *Am J Cardiol* 53:18-22, 1984.

55. Jones RH, Johnson SH, Bigelow C, et al: Exercise radionuclide angiocardiography predicts cardiac death in patients with coronary artery disease, *Circulation* 84(suppl I):I-52–I-58, 1991.

56. Lee KL, Pryor DB, Pieper KS, et al: Prognostic value of radionuclide angiography in medically treated patients with coronary artery disease: a comparison with clinical and

catheterization variables, *Circulation* 82:1705-1717, 1990.

57. Taliercio CP, Clements IP, Zinsmeister AR, et al: Prognostic value and limitations of exercise radionuclide angiography in medically treated coronary artery disease, *Mayo Clin Proc* 63:573-582, 1988.

58. Bonow RO: Prognostic implications of exercise radionuclide angiography in patients with coronary artery disease, *Mayo Clin Proc* 63:630-634, 1988.

59. Miller TD, Taliercio CP, Zinsmeister AR, et al: Risk stratification of single or double vessel coronary artery disease and impaired left ventricular function using exercise radionuclide angiography, *Am J Cardiol* 65:1317-1321, 1990.

60. Gibbons RJ, Zinsmeister AR, Ballard DJ, et al: Prognostic value of exercise radionuclide angiography in a community population, *Circulation* 78(suppl II):II-423, 1988.

61. Simari RD, Miller TD, Zinsmeister AR, et al: Capabilities of supine exercise electrocardiography versus exercise radionuclide angiography in predicting coronary events, *Am J Cardiol* 67:573-577, 1991.

62. Bonow RO, Bacharach SL, Green MV, et al: Prognostic implications of symptomatic versus asymptomatic (silent) myocardial ischemia induced by exercise in mildly symptomatic and in asymptomatic patients with angiographically documented coronary artery disease, *Am J Cardiol* 60:778-783, 1987.

63. Mazzotta G, Bonow RO, Pace L, et al: Relation between exertional ischemia and prognosis in mildly symptomatic patients with single or double vessel coronary artery disease and left ventricular dysfunction at rest, *J Am Coll Cardiol* 13:567-573, 1989.

64. Breitenbucher A, Pfisterer M, Hoffmann A, et al: Long-term follow-up of patients with silent ischemia during exercise radionuclide angiography, *J Am Coll Cardiol* 15:999-1003, 1990.

65. Miller TD, Taliercio CP, Zinsmeister AR, et al: Prognosis in patients with an abnormal exercise radionuclide angiogram in the absence of significant coronary artery disease, *J Am Coll Cardiol* 12:637-641, 1988.

66. Corbett JR, Nicod PH, Huxley RL, et al: Left ventricular functional alterations at rest and during submaximal exercise in patients with recent myocardial infarction, *Am J Med* 74:577-591, 1983.

67. Corbett JR, Nicod PH, Lewis SE, et al: Prognostic value of submaximal exercise radionuclide ventriculography after myocardial infarction, *Am J Cardiol* 52:82A-91A, 1983.

68. Dewhurst NG, Muir AL: Comparative prognostic value of radionuclide ventriculography at rest and during exercise in 100 patients after first myocardial infarction, *Br Heart J* 49:111-121, 1983.

69. Hung J, Goris ML, Nash E, et al: Comparative value of maximal treadmill testing, exercise thallium myocardial perfusion scintigraphy and exercise radionuclide ventriculography for distinguishing high- and low-risk patients soon after acute myocardial infarction, *Am J Cardiol* 53:1221-1227, 1984.

70. Murray DP, Rafiqi E, Murray RG, et al: Prognostic investigations after myocardial infarction: a comparison of radionuclide angiography and ^{201}T1 scintigraphy, *Eur J Nucl Med* 11:381-385, 1986.

71. Morris KG, Palmeri ST, Califf RM, et al: Value of radionuclide angiography for predicting specific cardiac events after acute myocardial infarction, *Am J Cardiol* 55:318-324, 1985.

72. Abraham RD, Harris PJ, Roubin GS, et al: Usefulness of ejection fraction response to exercise one month after acute myocardial infarction in predicting coronary anatomy and prognosis, *Am J Cardiol* 60:225-230, 1987.

73. Lavie CJ, Gibbons RJ, Zinsmeister AR, et al: Interpreting results of exercise studies after acute myocardial infarction altered by thrombolytic therapy, coronary angioplasty or bypass, *Am J Cardiol* 67:116-120, 1991.

74. Kent KM, Bonow RO, Rosing DR, et al: Improved myocardial function during exercise after successful percutaneous transluminal coronary angioplasty, *N Engl J Med* 306:441-446, 1982.

75. De Puey EG, Leatherman LL, Leachman RD, et al: Restenosis after transluminal coronary angioplasty detected with exercise-gated radionuclide ventriculography, *J Am Coll Cardiol* 4:1103-1113, 1984.

76. Jones RH, Floyd RD, Austin EH, et al: The role of radionuclide angiocardiography in the preoperative prediction of pain relief and prolonged survival following coronary artery bypass grafting, *Ann Surg* 197:743-754, 1983.

77. Kronenberg MW, Pederson RW, Harston WE, et al: Left ventricular performance after coronary bypass surgery: prediciton of functional benefit, *Ann Intern Med* 99:305-313, 1983.

78. Lewis RL, Videll JS, Strong MD, et al: Exercise radionuclide assessment of left ventricular function before and after coronary bypass surgery, *Angiology* 38:601-608, 1987.

79. Rozanski A, Berman D, Gray R, et al: Preoperative prediciton of reversible myocardial asynergy by postexercise radionuclide ventriculography, *N Engl J Med* 307:212-216, 1982.

80. Dilsizian V, Cannon RO, Tracy CM, et al: Enhanced regional left ventricular function after distant coronary bypass by means of improved collateral blood flow, *J Am Coll Cardiol* 14:312-318, 1989.

81. Candell-Riera J, Castell-Conesa J, Ortega-Alcalde D, et al: Diagnostic accuracy of radionuclide techniques in patients with equivocal electrocardiographic exercise testing, *Eur Heart J* 11:980-989, 1990.

82. Borges-Neto S, Coleman RE, Jones RH: Perfusion and function at rest and treadmill exercise using technetium-99m-scstamibi: comparison of one and two day protocols in normal volunteers, *J Nucl Med* 31:1128-1132, 1990.

83. Dilsizian V, Perrone-Filardi P, Cannon RO, et al: Comparison of exercise radionuclide angiography with thallium SPECT imaging for detection of significant narrowing of the left circumflex coronary artery, *Am J Cardiol* 68:320-327, 1991.

14 Stress Echocardiography

Electrocardiographic monitoring during upright treadmill exercise remains, by far, the most common screening test for the detection of coronary artery disease. Limitations of this technique, however, including both false-negative and false-positive test results, are well known and described in detail throughout this text. Accordingly, adjunctive imaging techniques have been applied during stress testing to increase both predictive accuracy and the amount of information obtained during such tests. Radionuclide imaging techniques, including rest and stress perfusion agents such as thallium 201 and radionuclide angiography, are described in detail elsewhere in this text. The focus of this chapter is the use of cardiac ultrasound during various forms of stress testing.

Echocardiographic imaging and cardiac Doppler velocity measurements have been applied both during treadmill and bicycle exercise stress tests and during pharmacological stress, induced by a variety of agents. During stress testing, myocardial segments in the distribution of a stenotic coronary artery may become ischemic. This ischemia often results in wall-motion abnormalities including hypokinesis and decreased wall thickening, which are apparent with two-dimensional echocardiographic monitoring. The relatively high sensitivity of echocardiography in recording these stress-induced wall-motion abnormalities makes it an excellent adjunctive imaging technique for stress testing.

HISTORICAL PERSPECTIVE

Echocardiographic monitoring of left ventricular wall motion during exercise was first reported in 1970.[1] However, this and several subsequent reports utilized M-mode echocardiography.[2-4] This technique was inherently limited by the inability to simultaneously image all but a small area of the ventricular septum and posterior left ventricular wall. In the early 1980s there were several reports assessing the use of two-dimensional echocardiography during exercise stress testing in the detection of coronary artery disease.[5-13] Although these studies were very promising, the limitations of cardiac ultrasound as a stress-imaging technique were quite apparent. Despite optimal patient selection, success rates remained consistently below 90%, limiting the widespread application of this technique. Many of the early studies focused on obtaining images during maximal exercise, thus compounding the low success rate in trying to obtain images in a moving patient. This, along with rapid respirations and tachycardia, made interpretation more difficult. At the same period of time, rapid advances in the field of radionuclide imaging blunted the incentive for further development of stress echocardiography techniques.

During the 1980s, however, there were several developments that led to a re-emergence of stress echocardiography as a viable technique. Advances in computer parallel-processing techniques led to development of higher quality equipment. Endocardiovisualization improved steadily with newer cardiac ultrasound machines, and advanced image processing led to a sharp decrease in the number of technically unsatisfactory studies (Table 14-1). In addition, several pharmacological stress agents became available during the past decade with which one could stress the heart up to the development of regional wall-motion abnormalities without exercise, also lowering the incidence of technically unsatisfactory studies. Similarly, it became evident that one need not obtain stress images during maximal exercise in all patients and that immediately after exercise images would more often than not provide similar information. Finally the widespread application and availability of digitally processed images enabled

Table 14-1 Exercise echocardiography success rate

Author	Year	Type of exercise	Number of patients	Success Rate (%)
Wann	1979	Supine bike	28	71
Morganroth	1981	Supine bike	55	78
Visser	1983	Supine bike	52	75
Crawford	1983	Upright bike	25	72
Maurer	1981	Treadmill	48	85
Heng	1984	Treadmill	54	87
Armstrong	1986	Treadmill	95	100
Labovitz	1989	Treadmill	73	94
Crouse	1991	Treadmill	228	100
Marwick	1992	Treadmill	150	100
Quinones	1992	Treadmill	292	99

one to obtain a single cardiac cycle of high quality after stress that could be displayed in an endless-loop format. This technique provided several advantages over studies recorded on tape, including a format by which comparison of rest and exercise images could be made side-by-side, thus enhancing the sensitivity of more subtle ischemic wall-motion abnormalities.

EXERCISE
Methodology

Exercise echocardiography has enjoyed increased popularity over the past several years for several reasons. In light of recent reports indicating sensitivities and specificity similar to radionuclide imaging techniques, clinicians have found echocardiography to be an examination easily performed in the office setting. This may be in part attributable to the presence of both treadmill and echocardiographic equipment now in the majority of cardiology office settings. The equipment requirements for echocardiographic image acquisition and interpretation appear to be much less cumbersome than those needed for radionuclide techniques.

The methods employed for the performance of a stress echocardiography examination include the acquisition of two-dimensional images both at rest and during maximal exercise. Although maximal exercise images can be obtained during bicycle exericse, most studies done in the United States involve the use of upright treadmill testing. Accordingly, exercise stress echocardiographic images are usually obtained immediately after exercise. A careful and comprehensive resting examination should be obtained before exercise. Parasternal long-axis and short-axis views, as well as apical four- and two-chamber views should be obtained at rest (Figure 14-1). It is helpful to mark the chest

for optimal transducer location so that electrocardiographic leads do not obscure these windows after exercise testing. The patient then exercises according to the standard protocol. The test is terminated upon the occurrence of symptoms (angina, shortness of breath, leg fatigue, and so on)

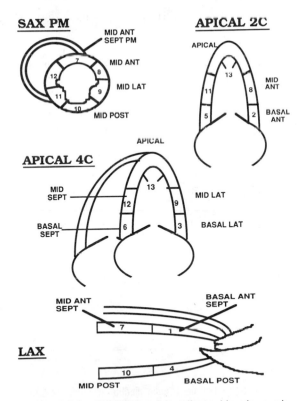

Figure 14-1 Standard echocardiographic views obtained for stress echo analysis usually include the short axis at the papillary muscle level (SAX PM), the apical two-chamber view (APICAL 2C), the apical four-chamber view (APICAL 4C), and the parasternal long-axis view (LAX). The basal, midventricular, and apical segments are identified in each view.

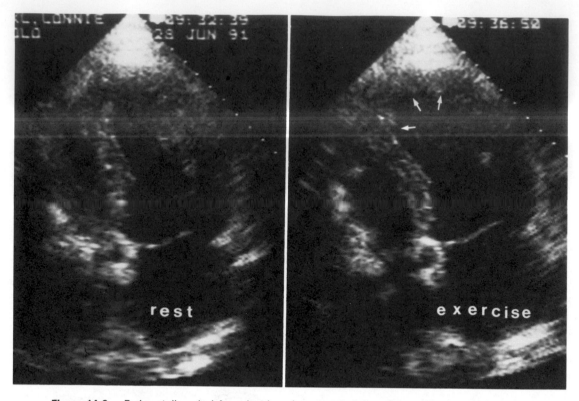

Figure 14-2 End-systolic apical four-chamber view at rest, *left*, and immediately after exercise, *right*. Although the apical region functions normally at rest, there is severe hypokinesis seen, *arrows*, immediately after exercise in this patient with a 90% stenosis in the middle of the left anterior descending coronary artery.

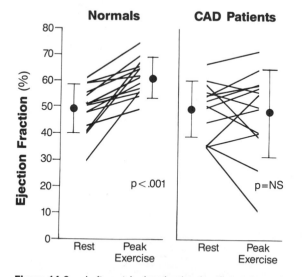

Figure 14-3 Left ventricular ejection fraction measured at rest and immediately after exercise by two-dimensional echocardiography in normal individuals and patients with coronary artery disease (CAD). Notice the blunted response, and even a fall, in the left ventricular ejection fraction in patients with significant exercise-induced ischemia. (From Mehdirad AA, Williams GA, Labovitz AJ, et al: *Circulation* 75:413-419, 1987.)

or other predetermined end points, including age-predicted maximal heart rate. Immediately after exercise, the patient needs to be positioned in the supine or left lateral decubitus position so that stress images can be obtained. These should be recorded as closely as possible to the levels obtained in the basal state. Bicycle exercise offers the potential of obtaining images during maximal exercise. However, the parasternal views are often suboptimal during this form of exercise. Preste and co-workers examined a group of patients at peak bicycle exercise using two-dimensional echocardiography and compared these results to those obtained immediately after exercise.[19] Up to one third of the patients studied had wall-motion abnormalities that resolved within 30 seconds of completing exercise. Caution must be used in extrapolating these data to those obtained immediately after treadmill exercise where ischemic wall-motion abnormalities may persist for a longer period of time.

Analysis

Analysis of stress echocardiographic images involves comparision of baseline and peak exercise

Table 14-2 Exercise echocardiography in the detection of coronary artery disease

Author	Year	Number of patients	Sensitivity	Specificity
Maurer	1981	48	80	92
Limacher	1983	73	91	88
Robertson	1983	30	100	75
Heng	1984	54	100	93
Berberich	1984	52	94	94
Armstrong	1986	95	81	87
Labovitz	1989	73	71	92
Crouse	1991	228	97	64
Marwick	1992	150	84	86
Quinones	1992	292	58	88

images. Although exact views may vary slightly from lab to lab, images obtained at rest and exercise will usually include the parasternal long axis and short-axis views as well as apical two- and four-chamber views. This will allow at least one and often two views of each myocardial segment. The most common method currently employed for evaluation of these images utilizes digitally displayed images at rest and stress in a side-by-side format (Figure 14-2). In general, a worsening of the contractility or inward endocardial motion of any segment is considered abnormal. Although the normal response usually includes increased contractility with exercise, many factors, including insufficient exercise capability and medications such as a beta-blocker, may blunt this response. Therefore a normally contracting segment that remains unchanged after stress is considered a normal response in most labs. Resting wall-motion abnormalities that remain unchanged after exercise, though not specific for stress-induced ischemia, often indicate underlying coronary artery disease and

are usually included in the final report. In addition, with high-quality image acquisition, wall thickening can be assessed as well as endocardial motion. Normal systolic wall thickening should be apparent in all myocardial segments visualized. A decrease in wall thickening is a specific sign of exercise-induced ischemia and is unaffected by situations such as right ventricular volume overload, postoperative motion, and conduction abnormalities that would lead to false-positive endocardial motion dynamics.

In general, most laboratories performing stress echocardiographic examinations will evaluate wall motion qualitatively by comparison of rest and stress echocardiographic images. One can use a semiquantitative wall-motion score in which segments are assigned a score from 0 to 3, depending on the presence of normal wall motion 0, hypokinesis 1, akinesis 2, or dyskinesis 3. Several off-line computer programs are now available by which quantitative regional wall-motion analysis may be accomplished. These include assessment

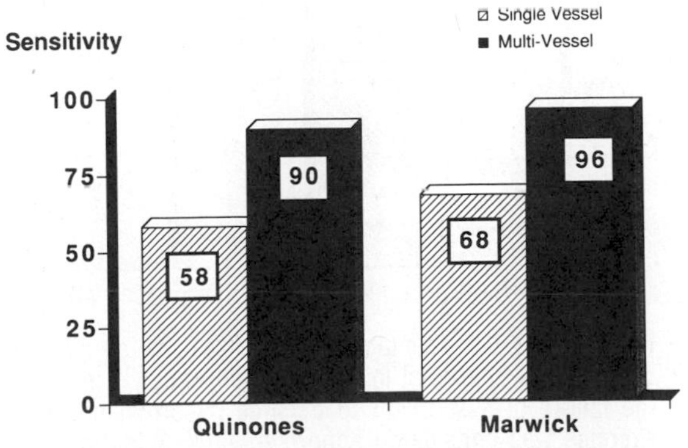

Figure 14-4 Sensitivity of exercise echo in the detection of single-vessel and multivessel coronary disease in two recent studies.[17,18] Notice the greatly enhanced sensitivity in patients with multivessel disease.

Table 14-3 Factors in influencing sensitivity of exercise echocardiography

Increased sensitivity
- Multivessel
- Resting wall-motion abnormality
- Lack of hypercontractility with exercise
- Peak exercise imaging
- Left anterior descending artery lesion
- Greater than 70% stenosis
- Reader experience

Decreased sensitivity
- Poor exercise effort
- Single-vessel disease
- Circulatory lesion
- Moderate stenosis (50% to 70%)

of both inward endocardial motion as well as wall-thickening programs in which baseline and poststress images are compared automatically. In addition, many centers routinely calculate left ventricular ejection fraction at rest and immediately after exercise. The normal response would include at least a 5% increase in the left ventricular ejection fraction. A blunted response or a fall in the left ventricular ejection fraction with exercise may be seen in patients with significant exercise-induced ischemic left ventricular dysfunction (Figure 14-3). This, however, is not a specific sign and could be seen in patients with idiopathic cardiomyopathy, valvular heart disease, or a variety of other cardiac disorders.

Diagnostic accuracy

Sensitivity or exercise echocardiography in the detection of coronary artery disease has been reported to range between 70% and 100%, depending on the characteristics of the patients studied and the methodology used for analysis of stress echocardiographic images (Table 14-2). Factors known to improve the sensitivity of stress echocardiography in the diagnosis of coronary disease include the presence of multi-vessel disease (Figure 14-4) and previous myocardial infarction (Table 14-3). Analysis of stress images that includes lack of increased contractility as in ischemic response will lead to increased sensitivity at the expense of increased false-positive results. Quinones reported on a group of 112 patients undergoing exercise echocardiography and coronary angiography.[18] The sensitivity of stress echocardiography in the detection of coronary artery disease was dependent on the extent of disease. Overall sensitivity was 74%, whereas in patients with single-vessel disease exercise echocardiograms were abnormal in only 58%. However, when only single-vessel disease with lesions greater than 70% stenosis were included, the sensitivity increased to 85%. With two- and three-vessel disease, sensitivities increased to 86% and 94% respectively. Armstrong, likewise, reported a lower sensitivity of exercise echocardiography in single-vessel versus multivessel disease (81% versus 93% sensitivity) and furthermore documented significantly enhanced sensitivity in patients with prior myocardial infarction and resting wall-motion abnormalities.[20] Stress echocardiography also appears to be of greater diagnostic value in patients with stenosis in the distribution of the left anterior descending coronary artery as opposed to lesions in the right or circumflex distribution. Sheikh and co-workers further demonstrated the relationship between exercise-induced ischemic wall-motion abnormalities and the degree of coronary stenosis in

a group of 34 patients with isolated single-vessel coronary lesions.[21] Although patients with high-grade as well as minimal coronary stenoses had diagnostic exercise echocardiograms, those with 50% stenoses had a variable response. With quantitative analysis of minimal luminal diameter, groups with ischemic wall-motion abnormalities had significantly smaller luminal diameter than those with normal responses.

Marik and co-workers recently reported a study of 150 consecutive patients who underwent both exercise echocardiography and cardiac catheterization.[17] Of the 114 patients who had significant coronary stenosis, 96 had an abnormal echocardiogram (sensitivity 84%). False-negative results were found in patients with submaximal exercise, single-vessel disease, and only moderate (50% to 70%) stenosis. In the 36 patients without significant coronary disease, exercise echocardiography had an overall specificity of 86%. As stated above, the manner in which the resting wall-motion abnormalities or stress responses are interpreted will influence both the sensitivity and specificity of stress echocardiography. Crouse and co-workers reported on a group of 228 patients evaluated by exercise echocardiography, all of whom underwent subsequent coronary angiography.[16] The exercise echocardiogram was abnormal if any segment failed to become hypercontractile with exercise. Using these criteria, overall sensitivity was 97% (92% in single-vessel disease, 100% in multivessel disease). The specificity, however, decreased to 64% according to these criteria (Figure 14-5). Therefore, utilizing the absence of hypercontractility with exercise or the presence of resting wall-motion abnormalities greatly enhances the

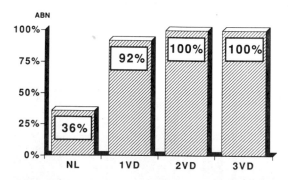

Figure 14-5   Percentage of exercise echo studies interpreted as abnormal in a recent publication[16] in which the failure of a segment to become hyperdynamic with exercise was considered abnormal, *ABN*. Although sensitivity is increased significantly for single-vessel disease, the specificity decreases proportionally (36% false-positive results). *NL*, Normal; *1VD*, single-vessel disease; *2VD*, two-vessel disease; *3VD*, three-vessel disease.

sensitivity of this examination at the expense of false-positive results. Finally, Picano and co-workers emphasized the importance of being expert in the evaluation of 50 patients undergoing stress echocardiographic examination.[22] Inexperienced observers identified stress-induced wall-motion abnormalities significantly less often than their experienced counterparts (61% versus 85%). They suggested that training including interpretation of 100 stress echocardiographic studies is adequate to build the individual learning curve and reach the plateau of diagnostic accuracy available from this test.

Comparision with radionuclide imaging

Although coronary angiography and the extent of coronary stenosis remains the anatomic standard in the quantitation of coronary artery disease, stress-induced perfusion abnormalities demonstrated by thallium-201 scintigraphy is the functional standard in the evaluation of ischemic heart disease. Although perfusion abnormalities that develop during exercise correlate well with the extent and location of coronary artery lesions, differences exist between the two techniques for several reasons. These include coronary reserve, collateral supply and loading conditions, and underlying metabolic demands. In the absence of relative hypoperfusion, it is unlikely that a myocardial segment will become dysfunctional and develop abnormalities of motion and thickening during systole. Recognizing therefore that thallium scintigraphy and two-dimensional echocardiographic imaging are examining different parameters of ischemia, one would not expect 100% concordance between the two techniques.

Several investigators have compared the techniques over the years and have reported good correlation between thallium scintigraphy and stress echocardiography. Mauer first reported in 1981 an excellent correlation between the two techniques, with a sensitivity of 74% for thallium and 83% for exercise echocardiography in a group of 36 patients with coronary disease and no previous myocardial infarction.[8] The specificity by both techniques was 92%. Heng and co-workers likewise showed a good correlation between the two techniques as well as good concordance in localizing the area of perfusion and wall-motion abnormalities.[12] More recently, larger series of patients have been examined and have provided more insight into the strengths and limitations of each technique. Pozzoli and co-workers reported on comparative studies in 75 patients with suspected coronary artery disease and normal resting electrocardiograms.[23] Perfusion imaging was performed with technetium-99 sestamibi SPECT (single-pho-

ton emission computerized tomography) and concordance found in 88% of the patients. Stress echocardiography was abnormal in 71% and SPECT 84% of the 49 patients with greater than 50% stenosis in a coronary artery. There was one false-positive stress echo and three false-positive SPECT results (96% versus 88% specificity respectively). Both tests were superior to standard electrocardiographic evaluation during exercise. SPECT imaging appeared to be superior to echocardiography in patients with single-vessel coronary disease. These were primarily abnormalities in the distribution of the circumflex coronary artery. Quinones and co-workers reported the results of treadmill stress testing with echocardiographic and SPECT thallium imaging in a group of 289 patients prospectively evaluated.[18] There was 88% agreement between the two techniques. Equal numbers of regional abnormalities were detected by one test when missed by the other. SPECT imaging detected more reversible abnormalities than echocardiography, whereas echocardiography detected more fixed abnormalities than SPECT. Sensitivity for the detection of coronary arter disease by angiography was similar for the two tests, ranging from 58% and 61% (echocardiography and SPECT respectively) for single-vessel disease to 94% for three-vessel disease. The specificities for echocardiography and SPECT were 88% and 81% respectively.

Several investigators have examined the change in left ventricular ejection fraction with exercise as an indicator of abnormal wall motion secondary to ischemia. Crawford examined the ability of bicycle exercise echocardiography to diagnosis the presence of coronary artery disease.[7] He compared changes in left ventricular ejection fraction to those measured by radionuclide ventriculography and found comparable results between the two techniques. Patients with multivessel disease more frequently had a blunted response with no change or a decrease in left ventricular ejection fraction with exercise than those with single-vessel disease. This typically occurs because of the compensatory hyperkinesis occurring in segments with normal coronary perfusion during maximal stress.

Exercise echocardiography offers certain advantages over radionuclide imaging as an adjunctive procedure in the diagnosis of coronary artery disease. Exercise echocardiography offers the ability to measure both global left ventricular function (ejection fraction) as well as regional wall-motion abnormalities in response to exercise. Nuclear licensing requirements, intravenous injections, and specialized equipment are not needed to the same extent with exercise echocardiography as they are with radionuclide stress testing. Since both rest and stress images are obtained at close temporal sequence with exercise echo, the throughput time for the patient in the laboratory is greatly decreased with this technique.

Clinical applications

Exercise echocardiography has been reported to be useful in several clinical settings. In addition to its predictive accuracy in the diagnosis of coronary artery disease, stress echocardiography is helpful in determining the functional significance of a known coronary stenosis. Segmental wall-motion analysis allows a quantitative assessment of the "ischemic burden" of a particular coronary lesion. One can rapidly assess whether wall-motion abnormalities develop in the distribution of a known coronary stenosis and determine how extensive this wall-motion abnormality might be. In this regard, stress echocardiography has been reported to be useful in the evaluation of the results of percutaneous balloon angioplasty.[24-26] In our own laboratory,[24] exercise two-dimensional echocardiography was superior to electrocardiographic stress testing in the evaluation of the results of angioplasty. Likewise, Crouse examined a group of patients by exercise echocardiography before and after angioplasty. All patients had abnormal findings on stress echo before angioplasty; 91% had improvement after angioplasty. Those patients with persistently abnormal test results were found to have early restenosis. Several other investigators have subsequently confirmed these findings.

Studies utilizing stress echocardiography after myocardial infarction have also indicated a role for this technique in the assessment of such patients.[27-29] The development of wall-motion abnormalities in areas remote from the site of infarction often indicates the presence of multivessel coronary disease. Furthermore, several investigators have reported an important prognostic role for stress echocardiography after myocardial infarction. Applegate and co-workers found that abnormal stress echo during low-level exercise early after uncomplicated myocardial infarction was highly predictive of late cardiac events.[27] Ryan and co-workers similarly examined a group of 40 patients prospectively by exercise echocardiography 10 to 21 days after myocardial infarction.[28] Stress echocardiograms were much more predictive of outcome than standard electrocardiographic exercise results. The exercise echocardiogram was negative in 19 of 20 patients with a good clinical outcome and abnormal in 16 of 20 patients with poor clinical outcomes. The use of stress echocardiography for risk stratification has also been recently utilized in patients undergoing noncardiac surgery and as a prognostic tool in patients with suspected coronary artery disease.[30]

Exercise echocardiography is indicated in many situations in which standard electrocardiographic stress testing is likely to be inadequate. Many of these indications include those in which radionuclide scintigraphy is frequently employed. Certainly patients who have had an equivocal electrocardiographic stress test are candidates for stress echocardiography evaluation. Likewise, patients with conduction abnormalities in whom electrocardiographic results may be difficult to interpret would be candidates for stress echocardiographic testing. In addition, patients with a high likelihood of false-positive stress tests, such as women, have been shown to have highly accurate results by stress echocardiography.[31]

PHARMACOLOGICAL STRESS ECHOCARDIOGRAPHY
General considerations

One of the most common causes for inconclusive or nondiagnostic exercise tests is the inability of the patient to exercise and achieve an adequate heart rate and blood pressure response. This is particularly prominent in older patients and those with poor general physical conditioning, as well as patients with significant lung disease or peripheral vascular disease. Accordingly, several agents have been developed by which cardiovascular stress may be simulated and information concerning the presence and significance of coronary artery disease can be evaluated. These agents are generally classified into two major categories: the coronary vasodilators, and beta-adrenergic receptor agonists or inotropic agents (Table 14-4). In general, the coronary vasodilators, with dipyridamole as the prototype, cause dilatation in the coronary vascular bed and an overall increase in coronary flow. Myocardium perfused by normal coronary vasculature will enjoy enhanced blood flow, whereas regions supplied by stenotic coronary arteries will have a blunted response and a relative decrease in coronary blood flow when compared to normal regions. The beta-agonists, on the other hand, will cause increased myocardial oxygen demand by an increase in the rate pressure product and hence ischemia in regions supplied by stenotic coronary arteries.

Echocardiography is ideally suited for use in pharmacological stress testing because it allows continuous or near-continuous monitoring of left ventricular function during the stress test. In contrast to exercise echocardiography, images are often of higher quality because the technical difficulty introduced by hyperventilation and motion

Table 14-4 Comparison of pharmacological stress echocardiographic agents

	Dipyridamole	Adenosine	Dobutamine
Mechanism	Vasodilator	Vasodilator	Inotropic agent
Dose	0.56-0.84 mg/kg	50-140 mg/kg/min	5-40 µg/kg/min
Contraindications	Unstable angina	Atrioventricular block	Hypertrophic cardiomy-opathy
	Asthma	Asthma	Uncontrolled hyperten-sion
		Unstable angina	Ventricular arrhythmia
Effect on heart rate	↑	↑	↑ ↑
Effect on blood pressure	→ ↓	→ ↓	→ ↑
Coronary flow	↑ ↑	↑ ↑	↑
Myocardial O_2 demand	→ ↑	→ ↑	↑ ↑

are not present during pharmacological stress testing. The general principles of wall-motion analysis applied during exercise echocardiography are utilized in the evaluation of pharmacological stress echocardiography. In general, baseline images are compared to those obtained at peak stress. The development of new wall-motion abnormalities at peak drug effect are abnormal and most consistent with the development of ischemia.

Dipyridamole

Intravenous dipyridamole is a potent coronary vasodilator that has been used extensively over the past several years as a stress agent. Dipyridamole is a complex, pyrimidine derivative that inhibits phosphodiesterase and increases endogenous cyclic AMP. The effect of dipyridamole on coronary blood flow is mediated by an increase in adenosine concentration in the arterial wall of resistance vessels. Dipyridamole will therefore increase coronary blood flow in nondiseased coronary vessels relative to coronary vessels with significant atherosclerotic disease. This will cause a relative hypoperfusion in the distal coronary bed beyond a stenotic lesion and, if the stenosis is severe enough, ischemia resulting in wall-motion abnormalities detectable by echocardiography.

Patients undergoing dipyridamole echocardiography typically need to have theophylline derivatives discontinued at least 2 days before the test and caffeinated beverages withheld as well. After one obtains a baseline echocardiogram, dipyridamole is infused at a rate of 0.14 mg/kg/min over a 4-minute period, for a total dose of 0.56 mg/kg. Continuous electrocardiographic monitoring should be obtained, in addition to 12-lead electrocardiograms at defined intervals. Two-dimensional echocardiograms should be continuously recorded during the dipyridamole infusion and up to 15 minutes after completion of infusion.

A peak dipyridamole effect is typically seen between 5 and 10 minutes after the infusion. Rest and stress images are compared. This is best accomplished by digital acquisition and display in a side-by-side continuous loop (cine) format. In the presence of considerable clinical suspicion and an inconclusive or negative test, Picano and co-workers recommend a high-dose protocol, which involves the additional infusion of 0.28 mg/kg of dipyridamole over 2 minutes for a cumulative dose of 0.84 mg/kg over 10 minutes.[32] Some investigators recommend the combination of isometric handgrip or leg-swings to enhance sensitivity of this test.[33]

Clinical applications. Dipyridamole echocardiography has been evaluated in terms of its predictive accuracy in the diagnosis of coronary artery disease[34-40] (Table 14-5). The sensitivity of dipyridamole echocardiography depends to a large extent on the degree of inducible ischemia. Sensitivities reported for one-, two-, and three-vessel disease are in the range of 40%, 70%, and 90% respectively. Specificity is reproducibly in the 90% to 100% range. We compared thallium scintigraphy and two-dimensional echocardiography after intravenous dipyridamole stress testing in a group

Table 14-5 Sensitivity of dipyridamole echocardiography in suspected coronary artery disease

	Patients	Sensitivity	Specificity
Picano	40	72	100
Picano	75	56	100
Bolognese	94	64	—
Picano	103	74	100
Labovitz	100	64	80
Previtali	35	57	100
Martin	40	56	67

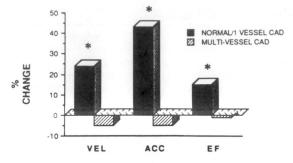

Figure 14-6 Aortic flow velocity parameters of peak acceleration, *(ACC)* and peak velocity *(VEL)* were as good as diffurunoou in oohooardiographioally moaourod loft ventricular ejection fraction (EF), and diagnosing those with multi-vessel coronary artery disease (CAD) after intravenous dipyridamole stress testing. (From Labovitz AJ: *Am J Cardiol* 62:1180-1185, 1988.)

of 100 consecutive patients.[35] There was diagnostic agreement in 76% of the patients studied by both techniques. The sensitivity and specificity of dipyridamole stress echocardiography was 64% and 80% respectively. Not surprisingly, sensitivity was much better in patients with multivessel coronary artery disease. Doppler evaluation of aortic flow velocity parameters after intravenous administration of dipyridamole also appears to be helpful in the diagnosis of coronary artery disease[35,41] (Figure 14-6).

Dipyridamole echocardiography has also been reported to be useful in the early assessment of coronary bypass graft patency[42] and restenosis after coronary angioplasty.[43] Parelli and co-workers found exercise electrocardiography and dipyridamole echocardiography similar in detecting asymptomatic restenosis after angioplasty (sensitivity is 71% for both techniques) but a much greater specificity (61% versus 90%) with dipyridamole.[43] In addition, dipyridamole stress echocardiography appears to be useful in predicting cardiac events, both in the population of patients with coronary artery disease,[44] and in the prediction of major cardiac events associated with peripheral vascular surgery.[45] Side effects are seen in up to 10% of patients studied and include angina pectoris, flushing, headache, dizziness, nausea, and epigastric pain. These are rapidly reversed by administration of aminophylline.

Adenosine echocardiography

Adenosine is another potent coronary vasodilator that when given by intravenous infusion and combined with thallium-201 perfusion imaging can produce defects in myocardial regions supplied by stenotic coronary arteries. Its very short half-life

makes it an attractive agent when compared to the coronary vasodilator dipyridamole. Several investigators have combined intravenous infusion of adenosine at a rate of 50 mg/kg/min, with incremental increases in dosages up to 140 mg/kg/min during two-dimensional echocardiographic monitoring.[38,46,47] Wall-motion abnormalities, presumably secondary to ischemia, develop in regions supplied by stenotic coronary arteries. The sensitivity of adenosine echocardiography has been reported to be 60% and 80% in patients with single-vessel and multivessel coronary disease. The side-effect profile appears to be somewhat better than that obtained with intravenously administered dipyridamole.

Dobutamine echocardiography

Dobutamine is a synthetic sympathetic amine first developed in 1975 that has both beta and alpha effects on cardiac smooth muscle. It is a potent positive inotrope and a relatively weak positive chronotrope. Dobutamine has a balanced effect on vascular smooth muscle, often resulting in a slight decrease in peripheral vascular resistance. Dobutamine, in pharmacological doses, causes an increase in the dp/dt, stroke volume, and cardiac output, with a resultant increase in myocardial oxygen consumption. This increase in myocardial oxygen demand in regions supplied by stenotic coronary arteries will result in ischemia and subsequent systolic wall-motion abnormalities identified by echocardiography. We and others have found that overall coronary flow is usually increased at least twofold in normal coronary vascular beds by dobutamine.[48] The drug is typically infused intravenously in a series of 3-minute stages, starting in a dose of 5 μg/kg/min and increasing incrementally up to 40 μg/kg/min. The test is terminated for the following end points: new wall-motion abnormality, greater than 2 mm of ST-segment depression, angina pectoris, precipitous drop in blood pressure, significant ventricular arrhythmia, or attainment of maximal dose (Table 14-6). Patients with significant coronary artery disease will typically have development of ischemia

Table 14-6 Dobutamine echocardiography

End points:
- New wall-motion abnormality
- ≥2 mm of ST-segment depression
- Angina pectoris
- Hypotension
- Arrhythmia
- Maximal dose
- Severe hypertension

at doses less than maximum. The typical side-effect profile apparent in approximately 5% to 10% of the patients studied include arrhythmias both ventricular and supraventricular, nauses, tremor, electrocardiographic changes, angina pectoris, palpitations, and headache. Reported sensitivities and specificities with dobutamine stress testing are dependent on the prevalence and extent of coronary disease present in the patient population and have ranged from 70% to 96% sensitivity, with specificities in the 60% to 80% range[49-54] (Table 14-7). Berthe first reported sensitivity of dobutamine echocardiography in predicting remote coronary disease in patients after a myocardial infarction, with an 85% sensitivity compared to 42% by standard exercise electrocardiography stress testing.[49] Sawada reported on a group of 103 patients in whom dobutamine stress echocardiography was used for the detection of coronary artery disease.[53] Sensitivity and specificity overall were 89% and 85% respectively. For patients with multivessel coronary disease, sensitivity was 100%. Marcovitz reported on the diagnostic accuracy of dobutamine stress echocardiography in 141 patients who underwent coronary arteriography and reported a sensitivity of 96% for the detection of coronary artery disease.[54] This was slightly less (87%) for the 53 patients with normal resting wall motion.

In addition to the detection of coronary stenosis, dobutamine stress echocardiography has been utilized for preoperative risk assessment,[55] assessment of the results of revascularization after angioplasty,[56] and, more recently, identification of viable myocardium after myocardial infarction.[57] Pierard and co-workers examined 17 patients after anterior myocardial infarction treated with thrombosis.[57] Dobutamine stress echocardiography and positron-emission tomographic (PET) scanning were performed before discharge from the hospital. Echocardiography and PET scanning were repeated an average of 9 months later. Concordant interpretation and identification of viable myocardium occurred in 79% of the patients studied (Figure 14-7). Myocardial thickening that im-

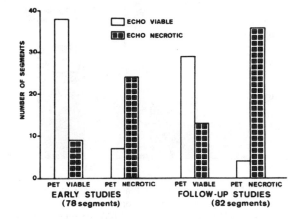

Figure 14-7   Comparison of dobutamine echo in metabolic position emission tomographic scans in allowing prediction of viable myocardium after myocardial infarction. There was a high concordance between the two techniques. (From Piérard LA: *J Am Coll Cardiol* 15:1021-1031, 1990.)

proved during intermediate stages of dobutamine infusion most often indicated viable myocardial segments. This promising application of dobutamine stress echocardiography is currently the subject of continuing investigation.

Dobutamine stress echocardiography has been compared with dipyridamole and adenosine with respect to determining the optimal pharmacological agent for stress echocardiography testing.[38] In a dog model, Fung and co-workers showed that wall-thickening abnormalities occurred in 100% of the myocardial segments supplied by a flow-restricted circumflex during dobutamine infusion.[58] Similar wall-motion abnormalities were observed by echocardiographic wall-motion analysis in only 55% of the animals during intravenous dipyridamole infusion. Previtali and co-workers demonstrated that both dipyridamole and dobutamine had equally high sensitivity (greater than 90%) in patients with multivessel disease, though dobutamine appeared superior in detecting wall-motion abnormalities in the presence of single vessel disease[39] (Figure 14-8).

Table 14-7   Dobutamine stress echocardiography

Author	Number of patients	Coronary artery disease (%)	Sensitivity		Specificity
			All	Multivessel disease	
Marcovitz	141	77	96	97	66
Sawada	103	64	89	100	85
Mazeika	50	72	78	86	93
Sagar	85	78	95	—	82
Cohen	70	75	86	96	95

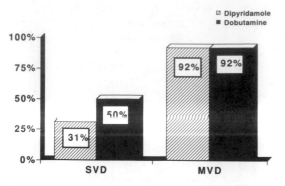

Figure 14-8 Comparison of the sensitivity of dipyridamole and dobutamine stress echo in patients with single-vessel (SVD) and multivessel (MVD) coronary artery disease in a recent study.[39]

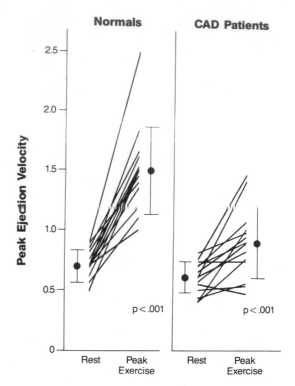

Figure 14-9 Peak aortic ejection velocity at rest and immediately after exercise in normal individuals and patients with coronary artery disease (CAD). Notice the blunted response in patients with significant exercise-induced ischemia. (From Mehdirad AA, Williams GA, Labovitz AJ, et al: *Circulation* 75:413-419, 1987.)

DOPPLER STRESS TESTING
Assessment of coronary artery disease

Doppler evaluation of aortic blood flow velocities in the absence of aortic stenosis provides information about left ventricular function. In the resting state, it has been demonstrated that peak aortic flow velocities, as well as peak aortic velocity acceleration, correlate with parameters of left ventricular function, including the left ventricular ejection fraction and stroke volume.[59,60] In fact, one may derive stroke volume from the aortic flow velocity tracing as the product of the total velocity integral and the cross-sectional area of the left ventricular outflow tract.[61] Evaluation therefore of aortic flow velocities during stress testing provides another method to evaluate left ventricular functional response to stress and stress-induced ischemia (Figure 14-9). In a study of 46 subjects using upright treadmill exercise, we initially described three types of Doppler aortic velocity response to exercise[62] (Figure 14-10):

- Type I is a normal response characterized by an increase in peak aortic velocity with exercise of at least 80% over the baseline measurements. This is seen in most normal individuals, as well as some patients with minimal coronary disease, most often single-vessel disease.
- Type II response is characterized by a blunted increase in peak aortic ejection velocities. It is the most common type of response seen in individuals with coronary disease.
- Type III response is characterized by an actual decrease in the peak aortic velocity over resting values. This response is seen almost exclusively in patients with multivessel disease and significant exercise-induced ischemia.

Furthermore, we have shown that there is a good correlation between the percent change in ejection fraction from rest to peak exercise and the percent change in the peak aortic velocity ($r = 0.64$)[63] (Figure 14-11). Teague and co-workers likewise compared exercise Doppler tracings and left ventricular ejection fraction as measured by exercise radionuclide angiography.[64] The Doppler velocity parameter of peak acceleration of aortic flow correlated well with radionuclide changes in left ventricular ejection fraction ($r = 0.89$). A decrease in aortic peak acceleration had a sensitivity and specificity of 90% and 88%, respectively, for the presence of significant coronary artery disease. Other investigators have found exercise Doppler tracings to correlate less well with thallium scintigraphy. Harrison studied 102 subjects and found peak velocities to be similar in patients with normal and abnormal thallium scan results.[65] Peak acceleration, however, was significantly decreased in patients with scintigraphic evidence of ischemia, with more pronounced abnormalities demonstrated in patients with multivessel disease. The use of

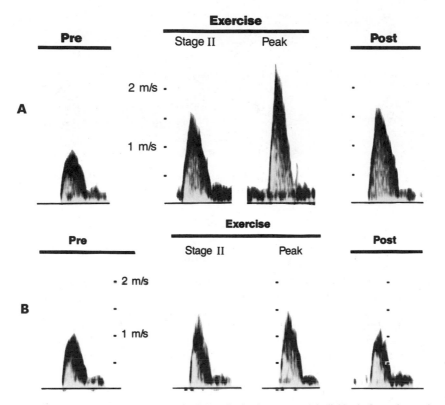

Figure 14-10   Doppler tracing of aortic flow velocity in a normal individual, **A**, and a patient with multivessel coronary artery disease, **B**.

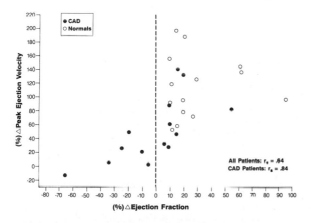

Figure 14-11   Correlation of the percent change in left ventricular ejection fraction and peak aortic ejection velocity with exercise in normal individuals and patients with coronary artery disease (CAD). r_s, Correlation coefficient. (From Mehdirad AA, Williams GA, Labovitz AJ, et al: *Circulation* 75:413-419, 1987.)

Doppler velocity measurements as an adjunctive diagnostic aid in the evaluation of coronary artery disease might be limited by the influence of a variety of factors on aortic flow velocity. Increasing age, concomitant use of beta-adrenergic receptor blockers or calcium-channel blockers, or both, and decreased resting ejection fraction are known to diminish aortic flow velocity parameters. Several reports have indicated that Doppler evaluation of aortic flow velocity parameters may provide useful information during pharmacological stress testing as well.

Doppler recordings of transmitral flow have been studied during stress testing. Stress-induced mitral insufficiency was highly predictive of multivessel coronary disease.[66] Other investigators have suggested that measurements of total mitral flow velocities or changes in the early and late components of transmitral flow may be characteristic of an ischemic response.[67] Confounding changes in left ventricular filling pressures, however, may limit the application of such measurements.

Valvular heart disease

Exercise Doppler tracing provides a method by which one can evaluate transvalvular hemodynamics, both in native and prosthetic heart valves. The ability to measure transvalvular peak and mean gradients at rest and after exercise noninvasively provides an additional diagnostic aid in the evaluation of patients with suspected valvular dis-

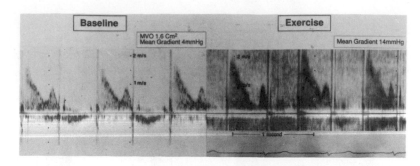

Figure 14-12 Continuous-wave transmitral Doppler recording in patient with moderately severe mitral stenosis. Mean transvalve gradient increases from 4 to 14 mm Hg with exercise. *MVO*, Mitral valve orifice.

ease in whom basal conditions are insufficient to provide clinical insight into the patient's set of symptoms. Hatle reported approximately a twofold increase in Doppler tracing–derived valve gradients in patients with mitral stenosis with exercise.[68] Sagar and co-workers demonstrated that catheter-derived mitral valve gradients at rest and during exercise correlated well with those obtained noninvasively by Doppler interrogation.[69] Exercise gradients have also been reported in patients with valvular aortic stenosis, as well as prosthetic mitral and aortic valves (Figure 14-12). Normally functioning prosthetic heart valves typically demonstrate a twofold increase in Doppler tracing–derived gradients immediately after exercise.[70]

ADDITIONAL STRESS ECHO AND DOPPLER METHODS

There has been a variety of other stress methods employed using either echo or Doppler techniques to assess for the presence and extent of coronary disease. Additional methods of exercise, including arm ergometry and isometric exercise with two-dimensional echocardiographic left ventricular monitoring and aortic Doppler recordings, have yielded results similar to those previously described.[71] Right atrial and transesophageal pacing have also been performed with the detection of wall-motion abnormalities occurring secondary to ischemia at increasing ventricular rates.[72,73] The superior resolution of transesophageal echocardiography has allowed measurement in selected cases of coronary flow and calculation of coronary flow reserve in normal individuals and patients with coronary artery disease in response to coronary vasodilators.[74] Newer echo contrast agents may very well allow future assessment of myocardial perfusion in the resting and stress states for comparision.[75,76]

SUMMARY

Two-dimensional echocardiographic monitoring of left ventricular function during various forms of exercise and pharmacological stress is a safe and cost-effective diagnostic test in the evaluation of patients with suspected coronary artery disease. This technique will provide information similar in predictive value to radionuclide imaging techniques. Echocardiography is ideally suited for the clinician's office as well as the hospital setting and is likely to assume an increasingly important role in the clinical evaluation of patients with coronary and valvular heart disease.

REFERENCES

1. Kraunz K, Kennedy J: Ultrasonic determination of left ventricular wall motion in normal man: studies at rest and after exercise, *Am Heart J* 79:36-43, 1970.
2. Crawford MH, White DH, Amon DW: Echocardiographic evaluation of left ventricular size and performance during handgrip and supine and upright bicycle exercise, *Circulation* 59:1188-1196, 1979.
3. Mason SJ, Weiss JL, Weisfeldt ML, et al: Exercise echocardiography: detection of wall motion abnormalities during ischemia, *Circulation* 59:50-59, 1979.
4. Sugishita Y, Kaseki S: Dynamic exercise echocardiography, *Circulation* 60:743-752, 1979.
5. Wann LS, Faris JV, Childress RH, et al: Exercise cross-sectional echocardiography in ischemic heart disease, *Circulation* 60:1300-1308, 1979.
6. Morganroth J, Chen CC, David D, et al: Exercise cross-sectional echocardiographic diagnosis of coronary artery disease, *Am J Cardiol* 47:20-26, 1981.
7. Crawford MH, Amon KW, Vance WS: Exercise two-dimensional echocardiography: quantitation of left ventricular performance in patients with severe angina pectoris, *Am J Cardiol* 51:1-6, 1983.
8. Maurer G, Nanda NC: Two-dimensional echocardiographic evaluation of exercise-induced left and right ventricular asynergy: correlation with thallium scanning, *Am J Cardiol* 48:720-727, 1981.
9. Visser CA, van der Wieken RFL, Kan G, et al: Comparison of two-dimensional echocardiography with radionuclide angiography during dynamic exercise for the detec-

tion of coronary artery disease, *Am Heart J* 106:528-534, 1983.

10. Limacher MC, Quinones MA, Poliner LR, et al: Detection of coronary artery disease with exercise two-dimensional echocardiography: description of a clinically applicable method and comparison with radionuclide ventriculography, *Circulation* 67:1211-1218, 1983.

11. Robertson WC, Feigenbaum H, Armstrong W, et al: Exercise echocardiography: a clinically practical addition in the evaluation of coronary artery disease, *J Am Coll Cardiol* 2:1085-1091, 1983.

12. Heng MK, Simard M, Lake R. Udhoji VH: Exercise two-dimensional echocardiography for diagnosis of coronary artery disease, *Am J Cardiol* 54:502-507, 1984.

13. Berberich SN, Zager JRS, Plotnick GD, Fisher ML: A practical approach to exercise echocardiography: immediate postexercise echocardiography, *J Am Coll Cardiol* 3:284-290, 1984.

14. Armstrong WF, O'Donnell J, Dillon JC, et al: Complementary value of two-dimensional exercise echocardiography to routine treadmill exercise testing, *Ann Intern Med* 105:829-835, 1986.

15. Labovitz AJ, Lewen MK, Kern MJ, et al: The effects of successful PTCA on left ventricular function: assessment by exercise echocardiography, *Am Heart J* 117:1003-1008, 1989.

16. Crouse LJ, Harbrecht JJ, Vacek JL, et al: Exercise echocardiography as a screening test for coronary artery disease and correlation with coronary arteriography, *Am J Cardiol* 67:1213-1218, 1991.

17. Marwick TH, Nemec JJ, Pashkow FJ, et al: Accuracy and limitations of exercise echocardiography in a routine clinical setting, *J Am Coll Cardiol* 19:74-81, 1992.

18. Quinones MA, Verani MS, Haichin RM, et al: Exercise echocardiography versus ^{201}Tl single-photon emission computer tomography in evaluation of coronary artery disease: analysis of 292 patients, *Circulation* 85:1026-1031, 1992.

19. Presti CF, Armstrong WF, Feigenbaum H: Comparison of echocardiography at peak exercise and after bicycle exercise in the evaluation of patients with known or suspected coronary artery disease, *J Am Soc Echocardiogr* 1:119-126, 1988.

20. Armstrong WF, O'Donnell J, Ryan T, Feigenbaum H: Effect of prior myocardial infarction and extent and location of coronary disease on accuracy of exercise echocardiography, *J Am Coll Cardiol* 10:531-538, 1987.

21. Sheikh KS, Bengtson JR, Helmy S, et al: Relation of quantitative coronary lesion measurements to the development of exercise-induced ischemia assessed by exercise echocardiography, *J Am Coll Cardiol* 15:1043-1051, 1990.

22. Picano E, Lattanzi F, Orlandini A, et al: Stress echocardiography and the human factor: the importance of being expert, *J Am Coll Cardiol* 17:666-669, 1991.

23. Pozzoli MMA, Fioretti PM, Salustri A, et al: Exercise echocardiography and technetium-99m MIBI single photon emission computed tomography in the detection of coronary artery disease, *Am J Cardiol* 67:350-355, 1991.

24. Labovitz AJ, Lewen MK, Kern MJ, et al: The effects of successful PTCA on left ventricular function: assessment by exercise echocardiography, *Am Heart J* 117(5):1003-1008, 1989.

25. Broderick T, Sawada S, Armstrong WF, et al: Improvement in rest and exercise-induced wall motion abnormalities after coronary angioplasty: an exercise echocardiographic study, *J Am Coll Cardiol* 15:591-599, 1990.

26. Aboul-Enein H, Bengtson JR, Adams DB, et al: Effect of the degree of effort on exercise echocardiography for the detection of restenosis after coronary artery angioplasty, *Am Heart J* 122:430, 1991.

27. Applegate RJ, Dell'Italia LJ, Crawford MH: Usefulness of two-dimensional echocardiography during low-level exercise testing early after uncomplicated acute myocardial infarction, *Am J Cardiol* 60:10-14, 1987.

28. Ryan T, Armstrong WF, O'Donnell JA, Feigenbaum H: Risk stratification after acute myocardial infarction by means of exercise two-dimensional echocardiography, *Am Heart J* 114:1305, 1987.

29. Jaarsma W, Visser C, Funke Kupper A: Usefulness of two-dimensional exercise echocardiography shortly after myocardial infarction, *Am J Cardiol* 57:86-90, 1986.

30. Sawada SG, Ryan T, Conley MJ, et al: Prognostic value of a normal exercise echocardiogram, *Am Heart J* 120:49-55, 1990.

31. Sawada SG, Ryan T, Fineberg NS, et al: Exercise echocardiographic detection of coronary artery disease in women, *J Am Coll Cardiol* 14:1440-1447, 1989.

32. Picano E, Lattanzi F, Masini M, et al: High dose dipyridamole echocardiography test in effort angina pectoris, *J Am Coll Cardiol* 8:848-854, 1986.

33. Brown BG, Josephson MA, Petersen RB, et al: Intravenous dipyridamole combined with isometric handgrip for near maximal acute increase in coronary flow in patients with coronary artery disease, *Am J Cardiol* 48:1077, 1981.

34. Picano E, Distante A, Masini M, et al: Dipyridamole-echocardiography test in effort angina pectoris, *Am J Cardiol* 56:452, 1985.

35. Labovitz AJ, Pearson AC, Chaitman BR, et al: Doppler and two-dimensional echocardiographic assessment of left ventricular function before and after intravenous dipyridamole stress testing for detection of coronary artery disease, *Am J Cardiol* 62:1180, 1988.

36. Margonato A, Chierchia S, Cianflone D, et al: Limitations of dipyridamole-echocardiography in effort angina pectoris, *Am J Cardiol* 59:225-230, 1987.

37. Picano E, Lattanzi F, Masini M, et al: Comparison of the high-dose dipyridamole-echocardiography test and exercise two-dimensional echocardiography for diagnosis of coronary artery disease, *Am J Cardiol* 59:539-542, 1987.

38. Martin TW, Seaworth JF, Johns JP, et al: Comparison of adenosine, dipyridamole, and dobutamine in stress echocardiography, *Ann Intern Med* 116:190-196, 1992.

39. Previtali M, Lanzarini L, Ferrario M, et al: Dobutamine versus dipyridamole echocardiography in coronary artery disease, *Circulation* 83(suppl III):III-27-32, 1991.

40. Bolognese L, Sarasso G, Araldaa D, et al: High dose dipyridamole echocardiography early after uncomplicated acute myocardial infarction: correlation with exercise testing and coronary angiography, *J Am Coll Cardiol* 14:357, 1989.

41. Agati L, Arata L, Neja CP, et al: Usefulness of the dipyridamole-Doppler test for diagnosis of coronary artery disease, *Am J Cardiol* 65:829-834, 1990.

42. Bongo AS, Bolognese L, Sarasso G, et al: Early assessment of coronary artery bypass graft patency by high-dose dipyridamole echocardiography, *Am J Cardiol* 67:133-136, 1991.

43. Pirelli S, Danzi GB, Alberti A, et al: Comparison of usefulness of high-dose dipyridamole echocardiography and exercise electrocardiography for detection of asymptomatic restenosis after coronary angioplasty, *Am J Cardiol* 67:1335-1338, 1991.

44. Picano E, Severi S, Michelassi C, et al: Prognostic importance of dipyridamole-echocardiography test in coronary artery disease, *Circulation* 80:450-457, 1989.

45. Tischler MD, Lee TH, Hirsch AT, et al: Prediction of major cardiac events after peripheral vascular surgery using dipyridamole echocardiography, *Am J Cardiol* 68:593-597, 1991.

46. Nguyen T, Heo J, Ogilby JD, Iskandrian A: Single pho-

ton computed tomography with thallium 201 during adenosine-induced coronary hyperemia: correlation with coronary arteriography, exercise thallium imaging and two-dimensional echocardiography, *J Am Coll Cardiol* 16:1375-1383, 1990.

47. Zoghbi WA, Cheirif J, Kleiman NS, et al: Diagnosis of ischemic heart disease with adenosine echocardiography, *J Am Coll Cardiol* 18:1271-1279, 1991.

48. Castello R, Ofili EO, St. Vrain JA, et al: Dobutamine stress echocardiography: effect on coronary flow and left ventricular function, presented at XIVth Congress of European Society of Cardiology (Barcelona, Spain), August 31, 1992. (In press.)

49. Berthe C, Piérard LA, Hiernaux M, et al: Predicting the extent and location of coronary artery disease in acute myocardial infarction by echocardiography during dobutamine infusion, *Am J Cardiol* 58:1167-1172, 1986.

50. Segar DS, Brown SE, Sawada SG, et al: Dobutamine stress echocardiography: correlation with coronary lesion severity as determined by quantitative angioplasty, *J Am Coll Cardiol* 19:1197-1202, 1992.

51. Cohen JL, Greene TO, Ottenweller J, et al: Dobutamine digital echocardiography for detecting coronary artery disease, *Am J Cardiol* 67:1311-1318, 1991.

52. Mazeika PK, Nadazdin A, Oakley CM: Dobutamine stress echocardiography for detection and assessment of coronary artery disease, *J Am Coll Cardiol* 19:1203-1211, 1992.

53. Sawada SG, Segar DS, Ryan T, et al: Echocardiographic detection of coronary artery disease during dobutamine infusion, *Circulation* 83:1605-1614, 1991.

54. Marcovitz PA, Armstrong WF: Accuracy of dobutamine stress echocardiography in detecting coronary artery disease, *Am J Cardiol* 69:1269-1273, 1992.

55. Lane RT, Sawada SG, Segar DS, et al: Dobutamine stress echocardiography for assessment of cardiac risk before noncardiac surgery, *Am J Cardiol* 68:976-977, 1991.

56. McNeill AJ, Fioretti PM, El-Said ESM, et al: Dobutamine stress echocardiography before and after coronary angioplasty, *Am J Cardiol* 69:740-745, 1992.

57. Piérard LA, De Landsheere CM, Berthe C, et al: Identification of viable myocardium by echocardiography during dobutamine infusion in patients with myocardial infarction after thrombolytic therapy: comparison with positron emission tomography, *J Am Coll Cardiol* 15:1021-1031, 1990.

58. Fung AY, Gallagher KP, Buda AJ: The physiologic basis of dobutamine as compared with dipyridamole stress interventions in the assessment of critical coronary stenosis, *Circulation* 76:943-951, 1987.

59. Sabbah HN, Khaja F, Brymer JF, et al: Non-invasive evaluation of left ventricular performance based on peak aortic blood acceleration measured with continuous-wave Doppler velocity meter, *Circulation* 74:323, 1986.

60. Sagar KB, Wann LS, Boerboom LE, et al: Comparison of peak and modal aortic blood flow velocities with invasive measures of left ventricular performance, *J Am Soc Echocardiogr* 1:194, 1983.

61. Labovitz AJ, Buckingham TA, Habermehl K, et al: The effects of sampling site on the two-dimensional echo-Doppler determination of cardiac output, *Am Heart J* 109:327, 1985.

62. Bryg RJ, Labovitz AJ, Mehdirad AA, et al: Effect of coronary artery disease on Doppler-derived parameters of aortic flow during upright exercise, *Am J Cardiol* 58:14, 1986.

63. Mehdirad AA, Williams GA, Labovitz AJ, et al: Evaluation of left ventricular function during upright exercise: correlation of exercise Doppler with post exercise two-dimensional echocardiographic results, *Circulation* 75:413, 1987.

64. Teague SM, Corn C, Sharma M, et al: A comparison of Doppler and radionuclide ejection dynamics during ischemic exercise, *Am J Cardiac Imaging* 1:145, 1987.

65. Harrison MR, Smith MD, Friedman BJ, DeMaria AN: Uses and limitations of exercise Doppler echocardiography in the diagnosis of ischemic heart disease, *J Am Coll Cardiol* 10:809, 1987.

66. Zachariah ZP, Hsiung MC, Nanda NC, et al: Color Doppler assessment of mitral regurgitation induced by supine exercise in patients with coronary artery disease, *Am J Cardiol* 59:1266, 1987.

67. Mitchell GD, Brunken RC, Schwaiger M, et al: Assessment of mitral flow velocity with exercise by an index of stress-induced left ventricular ischemia in coronary artery disease, *Am J Cardiol* 61:536, 1988.

68. Hatle L, Angelsen B: *Doppler ultrasound in cardiology: physical principles and clinical applications,* ed 2, Philadelphia, 1985, Lea & Febiger, p 110.

69. Sagar KB, Wann LS, Paulsen WJH, Levin S: Role of exercise Doppler echocardiography in isolated mitral stenosis, *Chest* 92:27, 1987.

70. Tatineni S, Barner HB, Pearson AC, et al: Rest and exercise evaluation of St. Jude Medical and Medtronic Hall prostheses: influence of primary lesion, valvular type, valvular size, and left ventricular function, *Circulation* 80(3 Pt 1):I16-23, 1989.

71. Bryg RJ, Lewen MK, Williams GA, Labovitz AJ: Effects of isometric handgrip exercise on Doppler-derived parameters of aortic flow in normal subjects, *Am J Cardiol* 63:1410-1412, 1989.

72. Kondo S, Meerbaum S, Sakamaki T, et al: Diagnosis of coronary stenosis by two-dimensional echographic study of dysfunction of ventricular segments during and immediately after pacing, *Am Col Cardiol* 2(4):689-698, 1983.

73. Chapman PD, Doyle TP, Troup PJ, et al: Stress echocardiography with transesophageal atrial pacing: preliminary report of a new method for detection of ischemic wall motion abnormalities, *Circulation* 70(3):445-450, 1984.

74. Iliceto S, Marangelli V, Memmola C, Rizzon P: Transesophageal Doppler echocardiography evaluation of coronary blood flow velocity in baseline conditions and during dipyridamole-induced coronary vasodilation, *Circulation* 83:61-69, 1991.

75. Kaul S, Kelly P, Oliner JD, et al: Assessment of regional myocardial blood flow with myocardial contrast two-dimensional echocardiography, *J Am Coll Cardiol* 13:468-482, 1989.

76. Sanders WE, Cheirif J, Desir R, et al: Contrast opacification of left ventricular myocardium following intravenous administration of sonicated albumin microspheres, *Am Heart J* 122:1660-1665, 1991.

15 | Effects of Exercise on the Heart and the Prevention of Coronary Heart Disease

The protective effects of chronic physical activity have been elucidated by many animal and human studies over the past 20 years. Although there have been some studies showing a lack of benefit, the majority have demonstrated that habitual physical exercise or physical fitness prolong life. As a result, many international health organizations have put forth recommendations regarding the quantity and quality of exercise needed to improve the health of the public.

DEFINITION OF EXERCISE TRAINING

Exercise training and physical conditioning are terms used for chronic exercise or an exercise program. Exercise training can be defined as maintaining a regular habit of exercise at levels greater than those usually performed. An exercise program can be designed for increasing muscular strength, muscular endurance, or dynamic performance. The type of exercise that results in an increase in muscular strength involves short bursts of activity against a high resistance. Isometric exercise involves developing muscular pressure against resistance without much movement. Although such an exercise results in an increase in muscular mass along with strength, they do not benefit the cardiovascular system. They cause a pressure load on the heart rather than a flow load because mean pressure is greatly elevated in proportion to the increase in cardiac output. Flow cannot be increased much because of increased pressure within the active muscle groups. Dynamic exercise, also called isotonic, involves the rhythmic movement of large groups of muscles and requires an increase in cardiac output, ventilation, and oxygen consumption. Such exercise is also called aerobic because it must be performed with sufficient oxygen present. This is the type of exercise that results in the cardiovascular changes that are described in this chapter.

The features of an aerobic exercise program that must be considered include the mode, the duration, the intensity, and the frequency of the exercise. In general, the mode of exercise must involve movement of large muscle groups such as that required by bicycling, walking, running, skating, cross country skiing, and swimming. The exercise should be carried out in at least three sessions a week and should be spread throughout the week. Duration should be 30 to 60 minutes. Intensity should be at least 50% of the maximal oxygen consumption and involve at least 300 kilocalories of energy expenditure per session. The percentage of maximal oxygen consumption being performed can be approximated by heart rate or by the level of perceived exertion.

The results of such an aerobic exercise program include hemodynamic, morphological, and metabolic changes. The hemodynamic consequences of an exercise program include a decrease in resting heart rate, a decrease in the heart rate and systolic blood pressure at any matched submaximal work load, an increase in work capacity and maximal oxygen consumption, and a faster recovery from a bout of exercise. It is argued whether these changes are attributable to peripheral or to cardiac adaptations, but they are probably attributable to both. Peripheral adaptations are more important in older individuals and in patients with heart or lung disease, whereas cardiac adaptations are more of a factor in younger individuals. Cardiac hemodynamic changes that have been observed in some instances include enhanced cardiac function and cardiac output.

The morphological changes that occur with an exercise program are age related. These changes occur most definitely in younger individuals and

323

may not occur in older individuals. The exact age at which the response to chronic exercise is altered is uncertain, but it would seem to be in the early thirties. Morphological changes include an increase in myocardial mass and left ventricular end-diastolic volume. Paralleling these changes are increases in coronary artery size and the myocardial capillary–to–fiber ratio. These changes are clearly beneficial, making it possible for the heart to function more efficiently and to have greater perfusion during any stress. In older individuals there can be a decrease in myocardial mass resulting in an improvement in capillary–to–muscle fiber ratio but no change in coronary artery size. No studies have shown an exercise program to decrease atherosclerotic plaques once they are present. However, a monkey study has shown that exercise can offset the effect of an atherogenic diet by increases in coronary artery size.

The metabolic alterations secondary to an aerobic exercise program are summarized below. Total serum cholesterol level is not affected, but high density lipoproteins (which remove cholesterol from the body) are increased, particularly when weight loss accompanies the exercise. Serum triglyceride and fasting glucose levels are decreased. In addition, it appears that there are favorable alterations in insulin and glucagon responses. Diabetics need less insulin if they maintain a regular exercise program. Also, after an exercise program, blood catecholamine levels are lower in response to any stress. The fibrinolytic system seems to be enhanced, and since coronary thrombosis is no longer a misnomer, such enhancement would seem to be beneficial in preventing myocardial infarction.

Although it is said that exercise enhances psychological well-being and can even produce the "runner's high," few convincing studies have been performed in this area. It would seem, however, that exercise does have a tranquilizing effect and increases pain tolerance, which may be beneficial in some individuals. This chapter presents the studies that have investigated the effects of chronic exercise on the heart, specifically regarding animals as well as human studies of hemodynamics, the echocardiogram, and the electrocardiographic response to exercise testing. The available body of literature concerning the effects of chronic exercise on the hearts of humans and animals is now substantial. Several excellent and more detailed reviews of this topic have been published recently.[1,2] In the following, only some of the classic articles are described to underscore each issue.

ANIMAL STUDIES RELATING EXERCISE TO CARDIAC CHANGES
Capillary changes

Animal studies provide some of the strongest evidence for the health benefits of regular exercise. The many effects listed in Table 15-1 have been demonstrated in various studies. Vigorous exercise has been shown to induce cardiac hypertrophy in animals. Heart-to-body ratios are invariably larger and the density of muscle cells and capillaries are greater in wild animals as compared with the domestic form of an animal species. In young animals, cardiac hypertrophy is secondary to fiber hyperplasia, whereas in older animals it is secondary to cellular hypertrophy. The capillary bed responds most dramatically to growth stimuli if applied at an early age.[3] There is an age-related response of the ventricular capillary bed and myocardial fiber width in rats. At autopsy, the myocardial fiber width is constant, whereas the capillary-fiber ratios are increased in the exercised rats over the controls in all age groups.[4]

Experiments have been performed to study the effects of chronic exercise on the heart at different ages in rats. Although the response of the rat heart to chronic exercise appears to vary with age, the capillary-fiber ratio increases at all ages. Capillary proliferation in the heart and skeletal muscle has been studied by radioautography after injection of radioactive thymidine in rats exercised by swimming.[5] Swimming led to hypertrophy of the myocardium and in muscle fibers of the limbs. There was also new formation of myocardial capillaries in swimming-induced cardiac hypertrophy.

Table 15-1   Results of animal studies investigating the effects of chronic exercise

Age dependent myocardial hypertrophy
Myocardial microcirculatory changes (increased ratio of capillaries to muscle fibers)
Proportional increase in coronary artery size
Mixed results when studying changes in coronary collateral circulation
Improved cardiac mechanical and metabolic performance
Favorable changes in skeletal muscle mitochondria and respiratory enzymes
Mixed results with myocardial mitochondria and enzyme changes
Little effect on established atherosclerotic lesions or risk factors
Improved peripheral blood flow during exercise

These results are strong support for the exercise hypothesis. Perhaps if people were as "compliant" as animals, the benefits of exercise to humans would be more apparent.

Coronary artery size changes

The effects of exercise on the coronary tree of rats has been studied by the corrosion-cast technique.[6] Two groups of rats were studied, one undertook a swimming program and one a running program. After the animals were killed, their hearts were weighed, and then the coronary arteries were injected with vinyl acetate. Compared with the controls, both exercise groups had an increased ratio of heart weight to body weight and an increased ratio of coronary tree cast weight to heart weight.

Coronary collateral circulation

Eckstein performed the classic study of the effect of exercise and coronary artery narrowing on coronary collateral circulation.[7] He surgically induced a constriction in the circumflex artery in approxi-

mately 100 dogs during a thoracotomy. After 1 week of rest, the dogs were put into two groups. One group was exercised on a treadmill 1 hour a day, 5 days a week, for 6 to 8 weeks. The other group remained at rest in cages. The extent of arterial anastomoses to the circumflex artery was then determined during a second thoracotomy. Moderate and severe arterial narrowing resulted in collateral development proportional to the degree of narrowing. Exercise led to even greater retrograde flow. This study is illustrated in Figure 15-1.

Coronary blood flow has been studied in exercised and sedentary rats using labeled microspheres during hypoxemic conditions.[8] Even though cardiac hypertrophy was found in the trained rats, this increase in perfused mass accounted for only one third the increase in total cor-

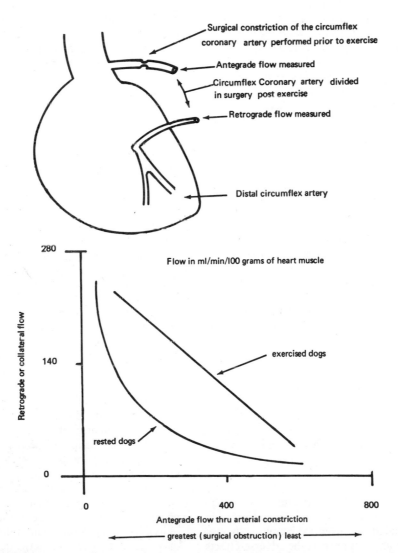

Figure 15-1   Description of Eckstein's study showing surgical procedure and results.

onary blood flow. Thus there was a greater coronary blood flow per unit mass of the myocardium in the trained rats.

The effects of endurance exercise on coronary collateral blood flow has been studied in miniature swine.[9] Coronary collateral blood flow was measured in 10 sedentary control pigs and in seven pigs that ran 20 miles a week for 10 months. Ten months of endurance exercise training did not have an effect on the development of coronary collaterals as assessed by microsphere blood flow measurements in the left ventricle of the pigs. When this was repeated after artificial partial occlusions were caused in the coronary arteries of their pigs (that is, ischemia was induced), exercise resulted in enhanced myocardial perfusion.

The effect of physical training on collateral blood flow in 14 dogs with chronic coronary occlusions revealed that myocardial blood flow to collateral dependent zones that were measured using injected radionuclide was increased by 39% in those exercised.[10]

The effects of exercise training on the development of coronary collaterals in response to gradual coronary occlusion in dogs has been studied.[11] After placement of an amaroid constrictor on the proximal left circumflex coronary artery, 33 dogs were randomly assigned to exercise or sedentary groups. After 2 months, the exercised dogs developed greater epicardial collateral connections to the occluded left circumflex, as judged by higher blood flow and less distal pressure drop. However, no difference in collaterals was found angiographically. Injection of microspheres demonstrated that exercised dogs were not better protected against subendocardial ischemia. Exercise promoted coronary collateral development without improving perfusion of ischemic myocardium. Thus, even if collateral development does occur, the question remains whether it significantly influences myocardial perfusion.

Ventricular fibrillation threshold

Ventricular fibrillation threshold studies in rats and dogs have found increased resistance to ventricular fibrillation after regular running possibly through mechanisms involving cyclic adenosine monophosphate and the slow calcium channel.[12]

Mortality

Holloszy reviewed the literature and his own data regarding the effects of exercise on longevity in rats and concluded that exercise increases the average life span and can prevent the adverse effects of overeating.[13]

Effects of exercise on atherosclerosis

Kramsch and colleagues randomly allocated 27 young adult male monkeys into three groups.[14] Two groups were studied for 36 months, and one group was studied for 42 months. Of the groups studied for 36 months, one was fed a vegetarian diet for the entire study whereas the other was fed the vegetarian diet for 12 months and then an isocaloric atherogenic diet for 24 months. Both were designated as sedentary because their physical activity was limited to a single cage. The third group was fed the vegetarian diet for 18 months and then the atherogenic diet for 24 months. This group exercised regularly on a treadmill for the entire 42 months. Total serum cholesterol remained the same but HDL cholesterol was higher in the exercise group. ST-segment depression, angiographic size of coronary artery narrowing, and sudden death were observed only in the sedentary monkeys fed the atherogenic diet. In addition, postmortem examination revealed considerable coronary atherosclerosis and stenosis in this group. Exercise was associated with substantially reduced overall atherogenic involvement, lesion size, and collagen accumulation. These results demonstrate that exercise in young adult monkeys increases heart size, left ventricular mass, and the diameter of coronary arteries. Also, the subsequent experimental atherosclerosis, induced by the atherogenic diet, was substantially reduced in the exercised group. Exercise before exposure to the atherogenic diet delayed the development of the manifestation of coronary heart disease.

HUMAN STUDIES SUPPORTING MORPHOLOGICAL CHANGES

The effects of an exercise program can be studied by the cross-sectional approach, comparing athletes to normal people, and by the longitudinal approach, comparing individuals before and after a training program. Both of these approaches have limitations and difficulties. The cross-sectional approach is the easier of the two because the trouble and expense of organizing a training program can be avoided. However, athletes are endowed with biological attributes and motivation that make them capable of superior performance. Also, they undergo long periods of physical training that usually begin at a young age when dimensional and morphological changes are more likely to occur. This fact makes comparison with normal people questionable, since most trained normal individuals cannot reach an athlete's level of cardiovascular function or performance. Beside the expense and difficulty in organizing and maintaining an exercise program, there are other problems encountered in longitudinal studies. Volunteers often are athletic and differ from randomly selected normal people. An exercise program can modify significant variables, such as body weight and smoking habits, and results can be biased by dropouts. In persons with coronary heart disease, a placebo effect on hemodynamics has been documented and a training program may select a healthier group.

In any training program, the result depends on several factors. These factors include the level of fitness, physical endowment, previous physical training, age, sex, and health of the individual entering the program. The changes are greater in sedentary individuals than in those somewhat physically fit and greater in younger individuals than in older individuals. The most important of these variables are evaluated in this review by inclusion of studies of normal trainees of different ages and of persons with coronary heart disease.

Prescription of exercise

The structure of an exercise program is important. Intensity and duration of the work periods must be considered, as well as the overall time of exercise. Individuals with coronary heart disease whose disease is stable must be selected. During training they follow a less demanding exercise protocol because of the danger of exercise-induced sudden death. An exercise program can be aimed at improving or increasing muscle strength and anaerobic or aerobic performance. Only the latter effect is dependent on the improvement of the oxygen-transporting system (that is, blood, lungs, heart, and blood vessels) and comes about mainly because of an improvement in the overall capacity of the cardiovascular system.

Muscle strength can be improved by repetitious isotonic or isometric muscle contractions of a duration of a few seconds and against resistance. This type of exercise does not improve cardiovascular function, as shown by relatively normal-sized hearts, normal resting and exercise heart rates, and unexceptional maximal oxygen intakes of athletes who train only in this manner. Anaerobic capacity is necessary for short activities of high intensity or for activities that require more energy than is available from the oxygen-transport system. Much of this energy is derived from high-energy phosphate compounds that result from breakdown of glycogen to lactic acid, which is oxygen independent. Athletes, such as sprinters, who require relatively infrequent short bursts of high-intensity activity acquire this capacity and often do not improve their overall cardiovascular function. Train-

ing aimed at developing anaerobic capacity should consist in near-maximal work periods of short duration (10 to 60 seconds). This type of training requires much motivation because it is difficult and painful. Aerobic performance depends on an increase in the oxygen transport system, which is developed principally through adaptations in the cardiovascular system and the skeletal muscles. Large muscle masses are active, and so the greatest demand for oxygen is made. Physical activity ranging from work periods of a few seconds repeated quickly to hours of continuous work may induce an improvement in aerobic performance. The following patterns are effective:

1. *Dash exercise training*—maximal effort (that is, running full speed preferably uphill) for 30 to 60 seconds and repeated 5 to 10 times with several minutes of low-level activity between each dash. This pattern also improves anaerobic performance.
2. *Interval exercise training*—slightly less effort than maximal (80% of dash effort), lasting 3 to 7 minutes repeated 3 to 7 times with low-level activity periods of 6 to 8 minutes between each interval.
3. *Continuous exercise training*—submaximal effort for 45 to 75 minutes. Heart rates should range from 130 to 170 beats/min depending on age and fitness.

These exercise training patterns are applicable to walking, running, bicycling, swimming, or isotonic arm exercises. Isometric exercises such as weight lifting are generally not aerobic, and they can be dangerous for heart disease patients with dilated ventricles because of the excessive level of myocardial pressure work associated with them. Modest resistance exercise programs for selected cardiac rehabilitation patients have gained popularity as a complement to aerobic activities, but guidelines issued by the Amercian Association of Cardiovascular and Pulmonary Rehabilitation should be considered before one recommends these activities to patients with heart disease. For healthy individuals, a recent increase in the popularity of "circuit" weight training has occurred, which involves high-repetition, low-resistance weight training at different stations interspersed with brief periods of rest, and aerobic benefits have been demonstrated.[15]

The exercise prescription for cardiovascular changes and fitness must consider the frequency, duration, and intensity of aerobic exercise. Three sessions a week for at least 30 minutes is recommended. Less exercise may be suitable for maintenance, and more exercise is associated with an increased incidence of injuries. For cardiac patients, a warm-up and a cool-down are important. Starting slowly can usually be substituted for the stretching routine in normal subjects. Intensity should be within 60% to 80% of maximal oxygen uptake. This level is most easily monitored by heart rate, which is linearly related to oxygen consumption. The Karvonen technique for determining training heart rate most closely approximates the appropriate exercise intensity. It is calculated by subtracting basal heart rate from maximal, multiplying by 75%, and adding the product to the basal value. Perceived exertion levels of 13 to 14 seem to approximate an exercise intensity for achieving a training effect. For cardiac patients taking beta-blockers or with symptoms or signs that are maximal end points, one can achieve an exercise effect by subtracting 5 to 10 beats from the heart rate at the end point (that is, at angina) or using the Borg perceived exertion scale.

Echocardiography before and after exercise training in normals

Ehsani and co-workers reported rapid changes in left ventricular dimensions and mass in response to physical conditioning and deconditioning.[16] Two groups of healthy young subjects were studied. The training group consisted of eight competitive swimmers who were studied serially for 9 weeks. Mean left ventricular end-diastolic dimension increased by a total of 3.3 mm and posterior wall thickness increased 0.7 mm by the ninth week of training. There was no significant change in the ejection fraction. The deconditioned group consisted of six competitive runners who stopped training for 3 weeks. End-diastolic dimension decreased 4.7 mm, and posterior wall thickness decreased 2.7 mm by the end of the 3-week period. Deconditioning did not influence ejection fraction. Exercise training induced rapid adaptive changes in left ventricular dimensions and mimicked the pattern of chronic volume overload, and modest degrees of exercise-induced left ventricular enlargement were reversible. Surprisingly, changes in left ventricular dimension occurred early during endurance training, but there was no significant increase in measured left ventricular posterior wall thickness until the fifth week of training. Estimated left ventricular mass significantly increased after the first week of training.

DeMaria and colleagues reported the results of M-mode echocardiography in 24 young normals before and after 11 weeks of endurance exercise training.[17] After training, they exhibited an increased left ventricular end-diastolic dimension, a decreased end-systolic dimension, and both an increased stroke volume and a shortening fraction.

An increase in mean fiber-shortening velocity was observed, as were increases in left ventricular wall thickness, ECG voltage, and left ventricular mass.

Stein and colleagues studied the effects of exercise training on ventricular dimensions at rest and during supine submaximal exercise.[18] Fourteen healthy students were studied using M-mode echocardiography at rest and in the third minute of 300 kilogram-meters/min of supine bike exercise. They were studied before and after a 14-week training program that resulted in a 30% increase in maximal oxygen consumption. The authors concluded that exercise training is associated with an increased stroke volume mediated by the Frank-Starling effect and enhanced contractility. Parrault and colleagues studied 14 middle-aged subjects with a chest x-ray film, electrocardiogram, vectorcardiogram, and echocardiogram before and after 5 months of training.[19] Maximal oxygen consumption increased 20%. The echocardiograms showed no significant changes, in contrast to those in studies in younger subjects. Wolfe and colleagues performed a similar study in 12 men with a mean age of 37 who exhibited 14% and 18% increases in aerobic capacity after 3 and 6 months of training, respectively.[20] They concluded that resting end-diastolic volume and stroke volume were increased but that left ventricular structure and resting contractile status are not altered by 6 months of jogging in healthy, previously sedentary men.

Adams and co-workers noninvasively studied the effects of an aerobic training program on the heart of healthy college-aged men.[21] Compared with a control group, echocardiography after training showed an increase in left ventricular end-diastolic dimension but no significant change in wall thickness or in ejection fraction. Although there was no change in myocardial wall thickness, the increase in end-diastolic dimension resulted in an increase in left ventricular mass.

Landry and co-workers evaluated 20 sedentary subjects and 10 pairs of monozygotic twins who were submitted to a 20-week endurance exercise program.[22] Maximal oxygen uptake increased significantly in both groups. Statistically significant increases in left ventricular diameter, posterior wall and septal thicknesses, as well as left ventricular end-diastolic volume and left ventricular mass were observed in the sedentary subjects but not in the monozygotic twins. After training, twin pairs differed more from each other than at the start. Concomitantly, within-pair resemblance was greater after training than before. Results indicate that cardiac dimensions are amenable to significant modifications under controlled endurance training conditions and that the extent and variability of the response of cardiac structures to training are perhaps genotype dependent. Tables 15-2 and 15-3 summarize these cross-sectional and longitudinal studies respectively.

Effect of exercise on risk factors

Marti and co-workers found that unsupervised jogging over a period of 4 months significantly improved high-density-lipoprotein cholesterol levels in nonsmoking males.[23] Data from the Framingham study showed that increasing levels of physical activity (as determined by a modified Minnesota Leisure Time Physical Activity questionnaire) were associated with higher levels of high-density-

Table 15-2   Cross-sectional echocardiographic studies comparing athletes to controls

Emory University echocardiographic study

	Controls	Athletes
LVPWT	9.8	10.9
LVVIED	62	72
VO$_2$	43	71
EF	72%	68%
Resting HR	62	51

University of Missouri echocardiographic study

	Controls	Athletes
LVPWT	9	11
LVEDD	52	57
LVESD	37	34
VO$_2$	47	74
EF	64%	78%
Resting HR	61	50
MVCFS	0.9	1.2

National Institutes of Health echocardiographic study

	Aerobic athletes	Isometric athletes	Normals
LVPWT	11	13.7	10
Septum	10.8	13	10.3
LVEDD	55	48	46

University of California, San Diego, echocardiographic study

	Controls	Athletes
RVEDD	13	21
Septum	13	14
LVPWT	10	11
LVEDD	50	54
LVESD	31	32
EF	76%	79%
MVCFS	1.13	1.18

All dimensions are in millimeters. *EF*, Ejection fraction; *HR*, heart rate (beats/min); *LVEDD* or *RVEDD*, left or right ventricular end-diastolic dimension; *LVESD*, left ventricular end-systolic dimension; *LVPWT*, left ventricular posterior wall thickness; *LVVIED*, left ventricular volume index at end diastole in ml; *MVCFS*, mean ventricular circumferential fiber shortening (contractions per seconds); *RVEDD*, see *LVEDD*; *VO$_2$*, maximal oxygen consumption (ml of O$_2$/kg/min).

lipoprotein cholesterol, lower heart rate, lower body mass index, and a decrease in smoking.[24] A recent excellent study by Blumenthal and co-workers failed to demonstrate a reduction in blood pressure in patients with mild hypertension.[25]

STUDIES IN PATIENTS WITH HEART DISEASE

Ehsani and colleagues reported their results after 12 months of intense exercise in a highly selected group of 10 patients with coronary heart disease.[26] The patients ranged in age from 44 to 63 years; nine had sustained a single myocardial infarction, one had severe three-vessel coronary artery disease, and all 10 had asymptomatic exercise-induced ST-segment depression. Eight comparable men were considered as controls. They completed 12 months in a high level exercise program. After 3 months of exercise training at a level of 50% to 70% of maximal oxygen consumption the level of training increased to 70% to 80%, with two to three intervals at 80% to 90% interspersed throughout the exercise session. The maximal amount of reported ST-segment depression was 0.3 mV, but most had 0.2 mV of depression, which was less at repeat testing 1 year later despite a higher double product, greater treadmill work load, and a 38% increase in maximal oxygen consumption. In addition, 0.1 mV of ST-segment depression occurred at a higher double product after the year of training. A weight loss from a mean of 79 to 74 kg occurred. The sum of the ECG voltage representing heart mass increased by 15%. Both left ventricular end-diastolic dimension and posterior wall thickness were significantly increased after training. This resulted in an increase in left ventricular mass from 93 to 135 g/m^2 of body surface area. These results cannot be generalized to the average cardiac patient population. These 10 men were a highly selected group, all with asymptomatic ST-segment depression (silent ischemia) and able to exercise at levels often even difficult for younger men. If applied to most patients with coronary disease, this intensity certainly could lead to a high incidence of orthopedic and cardiac complications. Rehabilitation patients with exercise-induced ST-segment depression who exceed standard exercise prescriptions are at increased risk of cardiac events.

Ditchey and co-workers obtained echocardiograms on 14 coronary patients before and after an average of 7 months (range 3 to 14 months) of supervised arm and leg exercise.[27] Each echocardiogram was interpreted jointly by two blinded observers, using three different measurement conventions and a semi-automated method of analysis

Table 15-3 Serial echocardiographic studies (longitudinal or prospective) evaluating the cardiac effects of exercise training

Washington University study (college athletes)	Eight swimmers trained for 9 weeks		Three runners detrained for 3 weeks	
	Before training	After training	Before detraining	After detraining
LVEDD	48.7	52	51	46.3
LVPWT	9.4	10.1	10.7	8.0
VO$_2$	52	60	62	57
Resting HR	70	63	57	64
EF	63%	63%	68%	63%

UCD study (policemen)	Before training	After training
LVEDD	48	50
LVESD	30	29
LVPWT	9.1	10.1
Resting HR	69	63
VO$_2$	36	41
EF	75%	80%
MVCFS	1.21	1.28

SUNY Downstate Medical Center study

	Before training		After training	
	rest	300 kpm	rest	300 kpm
LVEDD	47	46	50	50
LVESD	32	21	32	30
EF	70%	90%	73%	78%

Montreal Heart Institute (normal men ~40 years old)

	Before training	After training
VO$_2$	34	41
Septum	12.5	12.7
LVPWT	10	9.8
LVEDD	47.8	48.2
LVESD	33	33

Salt Lake City study (25 men exercised 3 months, mean age 22 years)

	Before training	After training
Resting HR	63	54
VO$_2$	49	56
% Body fat	17.2	13.7
R-wave lead V$_5$	1.7 mV	2.0 mV
LVEDD	45.8	49.6
EF	62%	66%
LVPWT	10.9	10.3
LVESD	32.3	33.5

Washington University Rehab study (9 post-MI patients, 1 year of exercise)

	Before training	After training
LVEDD	51	56
LVPWT	9	10
VO$_2$	26	35
Lead RV$_5$	1.7 mV	2.0 mV

All dimensions are in millimeters. *EF,* Ejection fraction; *HR,* heart rate (beats/min); *kpm,* kilogram-meters/minute; *LVEDD,* left ventricular end-diastolic dimension; *LVESD,* left ventricular end-systolic dimension; *LVPWT,* left ventricular posterior wall thickness; *mV,* millivolts; *MVCFS,* mean ventricular circumferential fiber shortening (contractions per second); *VO$_2$,* maximal oxygen consumption (ml or cc of O$_2$/kg/min).

to minimize errors of interpretation. Exercise training led to subjective improvement in all 14 patients and a 2 MET increase in estimated exercise capacity. However, this was not accompanied by any significant change in left ventricular end-diastolic diameter or wall thickness. Likewise, left ventricular cross-sectional area, an index of left ventricular mass that corrects for altered ventricular volume and theoretically reflects directional changes in mass despite nonuniform wall thickness, did not change significantly after training.

Exercise electrocardiographic studies

Since abnormal ST-segment shifts in coronary patients are most likely secondary to ischemia, lessening of such shifts would be consistent with improved myocardial perfusion. For purposes of comparison, only similar myocardial oxygen demands can be considered; therefore only ST-segment measurements at matched double products should be compared. The product of heart rate times systolic blood pressure is the best noninvasive estimate of myocardial oxygen demand during exercise. The studies of the effect of an exercise program on the exercise electrocardiogram are summarized in Table 15-4. In all the studies, training produced a lowering of heart rate for all submaximal exercise levels, permitting performance

of more work before the onset of angina or ST-segment depression (which occurred at the same heart rate before and after training) or both.

As part of a study to evaluate perfusion and function with exercise training (PERFEXT), 48 patients who exercised and 59 control patients had computerized exercise ECGs performed initially and 1 year later.[28] Obvious changes in exercise-induced ST-segment depression could not be demonstrated. Controversy now exists as to whether cardiac changes can occur in patients with heart disease and, if they do, whether these changes require high-intensity exercise. If high-intensity exercise is needed, exercise cannot be advocated as a public health measure during leisure time without medical supervision and the availability of medications and instrumentation for defibrillation.

EPIDEMIOLOGICAL STUDIES OF PHYSICAL ACTIVITY AND FITNESS
Studies relating physical activity to cardiac events

Since most animal, clinical, and pathological studies have not shown exercise to be directly related to the atherosclerotic process, it is reasonable to conclude that physical inactivity does not have a

Table 15-4 Effect of chronic exercise on the exercise electrocardiogram

Investigator[a]	Year	Male subjects	Training duration (months)	Results
Salzman	1969	100	33	ST-segment changes correlated with changes in functional capacity
Detry	1971	14	3	No change in computerized ST-segment measurements at matched double products
Kattus	1972	13	5	Thirteen percent improvement ST-segments in exercise and control groups
Costill	1974	24	3	No change in ST-segment response
Raffo	1980	12	6	Higher heart rate for similar degree of ST-segment
Ehsani	1981	10	12	Less ST-segment depression at matched double product and maximal exercise; higher double product at ischemic ST threshold (0.1 mV flat)
Watanabe	1982	14	6	Changes only in spatial analysis with coronary artery disease
Myers	1984	48	12	Less ST-segment depression at matched work load; no differences at matched heart rate or double product versus controls

*Salzman SH et al: In Blackburn H, editor: *Measurements in exercise ECG,* Springfield, Ill, 1969, Charles C Thomas. Detry J, Bruce RA: *Circulation,* 44:390, 1971. Kattus AA et al: *Chest* 62:678, 1972. Costill DL et al: *Med Sci Sports* 6:95, 1974. Raffo JA et al: *Br Heart J* 43:262, 1980. Ehsani AA et al: *Circulation* 64:1116-1124, 1981. Watanabe K et al: *Clin Cardiol* 5:27, 1982. Myers J et al: *J Am Coll Cardiol* 4:1094, 1984.

direct effect on atherosclerosis. Instead, the effects of regular exercise enable the body to better tolerate ischemia and lessen the manifestations of coronary heart disease. In addition, it can possibly alter other risk factors for atherosclerosis. The potential beneficial actions of regular exercise are multifactorial, which makes physical inactivity a complex risk factor to assess.

There are inherent difficulties in studying physical inactivity as a risk factor. An important consideration is that people often leave active jobs with onset of the first symptoms of heart disease, even without realizing the cause of the symptoms. That is, there is a premorbid transfer from an active job to a less active job, biasing the relationship of inactivity to coronary heart disease. There are other difficulties in studying this question, including the uncertainty of what type and quantity of exercise is protective. Although the most accurate way of assessing the physiological effect of an activity level would be an exercise test, only recent studies have had this luxury. Job title or class has often been used as a proxy variable for occupational energy expenditure and in some instances may be quite accurate. However, consideration of off-the-job activity, that is, leisure time, is important. Questionnaires have been used, but their reproducibility and accuracy are often doubtful. Parameters such as vital capacity, handgrip strength, and dietary assays have obvious limitations. The methods of diagnosing coronary artery disease have included death certificates, rest and exercise electrocardiograms, medical records, medical evaluations, and autopsy. All these methods have their shortcomings in terms of accuracy.

The question remains whether activity level or actual maximal oxygen uptake best predicts the risk for coronary heart disease. Leon has shown that in healthy men the results of resting measurements and a questionnaire correlate highly with treadmill time using a multivariate equation.[29] One hundred seventy-five apparently healthy men completed questionnaires about habitual physical activity, smoking, alcoholic beverage consumption, and sleep habits. Body mass index, heart rate and blood pressure at rest and during submaximal exercise, frequency of premature ventricular beats, handgrip strength, and serum cholesterol were measured. These characteristics were correlated with the duration of exercise using the Bruce protocol. Univariate analysis indicated that treadmill performance was significantly and positively correlated with leisure time activity and reports of sweating and dyspnea occurring regularly during such physical activity. Performance was negatively correlated with age, body mass index, resting heart rate, cigarette smoking, and consumption

of caffeine-containing beverages. A correlation of 0.75 was found between treadmill performance and 11 of the above variables, and it was increased to 0.81 when heart rate during submaximal exercise was included.

Morris has presented the data from the occupational-mortality records in England and Wales, interpreting the information as support for the hypothesis that occupational physical inactivity is risk factor for coronary artery disease.[30] Social class as used in these studies was based on the grading of occupation by its level of skill and role in production and its general standing in the community. The level of activity was based on the independent evaluation of the occupations by several industrial experts. The activity level of the last job held was found to be inversely related to the mortality from coronary artery disease, as determined from death certificates.

Morris and co-workers[31] presented data from a sequence of epidemiological studies to support the hypothesis that "men in physically active jobs have a lower incidence of coronary heart disease than men in physically inactive jobs." The first study dealt with the drivers and conductors of the London transport system. Thirty-one thousand white men, 35 to 64 years of age, were included for analysis over a period of 18 months from 1949 to 1950. The end points were coronary insufficiency, myocardial infarction, and angina as reported on sick leave records and listing of coronary artery disease on death certificates. The age-adjusted total incidence was 1.5 times higher in the more sedentery group of drivers than that in the conductor group, and the sudden and 3-month mortality was two times higher.

In their original study, Morris and co-workers did not investigate differences in selection in the two groups but did so in a subsequent study of postmen and clerks, the results of which also agreed with their hypothesis. In 1966, Morris also showed that the drivers had higher serum cholesterol levels and higher blood pressures than the conductors had. In addition, a study by Oliver documented that for some unknown reason even the recruits for the two jobs differed in lipid level and in weight.[32] These differences put the drivers at increased risk to coronary artery disease.

In 1958, Stamler and colleagues[33] began a prospective study of 1241 apparently healthy male employees of the Peoples Gas Company in Chicago. By 1965, there were 39 deaths from coronary disease among the groups. They found that the coronary disease mortality was higher in blue-collar workers (37 deaths per 1000 men) who had an estimated higher habitual activity at work than in the white-collar workers (20 deaths per 1000).

However, the population in general had a low level of physical activity and lacked a gradient between the groups, which limited the possibility of demonstrating an association of physical activity and mortality.

The Seven Countries Coronary Artery Disease Study included Japan, Yugoslavia, the United States, Finland, Italy, the Netherlands, and Greece.[34] This study minimized self-selection by complete coverage of all men 40 to 59 years of age in the geographically defined areas. Individuals were classified as sedentary, moderately active, or very active, as determined by a questionnaire for evaluating total physical activity. Data from 200,000 man-years observed, showed no difference in coronary disease incidence between physically active and sedentary men.

Epstein, and colleagues studied the relationship of cardiac events to vigorous exercise during leisure time in approximately 17,000 middle-aged male executive civil servants whose work was sedentary.[35] On a randomly selected Monday morning they recorded their leisure time activities over the previous weekend. An 8½ year follow-up study of this population demonstrated a 50% lower incidence of coronary events in those maintaining rigorous activity on the weekend.

Costas and colleagues,[36] reported a prospective study involving 8171 urban and rural men 45 to 64 years of age participating in the Puerto Rico Heart Program. A physical activity index was based on the number of hours spent at five different levels of physical activity as assessed by questionnaire. A slight increase in risk was found in the least active group of urban men. The level of physical activity was not related to the incidence of coronary heart disease.

Paffenbarger and colleagues[37] have reported numerous analyses of epidemiological data from San Francisco longshoremen, who work at relatively high activity levels under conditions well governed and documented by the longshoremen union. After a 22-year follow-up study of the longshoremen, one third of their energy expenditure was classified as high-energy work and the rest as low-energy work by analysis of their various jobs. An annual accounting of job transfers was taken so that the data on energy expenditures could be correlated to the occurrence of fatal myocardial infarction. Deaths from myocardial infarctions were assigned to the category in which the deceased had been employed 6 months before death to avoid selective bias because of premorbid job transfers. Age-adjusted frequencies of other risk factors among longshoremen were compared between the two energy-expenditure groups, and little difference was found. Three parameters were associated with increased risk for fatal myocardial infarction: low physical activity level, smoking cigarettes, and an elevated systolic blood pressure. Each of these factors posed approximately two times the risk. Paffenbarger concluded that physical activity is protective. The threshold of 5 kcal/min seemed to hold for strenuous bursts rather than for sustained activity.

Paffenbarger studied 36,000 Harvard University alumni who entered college between 1916 and 1950.[38] Alumnal offices and questionnaires were used to obtain information on adult exercise habits, morbidity, and mortality. A 6- to 10-year follow-up study during the period of 1961 to 1972 totaled 117,680 man-years of observation after the first questionnaire, and apparently healthy men were classified with specific measures of energy expenditure. They remained under study until heart attack occurrence, death from any cause, age 75, or the end of observation in 1972. Weekly updating of death lists by the alumnal office provided the means to obtain official death certificates. A physical activity index, devised to provide a composite estimate of total energy expenditure, was scaled in kilocalories per week and divided at 2000 kcal/wk, which produced a 60%-to-40% division of man-years of observation into low- and high-energy categories.

During the follow-up study, 572 men had their first myocardial infarction. Three high-risk characteristics were identified in this study: low physical activity index (less than 2000 kcal/wk), cigarette smoking, and hypertension. Presence of any one characteristic was accompanied by a 50% increase in risk of myocardial infarction, and the presence of two characteristics tripled the risk. Former varsity athletes retained a lower risk only if they maintained a high physical activity index as alumni. Maintenance of a high physical activity index reduced the heart attack risk by 26%.

In a second analysis of Harvard alumni, Paffenbarger and colleagues[39] examined the physical activity and other life-style characteristics of 16,936 alumni, 35 to 74 years of age, for relations to mortalities from all causes and for influences on length of life. A total of 1413 alumni died during 12 to 16 years of follow-up study (1962 to 1978). Exercise reported as walking, stair climbing, and sports play was inversely related to total mortality, primarily to death from cardiovascular or respiratory causes. Death rates declined steadily as energy expended on such activity increased from less than 500 to 3500 kcal/wk, beyond which rates increased slightly. Rates were one fourth to one third lower among alumni expending 2000 or more kilocalories during exercise per week than among less active men, when the study was controlled for hypertension, cigarette smoking, obesity or gains in body weight, or early parental death. Alumnal death rates were significantly lower among the physically active. Relative risk of death for individuals were highest among smokers and sedentary men. By 80 years of age, the amount of additional life attributable to adequate exercise, as compared with sedentary life-style, was from 1 to more than 2 years. In a third analysis, Paffenbarger and co-workers have reported that a change to a more active life style in these same men reduced their risk of cardiac events.

In Framingham, approximately 5000 men and women, 30 to 62 years of age and free of clinical evidence of coronary disease at the onset, have been examined regularly since 1949.[40] Coronary disease mortality was subsequently found to be higher in cohorts with indices or measurements consistent with sedentary life-style. However, physical inactivity did not have the predictive power of the three cardinal risk factors (smoking, hypertension, increased lipids). Kannel and Sorlie reanalyzed the Framingham data for the effects of physical activity on overall mortality and cardiovascular disease mortality. The effect of being sedentary on mortality was rather modest compared with the other risk factors but persisted when these other factors were taken into account. A low correlation was noted between physical activity level and the major risk factors.

The relationship of self-selected leisure-time physical activity to first major coronary disease events and overall mortality was studied in 12,138 middle-aged men participating in the Multiple Risk Factor Intervention Trial.[41] Total leisure-time physical activity over the preceding year was quantitated in mean minutes per day at baseline time by questionnaire, with subjects classified into tertiles (low, moderate, and high leisure-time physical activity). During 7 years of follow-up study, moderate leisure-time physical activity was associated with 63% of the fatal coronary heart disease events and sudden deaths, and low leisure-time physical activity was associated with 70% of the total deaths ($p < 0.01$). Mortalities with high leisure-time physical activity were similar to those in moderate leisure-time physical activity; however, combined fatal and nonfatal major coronary heart disease events were 20% lower with high that with low leisure-time physical activity. Leisure-time physical activity had a modest inverse relation to coronary heart disease and overall mortality in middle-aged men at high risk for coronary heart disease. The relationship of leisure time physical activity to mortality was investigated in 3043 white U.S. railroad workers followed for 20 years.[42] The Minnesota Leisure Time Physical Activity Ques-

tionnaire was used. After adjustment for age and other risk factors, the risk estimate for coronary heart disease deaths was 1.39 for sedentary men who expended 40 kcal/week compared with active men who expended 3632 kcal/wk.

A recent study represents an 8-year follow-up study of 7735 men 40-59 years of age in the general practice of each of 24 British towns.[43] Using a physical activity score, the overall level of physical activity was found to be an independent protection factor for heart attacks.

In the most extensive review up to 1987, Powell and co-workers performed a metanalysis of 43 such studies and concluded that an inverse relationship between physical activity and the incidence of coronary heart disease was observed in over two thirds.[44] Moreover, the relationship was strongest in those studies that best measured physical activity (Figure 15-2). Table 15-5 summarizes these studies.

Prospective studies relating exercise capacity to cardiac events

Is physical fitness or is physical activity necessary to achieve protection from coronary artery disease? This controversy is still debated in the literature[45] and may be as much of a rhetorical as a scientific question. Nonetheless, it is generally accepted that the maximum ventilatory oxygen uptake correlates with the level of physical fitness[46] and that this can be estimated as metabolic equivalents (METs) from the stage achieved on exercise testing.[47,48] This may be a more objective and reliable method of assessing a person's cardiovascular health than physical activity as reported by questionnaire. A few recent prospective studies have tried to assess physical fitness by these means and to make predictions about its effect on survival. Peters' prospective study[49] suggests that poor physical work capacity as measured by bicycle ergometry in apparently healthy Los Angeles County workers is related to subsequent myocardial infarctions. This was one of the first follow-up studies to measure exercise capacity directly rather than to estimate activity level. An adjusted relative risk of 2.2 was found only in men with certain other risk factors present, namely, above-median cholesterol level, smoking, above-median systolic blood pressure, or a combination of these.

Studies using exercise testing to relate exercise capacity to cardiac events (Table 15-6)

Investigations at the Aerobic Center in Dallas used treadmill performance to quantitate physical fitness. In a cross-sectional study of 753 men, treadmill performance was found to be inversely related to body weight, percent body fat, lipids,

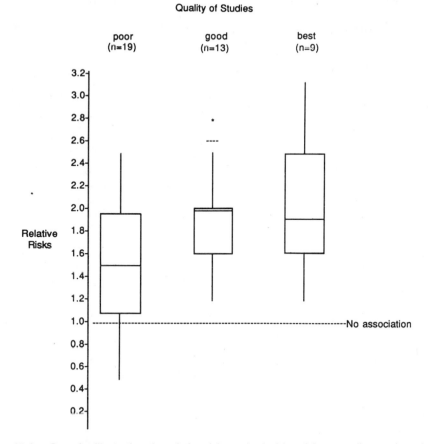

Figure 15-2 Box plot illustrating the relative risk or physical inactivity according to the scientific quality of the available studies. (From Williamson DF: *Ann Intern Med* 110:916-921, 1989.)

glucose, and systolic blood pressure.[50] In a longitudinal study, men who were treadmill tested both before and after an exercise program were analyzed to determine whether their performance had improved. Those men who reached the upper quartile of improved aerobic fitness exhibited decreases in lipids, diastolic blood pressure, serum glucose, uric acid, and weight. Regular exercise resulting in increased aerobic capacity was associated with decreased risk factors. In addition, they found in a study of 420 men who were broken up into groups of former athletes and nonathletes that prior athleticism had no significant effect on cardiovascular risk factors, physical fitness, and exercise habits.[51] This group also prospectively studied 10,224 men and 3120 women (99% of whom were white) who were all able to achieve 85% of manual-predicted heart rate.[52] They divided physical fitness levels into quintiles by estimating VO_2 max from a baseline treadmill test (using such a measurement as an estimation of a person's long-term physical fitness is not without controversy). With an average follow-up time of 8 years, they dem-

onstrated by multivariate analysis adjusted for age, other known cardiac risk factors, and length of follow-up time, that all cause mortality was inversely related to physical fitness. This study is quite important, being one of the only ones to study fitness in women prospectively, to include such a large sample size, and to document that gradations in physical fitness lead to significant differences in mortality.

The Lipid Research Clinics Mortality Follow-up Study also used a baseline treadmill test as their estimate of physical fitness in their study of 3106 men followed an average of 8.5 years.[53] They found a relative risk of cardiovascular death of 2.7 (95% confidence interval 1.4 to 5.1; $p = 0.003$) for the less physically fit men, none of whom had evidence of cardiac disease at entry.

An interesting study by Lie and co-workers in Norway prospectively followed for 7 years groups of men with no known cardiac disease at entry.[54] One group of 149 middle-aged élite athletes (Nordic skiers) had an extremely low incidence of death (1%) after 7 years. The other group was composed

Table 15-5 Epidemiological studies of physical activity as it relates to mortality

Investigator	Date/type	Activity level	Subjects	Conclusions
Morris	1958/Retro	Determined by social class	White men	Physical inactivity relates to class and occupation mortality from coronary artery disease
Blackburn	1970/Prosp	Questionnaire	Middle-aged	No difference between men physically active and sedentary men
Paffenbarger	1970/Retro	Job description	Longshoremen	Low physical activity level on the job doubles risk of fatal myocardial infarction
Epstein	1976/Prosp	Questionnaire	Middle-aged	Rigorous weekend sedentary activity protective for white men
Costas	1978/Prosp	Questionnaire	Middle-aged	Slight increase in mortality in the most inactive group of Puerto Rican men
Paffenbarger	1978/Retro	Questionnaire	Male Harvard alumni	Low physical activity alumni (<2000 kcal/wk) increases risk of myocardial infarction and death
Kannel	1986/Prosp	Questionnaire	Middle-aged	Low physical activity of men/women increases risk of cardiac mortality
Leon	1987/Prosp	Questionnaire	Middle-aged	Low physical activity of men moderately increases risk of mortality
Slattery	1989/Prosp	Questionnaire	White men	Near 50% increase risk of death from coronary artery disease in sedentary men (<40 kcal/wk)

Prosp, Prospective; *Retro*, retrospective.

Table 15-6 Epidemiological studies of exercise capacity assessed by research testing as it relates to mortality

Investigator	Year/type	Mean follow-up time (years)	Assessment	Subjects	Conclusions
Peters	1983/Prosp	4.8	Bicycle ergometry	2779 healthy middle-aged men	Adjust RR of 2.2 for low exercise capacity if other risk factors also present
Lie	1985/Prosp	7.0	Bicycle ergometry	149 middle-aged elite athletes 2014 middle-aged healthy men	Higher quintiles of physical fitness associated with decreased coronary middle-risk factors and mortality
Ekelund	1988/Prosp	8.5	Bruce treadmill	4276 males	RR of 2.7 for cardiovascular death in men with low exercise capacity
Blair	1989/Prosp	8	Bruce treadmill	10,224 men 3120 women	Exercise capacity inversely related to all-cause mortality

Prosp, prospective; *RR*, relative risk.

of 2014 middle-aged healthy men who were further subdivided into physical fitness quartiles based on their performance on a bike ergometry test upon entry (cumulative work, in kilogram-meters/minute, divided by body mass times body weight). This quartile grouping was also consistent with the subject's level of leisure activity determined by questionnaire. The highest quartile in this group had a 7-year mortality similar to that of the Nordic skiers, and a highly significant difference was found in survival between each of the quartiles. Physical fitness and leisure time physical activity in this study was found to be significantly inversely related to mortality.

INTERVENTION IN HEALTHY INDIVIDUALS

As part of the multifactorial 6-year randomized trial of risk-factor intervention 60,881 men in 80 factories located in Belgium, Italy, Poland and the United Kingdom, 40 to 59 years of age, were randomized.[55] The treatment group received advice regarding diet, smoking, weight, blood pressure, and exercise. The intervention group had a 6.9% reduction in fatal coronary heart disease, 14.8% nonfatal myocardial infarction, and 10.2% total coronary heart disease. These benefits were related to risk-factor change and the change being sustained.

POSTMORTEM STUDIES RELATING PHYSICAL INACTIVITY TO CARDIAC EVENTS

Mitrani and colleagues[56] reported the results of consecutive specialized cardiovascular autopsies on 172 European-born Jews who were victims of traumatic death. Each coronary artery was cross-sectioned at 1 cm distances to measure internal and external diameters. The percentage of narrowing of the vessels was calculated using these measurements. There was no significant difference between the active and inactive groups. The results of numerous other autopsy studies have failed to demonstrate a relationship between physical activity and atherosclerosis.

RECOMMENDATIONS ON PHYSICAL ACTIVITY

In 1989, the American Heart Association published a statement on exercise that was a position statement on goals for physical fitness.[57] They recommended (1) a physically active life-style for persons of all ages, (2) large muscle dynamic exercise for 30 to 60 minutes using at least 50% of a person's own exercise capacity, 3 to 4 times weekly, (3) physicians should participate in education and preparation of previously sedentary individuals for exercise programs. They also concluded that "daily low intensity activities may have some long-term health benefits in terms of lower risk of cardiovascular disease." The American College of Sports Medicine presented a position paper in 1989 that stated similar goals and in addition recommended strength training of moderate intensity ("one set of 8-12 repetitions of eight to ten exercises that condition the major muscle groups at least two times a week").[58] These recent recommendations that even moderate levels of activity are beneficial to health differ from the more rigid, earlier editions of these guidelines.

There is now some indication that a day's exercise can be broken up into thirds. DeBusk and colleagues showed that in lieu of the usually accepted 30 minutes of aerobic activity, short bursts of exercise (three episodes of 10 minutes each) can also significantly improve VO_2 max.[59]

DANGERS OF EXERCISE
Sudden death

Sudden death has been defined relative to onset of symptoms, that is, instantaneous or within 1, 6, or 24 hours. Autopsy findings in people dying instantaneously and those dying after 24 hours are different. Deaths occurring within 6 hours of onset of symptoms include all electrical deaths and are best defined as "sudden," since no anatomic change usually can be demonstrated. Most sudden deaths that occur during exertion do so within minutes of onset of symptoms. Sudden cardiac death is herein defined as "death occurring unexpectedly within 6 hours of onset of symptoms in a previously healthy person." The most frequent mode of death is sudden. The incidence of sudden death in the general population is high (15% to 30%) with the majority (80% to 90%) attributable to cardiovascular causes.

Coronary atherosclerosis in joggers and marathon runners

Interest in the causes of death in joggers and marathon runners was stimulated when claims were made that "marathon running provides complete immunity from coronary artery disease."[60] Over 90 cases of death in joggers and marathon runners have been reported. The most common cause of death has been coronary atherosclerosis (75%). The other reported causes of death have been automobile accidents (39%), amyloidosis, and tunnel coronary artery (2% each) and from myocarditis, congenital hypoplastic coronary arteries, heat stroke, prolapsed mitral valve, hypertrophic cardiomyopathy, and gastrointestinal hemorrhage

(1% each). In 10% of cases the cause of death was unknown.

Siscovick and colleagues reported a study of individuals who were reported by the paramedical immediate response system in Seattle to have had a sudden death.[61] They were compared to a matched sample randomly chosen by a special telephone dialing device. To examine the risk of primary cardiac arrest during vigorous exercise, they interviewed the wives of 133 men without known prior heart disease. They were classified according to their time of cardiac arrest and the amount of their habitual vigorous activity. Among men with low levels of habitual activity, the relative risk of cardiac arrest during exercise compared with that at other times was 56. The risk during exercise among men at the highest level was also elevated but only five times, and their overall risk of cardiac arrest at any time was 40% that of sedentary men. Although the risk of primary cardiac arrest is transiently increased during vigorous exercise, regular exercise decreases the risk of this event.

Waller and Roberts have reported the autopsies of five conditioned runners 40 years of age and over, all with severe coronary atherosclerosis.[62] The series by Thompson and co-workers described 18 joggers, with five "exercising regularly" for at least 1 year and nine exercising for 3 or more years.[63] Fifteen of 18 died suddenly while jogging, and, of them, 13 had coronary heart disease. Waller and co-workers described 10 patients over .30 years of age who ran 1 to 55 miles per week for 1 to 12 years. All had at least one artery severely narrowed by an atherosclerotic plaque and 6 had myocardial infarctions. As a sequel to his study of jogging deaths in California, Thompson has focused on Rhode Island.[64] From 1975 through 1980, 12 men died during jogging, and the cause of death in 11 was coronary heart disease. From a telephone survey, he found that 7.4% of adult male Rhode Islanders jogged at least twice a week. The incidence of death from jogging was one death per year for every 7620 joggers and only one death per 396,000 man-hours of jogging. This rate is seven times the estimated death rate from coronary heart disease during more sedentary activities in Rhode Island. Thompson and co-workers calculated the incidence of death during jogging for men between 30 and 64 years to be one per 7620 joggers, or approximately one death per 396,000 man-hours of jogging. Although the death rate is seven times the estimated death rate from coronary heart disease during more sedentary activity, the numbers are too small to draw any conclusions, since only 12 deaths occurred in 6 years.

Vander and colleagues conducted a 5-year retrospective survey of fatal and nonfatal cardiovascular events that occurred in community recreation centers.[65] Fifty-eight facilities reported 30 nonfatal and 38 fatal events. There was one nonfatal and one fatal event every 1,124,200 and 887,526 hours of participation, respectively. Although exercise contributes to sudden death in susceptible persons, its rare occurrence demonstrates that the risk of exercise is small and indicates that routine screening may not be justified.

What is the expected level of cardiovascular deaths among runners while running on the basis of chance alone? This is an important question because it is frequently assumed that exercise is the cause when a person dies of cardiovascular stresses during recreational running. Koplan used data from the National Center of Health Statistics and found that approximately 100 cardiovascular deaths per year in runners in the United States can be predicted on a purely temporal basis.[66] This is certainly higher than the number of deaths reported.

Morales and colleagues have reported three healthy individuals who died suddenly during strenuous exercise and were found to have a triad of pathological findings.[67] There were two men 34 and 54 years of age and one woman 17 years of age. The pathological triad was muscle bridging of the left anterior descending coronary artery, poor circulation to the posterior surface of the heart, and septal fibrosis. The angiographic finding of a coronary artery that passes underneath a band of myocardium is not that unusual, and it has been debated whether it has functional significance. Some studies of coronary blood flow have suggested that the constriction of a coronary artery by this myocardial band during systole results in decreased flow; however, most of coronary flow takes place during diastole. In regard to the second finding, there is great variability in the coronary artery distribution on the posterior surface of the heart around the crux and the posterior margin of the septum. In the most common situation, the right coronary artery branches into a posterior descending artery, which passes down the septum giving off septal perforators. Often though, there are normal variations where the left circumflex provides this branch or there are only small arteries in the area. Lastly, septal fibrosis could be attributable to chronic ischemia. These anatomic findings could be purely coincidental.

Noakes and colleagues presented four marathon runners with autopsy-proved coronary atherosclerosis.[68] The first individual was a 44-year-old white man who, after 14 months of training, had completed seven marathons in under 4 hours. He suddenly dropped dead halfway through a marathon. At autopsy he was found to have an old anteroseptal myocardial infarction and 90% lesions of his left anterior descending and circumflex coronary arteries. The second was a 41-year-old man who, after 2 years of running, had a symptomatic myocardial infarction. After release from the hospital, he returned to training and ran in five marathons. He was hospitalized with unstable angina, and coronary angiography was performed. He was found to have severe three-vessel coronary artery disease; while waiting for surgery, he died suddenly. The last two cases were 27- and 36-year-old athletes who had completed multiple marathons and were killed accidentally. Both had left anterior descending coronary artery lesions at autopsy; the younger a 50% and the older a 90% lesion.

An interesting review of this topic was later published by Noakes in which the deaths of 36 marathon runners previously reported in the medical literature were described.[69] This group had a mean age of 43.8 years (range 18 to 70), and 75% had a cardiovascular cause of death. Seventy-one percent of these runners with coronary disease had forewarning symptoms that they tended to ignore and continued training. Of the 26 runners from whom data were available, 50% died within 24 hours of a competitive running event. Thus, unlike what was believed for many years, it is clear that high levels of aerobic performance does not exclude the presence of significant coronary disease, and symptoms in such patients should be taken seriously.

Virmani reported findings in 30 joggers or marathon runners who died nontraumatic deaths.[70] Twenty-two men died with severe atherosclerosis; their ages ranged from 18 to 54 years (mean 36 years). The history of jogging was well documented in 18 patients who ran 7 to 105 miles per week (mean 33) and had been running 1 to 28 years (mean 10). Three were marathon runners, and the other 12 had been jogging for at least 6 months. Review of records revealed a family history of heart disease in 9, systemic hypertension in 9, and a total cholesterol greater than 200 mg% in 7. None were diabetic, and smoking history was uncertain. A history of coronary heart disease was present in 8 (27%); of these, 5 were from a retrospective review of medical records. Nineteen died suddenly, and 3 had a history of prolonged chest pain. In 6 patients, death occurred soon after jogging, and 2 were found dead in bed. At autopsy, the heart weight ranged from 345 to 600 grams (mean 432). In 16 patients, the heart weight was increased beyond the normal range. Twenty-two patients died of severe coronary atherosclerosis. Of the four major arteries examined for severe atherosclerosis, only one artery was involved in 9 patients (41%), two coronary arteries in 9 (41%); three and four coronary arteries in 1 each. Thrombi were noted in 6 (27%) patients. The most frequent single artery involved was the left anterior descending, and the most frequent combination was the left anterior descending and right coronary arteries. Virmani and colleagues found that of a total of 70 coronary arteries examined in 20 joggers, 34 (49%) were severely narrowed, and the average number of coronary arteries greater than 75% narrowed was 1.65 per jogger. Those with a history of coronary heart disease had a similar extent of coronary atherosclerosis as those without such histories (1.7 versus 1.6 coronary arteries narrowed per patient). In 6 of the 22 with severe coronary atherosclerosis, isolated healed myocardial infarction was present; acute MI with or without healed MI was present in 8. A total of 14 (64%) of 22 who died of severe coronary atherosclerosis had MI.

Virmani and colleagues studied another 11 male joggers with a mean age of 41 years (range 19 to 59 years). Sudden death occurred in 9 of 11 men while jogging. Available risk-factor history was as follows: two had hypercholesterolemia, one had systemic hypertension, and one had family history of premature coronary heart disease. Only two had a history of prior cardiac disease: one had angina, and one had undergone left ventricular aneurysmectomy with coronary bypass surgery. A 43-year-old man had been jogging 50 miles per week for 5 to 6 years and had participated in several marathons. His heart weighed 600 grams, an acute MI was found, and there was a greater than 75% cross-sectional-area luminal narrowing of the three major coronary arteries by atherosclerotic plaque also with thrombus in the left circumflex. Seven of the 11 had at least two vessels severely narrowed, one had one-vessel disease, and the other two had been described as having severe coronary atherosclerosis. Acute or healed MIs were in 6 of the 11.

Causes of death during or soon after exercise other than jogging or marathon running

Opie and co-workers reported sudden death in 21 athletes, 13 of whom took part in rugby or soccer. Eighteen were believed to be caused by coronary heart disease.[71] The Squash Rackets Association has estimated that there may be 2.5 million people in the United Kingdom playing squash once or more a month. The circumstances surrounding 60 sudden deaths associated with squash playing were described by Northcote and colleagues in Glasgow.[72] The mean age of those who died was 46 years (range 22 to 66 years). They were able to collate a series of 89 sudden deaths associated with squash that occurred between October 1976 and February 1984 by examining press reports and by a prospective mail survey of sports centers and squash clubs throughout the United Kingdom.

A recent study published by Corrado from Italy also found that sudden death in athletes occurs most often during or immediately after vigorous activity.[73] Their postmortem studies of 22 young athletes (mean age 23 years) showed arrhythmic cardiac arrest to be the most common cause of death (17 cases) and right ventricular dysplasia and atherosclerotic coronary artery disease to be the most frequent underlying cardiovascular disease (6 and 4 cases, respectively). Of note, many of the athletes had experienced premonitory signs or had abnormal baseline ECGs.

Maron and co-workers reported sudden unexpected death in 29 highly conditioned, competitive athletes 13 to 30 years of age (mean 19) drawn from news media reports, the registry of the cardiovascular division of the Armed Forces Institute of Pathology, and the pathology branch of the NIH.[74] All had been active, highly conditioned members of an organized athletic team for at least 2 years. The type of sport varied, but basketball and football were most common. In 28 of the 29 athletes, death occurred suddenly without warning and was virtually instantaneous, occurring on the playing field in 13. One athlete survived 12 hours after collapse. In 22 athletes, death occurred during or soon after severe exertion, in 2 after mild exertion, and in 5 during sedentary activities. Structural cardiovascular abnormalities were found in 28 athletes and were the cause of sudden death in 22. Of these, the most common anatomic abnormality was hypertrophic cardiomyopathy (HC), which was present in 14. HC was defined as asymmetric septal hypertrophy, with pronounced ventricular septal disorganization in another 2. Four athletes had anomalous origin of the left coronary artery from the right sinus of Valsalva, including one patient with hypertrophic cardiomyopathy. Four athletes had concentric left ventricular hypertrophy, 2 with and 2 without disorganization. Four athletes had anomalous orgin of the left coronary artery from the right sinus of Valsalva. Three athletes (24 to 28 years of age) had severe coronary atherosclerosis. Two died of aortic rupture, both had evidence of cystic medial necrosis and one had Marfan syndrome.

In 6 athletes the cardiovascular abnormality was considered probable evidence of cardiovascular disease: 5 had hypertrophied hearts (420 to 530 g), one had mild prolapse of anterior and posterior mitral leaflets, and one had normal heart weight with a hypoplastic right coronary artery. Several died

of coronary atherosclerosis, one after running a pass pattern in a professional football game. In this individual they hypothesized that a blow to the chest while he was being tackled caused a hemorrhage into a plaque in the left anterior descending coronary artery. Several others had congenital anomalies of the coronary arteries. Virmani and colleagues reviewed records of 32 individuals who died suddenly while engaging in either military training (6) or in other sports activity: basketball (6), running (8), racketball (2), volleyball (2), tennis (2), swimming (2), football (2), and one each in gymnastics and bowling. Their ages ranged from 14 to 60 with a mean age of 28 years; 31 were men and one was a woman. The anatomic abnormalities were varied: coronary disease in 8, idiopathic myocarditis in 4, congenital coronary abnormalities in 3, hypertrophic cardiomyopathy in 2, tunnel coronary artery in 2, floppy mitral valve in 2, intramural coronary thickening in 2, and one each with rheumatic heart disease and aortic dissection. Four had left ventricular hypertrophy of unknown cause (420- to 600-gram hearts) and were 17, 20, 21, and 32 years old. All died during exertion. Three who had sickle cell trait died while running and were only 17, 20, and 22 years old.

The cause of death in Virmani's subjects is considerably different from those of Maron and colleagues probably because symptomatic individuals are excluded from military service and none was highly trained, whereas Maron's population included only highly trained athletes. Virmani's subjects had a wide age range with only 25 being 30 years of age or younger, whereas Maron's athletes were 13 to 30 years of age, with a mean of 19 years. Prevalence of coronary heart disease is directly related to age. This has been confirmed in other studies of runners older than 40: CHD is their most common cause of death, and they usually have had symptoms of CHD before the event. Moreover, all these events are extremely unusual, and it would be difficult to screen for them. It is known that athletes frequently have abnormal ECGs and even echocardiographic hypertrophy. In addition, they have a higher prevalence of false-positive exercise test results. However, screening for lipid abnormalities would be a wise public health measure regardless of a lack of specificity, and it would be advisable to get an echocardiogram from an athlete with symptoms or signs of a hypertrophic cardiomyopathy.

EFFECT OF ENVIRONMENT

An important factor in sudden death among athletes and joggers is the climate in which exercise is being performed. Serious thermal injuries are preventable, and the American College of Sports Medicine recommends that long-distance races should not be conducted in termperatures that exceed 28° C (82.4° F). The amount of heat generated is directly related to the intensity of exercise. The body is only 25% efficient in converting calories generated into external work, and the remaining 75% of energy is converted into heat. Therefore a large amount of heat must be lost by the body to prevent raising the core temperature.

If no heat were being lost by the body, the core temperature would increase by 1 Celsius degree every 5 minutes. It is the efficient mechanisms of thermoregulation of the body that prevent hypothermia. These mechanisms include sweating and heat loss by radiation and by conversion. The factors that prevent heat loss are high ambient temperature, high humidity, dehydration (which prevents cutaneous vasodilatation), extremes of age, debilitation, excessive clothing, and drugs that may impair thermoregulation. The range of heat injury includes three well-recognized syndromes: (1) heat cramps, (2) heat exhaustion, and (3) heat stroke. Heat cramps are painful spasms in the muscles, whereas heat exhaustion is characterized by fatigue, hyperventilation, headache, light-headedness, nausea, and muscle cramps. Patients with heat exhaustion sweat and have chills despite the core temperature's being high. Heat stroke, the most serious of thermal injuries, is characterized by an altered state of consciousness, which may progress rapidly to unconsciousness and seizure activity. The heat stroke patient is hot and flushed and has dry skin because sweating has stopped. Dehydration and circulatory collapse soon follow. Body temperature is usually above 41° C (106° F), and the laboratory tests show hemoconcentration, leukocytosis, azotemia, acidosis, abnormal liver function tests, and abnormal muscle enzymes. Treatment includes submersion in ice water and intravenous administration of heparin to stop fibrinolysis. At autopsy, the findings usually are nonspecific and appear as petechial hemorrhages in the skin, mucous membranes, brain, lung, and heart. The hemorrhages in the heart are most pronounced in the epicardial and endocardial region, especially on the left side of the ventricular septum. Damage to myocardial filaments and intercalated discs have been described by electron microscopy in patients with malignant hyperthermia induced by anesthetic agents.

SUMMARY OF EXERCISE-RELATED DEATH IN ATHLETES

Cardiovascular diseases responsible for sudden unexpected death in highly conditioned athletes are largely related to the age of the patient. In most young competitive athletes (less than 35 years of age) sudden death is attributable to congenital cardiovascular disease. Hypertrophic cardiomyopathy appears to be the most common cause of such deaths, accounting for about half of the sudden deaths in young athletes. Other cardiovascular abnormalities that appear to be less frequent in young athletes include congenital coronary artery anomalies, ruptured aorta (caused by cystic medial necrosis), idiopathic left ventricular hypertrophy, and coronary atherosclerosis. Very uncommon causes of sudden death include myocarditis, mitral valve prolapse, aortic valve stenosis, and sarcoidosis. Cardiovascular disease in young athletes is usually unsuspected during life, and most athletes who die suddenly have experienced no cardiac symptoms. In only about 25% of those competitive athletes who die suddenly is underlying cardiovascular disease detected or suspected before participation, and rarely is the correct clinical diagnosis made. In contrast, in older athletes (≥35 years of age) sudden death is usually attributable to coronary artery disease. Currently available are noninvasive screening procedures that can detect many subjects at risk of sudden death but with an uncertain specificity. However, although some potentially lethal diseases can be excluded by a relatively simple screening program, other diseases require expensive procedures, such as echocardiography, exercise testing, and cardiac catheterization. This means that the sensitivity of detecting diseases leading to sudden death increases in proportion to the financial resources that can be applied to the screening program. Thus, when a screening program designed to identify all cardiac diseases that have the potential to cause sudden death is planned by a community, school, or non-professional athletic team, the costs will be prohibitive. The practicality of applying a community or school screening program can be questioned because of the very low incidence of sudden unexpected death in young healthy individuals. Comprehensive screening programs are confined to individuals or organizations with adequate financial resources. Less expensive, limited screening can be undertaken by individuals or groups to identify some subjects at risk of sudden death during athletic competition. An important consideration is the education of the team physician. Symptoms and family history of sudden death or syncope should not be overlooked. However, because of high vagal tone, young athletes often faint. In addition, ECG abnormalities, S_3 waves, and systolic murmurs are common.

The normal heart, even when subjected to vigorous forms of stress, is protected from lethal arrhythmias except in unusual conditions such as profound electrolyte derangement, thermal stress, or adverse drug reactions. Victims of sudden death almost always have underlying heart disease. Coronary artery disease is found in about 80% of victims of sudden cardiac death, whereas other abnormalities, such as cardiomyopathy, valvular heart disease, or primary arrhythmic disorders, may also cause unexpected cardiac arrest. Although exertion-related death appears to be confined to patients with structural heart disease, a third of these individuals may be asymptomatic. Mechanisms underlying sudden death in cardiac patients include ventricular fibrillation and myocardial ischemia. Ventricular fibrillation is the arrhythmia usually underlying the sudden cardiac death syndrome particularly in exertion-related events. In following patients resuscitated from out-of-hospital ventricular fibrillation, Cobb recognized three major clinical settings in which ventricular fibrillation occurs: (1) as a complication of typical acute myocardial infarction; (2) as a manifestation of transient myocardial ischemia, especially during or after exertion; and (3) as an event unassociated with ischemia and occurring while sedentary. In the last setting, ventricular fibrillation most often occurs in patients with prior myocardial infarction and left ventricular dysfunction.

Transient ischemia is a plausible cause for most episodes of exertion-related cardiac arrest in patients with coronary disease. In assessing resuscitated patients who collapsed during or after exertion, Cobb found that compared with persons with non–exertion related cardiac arrest these patients had less limitations and more often had no recognized preceding heart disease.[75] In addition, warning symptoms were noted in only about 25%, and less than one third had new Q-waves. These patients have few episodes of ventricular arrhythmia during ambulatory monitoring. Although there has been no large, prospective assessment of the role of exertion in precipitating cardiac arrest, some relevant information is available. In patients treated by the paramedic system in Seattle, 36 (11%) of 316 consecutive victims had collapsed during or immediately after exertion or stress. This incidence is similar to that of 17% of 150 patients reported in Miami. In autopsy registries, the incidence of exertion-related cardiac arrest was reported to be 10% to 30% of all sudden deaths. In studies of unexpected sudden death in younger persons, cardiac arrest commonly was associated with physical activity.

In a prospective 5-year survey by Hinkle involving approximately 270,000 men, 42% of the sudden coronary deaths occurred in persons without previously recognized coronary disease.[76] About one third of these deaths occurred within minutes of engaging in activities known to be associated with myocardial ischemia or in the setting of suspected sympathetic nervous system stimulation. In a report from the Cooper Clinic, in a predominantly normal population of middle-aged persons, one cardiac arrest occurred per 375,000 person-hours of exercise. In the Framingham Study, there was a significant association between the mode of death and activity; sudden death occurred more often in the setting of physical activity. Cobb and co-workers reported that in 133 men who experienced cardiac arrest in Seattle, the incidence of cardiac arrest was 5 to 56 times greater during high-intensity exercise than at other times. The persons considered in that study were 25 to 75 years of age and were without previously recognized cardiovascular disease. The estimated incidence of cardiac arrest during vigorous activity ranged from one case per 137,000 hours to one per 4.7 million hours at risk.

These studies serve to point out that physical exertion may precipitate cardiac arrest in the "normal" population and that prior recognition of susceptible individuals has not been possible. Exercise-induced cardiac arrest is a rare but real phenomenon, particularly in patients with known heart disease. However, the majority of sudden deaths are temporally associated with routine activities of daily life and not with exercise. Therefore the number of deaths attributable to strenuous physical exertion is relatively modest. Exertion-related cardiac arrest usually is attributable to ventricular fibrillation or tachycardia, and exercise may increase its risk by 100 times.

COMPLICATIONS OTHER THAN DEATH

There are numerous risks for amateur and professional athletes. Heat stroke can be avoided if one takes precautions for humid, hot environments including adequate oral replacement of dilute electrolyte solutions. There is no place for fluid restriction in order to limit sweating. Runners can have heat stroke and still be actively sweating, though once it was taught that heat stroke was always preceded by a cessation of sweating. Hematuria after a run can be attributable to bladder trauma, and proteinuria can even be normal. Diarrhea and other gastrointestinal complaints are fairly common in runners during and after events. Numerous episodes of anaphylaxis believed to be exercise-induced have been reported. Diagnosis by the findings of bronchospasm and urticaria is important because treatment with epinephrine and antihistamines can be lifesaving. This usually occurs in individuals who previously had an anaphylactic reaction to shellfish.

Orthopedic injuries

The popular concern with fitness is responsible for both general practitioners and sports-medicine specialists noticing an increase in sports-related injuries among weekend and after-work athletes. Basketball and soccer leagues, ski vacations, evening runs, dance classes, and tennis cause injuries once found chiefly among professional and college athletes.

The Center for Sports Medicine in San Francisco recently compiled statistics on over 10,000 injuries treated at the center. They found that nine activities—basketball, dance, football, gymnastics, running, skiing, tennis, soccer, and figure skating—accounted for nearly three fourths of the injuries. More than two thirds of the injuries were caused by overuse—problems such as shin splints and tendinitis that develop from a repetitive trauma to muscle and bone. Tennis, aerobic dance, and running frequently cause such problems. The remaining injuries were acute ones, incidents that happen instantly, such as a sprained ankle. These tend to occur in skiing, football, basketball, and soccer. Injuries to the knee cause the most visits, and skiers have the most knee problems. Aerobic dance causes more fractures than any other recreational activity. Many problems stem from acute injuries that occurred in the past. Unlike football injuries, most of the basketball injuries occur in participants over 25 years of age.

Is the recommended physical activity safe? De Loes and Goldie reported the incidence of injury from physical exercise as recorded by physician visits over the course of an entire year in a town with 31,620 inhabitants in Sweden.[77] They found that injuries from sports or physical exercise comprised 17% of all clinic visits for accidents. The types of physical activity were divided into two: (1) jogging or marathon running and (2) other athletic activities, that is, military training, all types of ball games, swimming, running, wrestling, mountain climbing, yachting. This compared to 26% home related and 19% work related. It should be noted that whereas the Swedes play a great deal of ice hockey (the sport they found causing the greatest incidence of injury), they do not play football.

Education regarding how recreational injuries happen and how to treat them is an important step in prevention. Treatment may include weight lifting for rehabilitation, shoe inserts to correct irregularities in stride or foot strike, ultrasound and electrical stimulation for muscle tears and stiffness, and compression and icing to control swelling. Rest, ice, compression, and elevation is still the best treatment for all acute injuries. There has been a trend toward active rehabilitation. For example, to treat a sprained ankle a program that focuses on muscle strengthening is used because if ligaments do not heal well, a tear may become a persistent problem. Prolonged rest can cause a decrease in muscle mass around the ankle, resulting in a loss of strength. The muscles lose their ability to move quickly and stabilize the ankle. Instead, strengthening surrounding muscles will avoid atrophy. In many cases, the strengthened muscles will compensate for the deficient ligaments, making the joint stable for further activities.

Knochel reported that "white collar rhabdomyolysis" (weekend competitive running in middle-aged moderately conditioned people leading to rhabdomyolysis) is much more common than currently believed.[78] One can avoid it by ensuring gradual conditioning and reasonable competition.

CONCLUSION

Animal studies have provided substantial evidence of the cardiovascular benefits of regular physical activity. Improved coronary circulation has been demonstrated in exercise-trained animals through increases in coronary artery size, capillary density, and collateral development in response to hypoxia. Studies utilizing various animal models have reported improvements in cardiac function secondary to exercise training. Improved intrinsic contractility, faster relaxation, enzymatic alterations, calcium availability, and enhanced autonomic and hormonal control of function have been suggested as reasons for these findings.

These animal studies demonstrate that there are morphological and metabolic changes that make the cardiovascular system better able to withstand stress, possibly even that imposed by atherosclerosis. The study by Kramsch and colleagues provides the strongest evidence yet for the favorable influence of exercise and diet on the primary prevention of coronary disease. However, although exercise lessened ischemic manifestations, only diet stopped the progression of coronary atherosclerosis. Although myocardial ischemia seems to be a necessary stimulus for the development of collateral vessels, exercise appears to enhance their development. Exercise does not affect the atherosclerotic process but instead enlarges coronary arteries to provide protection by increased flow. Precisely how these observations made among animals relate to the human heart is unknown, particularly since many of the changes are age related.

Echocardiographic studies have shown endurance training in young subjects to result in increased ventricular mass, wall thickness, volume, and function, but not all results have been conclusive, probably because of problems with measurement reproducibility. However, these increases in left ventricular mass may not occur in younger subjects unless higher levels of exercise are used and may never occur in older subjects. In cardiac patients, an exercise program may not lessen exercise-induced ischemia (as assessed by ST segment depression). In addition, patients with exercise-induced ST-segment depression who exceed their usually prescribed exercise limits are known to be at higher risk of cardiac events during and immediately after bouts of exercise.

The association between physical inactivity and the underlying atherosclerotic process is modest compared with other factors such as serum cholesterol, cigarette smoking, and hypertension. An inversely proportional association between the level of activity and degree of atherosclerosis has not been demonstrated. Although physical inactivity does not necessarily precede the atherosclerotic process, its relationship to cardiac events is certainly strong. The level of exercise necessary to lessen the risk of cardiovascular death differs from that required to obtain the hemodynamic and morphological benefits of more rigorous training. The latter requires careful attention to training intensity, duration, frequency, and mode. The prescription for good health however, can be less demanding. Vigorous walking for a half hour, four to five times per week, is probably sufficient to obtain health benefits.

Interestingly, activity surveys have demonstrated that more than 50% of the U.S. population exercises less than 20 minutes three times a week. This makes inactivity a very prevalent risk factor and increases the population with attributable risk of inactivity in modern society far above that of other risk factors. Recent studies of primary prevention support a life-style of regular physical activity to decrease one's risk for coronary heart disease. Such physical activity helps to decrease other risk factors as well.[79] Regular moderate exercise can improve one's quality of life by lessening fatigue and by increasing physical performance.

Although athletic deaths gather much interest, they are extremely rare—all the available screening techniques cause more harm than good because of their high false positive rates. Knowledge of the causes of such deaths, however, can help us focus our attention appropriately. Unfortunately, even an exercise test is not effective for predicting exercise-related deaths in asymptomatic populations. The public health prescription of physical activity rather than the higher levels of exercise needed for physical fitness carries hardly any risk.

Thus, both animal and human studies have shown beneficial effects on the heart from chronic exercise. Large epidemiological studies have shown significant benefits from improvements in physical fitness and activity, especially with regard to decreasing cardiac mortality. Specific recommendations have been put forth by various medical societies on the precise extent and duration of exercise needed to improve both quantity and quality of life. All that lies before us now is to convince 50% of the American public to step out of the ranks of the sedentary. They need not become Olympic athletes, but they must engage in at least moderate activity.

REFERENCES

1. Mary DA: Exercise training and its effects on the heart, *Rev Physiol Biochem Pharmacol* 109:61-144, 1987.
2. Froelicher VF: Exercise, fitness, and coronary heart disease. In *Exercise, fitness and health: a consensus of current knowledge,* Champaign, Ill, 1990, Human Kinetics, pp 429-450.
3. Poupa O, Rakusan K, Ostadal B: The effect of physical activity upon the heart of vertebrates: physical activity and aging, *Medicine and Sport* 4:202, 1970.
4. Thomanek RJ, Rounton CA, Liskop KS: Relationship between age, chronic exercise, and connective tissue of the heart, *J Gerontol* 27:33, 1972.
5. Ljungqvist A, Unge G: Capillary proliferation activity in myocardium and skeletal muscle of exercised rats, *J Appl Physiol* 43:306, 1978.
6. Tepperman J, Pearlman D: Effects of exercise and anemia on coronary arteries of small animals as revealed by the corrosion-cast technique, *Circ Res* 9:576, 1961.
7. Eckstein RW: Effect of exercise and coronary artery narrowing on coronary collateral circulation, *Circ Res* 5:230, 1957.
8. Spear KL, Koerner JE, Terjung RL: Coronary blood flow in physically trained rats, *Cardiovasc Res* 12:135-143, 1978.
9. Bloor CM, White FC, Sanders TM: Effects of exercise on collateral development in myocardial ischemia in pigs, *J Appl Physiol* 56:656-665, 1984.
10. Heaton WH, Marr KC, Capurro NL, et al: Beneficial effects of physical training on blood flow to myocardium perfused by chronic collaterals in the exercising dog, *Circulation* 57:575, 1978.
11. Cohen MV, Yipinstoi T, Scheuer J: Coronary collateral stimulation by exercise in dogs with stenotic coronary arteries, *J Appl Physiol* 52:664-668, 1982.
12. Billman GE, Schwartz PJ, Stone HL: The effects of daily exercise on susceptibility to sudden cardiac death, *Circulation* 69(6):1182-1189, 1984.
13. Holloszy JO: Minireview: exercise and longevity: studies on rats, *J Gerontol* 43(6):149-151, 1988.
14. Kramsch DM, Aspen AJ, Abramowitz BM, et al: Reduction of coronary atherosclerosis by moderate conditioning exercise in monkeys on an atherogenic diet, *N Engl J Med* 305:1483-1489, 1981.
15. American Association of Cardiovascular and Pulmonary Rehabilitation: *Guidelines for cardiac rehabilitation programs,* Champaign, Ill, 1991, Human Kinetics, p 11.
16. Ehsani AA, Hagberg JM, Hickson RC: Rapid changes in left ventricular dimensions and mass in response to physical conditioning and deconditioning, *Am J Cardiol* 42:52, 1978.
17. DeMaria AN, Neumann A, Lee G, et al: Alterations in

ventricular mass and performance induced by exercise training in man evaluated by echocardiography, *Circulation* 57:237-244, 1978.

18. Stein RA, Michielli D, Fox EL, et al: Continuous ventricular dimensions in man during supine exercise and recovery, *Am J Cardiol* 41:655, 1978.

19. Parrault H, Peronnet F, Cleroux J, et al: Electro- and echocardiographic assessment of left ventricle before and after training man, *Can J Appl Sports Sci* 3:180, 1978.

20. Wolfe LA, Martin RP, Watson DD, et al: Chronic exercise and left ventricular structure and function in healthy human subjects, *J Appl Physiol* 58:409-415, 1985.

21. Adams TD, Yanowitz FG, Fischer AG, et al: Noninvasive evaluation of exercise training in college-age men, *Circulation* 64:958, 1981.

22. Landry F, Bouchard C, Dumesnil J: Cardiac dimension changes with endurance training, *JAMA* 254:77-80, 1985.

23. Marti B, Suter E, Riesen W, et al: Effects of long-term, self-monitored exercise on the serum lipoprotein and apolipoprotein profile in middle-aged men, *Atherosclerosis* 81:19-31, 1990.

24. Dannenberg AL, Keller JB, Wilson PW, Castelli WP: Leisure time physical activity in the Framingham offspring study, *Am J Epidemiol* 129(1):76-88, 1989.

25. Blumenthal JA, Siegel WC, Appelbaum M: Failure to exercise to reduce blood pressure in patients with mild hypertension: results of a randomized controlled trial, *JAMA* 266:15:2098-2104, 1991.

26. Ehsani AA, Heath GW, Hagberg JM, et al: Effects of 12 months of intense exercise training on ischemic ST-segment depression in patients with coronary artery disease, *Circulation* 64:1116-1124, 1981.

27. Ditchey RV, Watkins J, McKirnan MD, et al: Effects of exercise training on left ventricular mass in patients with ischemic heart disease, *Am Heart J* 101:701-706, 1981.

28. Froelicher VF: The effect of exercise on myocardial perfusion and function in patients with coronary heart disease, *Eur Heart J* 8:1-8, 1987.

29. Leon AS, Jacobs DR, DeBacker G, et al: Relationship of physical characteristics of life habits to treadmill exercise capacity, *Am J Epidemiol* 653-660, 1981.

30. Morris JN, Crawford MD: Coronary heart disease and physical activity, *Br Med J* 2:1485, 1958.

31. Morris JN: Uses of epidemiology, London, 1975, Churchill Livingstone.

32. Oliver RM: Physique and serum lipids of young London busmen in relation to ischemic heart disease, *Br J Intern Med* 24:181, 1967.

33. Stamler J, Kjelsberg M, Hall Y: Epidemiologic studies on cardiovascular-renal diseases: analysis of mortality by age-race-sex-occuaption, *J Chronic Dis* 12:440, 1960.

34. Blackburn H, Taylor HL, Keys A: Coronary heart disease in seven countries, *Circulation* 41:154, 1970.

35. Epstein L, Miller GJ, Stitt FW, et al: Vigorous exercise in leisure time, coronary risk factors, and resting electrocardiogram in middle-aged male civil servants, *Br Heart J* 38:403, 1976.

36. Costas R, García-Palmieri MR, Nazario E, et al: Relation of lipids, weight and physical activity to incidence of coronary heart disease, *Am J Cardiol* 42:653, 1978.

37. Paffenbarger RS, Laughlin ME, Gima AS, et al: Work activity of longshoremen as related to death from coronary heart disease and stroke, *N Engl J Med* 282:1109, 1970.

38. Paffenbarger RS, Wing AL, Hyde RT: Physical activity as an index of heart attack risk in college alumni, *Am J Epidemiol* 108:161-167, 1978.

39. Paffenbarger RS, Wing AL, Hyde RT: Chronic disease in former college students: physical activity as an index of heart attack risk in college alumni, *Am J Epidemiol* 108:161-175, 1981.

40. Kannel WB, Belanger A, D'Agostino R, et al: Physical activity and physical demand on the job and risk of CV disease and death: the Framingham Study, *Am Heart J* 112:820-825, 1986.

41. Leon AS, Connett J, Jacobs DR, Rauramaa R: Leisure-time physical activity levels and risk of coronary heart disease and death, *JAMA* 258(17):2388-2395, 1987.

42. Slattery ML, Jacobs DR, Nichamann MZ: Leisure time physical activity and coronary heart disease death: the US Railroad Study, *Circulation* 79:304-311, 1989.

43. Shaper AG, Wannamethee G: Physical activity and ischaemic heart disease in middle-aged British men, *Br Heart J* 66:384-394, 1991.

44. Powell VK, et al: Protective effect of physical activity on coronary heart disease, *MMWR* 36(26):426-429, 1987.

45. Blackburn H, Jacobs DR: Physical activity and the risk of coronary heart disease, *N Engl J Med* 319:1217-1219, 1988.

46. Taylor HL, Buskirt E, Henschel A: Maximal oxygen intake as an objective measurement of cardiorespiratory performance, *J Appl Physiol* 8:73-80, 1955.

47. Bruce RA, Kusumi F, Hosmer D: Maximal oxygen intake and nomographic assessment of functional aerobic impairment in cardiovascular disease, *Am Heart J* 85:546-551, 1973.

48. Froelicher VF, Thompson AJ, Noguera I: Prediction of maximal oxygen consumption, *Chest* 68(3):331-336, 1975.

49. Peters RK, Cady LD, Bischoff DP, et al: Physical fitness and subsequent myocardial infarction in healthy workers, *JAMA* 249:3052-3056, 1983.

50. Blair SN, Cooper KH, Gibbons LW, et al: Changes in coronary heart disease risk factors associated with increased treadmill time in 753 men, *Am J Epidemiol* 118:352-359, 1983.

51. Brill PB, Burkhalter HE, Kohl HW, et al: The impact of previous athleticism on exercise habits, physical fitness, and coronary heart disease risk factors in middle-aged men, *Research Q Exerc Sport* 60(3):202-215, 1989.

52. Blair SN, Kohl HW, Paffenbarger RS, et al: Physical fitness and all-cause mortality, *JAMA* 262:2395-2401, 1989.

53. Ekelund LG, Haskell WL, Johnson JL, et al: Physical fitness as a predictor of cardiovascular mortality in asymptomatic North American men, *N Eng J Med* 319:1379-1389, 1988.

54. Lie H, Mundal R, Erikssen J: Coronary risk factors and incidence of coronary death in relation to physical fitness: seven year follow-up study of middle-aged and elderly men, *Eur Heart J* 6:147-157, 1985.

55. Kovat R: Prevention of CHD (WHO Multicenter Project), *Lancet* 1:216-224, 1986.

56. Mitrani Y, Karplus H, Brunner D: Coronary atherosclerosis in case of traumatic death, *Med Sports* 4:241, 1970.

57. McHenry PL, Ellestad MH, Fletcher GF, et al: Statement on exercise, *Circulation* 81(1):396-398, 1990.

58. American College of Sports Medicine: Position stand: the recommended quantity and quality of exercise for developing and maintaining cardiorespiratory and muscular fitness in healthy adults, *J Cardiopulmonary Rehabil* 10:235-245, 1990.

59. DeBusk RF, Stenestrand U, Sheehan M, et al: Training effects of long versus short bouts of exercise in healthy subjects, *Am J Cardiol* 65:1010-1013, 1990.

60. McManus BM, Waller BF, Graboys TB, Froelicher VF, et al: Exercise and sudden death, Parts I and II, Chicago, 1983, Year Book Medical Publishers (St. Louis, Mosby).

61. Siscovick DS, Weiss NS, Fletcher RH, Lasky T: The incidence of primary cardiac arrest during vigorous exercise, *N Engl J Med* 311:874-877, 1984.

62. Waller BF, Roberts WC: Sudden death while running in

conditioned runners aged 40 years or over, *Am J Cardiol* 45:1291, 1980.

63. Thompson PD, Stern MP, William P, et al: Death during jogging or running (in California), *JAMA* 242:1265, 1979.

64. Thompson PD, Funk EJ, Carleton RA, Sturner WQ: Incidence of death during jogging in Rhode Island from 1975 through 1980, *JAMA* 247:2535-2538, 1982.

65. Vander L, Franklin B, Rubenfire M: Cardiovascular complications of recreational physical activity, *Physician Sports Med* 10:89-98, 1982.

66. Koplan JP: Cardiovascular deaths while running, *JAMA* 242:2578-2579, 1979.

67. Morales AR, Romanelli R, Boucek RJ: The mural left anterior descending coronary artery, strenuous exercise and sudden death, *Circulation* 62:230-237, 1980.

68. Noakes TD, Opie LH, Rose AG, et al: Autopsy-proved coronary atherosclerosis in marathon runners, *N Engl J Med* 301:86-89, 1979.

69. Noakes TD: Heart disease in marathon runners: a review, *Med Sci Sports Exerc* 19(3):187-194, 1987.

70. Virmani R, McAllister HA: Coronary heart disease at young age: a report of 187 autopsy patients who died of severe coronary atherosclerosis, *Cardiovasc Rev Rep* 5:799-809, 1984.

71. Opie LH: Sudden death and sport, *Lancet* 1:263-266, 1975.

72. Northcote RJ, Evans ADB, Ballantyne D: Sudden death in squash players, *Lancet* 1:148-151, 1984.

73. Corrado D, Thiene G, Nava A, et al: Sudden death in young competitive athletes: clinicopathologic correlations in 22 cases, *Am J Med* 89:588-595, 1990.

74. Maron BJ, Epstein SE, Roberts WC: Causes of sudden death in competitive athletes, *J Am Coll Cardiol* 7:204-214, 1986.

75. Cobb LA, Weaver D: Exercise: a risk for sudden death in patients with coronary heart disease, *J Am Coll Cardiol* 7:215-219, 1986.

76. Hinkle LE, Whitney LA, Lehman EW, et al: Occupation, education, and coronary heart disease, *Science* 161:238, 1968.

77. De Loes M, Goldie I: Incidence rate of injuries during sport activity and physical exercise in a rural Swedish municipality: incidence rates in 17 sports, *Int J Sports Med* 9:461-467, 1988.

78. Knochel JP: Catastrophic medical events with exhaustive exercise: "white collar rhabdomyolysis," *Kidney Int* 38:709-719, 1990.

79. Leon AS: Physiological interaction between diet and exercise in the etiology and prevention of ischaemic heart disease, *Ann Clin Res* 20:114-120, 1988.

16 | Cardiac Rehabilitation

Before the 1970s, the patient who suffered a myocardial infarction (MI) was almost completely immobilized for 6 weeks or more and was even washed, shaved, and fed in order to keep the work that the heart had to do to a minimum. It was believed that this approach provided the heart with the opportunity to form a firm scar. Also, the patient was told not to expect to be able to return to a normal life. These were incorrect beliefs particularly in the situation of an uncomplicated MI. Prolonged immobilization not only did not speed healing but exposed the patient to the additional risks of venous thrombosis, pulmonary embolism, muscle atrophy, lung infections, and deconditioning. Equally serious was the psychological result of such an approach, often leading to psychological impairment. We now know that most patients can return to a normal life and most even have a normal life expectancy.

It is interesting to consider that following today's standard of care for the patient with acute MI 20 years ago would have been malpractice and vice versa (Table 16-1). Today, the physician's approach to the acute MI has completely changed.[1] A relatively brief period of time monitored by the high technology in the coronary care unit is followed by early mobilization, sitting at the bedside, carefully graduated exercise, and, in the uncomplicated patient, discharge from the hospital within a week.

Although the current policy has been shown by randomized trials to be safe from the point of view of cardiac complications, it has nevertheless generated problems for the physician, other health care personnel, and the entire health care system. It also puts a drain on already limited resources, since modern health care must include mechanisms for the prescribing of safe exercise and for education and psychological rehabilitation. The shortened length of stays dictated by the DRG (diagno-

sis-related groups) approach leaves very little time for patient education and other rehabilitative services. Certainly all patients do not need all rehabilitative interventions, but exercise programs, educational sessions, group therapy, and psychological and vocational counseling should be available to those who need them.

Hospital admission for an acute MI is a stressful experience with a powerful influence. But it must be remembered that hospital discharge, though less dramatic, can be equally stressful after one relies on the highly protective hospital support systems. Discharge into an uncertain future and to a home and work setting in which one is considered a helpless invalid can be as damaging to one's self-esteem as the acute event itself. The physician is faced with the difficult task, not only of supervising the physical recovery of the patient, but also of maintaining morale, providing education, helping the family cope and provide support, and facilitating the return to a gratifying life-style. Cardiac rehabilitation can be considered the conservation of human life. Its goal is to restore the patient to optimal physiological, psychological, and vocational status. As a preface to discussing cardiac rehabilitation, it may be worthwhile initially to review how the clinical approach to acute myocardial infarction has evolved over the years, particularly since we are now in an entirely new era of thrombolytic therapy.

PATHOPHYSIOLOGY OF AN ACUTE MYOCARDIAL INFARCTION

The pathophysiology of acute myocardial infarction has become better understood. In the 1970s we were taught not to call an MI a "coronary thrombosis" as it was called previously. The reason was that a thrombosis was not found in the acute phase of a recent MI, but only in older in-

347

Table 16-1 Review of previous recommendations for bed rest in acute myocardial infarction

Lewis T (*Diseases of the heart*, New York, 1937, Macmillan Co.)	8 weeks of bed rest
White PD (*Heart disease*, ed 3, New York, 1945, Macmillan Co.)	4 weeks of bed rest
Wood P (*Diseases of the heart and circulation*, ed 2, London, 1960, Eyre & Spottiswoode)	3 to 6 weeks in bed
Friedberg CK (*Diseases of the heart*, ed 3, Philadelphia, 1966, WB Saunders Co.)	2 to 3 weeks minimum of bed rest
Wood P (*Diseases of the heart and circulation*, ed 3, London, 1968, Eyre & Spottiswoode)	2 weeks in bed

farctions. It was believed that the thrombosis was caused by the MI and did not precipitate it. However, studies utilizing coronary angiography at the time of infarction have shown that a thrombosis is usually seen in the acute stage. This feature has led to the current therapeutic approach to lyse clots with streptokinase, urokinase, or thrombolysin plasminogen activator (TPA) or remove them with catheters. Multiple trials have convincingly demonstrated that mortality can be lowered with this approach, particularily when aspirin and heparin are added to stop the thrombus from reforming. It appears that thrombolysis is most effective if the drugs are given within 4 hours of onset of pain for large anterior Q-wave infarcts or for MIs that are extending. But even when the thrombosis is lyzed, the patient can proceed to infarct. The substrate (that is, "dirty" plaque or critically narrowed artery) remains, and another thrombosis quickly forms unless followed by aspirin and coumadin. This chemical débridement must be followed by percutaneous transluminal coronary angioplasty (PTCA) or coronary artery bypass surgery (CABS) only in a small number of patients. Several randomized trials have demonstrated the dangers of proceeding directly to PTCA to abort an evolving infarction. Randomized trials using thrombolysis have demonstrated decreased mortality and less myocardial damage when the thrombolytic agents are given early. The time required for myocardial cell death appears to be 3 hours of ischemia, but this has considerable variability, and treatment as much as 12 hours late may still be beneficial.

Currently, there is no good indicator of irreversible cell death—even the electrocardiogram can be very misleading. However, once this time has passed, intervention to restore blood flow may still be beneficial. A patent vessel may still be advantagous in an infarcted area possibly because of surrounding and residual tissue.

Infarct severity

Myocardial infarctions are divided basically into those that evolve Q-waves and result in transmural myocardial cell death and those that do not evolve Q-waves and result only in subendocardial cell death.[7] Even though Q-wave infarcts are not always transmural and non–Q wave infarcts can be transmural, the ECG pattern allows one to predict the clinical course and outcome surprisingly well. Subendocardial MI cannot be localized, whereas transmural MI can be roughly localized by the Q-wave pattern. Attempts have been made to judge MI severity or size electrocardiographically by Q-wave and R-wave scores and even by utilizing body surface mapping, but these methods provide only rough estimates. In general, the greater the number of areas with Q-waves and the greater the R-wave loss, the larger is the MI. Non–Q wave MIs are usually less associated with complications such as congestive heart failure or shock, but they can be complicated particularly when a prior MI has taken place. Their prognosis is particularly good if it's not associated with prior MIs and a decreased ejection fraction. Because more myocardium has survived, patients with non–Q wave MIs are more likely to suffer ischemic events. Their risk can be estimated by rest or exercise ST-segment depression.

Enzymatic marker of infarct size

MI size can be judged by the creatine phosphokinase (CPK) levels particularly by the amount of the MB band released. This enzyme has improved the laboratory diagnosis of myocardial infarction, since it is highly specific for myocardium. Although careful sampling of CPK over time has enabled construction of a CPK-MB curve and the integrated area of the curve correlates with MI size, this has not been very helpful clinically. Unfortunately, many infarcts do not yield a smooth curve. In general, however, the higher the amount of MB released and the longer the CPK stays elevated, the larger is the infarction. Successful thrombolysis is characterized, however, with high CPK values and arrhythmias. Elevations of the white blood cell count and sedimentation rate and pericarditis are also indicators of a relatively large MI.

A better understanding of the anatomic substrate

of MI has occurred in recent years. An inferior Q-wave infarct is more likely to have associated multivessel disease than an anterior wall infarct. The reason is that occlusion of the right or left circumflex coronary arteries alone usually is "silent" because of the dual circulation to the posterior surface of the heart. Inferior infarcts usually occur only when both arteries are occluded. Inferior infarcts are more commonly associated with right ventricular infarction because of the common coronary artery supply. Inferior infarcts are usually smaller and less severe and less likely to be associated with shock or congestive heart failure. They are usually accompanied by bradycardia and sometimes temporary heart block. The associated pain is usually less severe and often imitates indigestion. When an inferior infarct is associated with heart block or right ventricular infarction, there is a higher risk.

Anterior Q-wave MIs are usually larger than inferior infarcts and are more likely to be associated with congestive heart failure and cardiogenic shock. Anterior infarcts are more likely to cause aneurysms and a greater decrease in ejection fraction. Surprisingly however, in follow-up study they have a similar or not much poorer prognosis than Q-wave inferior MIs have.[3] Fifteen percent of patients with Q-wave MI lose their Q-waves over the following year but still have the same prognosis as those who do not lose their Q-waves.

Interventions

Much work has been done to try to limit myocardial infarction size. This is extremely important, since prognosis after MI is largely predicted in regard to the amount of remaining myocardium. Randomized trials indicate that pharmacological intervention can be applied in a logical fashion to possibly limit infarction size. An unresolved question is whether this then leaves the patient with relatively more jeopardized myocardium, ready for another myocardial infarction, or with angina pectoris. In most cases, nitrates and beta-adrenergic receptor blockers can be useful in limiting MI size. Nitrates reduce preload and myocardial wall tension, which are important determinates of myocardial oxygen demand and lessen coronary artery spasm, which can occur during an MI. However, they can cause hypotension and headache. Beta-blockers must be used cautiously when congestive heart failure or heart block are present. However, when properly used, they rarely cause heart failure and definitely decrease myocardial oxygen consumption. Nitroprusside appears to be the choice for preload and afterload reduction in patients with heart failure and hypertension. When a dropping systolic blood pressure

is not attributable to hypovolemia, pressor agents can be helpful in shock, but the dismal prognosis in cardiogenic shock often necessitates artificial assisting devices and intervention with PTCA or CABS. Neck vein distension, a sign of congestive heart failure, can also be caused by right ventricular infarction. This must be considered in patients with an inferior infarct with neck vein distension that do not have rales. Often intravenous fluids can help such patients. Calcium-channel antagonists have been studied in randomized fashion and may be associated with a worse outcome except in the non–Q wave group. They can cause hypotension and reduce coronary perfusion in the acute MI patient. ACE inhibitors appear to be effective in limiting infarct expansion, which often occurs with large infarcts.

Thrombolysis

Although streptokinase has been availabile for 30 years, a major breakthrough in the 1980s has been the demonstration of its effect on the mortality associated with MI. The application of aspirin both in acute and chronic treatment of ischemic heart disease has also been monumental. Imagine the reaction of the medical community 10 years ago if a physician would prescribe aspirin for an MI or unstable angina. Now it is malpractice not to do so. The widespread use of thrombolysis has been complicated by debate over which agent to use, risk of stroke, if and when to follow with heparin, and who to exclude from treatment. Thrombolysin plasminogen activator (TPA) appears to lyse clot more quickly and effectively but its effect is briefer than that of streptokinase. Most comparison trials have shown them to be equally effective on mortality, and TPA costs 10 times more than streptokinase. The concerns with stroke have been lessened by appropriate dosing and by demonstration of comparable stroke rates in the placebo group. These studies have highlighted the 1% to 2% stroke rate associated with MI as well as the high mortality in this group. Heparin appears to be advantagous in low doses after the use of thrombolysis. Thrombolysis should in general be extended to the elderly, inferior MIs, and patients who have had CABS and be given up to 12 hours after the onset of chest pain. Most studies have shown that only 15% to 20% of patients with an acute MI are receiving thrombolytics.[4] Therefore the thrombolytic era does not affect 85% of new MI patients, and even those affected still need cardiac rehabilitation.

Risk prediction

It is well known that morbidity and mortality in postinfarction patients who have complicated courses are much higher than in those with uncomplicated MIs. The criteria for a complicated MI are listed in Table 16-2. Early ambulation is not appropriate for the patient with a complicated infarct. The progressive ambulation program should be delayed until such individuals reach an uncomplicated status, and even then progressive ambulation should be slower.

There has been some controversy over the relative long-term risk of subendocardial versus transmural myocardial infarction. Some of this difficulty has been attributable to whether prior MIs occurred. An infarct with evolving Q-waves on the ECG is "transmural" and considered to be large, whereas an infarction with only ST-segment and T-wave changes has been called "subendocardial" and considered to be small. Estimation of the severity of a MI requires consideration of clinical findings and test results other than the ECG to judge a patient's risk and infarct size. The presence of Q-waves does not prove the occurrence of a transmural MI, and a transmural MI can occur with only ST-segment and T-wave changes. The severity of an infarction should be judged by clinical findings, hemodynamic monitoring, the level of creatinine kinase elevation, and the presence of congestive heart failure or shock or both. The concept that a subendocardial infarction is "uncompleted" and poses an increased postdischarge risk has not been substantiated; however, they are more likely to be associated with postinfarction angina. The Mayo Clinic study demonstrated that in the patient with a first MI, prognosis is much better in follow up for a non Q–wave MI than for a Q-wave MI.[5] Patients with Q-wave MIs, particu-

Table 16-2 The presence of any one or more of the following criteria classifies a myocardial infarction as complicated

Prior MI
Continued cardiac ischemic (pain, late enzyme rise)
Left ventricular failure (congestive heart failure, new murmurs, chest x-ray changes)
Shock (blood pressure drop, pallor, oliguria)
Important cardiac dysrhythmias (premature ventricular contractions greater than 6/min, atrial fibrillation)
Conduction disturbances (bundle branch block, atrioventricular block, hemiblock)
Severe pleurisy or pericarditis
Complicating illnesses
Pronounced creatine kinase rise without a noncardiac explanation
Age greater than 75 years
Stroke or transient ischemic attacks

larly anterior wall infarcts, have a higher inhospital morbidity and mortality, just as patients with a history of multiple MIs. Controversy surrounds the impression that calcium-channel antagonists are specific therapy for non–Q wave MIs. Yosuf makes a strong argument for the use of beta-blockers in this group.

Certain clinical features during a patient's immediate post–myocardial infarction convalescence identify a higher risk for future cardiac events or death and mandate coronary angiography for consideration of coronary revascularization (PTCA or CABG) (see Table 16-2). Ross and colleagues have developed a scheme for deciding which patients should undergo coronary angiography after myocardial infarction by studying 1848 patients and testing it on another 780 patients.[6] If a patient manifests any spontaneous ischemia during hospitalization, he or she then has an increased risk of 18% to 20% mortality in the first year after myocardial infarction and should be referred for diagnostic coronary angiography before discharge. If a patient has had a previous myocardial infarction and clinical or radiographic evidence of left ventricular failure, his or her projected mortality risk is 25% in the first year and should undergo coronary angiography as well. In those patients who are unable to exercise, a resting radionuclide evaluation of ventricular function is recommended. Given that ventricular function is the most powerful predictor of prognosis in patients under 70 years of age, patients with left ventricular ejection fractions between 20% and 40% would be classified as high risk (12% first-year mortality).[7] Finally, the low-level predischarge exercise test completes the stratification work-up, and poor work load or evidence of inducible ischemia with ST-segment depression or angina identifies an annual mortality of 11% to 15%. A review by DeBusk estimates that for every 100 people who suffer an acute myocardial infarction and survive their hospitalization, 10 will manifest spontaneous ischemia or angina, 20 will have evidence of diminished ventricular function, and an additional 10 patients will have probable ischemia on predischarge exercise testing and be identified at higher risk.[8] Krone has recently reviewed this subject, and the strategies he recommends are outlined in the chapter on post-MI exercise testing.[9] Miranda and co-workers have attempted to consolidate these guidelines in a form specifically for practitioners involved in cardiac rehabilitation, and these are illustrated in Figures 16-1 and 16-2.[10]

Nicod and associates have recently reconfirmed in a large patient population that the overall 1-year mortality for patients with a non–Q wave myocardial infarction is nearly equal to that of patients

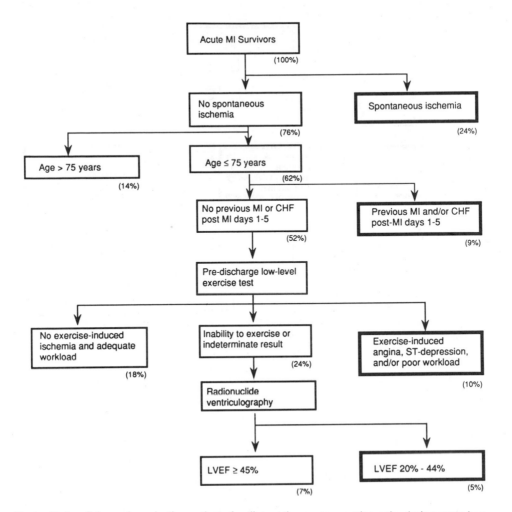

Figure 16-1 Scheme for selecting patients for diagnostic coronary angiography during acute hospitalization. Coronary angiography recommended for groups in dark boxes at right. Numbers under boxes are percentages of patients from entire group derived from test population in Ross et al. (*Circulation* 79:292-303, 1989) from which this scheme is adapted. Patients not included in stratification are patients greater than 75 years of age or with LVEF < 20%. It is assumed that these groups of patients are evaluated on an individual basis. Some centers may substitute an echocardiographic evaluation of ventricular function instead of radionuclide ventriculography. (*CHF,* Congestive heart failure; *LVEF,* left ventricular ejection fraction; *MI,* myocardial infarction.) (From Miranda C, Froelicher V: *Eurorehab* 1:5-23, 1991.)

who suffer a Q-wave infarction.[11] They should therefore undergo similar risk stratification. Klein and colleagues studied 198 patients who survived a myocardial infarction and underwent predischarge submaximal exercise testing and followed them for 2 years.[12] They found that patients who had exercise-induced ST-segment depression had a risk ratio of two times for suffering reinfarction or death compared to patients without ST-segment depression. However, if the pretest electrocardiogram did not have diagnostic Q-waves, the risk increased to 11 times for an abnormal ST-segment response. This indicates that the predischarge ex-

ercise test is an even more powerful predictor of risk in the patient who has suffered an acute non–Q wave myocardial infarction. This is in agreement with the work done by Krone and co-workers who found that non–Q wave myocardial infarction patients with exercise induced ischemia (angina or ST-segment depression, or both) had a threefold higher incidence of cardiac events in the year after their infarction compared to those with a normal predischarge exercise test.[13]

The invasive strategy of predischarge diagnostic coronary angiography to consider PTCA in patients with clinical evidence of reperfusion by

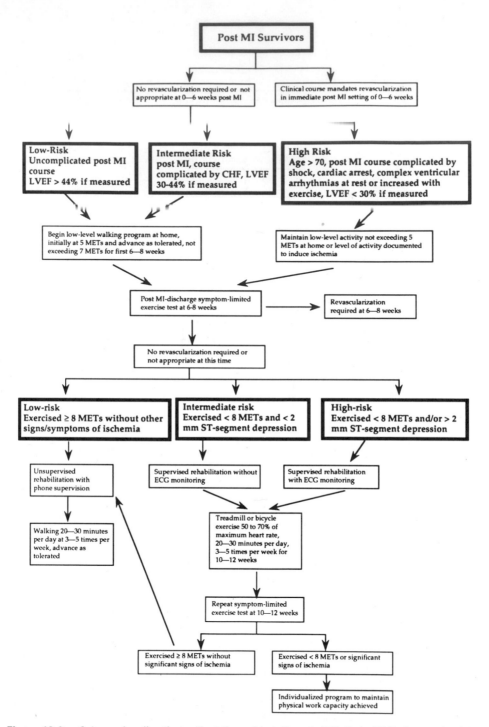

Figure 16-2   Scheme for directing patient through cardiac rehabilitation. (*CHF*, Congestive heart failure: *ECG*, electrocardiogram; *LVEF*, left ventricular ejection fraction; *1 MET*, metabolic equivalent = 3.5 cc of O_2 consumed/kg/minute.) (From Miranda C, Froelicher V: *Eurorehab* 1:5-23, 1991.)

thrombolytic therapy, but no evidence of spontaneous or residual ischemia, has been found to offer no benefit over a conservative strategy. In this latter approach, only patients who manifest residual ischemia by routine noninvasive stratification work-up are referred for coronary angiography.[14-16]

One of the benefits of thrombolytic and mechanical reperfusion therapy for myocardial infarction may be earlier discharge from the hospital. Topol and associates studied 80 patients with uncomplicated myocardial infarctions, 76 of whom were treated initially with thrombolytic therapy or PTCA, or both.[17] The patients were randomly assigned to either routine 7-day hospital care or discharge or to low-level predischarge exercise testing on the third day of hospitalization and discharge at that time if the exercise test was normal. There were no deaths and no significant differences in reinfarction rate or rehospitalization rate for unstable angina in either group in 6 months of follow-up study. The early discharge group had lower hospital charges, professional fees, and also returned to work earlier. It should be noted that only 18% of the patients with acute myocardial infarctions were eligible for early discharge by their criteria and 63% of the early discharge patients had inferior myocardial infarctions.

Clinical practice has evolved to the point that we now have the capability of recognizing the relative size of an MI and the risk that it represents for subsequent morbidity and mortality. It is now possible to assess risk at different temporal points from presentation in the emergency room, through the coronary care unit and predischarge time, and during later follow-up examination. However, the clinical picture changes over time and a low-risk patient can become a high-risk patient and vice versa. This changing risk is partially attributable to the vicissitudes of the atherosclerotic process, reformation of thrombus after interventions, and disease-host interactions. For instance, a patient may present with premature ventricular contractions (PVCs) but then such PVCs can disappear or worsen, chest pain may come and go, the electrocardiographic pattern may change, or the enzymes may have a late peak. All of this makes it difficult to strictly classify a patient as having a high or low risk—it is only the patient's physician who can determine the relative risk, aided by the nursing staff. However, such attempts at determination can lead to a great deal of frustration for the patient and the nurses. Often promises by the discharging physician from the coronary care unit or other changes signifying progress must be superseded by the day's findings. The progressive steps very often must be adjusted, sometimes even several times in a day. Table 16-3 lists a practical step approach.

CARDIAC REHABILITATION
Early ambulation

Before 1970, patients with acute MI were believed to require prolonged restriction of physical activity. The concern was that physical activity could lead to complications such as ventricular aneurysm formation, cardiac rupture, congestive heart failure, dysrhythmias, reinfarction, or sudden death. This approach was based on pathological studies indicating that at least 6 weeks were required for necrotic myocardium to form a firm scar and for checking on the increased prevalence of cardiac rupture reported among patients who had an infarct in mental hospitals where bed rest could not be enforced.

Animal experiments. Hammerman designed a study to evaluate the effect of early exercise on late scar formation in an MI animal model.[18] After occlusion of the proximal left coronary artery, the infarct extent was assessed 24 hours later by ECG criteria. The rats were divided into two groups: 8 were subjected to daily graded swimming for up to 45 minutes a day for a week followed by 2 weeks of nonswimming; 7 served as a control group. Twenty-two days after coronary occlusion, their hearts were excised and the wall thickness was determined histologically. A ratio for transmural infarcts was obtained from multiple measurements when scar thickness was divided by noninfarcted septal wall thickness. In the exercise group, there was considerable scar thinning. Infarct extent was similar in both groups. They concluded that short-term swimming during the first week after an MI had effects on scar formation when assessed 2 weeks later. A similar study by Kloner and Kloner with rats forced to swim 7 days after an MI reported the same results.[19] However, the relevance of rats forced to swim to the clinical situation is uncertain. Hochman and Healy performed similar experiments and found no signs in their rats of myocardial thinning or aneurysm formation.[20]

Controlled clinical studies of early mobilization have not found a greater incidence of death or other complications in patients mobilized early compared to patients who remain at bed rest longer. The promising results of these studies led to recommendations of gradual mobilization during the early post-MI stages. In certain patients, the major cause of decreased exercise capacity is enforced bed rest. The exercise prescription for MI patients in the coronary care unit can avoid iatrogenically induced deconditioning.

Chair treatment. A revolutionary approach to treatment occurred in the 1940s when Levine recommended "chair treatment" for the post-MI patient.[21] This emphasized the benefits of the sitting versus the supine position for increasing peripheral venous pooling and reducing preload on the myocardium. Levine theorized correctly that such a reduction would lead to a decrease in resting left ventricular wall tension and to a decrease in myocardial oxygen demand, in addition to decreasing the risk of thrombosis and pulmonary embolism. Physiological studies performed since have documented the hemodynamic alterations caused by deconditioning. After prolonged bed rest, tachycardia and hypotension are common upon standing. This is most likely attributable to alterations in the baromotor reflexes and to hypovolemia that occurs with bed rest. Clearly, the disability secondary to most MIs is attributable both to

bed rest and to myocardial dysfunction. The spontaneous hemodyamic improvement usually seen is attributable both to improving function (scar formation and possibly compensatory hypertrophy) and to a return to normal activities. An additional change was the use of a bedside commode, which is less of a hemodynamic stress than using a bed

Table 16-3 Post–myocardial infarction (MI) protocol—eight levels of activity*†

Level	Activities	Nursing	Exceptions
ICCU	Strict bed rest Commode vs. bedpan Feed self if set up	Complete bed bath (pt. may wash genitalia) *Exercises:* 5 × each BID: exercises 1-4 (see below)	Chest pain DOE Frequent PVCs HR greater than 100 Dizziness Diaphoresis

<2 METs
Teaching: simple explanations of equipment and procedures. Reassurance!

Level	Activities	Nursing	Exceptions
II CCU	Bed rest, up in chair 1 × vs. dangle Bedside commode	Bed bath; pt. may wash hands, face, genitalia *Exercises:* Passive ROM BID 5 × each BID: exercises 1-5	Chest pain, DOE Frequent PVCs HR greater than 100 Dizziness Diaphoresis

<2 METs   Feed self
Teaching: if diagnosis known—simple explanation, "You had a heart attack," and the role cardiac rehabilitation team will play in education and increasing activity.

Level	Activities	Nursing	Exceptions
III CCU or ward	Bed rest—up in chair 20 min TID Bedside commode Meals in chair	Bed bath—pt. may wash hands, face, genitalia *Exercises:* Active ROM all extremities 5 × each BID: Exercises 1-6	Chest pain, DOE Frequent PVCs HR greater than 100 Dizziness Diaphoresis

2 METs
Teaching: restate diagnosis with healing time: 3 months. Activity progression to be slow and steady with attention to pacing convalescence.
Stress: report any cardiac symptoms—e.g., chest, neck, jaw, arm, or abdominal discomfort

Level	Activities	Nursing	Exceptions
IV ward	Bed rest—bathroom privileges Up in chair as desired Walk about room	Partial bath (in bed or at sink)—Pt. not to wash back, legs, or feet *Exercises:* Active ROM BID 10 × each BID: 1-6 Add 5 × each BID: 7	Chest pain, DOE HR greater than 110 Frequent PVCs Dizziness Diaphoresis

<3 METs
Teaching: rehabilitation group discussion—family invited.
1. Anatomy and physiology of heart in relation to MI.
2. Convalescent care, activity progression, and risk factor management—hypertension, diet, activity, smoking, stress reduction.
3. Diet class low sodium and low cholesterol.
Reexplain class information on one-to-one level. Begin medication teaching including use of nitroglycerin.

Level	Activities	Nursing	Exceptions
V ward	Up in room Walk to TV room and back after warm-up exercises	Chair shower *Exercises:* Active ROM BID 10 × each BID 1-7 5 × each BID: exercise 8	Chest pain DOE HR greater than 110 Frequent PVCs Dizziness Diaphoresis

*Composite developed by Barbara Kellerman, RN, for use in Veterans Affairs Medical Centers.
†Primary physician is to draw a line down through levels, date, and initial order. Patient may be held at *any* level.
MI date _____ Highest CK _____

pan. The Valsalva maneuver, common when an individual is straining with a bowel movement, can lead to elevations of systolic blood pressure. However, in the sitting position, it is less forceful.

Bed rest: lack of activity or gravity. There are definite hemodynamic alterations caused by deconditioning. Young men maintained at bed rest for 3 weeks demonstrated a 20% to 25% decrease in maximal oxygen uptake.[22] Other than decreased functional capacity, prolonged bed rest can result in orthostatic hypotension and venous thrombosis through a loss of blood volume, in which plasma

Table 16-3   Post–myocardial infarction (MI) protocol—eight levels of activity*†—cont'd

Level	Activities	Nursing	Exceptions
4 METs	Up in chair		

Teaching: taking pulse. Explain medications, beta-blockers and digitalis (if applicable), action of medications. Reasons for slow, steady activity increase over 3-month period. Report any problems noted as activity increases—e.g., (1) chest, neck, jaw, arm, abdominal pain, or pressure or discomfort; (2) shortness of breath

Level	Activities	Nursing	Exceptions
VI ward	Ward ambulation Work toward walking around floor square nonstop (⅙ mile) Start with 1 leg of square—gradually increase pace before distance (12 × around = mile)	Chair shower *Exercises:* 10 × each BID: exercises 1-8	Chest pain DOE HR greater than 110 Frequent PVCs Dizziness Diaphoresis
<5 METs			

Teaching: reinforce activity progression. Patient does not leave ward unless pushed in a wheelchair (needs ward nurse knowledge to leave ward). No heart patient is to push another patient!

Level	Activities	Nursing	Exceptions
VII ward	Ambulate off ward Walk up one flight of stairs with rehab team member	Shower *Exercises:* 10 × each BID: exercises 1-9	Chest pain DOE Frequent PVCs HR greater than 120 Dizziness Diaphoresis
5 METs			

Teaching: review any questions.

Stress: treadmill test is not a pass/fall situation.

Level	Activities	Nursing	Exceptions
VIII	Submaximal treadmill test (5 MET) for discharge. If held in hospital for problems, return to level as indicated. If held in hospital for elective procedure (i.e., angiogram), stress the need to continue warm-up exercises and increase number of times around floor for training walk as in Level VI.		

5 METs

Exercises for post-MI protocols (numbers used above in "Nursing" column)
1. Foot circles
2. Ankle pumps
3. Toe flexion and extension
4. Neck exercises
   a. Head nod, chin on chest, then look to sky
   b. Head tilt: lean left ear to left shoulder, and then right ear to right shoulder
   c. Head turn: look to left and then right with chin over shoulder
   d. Five complete head circles, both right and left
5. Quadriceps setting, thigh press with knee locked
6. Shoulder exercises
   a. Shrug both shoulders up toward ears
   b. Move each shoulder in a circle forward and then backward
   c. Lift arms straight up over head until elbow is straight; alternate arms
7. Bring alternate knee to chest
8. Straight leg lifts, alternate legs
9. Side bends

loss exceeds red blood cell mass loss. Pulmonary function is decreased, and the patient can be in negative nitrogen and calcium balance.

The question has been raised whether the deleterious hemodynamic effects of bed rest, including decreased exercise capacity, are attributable to inactivity or to the loss of the upright exposure to gravity. There are at least four reasons supporting the concept that much of these alterations are attributable to loss of the upright exposure to gravity: (1) supine exercise does not prevent the deconditioning effects of being in bed; (2) there is both less and a slower decline in maximal oxygen consumption with chair rest than with bed rest; (3) there is a greater decrease in maximal oxygen uptake after a period of bed rest measured during upright exercise versus supine exercise; and (4) a lower body positive pressure device decreases the deconditioning effect of bed rest. Perhaps intermittent exposure to gravitational stress during the bed rest stage of hospital convalescence from surgery or MI may obviate much of the deterioration in cardiovascular performance that can follow these events. Previous efforts to limit the decrease in functional capacity after myocardial infarction or surgery have emphasized low-level exercise training, but these data indicate that simple exposure to gravitational stress substantially accomplishes this purpose.[23]

Progressive activity

A consideration often forgotten when one is dealing with an older patient or one with complicating illnesses is the level of activity that such a patient maintained before the MI. If a patient was physically limited before the event, the plan for progressive ambulation must be modified. It is generally inconceivable to expect a patient to be more physically active after an MI than before, unless previously limited by angina that disappeared later. It is important to assess the exercise capacity and activity level that existed before the myocardial infarction.

In addition to the oxygen cost and the heart rate achieved during activity, the duration of the activity must be considered. The effect of prolonged exercise on myocardial scar formation has not been carefully studied, but it is known that during prolonged steady-state dynamic exercise, heart rate increases, myocardial contractility declines, and left ventricular volume increases. It is apparent then that even though certain work levels can be achieved by a patient they should not be maintained for long periods of time in the acute recovery phase. Probably the safest recommendation is to tell patients not to fatigue themselves and to limit the duration of exercise by their fatigue level and perceived exertion.

Postdischarge activity recommendations have had little basis for their enforcement. Return to work, return to driving, and return to sex have been based on clinical judgments rather than physiological assessments. Because of this, physicians have left much of this up to their patients—allowing them to see how they respond symptomwise—rather than the older very conservative approach, which can foster invalidism. These decisions should be made in consideration of the consequence of the coronary event (ischemia or symptoms of congestive failure, or dysrhythmias) and the nature of the activities (manual labor versus desk work, light driving versus congested freeway driving, sex with an established partner versus other relationships).

In 1961, Cain and colleagues[24] reported on the use of a progressive activity program for acute MI patients. They had difficulty getting this report accepted for publication because the approach was considered dangerous. They reported 335 patients with an uncomplicated myocardial infarction who were at least 15 days after infarction. The patients had been restricted to bed, chair, and commode. The electrocardiogram was monitored after the patient performed activities such as climbing stairs and walking up a grade.

In 1964, Torkelson[25] reported results in 10 patients with an uncomplicated MI. On the sixth week of his inhospital rehabilitation program, a low-level treadmill test was performed using 1.7 mph at a 10% grade. He concluded that the treadmill test was a valuable procedure for the documentation of the specific exercise response of patients recovering from an acute MI.

Most later publications do not include ECG monitoring as part of progressive ambulation. Instead, generalized statements as to the activities on each postinfarct day are made for all patients, rather than individualized activity progression. Sivarajan, Bruce, and colleagues described 12 patients with an acute MI whose symptoms, signs, and hemodynamic and ECG responses during and after three activities were assessed. These activities included sitting upright, walking to the toilet, and walking on a treadmill. Studies of these activities were done at 3, 6, and 10 days after infarction. They concluded that successful performance of these three activities provided useful criteria for discharge.[26]

Hayes and colleagues studied 189 patients with an uncomplicated myocardial infarction selected at random for early or late mobilization and discharge from the hospital.[27] Patients were admitted to the study after 48 hours in a coronary care unit if they were free of pain and showed no evidence of heart failure or significant dysrhythmias. One group of patients was mobilized immediately and discharged home after a total of 9 days in the hospital, and the second group was mobilized on the ninth day and discharged on the sixteenth day. Outpatient assessment was carried out 6 weeks after admission. No significant differences were observed between the groups in terms of morbidity or mortality.

In a randomized study, Bloch and colleagues studied the effects of early mobilization after uncomplicated MI.[28] One hundred fifty-four patients under 70 years of age who were hospitalized for an acute MI and had no complications on day 1 or day 2 were randomly assigned to two treatment groups. In the early mobilization group, patients were treated by a physical therapist with a progressive activity program that began on day 2 or day 3 after infarction. In the control group, the patients underwent the traditional hospital regimen of strict bed rest for 3 or more weeks. The mean duration of hospitalization was 21 days for active patients and 33 days for the control group. The follow-up period ranged from 6 to 20 months, with an average of 11 months. There were no significant differences between the two groups with regard to hospital or follow-up mortality, to rates of reinfarction, dysrhythmias, heart failure, angina pectoris, or ventricular aneurysm, or to the results of an exercise test. On follow-up examination there was actually greater disability in the control group than in the active group.

Sivarajan and colleagues have reported the effects of early supervised exercises in preventing deconditioning after an acute MI.[29] Eighty-four patients were randomized to a control group, 174 to an exercise group. The exercise program began at an average of 4.5 days after admission. The mean discharge was 10 days after admission for both groups. There were no differences between the two groups in the clinical, hemodynamic, or ECG responses to a low-level treadmill test performed on the day before hospital discharge, nor was there any significant difference between the two groups for the incidence of complications or death. By the time this well-designed study was funded, the standard of community medical care in Seattle included early ambulation and discharge. Therefore the control group received treatment that was hardly different from the exercise group. Also, for safety reasons the sicker patients who most needed rehabilitation were excluded from this study. Six patients needed cardiac surgery before discharge in the exercise group, but none required it in the control group, which can be explained by chance distribution (failure of randomization) rather than by the mild exercises employed. These three randomized studies of patients with uncomplicated infarctions have demonstrated that the risks of early ambulation are minimal and that progressive mobilization during the early stages of an acute MI is recommended.

Exercise testing before hospital discharge. The low-level exercise test early after an acute MI (from 3 days to 3 weeks) has been shown to be safe. Today, it is a standard part of the treatment for MI patients in many hospitals. This test has many benefits including clarification of the response to exercise and the work capacity, determination of an exercise prescription, and recognition of the need for medications or surgery. It appears to have a beneficial psychological effect on recovery and is an effective part of rehabilitation.

Exercise prescription

Exercise training can be an important part of cardiac rehabilitation for returning a patient to his or her formerly active life-style or as functional a life-style as possible after an acute cardiac event. Cardiac rehabilitation is defined by the World Health Organization as "the sum of activities required to ensure them the best possible physical, mental, and social conditions so that they may, by their own efforts, resume as normal a place as possible in the life of the community . . . and that . . . rehabilitation cannot be regarded as an isolated form of therapy, but must be integrated into the whole treatment of which it constitutes only one facet."[30] The explicit details of exercise protocols and equipment, absolute and relative contraindications to exercise, warm-up and cool-down periods, and guidelines for terminating exercise are all outlined by the American College of Sports Medicine[31] and the American Association of Cardiovascular and Pulmonary Rehabilitation[32] and should be specifically tailored to each individual patient.

In prescribing exercise, one should consider two basic physiological principles. Myocardial oxygen consumption is the amount of oxygen required by the heart to maintain itself and do the work of pumping blood to the other organs. It cannot be measured directly without catheters but can be estimated by the product of systolic blood pressure and heart rate (double product). The higher the double product, the higher the myocardial oxygen consumption is and vice versa. Patients usually have their angina at the same double product, unless affected by other factors such as catecholamine level, left ventricular end-diastolic volume, hemoglobin-oxygen disassociation as affected by acid-base balance, and coronary artery spasm.

The second consideration is ventilatory oxygen consumption (VO_2), which is the amount of oxygen taken in from inspired air by the body to maintain itself and to do the work of muscular activity. Measuring VO_2 requires the collection of expired air, gas analyzers, and skilled technical help.

However, it can be estimated from knowing the work load of various activities. Since the body's mechanical efficiency is relatively constant, estimates of the oxygen cost of various activities without using gas analysis can be applied between individuals. There are many tables giving the approximate oxygen cost of different activities. Since oxygen consumption is equal to an arteriovenous oxygen difference (a-vO_2) times cardiac output, and an a-vO_2 difference is roughly a constant at maximal exercise, maximal oxygen consumption can be an approximation of maximal cardiac output. However, patients with diseased hearts will often have a wider a-vO_2 difference, a lower cardiac output, and a lower VO_2 than normal subjects performing the same submaximal work load.

Another important physiological concept of exercise is the type of work the body is performing. Dynamic work (bicycling, running, jogging) requires the movement of large muscle masses and requires a high blood flow and increased cardiac output. Since this movement is rhythmic, there is little resistance to flow, and in fact there is a "milking" action that returns blood to the heart. The other type of muscular work is isometric work such as lifting a weight or squeezing a ball. Isometric activities involve a constant muscular contraction, which limits blood flow. Instead of a cardiac response to increased cardiac output and blood flow, as during dynamic exercise, blood pressure must be increased in order to force blood into the active, contracting muscles. Pressure work demands much more oxygen by the heart than flow work,

and since coronary artery blood flow depends on cardiac output, the myocardial oxygen supply can become inadequate. Also, dynamic exercise is more easily controlled or graded so that myocardial oxygen consumption can be gradually increased, whereas isometric exercise can increase myocardial oxygen consumption needs very quickly. In addition, although isometric exercise is good for peripheral muscle tone and function, it does not result in the same beneficial cardiac and hemodynamic effects as dynamic exercise does.

Circuit training. Kelemen and colleagues[33] performed a prospective, randomized evaluation of the safety and efficacy of 10 weeks of circuit weight training in coronary disease patients, 35 to 70 years of age. Circuit weight training consisted in a series of weight-lifting exercises using a moderate load with frequent repetitions. Patients had participated in a supervised cardiac rehabilitation program for a minimum of 3 months before the study. Control patients ($n = 20$) continued with their regular exercise, which was in the form of a walk/jog and volleyball program, whereas the experimental group ($n = 20$) substituted circuit weight training for volleyball. No sustained arrhythmias or cardiovascular problems occurred. The experimental group significantly increased treadmill time 12%, whereas there was no change in the control patients. Circuit weight training was safe and resulted in significant increases in aerobic endurance and musculoskeletal strength compared with traditional exercise used in cardiac rehabilitation programs. Sparling and co-workers

Table 16-4 Summary of the randomized trials of cardiac rehabilitation

| Investigator | Year | Population randomized | | | | | Mean no. months entry after MI | Mean age |
		Total	Controls	Exercised	Exclusions	% women		
Kentala	72	158	81	77	150		2	53
Palatsi	76	380	200	180	>65	19%	2.5	52
Wilhelmsen	77	313	157	158	27%, >57	10%	3	51
Kallio	79	357	187	183	>65	19%	3	55
NEHDP	81	651	328	323	280	0%	14	52
Ontario	82	733	354	379	28, >54	0%	6	48
Bengtsson	83	171	90	81	45, >65	0%	1.5	56
Carson	83	303	152	151	>70	0%	1.5	51
Vermeulen	83	98	51	47		0%	1.5	49
Roman	83	193	100	93		10%	2	55
Mayou	83	129	42	44	>60	0%	1	51
Froelicher	84	146	74	76		0%	4	53
Hedback	85	297	154	143	>65	15%	1.5	57
AVERAGES								

have also demonstrated the safety and efficacy of circuit weight training in cardiac patients. In a 6-month study of 16 men, there was a 22% gain in strength without an increase in blood pressure.[34] Numerous other investigators have recently repeated this type of investigation with similar results. The AACVPR guidelines have even outlined recommendations on weight training for low-risk patients, an activity once believed to be far too dangerous for this population.

Intervention studies (Table 16-4)

Kallio and colleagues were part of a World Health Organization coordinated project to assess the effects of a comprehensive rehabilitation and secondary prevention program on morbidity, mortality, return to work, and various clinical, medical, and psychosocial factors after an MI.[35] The study included 375 consecutive patients under 65 years of age treated for acute MI from two urban areas in Finland between 1973 and 1975. General advice on rehabilitation and secondary preventive measures was given to all patients who were discharged from the hospital. On discharge, the patients were randomly allocated to an intervention or to a control group, both of which were followed for 3 years. Patients in the control group were followed by their own doctors and were seen by the study team only once a year during the 3-year follow-up study. The program for the intervention group was started 2 weeks after hospital discharge. An exercise prescription was determined from a bicycle test, and for most patients the program was supervised.

After the 3-year follow-up study, the cumulative coronary mortality was significantly smaller in the intervention group than in the controls (18.6% versus 29.4%). This difference was mainly attributable to a reduction of sudden deaths in the intervention group (5.8% versus 14.4%). The reduction was greatest in the first 6 months after infarction. Of the intervention group and the controls, 18.1% and 11.2%, respectively, presented with nonfatal infarctions. Total mortality was 21.8% in the intervention group and 29.9% in the control group. Although this was a landmark study, two weak points were that more patients in the intervention group than in the control group took antihypertensives and beta-blockers and that the exercise capacity measured at 1, 2, and 3 years after acute infarction was similar in both groups.

Kentala studied 298 consecutive males less than 65 years of age admitted to the University of Helsinki Hospital in 1969 with a diagnosis of acute MI.[36] They were divided by the year of birth: controls were from odd-numbered years ($n = 146$) and exercisers were from even-numbered years ($n = 152$). The average age was 53 years. Exclusions for controls included: 10 with uncertain diagnosis, 24 who died in hospital, 5 who refused or were not informed, 4 who had other severe disease, and 22 who lived too far away. Exclusions for the exercise group included: 12 with uncertain diagnosis, 21 who died in hospital, 3 who were not informed, 3 with other severe diseases, and 36 who lived too far away. Eighty-one controls and 77 exercisers were accepted for the study. Of the 81 controls, 4 died, 3 were hospitalized, and 1 refused, leaving 73. Of the 77 randomized to exercise, 5 died, 3 were hospitalized, and 1 refused,

| Years F-U | Dropouts Cntrl Ex | | Return to Work | | Percent mortality | | | | | | | |
| | | | | | Re-MI | | Sudden | | Cardiac | | Total | |
	Cntrl	Ex	Cntrl	Ex	Cntrl	Ex	Cntrl	Ex	Cntrl	Ex	Cntrl	Ex
1			5%	8%							22%	17%
2.5		35%	33%	36%	15%	12%	3%	6%	14%	10%	14%	10%
4		46%					18%	16%			22%	18%
3					13%	20%	14%	6%	29%	19%	30%	22%
3	31%	23%			7%	5%			6%	4%	7%	5%
4	45%	46%			13%	14%					7%	10%
1			73%	75%	4%	2%					7%	10%
3.5	6%	17%	81%	81%	7%	7%					14%	8%
5					18%	9%			10%	4%	10%	4%
9	4%	4%			5%	4%	7%	4%	5%	3%	6%	4%
1.5	25%	25%	30%	57%								
1	14%	17%			1%	1%					0%	1%
1		45%	59%	66%	16.2%	5.4%			7.8%	8.4%	7.8%	9.1%
	21%	29%	47%	54%	10%	8%	11%	8%	12%	8%	12%	10%

leaving 69 at 1 year of follow-up observation. Unless contraindicated, patients were kept on anticoagulation; beta-blockers were avoided. Both groups made their own decision on smoking and diet information was given. The training group was also urged to increase home activites after the exercise program daily, especially walking.

There were two training sessions weekly, later increasing to 3 per week, with a 20-minute warm-up and a 20-minute exertion (bicycle, rowing, stairs) followed by a cool-down phase. The exercise heart rate was optimally set at 10 beats less than the maximal heart rate from exercise testing. Attendance decreased to only 10 patients in the exercise group between the sixth and twelfth month. However, 16 trained on their own. Eleven controls were at a full training level after 1 year. There was no difference in morbidity or mortality between the groups. Both groups showed clear decreases in heart rate for given work loads, and both groups showed improved maximal work load, especially in those patients with greater than 70% attendance. Return to work was not influenced by training; 68% who worked before MI returned to work after 1 year.

Palatsi's study was a nonrandomized trial of 380 patients less than 65 years of age recovering from MI.[37] The patients were excluded if they had locomotive limitations, psychological problems, or congestive heart failure. The first 100 patients were allocated to an exercise program, and the second were the controls. The next 50 patients entered the exercise group, and then 50 entered the control group. The final total included 180 patients for exercise including 37 women and 200 controls including 34 women. Patients with non–Q wave MIs were treated with bed rest for 3 days, allowed to sit for 1 week, were allowed to walk on the tenth day, and were discharged on the twelfth day. Q-wave MI patients were bed rest for 7 days, sitting for 1 week, allowed to walk on the fourteenth day, and discharged on the sixteenth day.

Exercise training was begun 10 weeks after the MI and included breathing and relaxation exercises, calisthenics of all muscle groups, and walking, which progressed to running in place. Heart rate was at least 70% of the maximum rate during 30-minute sessions performed at home daily. Once a month, the patients returned for progression of their exercise program. No effort was made to change smoking habits. The authors concluded that home training was not so effective as continual supervised programs but still accelerated recovery of aerobic capacity. Rehabilitation had no effect on the clinical condition of the trainees. There was no group difference in symptoms, smoking habits, serum cholesterol, or return to work.

Wilhelmsen's study included patients born in 1913 or later and hospitalized for an MI between 1968 and 1970 in Göteborg, Sweden.[38] Patients were randomized to a control group ($n = 157$) or an exercise group ($n = 158$). Fifteen of the controls and 20 of the exercisers were females. The only criterion was an age of 60 years or older, but 27% of patients were excluded for cardiac complications. The two groups were comparable for hypertension, diabetes mellitus, treatment with digoxin, smoking status, congestive heart failure, and previous MI. The exercise group trained three times a week for 30 minutes a session. Calisthenics, cycling, and running were performed at 80% of the maximal age-predicted heart rate. All follow-up treatments were the same except for the exercise program. After 1 year the exercise group showed increased work capacity, lower blood pressure, but no difference in blood lipids. At 1 year only 39% continued to come to the hospital to exercise, whereas 21% trained elsewhere. Initially, 81% of the training opportunities were utilized. At 1 year only 63% of the sessions were utilized. Smoking after MI was found to be a significant predictor of fatal recurrent MI. There was also an association between smoking cessation and attending the exercise program. No significant differences were seen with respect to cause of death, type of death, or place of death. They concluded that antismoking advice and treatment with beta-blockers deserve higher priority than exercise training in the secondary prevention of MI.

The National Exercise and Heart Disease Project (NEHPD) included 651 men who had a myocardial infarction enrolled in five centers in the United States.[39] It was a randomized 3-year clinical trial of the effects of a prescribed supervised exercise program starting 2 to 36 months after an MI (80% were more than 8 months after infarction). In this study, 323 randomly selected patients performed exercise three times a week that was designed to increase their heart rate to 85% of the individual maximal heart rates achieved during treadmill testing, and 328 patients served as controls. This study was carefully designed by experts who took 2 years to complete the protocol. An initial low-level exercise session in both groups to exclude the faint of heart who would not comply with an exercise program was suprisingly effective in improving performance.

The three-year mortality was 7.3% (24 deaths) in the control group versus 4.6% (15 deaths) in the exercise group. Deaths from all cardiovascular causes (acute MI, sudden death, arrhythmias, congestive heart failure, cardiogenic shock, and stroke) for the 3-year follow-up study were 6.1% (20 deaths) in the control group versus 4.3% (14 deaths) in the exercise group. Neither difference was statistically significant. However, when deaths attributable to acute MI were considered as a separate category, the exercise group had a significantly lower rate: one acute fatal MI per 3 years (0.3%) in the exercise group versus eight fatal MIs (2.4%) in the control group ($p < 0.05$). The rate of all recurrent MI per 3 years, fatal and nonfatal, did not significantly differ between groups—23 cases (7.0%) in the control versus 17 cases (5.3%) in the exercise group. The number of rehospitalizations for reasons other than MI were identical in the two groups (27.4% versus 28.5% per 3 years). The need for coronary artery surgery was also equal in both groups—16 controls and 17 exercisers underwent surgery in the 3-year period. This study indicates a beneficial effect of cardiac rehabilitation, but insufficient participants because of financial limitations and dropouts prevented a definitive conclusion.

Unfortunately, this study could not be definitive but instead demonstrated the feasibility of resolving this important issue. It is unfortunate that it was discontinued, especially since the results are so encouraging. Only 1400 patients would be required to demonstrate a statistically significant reduction in mortality in the exercise group if the reported trend persisted. The patients in the exercise group who suffered a reinfarction had a lower mortality, an indication that an exercise program increases an individual's ability to survive an MI.

The Ontario Study included seven Canadian centers that collaborated in a randomized prospective trial.[40] Seven hundred thirty-three post-MI men underwent random stratified allocation to either a high-intensity group or a low-intensity exercise group. Patients were excluded for cardiac failure, insulin-dependent or uncontrolled diabetes, diastolic hypertension, orthopedic problems, or severe lung disease. The two groups were comparable for initial MI, angina, hypertension, type A personality, smokers, ex-smokers, and cholesterol level. Stratifying variables included (1) the presence or absence of hypertension, (2) blue- versus white-collar employment, (3) presence or absence of angina, (4) type A and B personality. The high-intensity group trained by walking or jogging 65% to 85% of their maximal oxygen uptake twice a week for 1 hour each session. This continued for 8 weeks after which they trained four times a week on their own. The low-intensity group trained once a week with relaxation exercises, volleyball, bowling, or swimming for 1 hour. They attempted to keep their heart rate at less than 50% of maximal oxygen uptake. Both groups were encouraged to stop smoking and control their weight. Less than 5% of the low intensity group regularly exercised vigorously. The dropout rate was 47%. The rate of reinfarction in the high-intensity group was 14%

and 13% in the low-intensity group. They found that the high-intensity exercise program had similar results to one designed to produce a minimal training effect and did not reduce the risk of reinfarction.

Bengtsson reported on 171 MI patients under 65 years of age who were randomized to a control and exercise group.[41] Patients were excluded for congestive heart failure, post-MI syndrome, aortic insufficiency, hepatitis, poliomyelitis, diabetes, new MI, thyroid disorders, stroke, or psychological problems. The rehabilitation program consisted of an outpatient exam, supervised exercise (large muscle group interval training by use of bicycles, calisthenics, and jogging for 30 minutes, 2 days a week for 3 months at 90% of the maximal heart) and counseling. There were no reported differences between groups for age, sex, number of infarcts, highest enzyme level, heart size, number of days in the hospital, number of admissions, angina, congestive heart failure, arrhythmias, or depression or hypochondriasis on the Minnesota Multiphasic Personality Inventory. The authors reported 100% compliance to the program. The exercisers showed lower mean systolic blood pressure at rest and lower diastolic blood pressure at high work loads than controls. Equal percentages of the exercise group and of the controls (74%) returned to work. The exercisers performed 31% heavier work at the end of training and 63% at the end of the follow-up study. They concluded that at 1 year all patients were less physically and socially active than before their MI. They were more dependent on their relatives than before, and they had a poor understanding of their illness. The rehabilitation program, including exercise, education, counseling, and social measures during the first 5 months after an acute MI, did not change the outcome 8 to 19 months after the MI compared to controls when one considers physical fitness, return to work, psychological factors, and an understanding of their illness.

Carson and co-workers performed their 3½ year study in a population of 1311 male MI patients.[42] Of these, 12.5% died in the hospital, 4% died after discharge but before the follow-up time, and 4.8% failed to attend follow-up appointments. Thus 70% of the original admissions remained. Patient exclusions included those greater than 70 years of age, congestive heart failure, cardiac enlargement, lung disease, hypertension, insulin, angina, orthopedic or medical problems, or personality disorders. After these exclusions, 442 patients were considered suitable, and 139 of these declined leaving 303. These patients accepted and were randomized to either a control or an exercise group. There was no group difference with regard to site of MI, number of MIs, highest enzyme level, smoking habits, known diabetes, previous angina or MI, cholesterol levels, family history, left ventricular failure, or occupation. The exercise group trained in a gym two times a week for 12 weeks at 85% of the exercise-test determined maximal heart rate or until symptoms of angina, shortness of breath, or a poor systolic blood pressure response occurred. Isometric exercise was avoided. The dropout rate was 17% in the exercise group and 6% in the controls. Mean age at death was significantly different in the two groups: 50 in the exercise group and 57 in the control group. Return to work was 81% in both groups, and both groups showed a similar decrease in smoking after their MI. They concluded that the difference in fitness between the exercise and control patients after completion of the study was highly significant. There was no significant decrease in mortality for the exercise group except for those with an inferior wall MI.

Vermeulen described a prospective randomized trial with a 5-year follow-up period.[43] Approximately 1 month after MI, patients underwent a symptom-limited exercise test. There was no total population description, no training description, no dropout rate reported, and no return to work described. Both the control and exercise groups received the same dietary advice. They found that rehabilitation did not influence smoking habits but lowered serum cholesterol. Their 6-week rehabilitation program was associated with a 50% decrease in progressive coronary artery disease when compared to the control group. Mortality and morbidity was 50% lower in the rehabilitation group. The incidence of progression of CAD was significantly decreased in patients smoking less than 20 cigarettes a day. They concluded that cardiac rehabilitation is a safe procedure and of benefit to patients with MI attributable to direct effects on myocardial perfusion and to lowering of cholesterol levels.

Roman reported on 139 patients including 19 women who entered their cardiac rehabilitation study.[44] A control and exercise group were comparable for age, sex, and MI location. The exercisers trained 30 minutes, three times a week at 70% of maximum heart rate for an average of 42 months. At the 9-year follow-up time, the control group had 24 cardiac deaths including 15 acute MIs, 7 sudden deaths, and 2 with congestive heart failure. The trained group had 13 deaths, which included 7 acute MIs, 4 sudden deaths, and 2 patients with CHF. The mortality was 5.2% for the control group and 2.9% for the rehabilitation group. There were 23 recurrent MIs in the control group (4.9% per year) and 16 recurrent MIs in the rehabilitation group (3.6% per year). There was no

difference in the incidence of myocardial ischemia, severe arrhythmias, or cardiovascular accidents between the two groups. There was a significant decrease in angina in the exercise group. The overall attendence was 76%, and the dropout rate was 4.1% of the exercise group and 3.9% among controls.

Mayou and colleagues studied 129 men, 60 years of age or less, admitted with an MI.[45] They were sequentially allocated to either normal treatment, exercise training, or counseling groups. The control group received standard inpatient care, advice booklets, and one or two visits as outpatients. They had no other education, walking program, or instructions for exercise. The exercise group received the normal treatment and eight sessions (two times a week) of circuit training in groups, written reminders, and reviews of their results. The "advice group" received normal treatment and discussion groups, kept a daily activity diary, had couples therapy, and had three or four follow-up sessions. The three groups were comparable socially, medically, and psychologically. Patients excluded were 13 who died and 1 with a stroke. Evaluation was performed after 12 weeks using exercise testing and standard tests of psychological state and social adjustment. There were no differences among the groups in psychological outcome, physical activity, or satisfaction with leisure or work. The exercise patients were more enthusiastic about their treatment and achieved higher work loads on exercise testing. At 18 months the only significant findings were a better outcome in terms of overall satisfaction, hours of work, and frequency of sexual intercourse for the counseled group. The dropout rate was 25% overall. There was no difference in exercise capacity at 6 weeks, but at 12 weeks there was a nonsignificant increase in the exercise group. The groups were similar for return to work, activities, sexual activity, and ratings of quality of life. There was no group difference with compliance to advice in smoking, diet, or exercise. They concluded that exercise training increased confidence during exercise in the early stages of convalescence but that the exercise program had little value in regard to cardiac performance, daily function, or emotional state.

Hedback's study in Sweden was retrospective with a control group of 154 patients and an intervention group of 143 patients; 23 of the controls and 22 of the exercisers were women.[46] There was no group difference regarding age, sex, risk factors for MI, rate of employment, income level, MI location or size, arrhythmias, medications, or heart size on discharge chest x-ray film. Exclusions for the training group included severe congestive heart failure, arthritis and stroke. Thirty-one declined to enter the program. Seventy-eight of the 84 who began completed the training program. Both groups were treated the same during their acute hospitalization. Training began 6 weeks after MI following a bicycle test. Training was performed on a bicycle to a maximum heart rate of 5 beats below maximal heart rate as determined during the exercise test. If symptoms or signs occurred, the heart rate was limited to 15 beats below maximal HR. Sessions were 25 to 30 minutes long. This was done for 4 weeks and then replaced by calisthenics and jogging as well as a home program. Patients with a cholesterol level of 8 mmol/L were referred to the dietician. Beta-blockers were administered to 60% of the patients. One year after the MI there was no group difference in mortality, but the exercise group had a significantly lower rate of nonfatal reinfarction, fewer uncontrolled hypertensives, and fewer smokers. Goble and coworkers in a recent study, found similar benefits from a low-level program compared to a high level.[47]

Metanalysis

Although not every single-center study has shown definitive differences between participants in exercise programs compared with controls in regard to physiological or psychosocial variables, the overall benefits of cardiac rehabilitation are now well accepted. More comprehensive reviews confirming these benefits are now available.[48] Because of the time and expense involved in conducting controlled studies with large numbers of patients, few such trials have been performed. We are left with numerous studies showing significant benefits in exercise capacity and often psychosocial benefits but frequently only trends toward improved morbidity and mortality. Metanalysis has gained popularity in recent years as a method of combining separate but similar studies, and this

approach has recently yielded some very important information on the efficacy of cardiac rehabilitation. May and colleagues have presented an excellent review of the long-term trials in secondary prevention after MI[49] (Table 16-5). Trials reported before November 1981 in which both intervention and follow-up study were carried out beyond the time of hospital discharge were considered. Random assignment and at least a total sample size of 100 were required. Total mortality was used whenever possible in order to minimize bias. All patients randomized were included in the mortality estimates to reduce the bias of differential withdrawal. Effectiveness was calculated by considering the percent reduction in deaths that would have occurred if the intervention had been applied to the control group. Although few of the interventions resulted in a significant difference, all of them except for the antidysrhythmics show a trend toward efficacy. The 19% reduction in death rate from exercise training indicates that exercise is as safe and effective as other available means of secondary prevention.

To circumvent the problem of inadequate sample sizes, O'Connor and colleagues performed a metanalysis of 22 randomized trials of cardiac rehabilitation involving 4554 patients.[50] They found a 20% reduction of risk for total mortality, a 22% reduction for cardiovascular mortality, and a 25% reduction in the risk for fatal reinfarction. Oldridge an associates performed a similar metanalysis with 10 randomized trials including 4347 patients and found a similar reduction for all-cause death and cardiovascular death in the patients undergoing cardiac rehabilitation.[51] Criticisms of these analyses are that each evaluated pooled study was not uniform in its treatment of patients, and a nonexercise intervention done in the different trials may have biased the results.

Table 16-5 Follow-up randomized intervention trials after myocardial infarction considered epidemiologically valid*

Intervention	Number of studies (with significant difference)	Number of patients randomized	Length of follow-up (range of means)	% mortality controls	% mortality intervention	Effectiveness (% reduction, in deaths)
Antidysrhythmics	6 (0)	1,675	4 mo-2 yr	10.3	10.8	−4.6
Lipid lowering	9 (1)	19,834	21 mo-11 yr	23.6	19.4	17.8
Anticoagulants	5 (0)	2,327	2-6 yr	17.7	13.7	22.6
Platelet active drugs	7 (0)	13,298	1-3 yr	10.5	9.7	7.6
Beta-blockers	11 (4)	11,325	9 mo-2 yr	11.5	8.8	23.5
Exercise	6 (1)	2,752	1-4.5 yr	14.7	11.9	19

*Adapted from May GS et al: *Prog Cardiovasc Dis* 24:331-352, 1982.

COMPLICATIONS OF AN EXERCISE PROGRAM
Risk of exercise testing

There is a small but definite incidence of cardiac arrest associated with exercise testing of cardiac patients, particularly in the early minutes of recovery. A large multicenter survey of complications of exercise testing by Rochmis and Blackburn showed a combined mortality and morbidity rate of four events per 10,000 tests.[52] In a retrospective review by Irving and Bruce of 10,751 symptom-limited exercise tests, five cardiac arrests were reported.[53] All occurred in the first 4 minutes of recovery, and all five patients survived after defibrillation (one arrest per 2000 tests). The relative risk of developing cardiac arrest with exercise testing (lasting 15 minutes) can be estimated to be one arrest per 538 hours of treadmill exercise, or 160 times greater than what might be expected to occur spontaneously (one death per 88,000 hours if one assumes a 10% yearly rate of sudden death).

Perhaps because of an expanded knowledge concerning indications, contraindications, and end points, maximal exercise testing appears safer today than 20 years ago. Gibbons and co-workers[54] recently reported the safety of exercise testing in 71,914 tests conducted over a 16-year period. The complication rate was 0.8 per 10,000 tests. This is greatly lower than earlier studies, but it was conducted in a population that was generally healthier. The authors also suggested tht the low complication rate might be attributable to the use of a cool-down walk, which may make the recovery period safer. However, we have found that out of 3351 tests in our laboratory, no cardiac arrests occurred, and sustained ventricular tachycardia occurred in only 5 patients.[55] In general, our population is a higher risk group, and all patients are placed supine immediately after the test for diagnostic purposes.

Complications during exercise training

Haskell surveyed 30 cardiac rehabilitation programs in North America using a questionnaire to assess major cardiovascular complications.[56] This survey included approximately 14,000 patients for 1.6 million exercise-hours. Of 50 cardiopulmonary resuscitations (CPR), 8 resulted in death, and, of 7 MIs, 2 resulted in death. Exercise programs resulted in four other deaths occurring after hospitalization. Thus there was one nonfatal event per 35,000 patient-hours and one fatal event per 160,000 patient-hours. The complication rates were lower in ECG-monitored programs. These programs reported a 4% annual mortality during exercise, which is a rate not different from that expected for such patients. Other programs have reported rates of cardiopulmonary resuscitations

ranging from 1 in 6000 to 1 in 25,000 man-hours of exercise. Such events are difficult to predict, can occur in patients with only single-vessel disease, and can occur at any time after a patient is in a program.

A Seattle cardiac rehabilitation program (CAPRI) reported the highest rate of 1 CPR in 6000 exercise hours.[57] Of 15 patients requiring defibrillation, the CAPRI group successfully resuscitated all of them. Eleven had angiography, which showed single-vessel disease in 4 patients and multivessel disease in 7. Subsequently, the CAPRI record improved, and they have had experience with defibrillating two patients simultaneously, on another occasion, a physician monitoring an exercise class was defibrillated. Of 2464 patients observed during a 13-year period, 25 cardiac arrests occurred during 375,000 hours of supervised exercise, a rate of 1 arrest per 15,000 hours. The same incidence rate was reported in Toronto and in Atlanta where five arrests occurred in 75,000 hours of exercise, and a similar rate of one arrest per 12,000 hours (total of 36,000 gymnasium hours) was reported in Connecticut. In CAPRI, 12 of the 25 victims had been enrolled for 12 or more months. Fibrillation was recorded in 23 cases and ventricular tachycardia in 2. Prompt defibrillation was carried out, and all patients survived. Each cardiac arrest was a "primary" arrhythmic event, and none were associated with acute MI. Eighteen of the 25 patients had ST- segment depression, and 5 had developed hypotension with prior exercise testing.

Fletcher and Cantwell reported five coronary disease patients resuscitated after ventricular fibrillation in an exercise program.[58] Multivessel coronary disease that could be treated with bypass surgery was present in four of them. Resuscitation was required unexpectedly and at unpredictable times, occurring 2 to 48 months after being in the exercise program.

Van Camp and Peterson obtained statistics from 167 randomly selected outpatient cardiac rehabilitation programs and found that the incidence rate for cardiac arrest was 8.9 per million patient-hours.[59] Of these cardiac arrests, 86% were successfully resuscitated, giving an incidence rate for death of 1.3 per million patient hours. This compares favorably with the estimated death rate for unselected joggers at 2.5 per million person-hours of jogging.[60] There also was no significant difference in cardiac event rate between rehabilitation programs with or without electrocardiographic monitoring. Their data have been widely cited to document that the risk of exercise training is quite small.[61]

The incidence of exertion-related cardiac arrest in cardiac rehabilitation programs is small, and because of the availability of rapid defibrillation, death rarely occurs. Using an annual 10% incidence rate of sudden arrhythmic deaths during any activity (one per 88,000 man hours), the risk is one sixth that observed during participation in exercise programs. Using a more conservative 3% to 5% annual incidence rate of sudden death would increase the risk. In an earlier review of survival in the CAPRI population, 85% of cardiac arrests took place during exercise classes that the subjects attended for about 3 hours each week. However, the majority of sudden deaths are temporally associated with routine activities of daily life and not with exercise. Therefore the number of deaths attributable to strenuous physical exertion is relatively modest. Exertion-related cardiac arrest is usually attributable to ventricular fibrillation or tachycardia, and exercise may increase its risk by 100 times.[58,62]

CURRENT PRACTICES

To determine changes in American health care delivery over the past decade for patients with an uncomplicated MI, questionnaires were sent to 6000 physicians in 1979.[63] Responses were compared to a similar survey taken in 1970. Almost all physicians in 1979 reported the use of a coronary care unit with continuous electrocardiographic monitoring. The average hospital stay dropped from 21 days to 14 days over the decade. Patient education materials were used more frequently than in 1970. Exercise tests were more commonly used and usually at 6 weeks after infarction. Early ambulation and return to work were more common; most physicians recommended progressive physical activity after hospitalization.

Spontaneous improvement after myocardial infarction

To document spontaneous improvement in aerobic capacity, the Stanford group has measured VO_2 max within the first 3 months after an uncomplicated MI.[64] Forty-six men underwent symptom-limited maximal treadmill tests 3 and 11 weeks after an MI. There was a significant increase between the two periods in heart rate, rate pressure product, and oxygen consumption during submaximal exercise. The mean maximal heart rate increased from 137 to 150, VO_2 max increased from 21 to 27 cc of O_2/kg/min, and maximal systolic blood pressure, double product, and oxygen pulse also increased.

To evaluate hemodynamic changes after MI, Kelbaek and colleagues measured VO_2 max and performed invasive studies at rest and during two submaximal exercise levels.[65] Thirty men were studied 2, 5, and 8 months after an uncomplicated MI. Fourteen patients participated in an exercise program during the first 3 months of the study, whereas the other 16 patients attended the training during the second 3-month period. An increase in VO_2 max occurred at the fifth month in both groups, 16% and 11%, respectively, along with an increase in cardiac index at the same relative submaximal work load. Later in the study, only slight increments in VO_2 max and no changes in hemodynamics were recorded within or between the two groups. They concluded that poor medical advice and pensions appeared to be the major factors responsible for unnecessary unemployment after an acute MI.

The Davis group studied the effects of walking for 14 weeks on 9 patients with coronary heart disease.[66] Each patient was tested after training at the individually determined horizontal treadmill speed that induced ST-segment depression in the pretraining test. Although VO_2 max did not increase significantly with training, submaximal heart rate and the double product were reduced by 10% and 16% respectively. Naturally, none of the patients had the same amount of ST-segment depression as in the first test. The patients became more efficient walkers with a 10% decrease in their oxygen consumption requirements. Although the authors proposed this was caused by the walking program, it has previously been shown that just serial treadmill testing results in improved efficiency.

In a comprehensive review, Greenland and Chu analyzed eight controlled studies of supervised exercise programs and their effect on physical work capacity.[67] In all the studies reviewed, exercise capacity improved after the intervention, whether the patients were in a control or active intervention group. This indicates that either a patient's exercise capacity may be artificially limited by the patient himself or by the physician's caring for them (such as a low-level predischarge exercise test), or there is a spontaneous improvement in exercise capacity as time passes from time of infarction. However, the exercise groups always had a greater exercise capacity than the control groups after the interventions—on the order of 20% to 25% better. Studies that failed to show that any benefit may have been limited by exercise programs of inadequate duration because it probably takes longer than 3 to 6 months for any improvement in cardiac adaptation and also by compliance with the exercise prescription

CARDIAC CHANGES IN PATIENTS WITH CORONARY HEART DISEASE

Many favorable physiological changes have been documented in patients with coronary heart disease who have undertaken an aerobic exercise program.

These include lower submaximal and resting heart rate, decreased symptoms, and increased maximal oxygen uptake. Peripheral adaptations are at least partially responsible for these changes, and controversy exists as to the effects of chronic exercise on the heart. In a review of the effects of exercise training on myocardial vascularity and perfusion, Scheuer concluded that in the normal animal heart there is strong evidence that chronic training promotes myocardial capillary growth and enlargement of extramural vessels.[68] However, it is unclear if these changes actually increase perfusion or protect the heart during ischemia. Controversy still remains whether exercise training can promote coronary collaterals in the animal model subjected to chronic ischemia, even though Bloor's landmark ischemic pig study supports this contention.[69]

There have been several attempts to demonstrate the effects of exercise training on the hearts of patients with coronary heart disease. Ferguson and colleagues performed coronary angiography on 14 patients before and after 13 months of exercise.[70] Despite a 25% increase in maximal oxygen uptake, collateral vessels were observed in only two coronary arteries and four of 14 patients demonstrated progression of disease. Nolewajka and co-workers studied 10 male patients before and after 7 months of exercise training.[71] Neither the exercisers nor the 10 control patients showed any changes in coronary angiograms, myocardial perfusion as assessed by intracoronary injection of radionuclides, or ejection fraction. Sim and Neill also failed to demonstrate cardiac changes in trained angina patients including assessment of myocardial blood flow and oxygen consumption.[72] Whether these negative findings can be explained by limitations in the techniques, patient selection, inadequate intensity, or length of training is uncertain.

Assessment of cardiac changes using radionuclides

The radionuclide techniques have been employed before and after exercise training in normals and cardiac patients. Verani and colleagues used radionuclide ventriculography and thallium scintigraphy to evaluate 16 coronary patients before and after 12 weeks of exercise training.[73] Thirty patients entered the study, but only 16 completed it. Ten patients had a documented MI at least 2 months previously, and all but one of the others had angiographic documentation of coronary disease. Nine patients received propranolol throughout the exercise period. Both posttraining exercise studies were performed at the same double product as in the pretraining studies. For the ventriculography, a multicrystal camera was used and scintigraphy

accomplished within 10 seconds of completion of exercise. After the training program, 15 of the 16 patients had improved exercise tolerance. Resting mean left ventricular ejection fraction increased from 52% to 57%, but no change was noted in exercise ejection fraction or regional wall motion abnormalities. The thallium studies were also unchanged.

The Duke group has reported the effects of 6 months of exercise training on treadmill and radionuclide ventriculography performance in 15 patients, all less than 6 months after MI.[74] A training effect was demonstrated by a lower heart rate at a submaximal work load and longer treadmill time despite a wide range of resting ventricular functions (ejection fractions from 17% to 67%). The mean ejection fraction, end-diastolic volume, and wall motion abnormalities during rest and at matched work loads and heart rates, were not significantly different after training. DeBusk and Hung randomized 11 patients with coronary heart disease to a home exercise program and 10 to a control group 3 weeks after myocardial infarction.[75] There was no significant difference in resting or exercise ejection fraction or thallium perfusion images between the two groups after 8 weeks. Recently, Todd and co-workers from Scotland reported improvement in thallium scores among 40 male patients with stable angina after 1 year of following the Canadian Air Force plan for physical fitness.[76]

PERFEXT

Our group at the University of California, San Diego preformed a study called PERFEXT (PERFusion, PERFormance, EXercise Trial).[77] The San Diego community was informed that we were recruiting male coronary heart disease patients between 35 and 65 years of age for a free exercise program. The responding volunteers were a select group because they were highly motivated to be in such a program. They were encouraged to accept randomization by being promised that if randomized to the control group they could join the exercise classes after the 1-year study was completed. Potential subjects were screened to determine if they (1) had coronary heart disease, (2) were willing to be randomized and comply with either a low-level home walking program or a medically supervised exercise program at UCSD Hospital, (3) could discontinue their medications for testing, (4) had no complicating illnesses or locomotive limitations, (5) had not recently been in an exercise program, and (6) had the approval of their physician. The patients were classified by the following criteria: (1) history of myocardial infarction, (2) stable exertional angina pectoris, or (3) coronary artery bypass surgery. Disease stability was assured by careful history taking and by not allowing the patient to enter the study until at least 4 months after a cardiac event, a change in symptoms, or surgery.

One hundred sixty-one patients were interviewed, signed consent forms, and agreed to randomization. The patients were then scheduled for three entry exercise tests done on separate days usually within a 2-week period. The thallium treadmill test was done first, for familiarization, followed by a maximal oxygen uptake treadmill test and finally a supine bicycle radionuclide study. Of 146 patients randomized, 72 were in the training group and 74 in the control group.

A modified Balke-Ware protocol was used for both the thallium scintigraphy and maximal oxygen uptake procedures. The ECG data were digitized on-line and later computer processed. The tests were maximal, except that the end point for the 1-year thallium treadmill test was the maximal rate pressure product achieved at the initial thallium study. Radionuclide angiography was accomplished by the gated equilibrium technique with the subject in the supine position with the legs horizontal and not elevated. With the axis of the pedals at the same level as the body, the patient performed 3 stages of supine bicycle exercise each 3 minutes in duration.

The patients randomized to the exercise intervention group began training in a continuous electrocardiographic monitored class. The initial training intensity was set at a minimum and duration of 60% of the estimated maximal oxygen uptake from the initial treadmill test and training intensity was progressed in standard fashion throughout the year. Patients randomized to the control group were offered a low-intensity walking program. Once randomized to control or intervention, a patient was always considered a member of that group regardless of his adherence to the protocol. The distribution of patients is illustrated in Figure 16-3. Randomization was successful in equally distributing the clinical, treadmill, radionuclide ventriculography, and thallium imaging parameters between the two groups. During the course of the study year, there were 5 medical dropouts in the control group: 2 for coronary artery bypass surgery, 1 for MI, 1 with both myocardial infarction and coronary artery bypass surgery, and 1 death. There were 6 medical dropouts from the exercise intervention group: 1 for coronary artery bypass surgery, 1 for MI, 1 for alcoholism, and 3 who became unstable medically. One of these three had the only complication during testing. He required defibrillation for ventric-

ular tachycardia during an extra treadmill test but suffered no sequelae. Of the 66 remaining in the exercise intervention group, 7 dropped out of exercise classes because of job conflicts or lack of motivation and refused further testing. Repeat 1-year testing was therefore performed on 59 of the 72 patients from the exercise intervention group and on 69 of the 74 controls.

After the completion of the study, the exercise records of the 59 exercise intervention patients who had 1-year testing were extensively reviewed. Average intensities for the entire year were as follows: percent maximal estimated oxygen uptake and percent maximal heart rate by the Karvonin method was approximately 60% ± 10% (ranging from 40% to 100%). Percent of maximal heart rate and measured maximal oxygen uptake was approximately 80%. The average caloric expenditure per session was 319 ± 104 (130 to 719 kilocalories). The mean attendance at exercise sessions was 76% ± 18% (23% to 97%).

Over the year of study, 1 control and 1 trained patient gained both abnormal treadmill-induced ST-segment depression by visual interpretation and angina, 1 trained lost both, and 3 controls and 1 trained patient gained angina but lost the criterion for abnormal ST-segment depression. Nine controls and 6 trained patients lost abnormal ST-segment depression, and 4 controls and 3 trained gained it. Ten trained and 4 controls lost or decreased treadmill-induced angina, and 4 controls and 3 trained gained it.

A significant training effect in the intervention group is evidenced by the decrease in their resting and submaximal heart rates, as well as the significant increase in the measured and estimated maximal oxygen uptake (Table 16-6). The control group showed a significant decrease in exercise capacity at least partially because of the lower maximal heart rate obtained at 1 year. There was also a small but significant decline in the submaximal heart rate and rate pressure product in the control group probably because of habituation. No changes were observed in maximal perceived exertion, respiratory quotient, or systolic blood pressure between the two groups initially or at 1 year, or between the initial and 1-year tests. Thus the 1 year of exercise training in our patients elicited the expected training response. The significant increase in estimated (18%) and measured (8.5%) VO_2 max is similar to most studies.

Analysis of variance testing confirmed that the training effect, including an increase in measured oxygen uptake, occurred in subgroups of the exercise-intervention patients relative to controls. These subgroups included those with and without the following features: a history of a Q-wave MI,

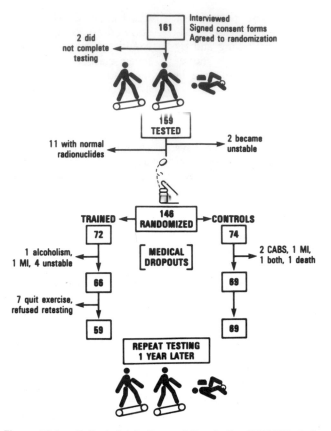

Figure 16-3 Patient distribution and flow in the PERFEXT study.

treadmill test–induced angina, ejection fraction less than 0.40 or 0.50, abnormal exercise test–induced ST-segment depression, beta-blocker administration, or a dropping ejection fraction response. However, three-way analysis of variance revealed that those with angina pectoris but without a Q-wave MI in the intervention group did not increase their estimated oxygen uptake relative to controls.

Radionuclide ventriculography demonstrated a baseline increase in both end-systolic and end-diastolic volume in response to supine exercise. We examined the effect of training relative to controls on the following variables: heart rate, ejection fraction, end-diastolic and end-systolic volumes, stroke volume, and cardiac output at rest and at each of three stages; and percentage change of each from rest to each of three stages. The statistical method used was ANACOVA (analysis of covariance). The model employed the 1-year value as the dependent variable and the initial value as the covariate and allowed for effects caused by training, angina, and Q-wave MI. Differences from angina or Q-wave MI, or from both, are not reported.

There were no significant differences at rest, during the three stages of exercise or the percent change from rest to exercise between the control and trained group at 1 year in ejection fraction, end-diastolic volume, stroke volume, or cardiac output. However, the intervention group, relative to controls, had significantly lower percentage changes in end-systolic volume at all three work loads. The data indicated that the magnitude of the intervention effect differed in the MI and non-MI groups though this was not statistically significant; the intervention effect appeared consistently stronger in the non-MI group than in the MI group.

The PERFEXT exercise intervention group experienced a significant improvement in the exercise thallium images following the year using the Atwood scoring system[78] as well as using computer techniques.[79] However, comparing thallium scans side by side, which has been done effectively to evaluate surgical intervention, was not successful in the clinical assessment of changes in myocardial perfusion following an exercise program. Disappointingly, the ST-segment changes neither showed an improvement nor matched the thallium changes.

Table 16-6 Initial and 1-year measurements from the maximal treadmill test showing the changes

Test	Control (n = 69)	Exercise-intervention group (n = 59)
Heart rate, beats/min		
Supine		
Initial	66 (9)	69 (12)
1 year	69 (11)	65 (11)
Mean difference	2.2 (10)	−3.8 (10)†‡
Submaximal, 3.3 mph/5%		
Initial	125 (15)	126 (16)
1 year	121 (16)	118 (15)
Mean difference	−3.1 (11)†	−9.3 (12) †‡
Maximal		
Initial	154 (19)	156 (22)
1 year	149 (23)	154 (22)
Mean difference	−5.2 (13)†	−2.2 (11)
Rate pressure product*		
Submaximal, 3.3 mph/5%		
Initial	209 (44)	215 (47)
1 year	199 (49)	196 (42)
Mean difference	−8 (35)‡	−19 (34)†
Maximal		
Initial	279 (57)	286 (59)
1 year	273 (60)	289 (67)
Mean difference	−6 (46)	3 (50)†
Maximal oxygen uptake		
Estimated, cc/kg/min		
Initial	33 (8)	33 (9)
1 year	32 (8)	37 (9)
Mean difference	1.3 (5)	4.7 (6)†‡
% change	−3 (18)	18 (24)†‡
Measured, L/min		
Initial	2.1 (.5)	2.2 (.6)
1 year	2.0 (.5)	2.3 (.6)
Mean difference	−0.1 (.3)†	0.1 (.3)†‡
% change	−4 (17)†	8.5 (17)†‡

*HR × SBP.
†Significant change from rest.
‡Significant difference between groups.

One of the only changes in ventricular function or volume of a consistent nature was the significantly lower percent of change of end-systolic volume in the exercise-intervention patients. There were no significant differences in blood pressure at any stage of bicycle exercise, and so there is no evidence that decreased afterload would explain this. It would appear that the trained heart calls on the Frank-Starling mechanism to a lesser extent than the untrained heart probably because of lessened ischemia or improved contractility. This response may not have been seen had the patient's legs been elevated during supine exercise testing (Table 16-7).

The other significant change was the effect of the intervention on stroke volume and maximal cardiac output. Training is known to increase both,

but the differential effect of angina was surprising. The decrease in stroke volume and cardiac output in the angina patients was accompanied by a lessening of ischemia and an increase in end-systolic volume in response to supine exercise. This indicates that absolute volume changes that could not be detected because of the variability of the volume technique had to occur. Future studies need to address the mechanism of this response.

In routine clinical practice, cardiac rehabilitation is begun as soon as possible after a cardiac event. However, given our study design and sample-size limitation, we chose only to deal with patients with stable coronary heart disease. Studying patients more acutely after MI is complicated by the degrees of severity and by the variable rate of spontaneous improvement. Our results may not be

Table 16-7 Estimated changes in stroke volume and cardiac output during supine bicycle exercise after 1 year

| Category | Exercise-intervention group | | p value |
	With angina ($n = 20$)	Without angina ($n = 39$)	
Resting supine stroke volume	−9.9 mL	7 mL	0.06
Stroke volume, stage 2	14.9 mL	11.3 mL	0.02
Maximal stroke volume	−10.9 mL	10.3 mL	0.03
Maximal cardiac output	−1.0 L/min	1.3 L/min	0.048

applicable to the cardiac population immediately after the event.

One criticism might be that our patients did not exercise hard enough and that, if they had, more definite improvements might have been possible. However, even if we chose those who trained the most intensely or had the highest exercise class attendance, we did not find greater changes. Surprisingly, there was a poor correlation between the intensity or attendance and the change in aerobic capacity or the radionuclide changes; in fact, there was a poor correlation between the change in aerobic capacity and changes in the radionuclide tests. A paradox now exists regarding this. Ehsani and colleagues have reported impressive cardiac changes in a highly selected group of cardiac patients with asymptomatic ST-segment depression exercised at very high levels.[80] Hossack and Hartwick have reported an increased risk for exercise-induced events in similar patients. The question remains whether the usual cardiac patient can be exercised safely at higher levels than we utilized and, if so, whether more definite cardiac changes can be demonstrated.

EFFECT OF AN EXERCISE PROGRAM ON THE VENTILATORY THRESHOLD

For documentation of the benefits of chronic exercise during submaximal levels, the noninvasive measurement of the ventilatory or lactate threshold has been considered. The PERFEXT study results were reviewed to evaluate alterations in the ventilatory threshold before and after 1 year of moderate exercise training in patients with coronary heart disease. Forty-one coronary patients out of 156 had complete continuous gas-exchange data.[81] The ventilatory threshold was identified as the oxygen uptake before a systematic increase in VE/VO_2 without an increase in VE/VCO_2. Agreement by two of three independent, blinded observers was the criterion needed to determine the ventilatory threshold. This criterion was met in all but five tests, in which case it was determined by the three observers collectively.

Supine resting and submaximal heart rates were reduced in the exercise group, and such reduction was suggestive of a trailing effect. However, the exercise group's peak VO_2 (L/min) increased only 1%, which was significantly different from the controls largely because of the 7% decrease in peak VO_2 (L/min) in the control group. Although there was no statistically significant difference between groups with respect to change in peak VO_2 (ml/kg/min), there was a significant difference in total treadmill time. With regard to the ventilatory threshold, there was no significant difference between groups when this variable was expressed in L/min or cc/kg/min or as a percentage of peak VO_2. However, there was a trend in the control group to decrease these variables. A significant correlation ($r = 0.45$; $p < 0.05$) between the absolute change in peak VO_2 (L/min) and the absolute change in VO_2 at the ventilatory threshold (L/min) was observed in the exercise group. In addition, there was a similar correlation ($r = 0.46$; $p < 0.05$) between the percent change in the VO_2 at the ventilatory threshold and the percent training intensity relative to the ventilatory threshold. It is frequently suggested that exercise training must occur at intensities above the ventilatory threshold to ensure increases in cardiorespiratory variables such as peak VO_2 or VO_2 at the ventilatory threshold. The relationship betwen percent training intensity and changes in VO_2 at the ventilatory threshold and peak VO_2 support this contention.

PERFEXT demonstrates that in patients with coronary heart disease, exercising two to three times per week at an intensity approximately equal to the ventilatory threshold is adequate for altering the hemodynamic response to exercise and for maintaining a state of conditioning. Their improved exercise capacity (that is, greater treadmill time) cannot be explained by an increase in the ventilatory threshold. It would appear that when an increase in peak VO_2 or the ventilatory threshold is desired the exercise intensity should be at a level above an individual's ventilatory threshold. However, in some patients with coronary disease this exercise intensity may be contraindicated because of signs or symptoms of their disease.

Care must be taken in interpreting many of the studies evaluating the effect of chronic exercise in cardiac patients. Often initial testing is submaximal, whereas follow-up tests are at a higher level because of increased patient and technician confidence and enthusiasm. This should be suspected when there are large increases in maximal heart rate, blood pressure, respiratory exchange ratio, or perceived exertion. Our study did not show significant changes in these parameters because we took care to encourage patients to perform a maximal effort in their initial test. Also, if oxygen consumption is estimated from treadmill time rather than measured, the changes are very much exaggerated.

Changes in the exercise ECG

It is attractive to think that myocardial perfusion could be evaluated noninvasively during exercise by the exercise ECG; there have been several efforts at this. As part of PERFEXT, 48 patients who exercised and 59 control patients had computerized exercise ECGs performed initially and 1 year later.[82] ST-segment displacement was analyzed 60 msec after the end of the QRS complex in the three-dimensional X, Y, and Z leads and utilizing the spatial amplitude derived from them. There were no significant differences between the groups except for less ST-segment displacement at a matched work load, but this could be explained by a lowered heart rate. Previous studies in this area have had mixed results; these are reviewed in Table 14-4.

Effect of beta-blockers on exercise training

There is evidence that a functioning sympathetic nervous system may be necessary to achieve the beneficial hemodynamic alterations of training. In addition, the limitation in cardiac output because of beta-adrenergic receptor blockade may result in fatigue and reduce the intensity of training or compliance to exercise. Also, if ischemia (the major stimulus for collateral development) is lessened by beta-blockade, this potential benefit of training could also be impeded. Beta-adrenergic receptor blockade is widely used to treat patients with coronary heart disease, and aerobic exercise is now commonly prescribed as part of cardiac rehabilitation. However, one of the beneficial hemodynamic effects of both regular exercise and beta-blockade is that the heart rate at rest and submaximal work loads are decreased. If beta-adrenergic stimulation is needed for the effects of exercise training to occur or if beta-blockade lessens the ischemia necessary to promote collateralization, beta-blockade might be expected to interfere with the beneficial

results of exercise. Beta-blockade could also increase perceived exertion and fatigue, thus lessening the tolerance for higher exercise levels and adherence to an exercise program. Therefore a pharmacologically imposed limitation in heart rate and cardiac output during exercise may prohibit obtaining an optimal training effect.

The mechanisms by which the hemodynamic changes occur secondary to regular exercise are poorly understood. High levels of sympathetic stimulation are present during aerobic exercise. It has been shown that regular intermittent infusions of dobutamine in dogs result in cardiovascular changes similar to those induced by an exercise program. However, the dogs did not get a true "training" effect. Other support for the importance of sympathetic stimulation for achieving the changes induced by exercise is that prolonged infusion of epinephrine has enhanced myocardial contractility and induced hypertrophy in dogs and that sympathectomy abolishes the increase in the heart–to–body weight ratio produced by exercise in rats. Hossack and colleagues found ventilatory changes during exercise in response to a single 40 mg oral dose of propranolol. They hypothesized that the changes were attributable to inhibited glucose metabolism, which could impede the training effect, but this has not been substantiated. These observations indicate that repeated, sustained sympathetic stimulation might be an important factor in exercise training. If beta-adrenergic sympathetic stimulation is needed for an exercise effect to occur, beta-blockade might be expected to interfere with this process.

In 1974, Malmborg and colleagues first reported that a training effect could not be obtained in coronary patients with angina on beta-blockers.[83] However, their exercise program was only two times a week for a duration of 18 minutes. Obma and colleagues reported a conflicting result in 1979.[84] Their patients were limited by angina but demonstrated a significant increase in estimated oxygen consumption after an 8 week, 30 to 60-minute, 5 to 7-days-per-week exercise program. Pratt and colleagues retrospectively studied 35 patients with coronary heart disease who underwent a 3-month walk-jog cycle training program.[85] Fourteen patients had received no beta-blocker, 14 received propranolol 30 to 80 mg/day, and 7 patients received propranolol 120 to 240 mg/day at the discretion of their physicians. Training consisted in three 1-hour periods per week at 70% to 85% of maximal pretraining heart rate. Each group's estimated oxygen uptake was assessed while they were receiving medications increased after training: by 27% in those not taking beta-blockers, by 30% in those taking a low dose, and by 46% in those taking a high dose.

Vanhees and colleagues compared two groups of post-MI patients without angina pectoris; 15 were receiving beta-blockers and 15 were not receiving them.[86] Propranolol and metoprolol were the beta-blockers most commonly used, at daily doses ranging from 30 to 120 and 75 to 200 mg, respectively. Exercise training was performed between 60% to 80% of their maximal capacity for 3 months. Both groups showed lower heart rates, systolic blood pressures, and rate pressure products after training, at rest, and during submaximal exercise. Testing was done while they received beta-blockers, but surprisingly the maximal heart rate was only about 13 beats/min higher in the group not using beta-blockers. Heart rate decreases were significantly less in the group having beta-blockade, whereas systolic blood pressure decreases were less pronounced in the other group. Peak measured oxygen uptake increased an average of about 35% in both groups, but maximal heart rate and rate pressure product were also higher.

Controversy even exists among studies of normals and the effects of beta-blockade. Ewy and colleagues studied 27 healthy male adults (mean age 24) who first underwent two maximal treadmill tests.[87] They were then randomly assigned to either a placebo group or to Sotalol 320 mg/day. A third maximal treadmill test was performed 1 week after the administration of the agents. Subjects then participated in a 13-week training program in which they exercised 45 minutes five times a week at a training heart rate equivalent to 75% of measured maximal oxygen uptake. A fourth maximal treadmill test was performed at the conclusion of the training program while they were taking the agent, and 7 days after cessation of medication a fifth maximal treadmill test was performed. Measured VO_2 max was increased after training in both groups; however, in the beta-blocked group this was demonstrated only when beta-blockers were not received. These findings indicate that stroke volume had attained its maximal physiological capacity during beta-blockade, and the reduction in maximal heart rate with beta-blockade prevented cardiac output to increase optimally after training. These observations are supported by Tesch and Kaiser who observed greatly reduced VO_2 max values in highly trained athletes after acute administration of propranolol.[88]

Sable and colleagues studied normal young men before and after 5 weeks of aerobic training.[89] In double-blind fashion, 8 received placebo and 9 propranolol throughout the period while training at the same intensities. Maximal exercise tests were performed before either drugs or training were started and then were repeated 3 to 5 days after completion of the exercise program when beta-blockade was no longer present. The subjects who received propranolol had no increase in measured VO_2 max, whereas the placebo group changed from a mean of 44 to 53 cc of O_2/kg/min. Maximal heart rate was unchanged in either group. High levels of propranolol were maintained by monitoring plasma levels with daily doses ranging from 160 to 640 mg. This certainly disagrees with what we and most others have found possibly because of the high levels of beta-blockade achieved. However, this same group has repeated this protocol using low doses of beta-blockers and reported the same attenuation of changes in VO_2 max.

The work of Gordon and co-workers at Stanford who randomized normals to drug or placebo and then trained them has shown particularly interesting results.[90] Beta-blockade eliminated the echocardiographic changes in left ventricular posterior wall and septal thickening that was found in the placebo group who underwent training. Other investigators who have done studies of cardiac patients have not randomized the patients to beta-blockade but have instead taken patients selected by their physicians to be receiving or not receiving beta blockade. Naturally, this can bias the findings. Other possible explanations for the different results obtained in studies of the effects of beta-blockers on training include (1) inadequate total time in training, (2) high initial levels of training or fitness, (3) differences in the suppression of maximal heart rate by beta-blockade, (4) only some studies have successfully blinded the subjects as to drug treatment, and (5) considerable differences in the altitude at which training occurred.

To help resolve these questions, we performed an analysis of patients in PERFEXT who exercised for 1-year versus controls in which patients were given beta-blockers at the prerogative of their physicians.[91] The patients medical records were reviewed to see who had taken beta-blockers prescribed by their physicians during the year of training for the exercise group and the year of observation for the controls. This information was then used to separate them into four groups: (1) controls using beta-blockers, (2) controls not taking beta-blockers, (3) trained patients using beta-blockers, and (4) trained not taking beta-blockers. All testing was performed after beta-blocker withdrawal. More of the patients in the exercise group using beta-blockers had exercise test-induced angina than those not using beta-blockers (64% versus 16%, $p < 0.01$), and they tended to have more ST-segment depression and higher thallium ischemia scores. Also, there was a trend for a higher prevalence of prior bypass surgery in those not receiving beta-blockers. These differences are probably attributable to exercise training making limitations caused by angina more obvious and leading to beta-blocker administration. Average exercise intensities in the beta-blocker group for the year were as follows: percent maximal estimated oxygen uptake was 60% ± 12% (ranging from 40% to 100%), percent measured maximal oxygen uptake was 77% ± 14% (ranging from 42% to 100%), average calories expended per session was 323 ± 104 (ranging from 130 to 719). There were no significant differences between those using or not using beta-blockers. The mean values were 62% versus 59% for estimated, 74% versus 79% for measured maximal oxygen uptake, and 305 versus 335 calories for the on and off beta-blocker groups respectively. Attendance at exercise sessions was a mean of 76% ± 18% (ranging from 23% to 97%) with no difference between those using or not using beta-blockers (73% for those using versus 78% for those not using beta-blockers).

Changes in treadmill performance. Two-way analysis of variance revealed highly significant changes in the treadmill parameters because of the exercise intervention. No interaction was detected attributable to beta-blocker status during the year. There was no correlation between beta-blocker dosage and the change in measured oxygen uptake in the exercise group. No other changes in treadmill parameters including maximal heart rate, blood pressure, perceived exertion, or respiratory quotient were detected. The changes in submaximal heart rate were significant despite the rebound effect of beta-blocker withdrawal.

Changes in thallium scintigrams. Two-way analysis of variance in consideration of the clinical classifications of angina, prior MI, and CABS revealed significant ($p < 0.01$) improvement in only the thallium scintigrams of the patients in the exercise program with exercise test-induced angina. Therefore, three-way analysis of variance for angina, beta-blockers, and intervention was performed. Although there was a trend for this improvement to be concentrated in angina patients not taking beta-blockers, this did not reach statistical significance.

By design, patients were selected by their physicians to be using or not using beta-blockers, and the effects of beneficial exercise training were demonstrated. This clinical question is different from studying the effects of beta-blockers on exercise training. However, this latter uncertainty has not been resolved, since conflicting results exist as to the effects of being randomized to beta-blockade in normal subjects engaged in exercise training. In coronary patients selected for beta-blockade treatment by their physicians the answer

regarding the beneficial effects of exercise is more definitive. From previous studies it has been demonstrated that expected changes in oxygen uptake, submaximal heart rate, and exercise duration usually occur in patients who engage in exercise training. Our study supports this but also demonstrates no preferential difference between those patients trained with or without beta-blockers. In addition, the present study has shown an increase in myocardial perfusion implied by improved thallium scintigrams in patients with angina in an exercise program. These findings and those summarized above support the beneficial effects of exercise training in coronary patients taking beta-blocker medication.

COMPLIANCE

The success and benefits of any exercise training program are obviously directly related to the amount of exercise actually performed by the patient; in other words, their compliance with the exercise prescription. Kentala reported that only 13% of his patients carried out their assigned exercise prescription at least 70% of the time. As time progresses, compliance fell. At 3 months, compliance was 80%; 1 year later compliance was only 45% to 60%, and at 4 years it was only 30% to 55%.[92] Several options are available to improve compliance behavior—reduce the waiting time, expert supervision, tailoring of the exercise prescription to avoid physical discomfort or frustration, use of variable activities including games, incorporation of social events, recalling absent patients, involving the patient's family or spouse in the program, and involving the patients in monitoring themselves and their progress.

PATIENTS WITH LEFT VENTRICULAR DYSFUNCTION

Not long ago, patients with left ventricular dysfunction were believed to be poor candidates for exercise programs. This was out of concern for safety and the general thinking that they were unable to benefit from training. This has been dispelled, however, by several studies performed over the last decade. Squires and colleagues studied 20 post-MI patients with left ventricular ejection fractions less than 25% in a supervised cardiac rehabilitation program. There was substantial improvement in exercise capacity in most patients, and a favorable trend was observed in performing desired activities and returning to work.[93] Conn and associates studied 10 patients with a history of prior myocardial infarction and left ventricular ejection fractions of less than 27% and found that with a cardiac rehabilitation program their exercise capacity increased from a mean of 7.0 to 8.5 METs and there was no exercise-related morbidity or mortality.[94]

Judgutt and co-workers studied 13 patients with anterior Q-wave myocardial infarctions using echocardiography before and after supervised low-level exercise training.[95] They found that patients with evidence of greater left ventricular asynergy (akinesis or dyskinesis) had more detrimental ventricular shape distortion, with expansion and thinning of their left ventricle after exercise training. This was believed to be secondary to remodeling of an incompletely healed infarct zone. Until this is confirmed, it should be stressed that, in general, patients with ventricular dysfunction do benefit from cardiac rehabilitation, and in fact an unpublished Italian randomized trial did not support these findings. Table 16-8 summarizes the improvement noted in exercise capacity in four studies. These studies are consistent and advocate that severely depressed left ventricular function is not an absolute contraindication to cardiac rehabilitation and that these patients can also attain a beneficial cardiovascular training effect safely. The most elaborate of these studies was recently reported from Duke.[96] Extensive hemodynamic measurements were performed in 12 patients with severely depressed left ventricular dysfunction before and after 4 to 6 months of training. An increase in maximal cardiac output of 1 liter led to a 23% increase in maximal oxygen uptake. However, central hemodynamics, including ventricular volumes, ejection fraction, pulmonary artery pressure, and pulmonary wedge pressure at rest and during exercise were not different after training. However, peak exercise and systemic and leg arteriovenous VO_2 differences were greater, and arterial and leg lactate levels were reduced greatly. These investigators suggested that the training adaptations were attributable to peripheral metabolic factors that appeared to be independent of central hemodynamics.

PATIENTS WITH RIGHT VENTRICULAR DYSFUNCTION

Haines and colleagues studied 61 patients after they had suffered an acute inferior or true posterior myocardial infarction.[97] Right ventricular dysfunction was determined to be none, moderate, or severe by blinded, subjective readings of gated equilibrium blood pool images at rest. They found no significant differences in exercise tolerance as assessed by treadmill time or METs, at predischarge or 3 months after discharge testing, and between patients with and without right ventricular dysfunction. There also was no difference in exercise-induced ST-segment depression, chest pain, thallium-201 defects, medically refractory angina, reinfarction rate, or cardiac mortality. No attempt was made to standardize cardiac rehabilitation, other than usual care by the patient's own physician. Crosby and associates more recently studied five patients who had suffered a hemodynamically significant right ventricular infarction and found an improvement in exercise capacity with cardiac rehabilitation similar to that of patients without right ventricular infarction.[98]

Table 16-8 Studies of cardiac rehabilitation after myocardial infarction in patients with left ventricular dysfunction

Study	No.	Patient characteristics	Entry time after MI	Program duration	Pre-rehab work capacity (average)	Post-rehab work capacity (average)	% change
Arvan	25	LVEF < 40%	Within 12 weeks after MI	12 weeks	6.4 METs	8.5 METs	+33
Conn	10	LVEF < 27%	>3 months after MI	Mean 12.7 months	7.0 METs	8.5 METs	+21
Lee	18	LVEF ≤ 40%	>6 weeks after MI	19 months	FAI 32%	FAI 23%	+28
Squires	20	LVEF ≤ 25%	16 patients within 3 weeks after MI Four patients at a mean of 2.8 years after MI	8 weeks	6.5 METs	8.9 METs	+37
Costs	11	LVEF = 20%	All with CAD	8 weeks	4 METs	5 METs	+25
TOTAL	84					MEAN	+30

FAI, Functional aerobic impairment; *LV;* left ventricle, *LVEF,* left ventricular ejection fraction; 1 MET = metabolic equivalent = 3.5 cc of O_2/kg/min.

ELDERLY PATIENTS

Williams and associates studied 361 patients grouped according to age with 76 patients being 65 years of age or older, all of whom had acute myocardial infarction or CABG enrolled in a 12-week exercise program. They found that the improvement in physical capacity by the elderly group was the same as for the younger groups and that benefits from cardiac rehabilitation were unrelated to age.[99] This is a very important result because, as was mentioned earlier, the majority of myocardial infarctions occur in this age group.

EXERCISE PROGRAMS FOR PATIENTS AFTER CABS

Coronary artery bypass surgery (CABS) has been shown to prolong life and relieve angina in selected groups of patients with coronary artery disease. Advances in operative techniques including cardioplegia, the use of the internal mammary artery, and more complete revascularization have improved operative results. Attention must now be turned to other methods for further improvement of the functional result in these patients and for management of those with a less favorable result. Postoperative exercise programs are one means of optimizing the surgical result and helping those with inadequate revascularization. Because of the large number of patients undergoing coronary artery bypass and their potential for rehabilitation, these patients have been included in exercise rehabilitation programs. However, less than 200 CABS patients in postoperative exercise programs in a total of seven studies have been reported. Most previous studies have considered only patients with successful surgery that alleviated angina pectoris, whereas our study group included approximately one third with signs or symptoms of ischemia.

Adams and colleagues were the first to report a study of exercise training for CABS patients.[100] They entered four male CABS patients into a training program with 45 sedentary normal males and 11 post-MI patients. After 3 months of walking and jogging at least 3 days a week, 40 minutes a day, at a heart rate 75% to 85% of maximum, the bypass patients had exercise capacities equal to the trained postinfarction patients and had shown an 11% increase in maximal oxygen uptake. As expected, the sedentary normal men out-performed both groups.

Oldridge and colleagues conducted a study of the effects of an exercise program of 32 months duration among post-CABS patients.[101] Twenty-one patients with angina were given maximal treadmill tests 1 week before CABS and again 16 weeks after surgery. Six of these patients then entered a program of 45 to 60 minutes of exercise, three times a week, at heart rates 65% to 75% of their postoperative functional capacity. A control group of six subjects from the remaining group of bypass patients was chosen. These men were matched "as closely as possible" to the exercising patients. The control group had participated only in sporadic physical activities such as tennis or walking since surgery. Treadmill tests were performed on the exercise subjects 32 months after training began and 28 to 34 months after surgery in the control group. No significant change in resting heart rate or blood pressure was found in either group. Maximal oxygen uptake increased by 28% in the exercisers, with only a 3% increase observed in the controls. The exercise group had also been tested after 4 months of exercise, and by that time 90% of the total improvement in functional capacity observed at the end of 32 months had already occurred.

Soloff conducted a nonrandomized study of the effect of rehabilitation on mood and physical performance in 27 postbypass and 18 postinfarction patients.[102] The postbypass patients significantly improved maximal oxygen uptake and maximum heart rate after an inpatient program of bedside exercise and early ambulation, followed by 6 weeks of monitored, three times weekly calisthenics and 20 minutes of bicycle ergometry.

In Ireland, Horgan and colleagues exercised 51 patients three times a week in a program that began 8 to 10 weeks after CABS.[103] These patients exercised 16 minutes each session at 85% of their maximal heart rate. After 8 weeks of exercise, the duration of exercise and maximum work load were increased. Similar results were seen in a group of postinfarction patients exercised simultaneously.

Hartung and Rangel reported their findings in 10 CABS patients who participated for 3 to 6 months in an exercise program.[104] They exercised three times a week in 20- to 40-minute sessions of walking, jogging, or bicycle ergometry at an intensity 70% to 85% of maximum heart rate beginning 10 months after surgery. Maximal oxygen uptake increased significantly at the conclusion of the study. Increased maximal oxygen uptake was also seen in 24 postinfarction patients and 16 high-risk asymptomatic individuals. No significant difference was found among the three groups in any of the variables evaluated.

Dornan and co-workers reported 210 men who were referred consecutively to a rehabilitation program after CABS.[105] The program involved submaximal exercise testing at 8 weeks with an intervening 12-week exercise program and a repeat exercise test. A retrospective analysis showed 50%

of the patients to be receiving no medication throughout their rehabilitation whereas the others were receiving medications likely to affect cardiac performance. Age and the extent of revascularization did not appear to influence exercise tolerance. After the 12-week exercise program, patients in both groups had improved significantly, but the initial and final performance of the cohort of patients requiring cardiac drugs was significantly poorer than those on no medication.

Fletcher retrospectively studied 22 patients who had undergone CABS.[106] Group I (mean age 53 years) was currently enrolled in the rehabilitation program. Group II (mean age 56 years) had begun but discontinued the program for nonmedical reasons. There was no difference in entry exercise tests, or presurgical catheterization data between the groups. Group I had a higher maximal oxygen uptake (31 versus 24 cc/kg/min) and greater treadmill time (11 versus 8 minutes). Nine of 11 in group I were fully employed versus four in group II. One in group I had been rehospitalized versus five in group II. No one in group I smoked, whereas 4 of the 11 subjects in group II smoked. They concluded that the CABS patients in their program had greater maximal oxygen uptake, smoked less, were less often rehospitalized, and were more often fully employed than those who dropped out.

A study by Nakai and associates showed that physical exercise improved graft patency rate at 7 weeks after CABS (98% patency in exercise group versus 80% patency in control group) documented by coronary angiography.[107] Perk and co-workers demonstrated less medication use and hospitalizations in CABS patients who participated in an exercise program.[108]

PERFEXT CABS patients. Analysis of the CABS patients in our randomized exercise trial, who represented a third of the total study group included 53 CABS patients who were randomized, resulting in 28 in the exercise-intervention group and 25 in the control group. This was a unique opportunity to evaluate the effects of CABS in rehabilitation because the numbers were fairly high, radionuclide changes were assessed, and, unlike most studies, it was a controlled trial. The mean time from surgery until entry into the study was 2 years with a standard deviation of 2 years and a range of 6 months to 9 years. This was rather long, and exercise training has a greater effect if applied sooner. Favorable training effects were observed, however, and they were similar to those in the larger group, but no radionuclide changes were significant.

The effects of revascularization vary, but many patients are presently 10 years past CABS; there is a recurrence rate of angina of 5% or less 1 year after surgery. A randomized trial of aspirin has demonstrated improved graft patency, and so efficacy could even be improved. The available studies, though limited by methodology, patient numbers, and highly variable details of the rehabilitation programs employed, demonstrate that exercise programs can improve the exercise capacity of patients who have undergone CABS.[109,110]

REHABILITATION AFTER PTCA

The exponential growth in percutaneous transluminal coronary angioplasty (PTCA) since its first clinical application in 1977 by Andreas Gruentzig has been dramatic to the point that over 150,000 procedures were performed in 1987. Despite improvements in equipment and techniques, late vessel restenosis occurs frequently within 3 to 6 months of the procedure. Depending on the types of patients studied and the definition of restenosis, it occurs in 12% to 48% of patients.[111] Because an average of 30% of patients will undergo restenosis, this constitutes a significant number of patients who are destined to have recurrence of their ischemia, and cardiac rehabilitation can assist them physically and mentally in coping with their coronary disease. Fitzgerald and associates have shown that despite the minimal invasiveness of PTCA and lack of any physical contraindications, some patients have found it difficult to return to work because of low self-confidence,[112] and only 81% of PTCA patients actually return to work.[113] It would therefore seem practical to offer cardiac rehabilitation to these patients in order that they too can benefit from the improvement in exercise capacity.

Ben-Ari and co-workers studied the effects of cardiac rehabilitation in patients after PTCA and compared them to a group of matched patients who received usual care after PTCA without rehabilitation.[114] They found a higher physical work capacity and ejection fraction in the rehabilitation group compared to controls, and a lower total cholesterol, lower low-density lipoproteins, and higher high-density lipoproteins as well. There was no difference in the rate of restenosis, though, at 5.5 months of follow-up time. Further work by this group documented a higher return to work after their program.[115]

RETURN TO WORK

The presumed inability to resume gainful employment can contribute greatly to a patient's loss of self-esteem and perceived economic impotence. A concerted effort by the medical and rehabilitation team must be directed to allay these concerns.[116] A symptom-limited exercise test, if normal, can do much to encourage and reinstill confidence in the patient to resume his or her job-related activities. On the other hand, an exercise test showing a lower exercise capacity can be used to guide a patient's level of activity at work.

Occupational evaluation and counseling was shown to be of benefit by Dennis and co-workers who decreased the time interval between infarction and return to work by an average of 32% with counseling low-risk patients.[117] Cost-benefit analysis of these same patients revealed that total medical costs per patient in the 6 months after myocardial infarction were lower by $502, and their occupational income in this same period was $2,102 greater.[118] The fact that people are working longer into their later years, and 80% of patients under 65 years of age eventually return to work after their myocardial infarction underscores that the majority of post–myocardial infarction patients can benefit from this type of counseling. A rehabilitation program has also been found to lower rehospitalization costs in 580 patients (58% after CABS and 42% after MI) followed over 3 years.[119]

RISK-FACTOR MODIFICATION

Given the recurrence rate of reinfarction and overall cardiovascular mortality in survivors of myocardial infarction, theoretical benefits of risk factor modification, in this selected high-risk population, could be very significant.[120] As part of a WHO study, Kallio and associates performed a multifactorial intervention combined with cardiac rehabilitation in post–myocardial infarction patients beginning 2 weeks after their event. They found in the treated group a decrease in blood pressure, lower body weight, and improved serum cholesterol and triglycerides; smoking decreased by 50% in both the treated and control groups. The National Exercise and Heart Disease Project showed a reduction in low-density lipoprotein (LDL) fractions.[121] The recent analysis of 10-year mortality from cardiovascular disease in relation to cholesterol level by Pekkanen and colleagues demonstrated the importance of serum cholesterol in men with preexisting cardiovascular disease.[122] Hämäläinen and colleagues noted a reduction in sudden deaths by almost 50% in patients enrolled in an aggressive, multifactorial intervention program for 10 years after myocardial infarction.[123] Their interventions included control of smoking,

hypertension, and lipids and the use of antiarrhythmic agents in addition to beta-blockers.

Previously it was argued that when atheroma were well established and causing symptoms, alterations in serum cholesterol would have little effect. These findings are encouraging, and evidence is beginning to accumulate that the progression of coronary atherosclerosis may be arrested and actually reversed with aggressive dietary and medical therapy.[124,125] Metanalysis of the lipid lowering trials using digital coronary angiography now consistently confirm that this is the case. Recommendations are now that all patients should have aggressive managment to lower their LDL cholesterol below 100. The interaction of triglycerides with gene-site activity, typing of apo-B, ultracentrifugation of LDL, and other new findings are leading to an exciting new hope that atherosclerosis can be treated more effectively. These studies are promising and emphasize the medical rehabilitation teams' responsibility to encourage patients to alter life-styles that could be deleterious to their health and institute medical therapy as necessary to control cardiac risk factors.

PREDICTING OUTCOME IN CARDIAC REHABILITATION PATIENTS

Cardiac rehabilitation programs are expensive and carry a risk. If a patient's likelihood of improving his or her work capacity could be predicted on the basis of initial data, much time and money could be saved. Considering VO_2 max and other indicators of a training effect,[126] we asked the following questions: (1) Can clinical features before training allow one to predict whether beneficial changes occur with training? (2) Do initial treadmill or radionuclide measurements contribute information to improve this prediction? (3) Does the intensity of training over the year predict beneficial changes? Our major finding was that a patient's success or failure in improving aerobic capacity after a 1-year aerobic exercise program was poorly predicted on the basis of initial clinical, treadmill, or radionuclide data. Correlations between initial parameters and outcome were poor. Training intensity had little to do with outcome. Those with ischemic markers (exercise test–induced angina, ST-segment depression, or dropping ejection fraction) did not show a different degree of training effect from that of patients without ischemia; neither did those with markers of myocardial damage. History of CABS or MI had no bearing on whether a patient's work capacity would improve after the training period.

There was a trend for those who initially showed

evidence of the poorest state of fitness (high resting or submaximal heart rate, low estimated maximal oxygen uptake) or high thallium ischemia scores to have the most improvement in the same respective parameter. However, initial measured maximal oxygen uptake, the best measure of aerobic capacity on entry, showed no relationship to any measure of training effect at the end of the year of training. Older patients showed only slightly less benefit than younger ones. Those with characteristics suggestive of larger amounts of scar or ischemia did not have significantly different results from those with less. Multivariate analysis did not greatly improve the ability to predict outcome.

Previous studies have found that those with the lowest initial measured oxygen consumption often have the largest improvement with an exercise program. In our study, the correlation between initial measured oxygen consumption with any measure of training effect was always nonsignificant, and it was never selected by multivariate analyses. The lack of correlation between training intensity and change in oxygen uptake over the year is difficult to explain. In healthy men this relationship has been shown to be good ($r = 0.80$); it is not clear from our study why the correlations were so poor ($r < 0.20$). It may well be that setting exercise prescriptions using exercise tests limited by signs or symptoms gives too low of an exercise intensity. The changes in test end points were moderately correlated to changes in oxygen uptake. This raises the question as to what portion of the changes were attributable to the patients being encouraged to perform better on the 1-year tests by those administering the tests or by their own faith in the exercise program. Even maximal testing appears of questionable reliability and argues for using a different technical staff for initial and final testing.

A very detailed initial evaluation did not allow accurate prediction of who would train and who would not. Even those patients whose characteristics indicated that they had the most ischemia or scar showed as much improvement from training as patients without such characteristics. Thus it would appear that using angina, a low resting ejection fraction, ST-segment depression, or a dropping ejection fraction with exercise, as contraindications to an exercise program is unjustified. Since many of the benefits obtained from an exercise program are intangible, it seems inappropriate to eliminate any patient from an exercise program on the basis of clinical, treadmill, or radionuclide data. Van Dixhoorn added psychosocial variables and was able to better predict "failure" to improve than success.[127] Mixed results have been observed by other investigators on this issue,[128] and we need

more data, which should include hemodynamic, exercise, clinical, and psychosocial variables.

SUMMARY: CHANGES ATTRIBUTABLE TO ECONOMIC FORCES

There are significant changes coming about in the United States regarding exercise testing and cardiac rehabilitation.[129] We are at a time when scientific advances are merging with economic and societal forces to alter medical practice dramatically. Some of the advances include the use of metanalysis to provide accurate study summaries,[130,131] the demonstration of regression and retarding progression of coronary artery disease,[132,133] the demonstration of cardiac changes attributable to diet and exercise,[134,135] the improvement of risk stratification,[136,137] and the development of the public health recommendations for physical activity rather than physical fitness.[138]

The current wave of changes also include care provider assessment by regulatory bodies and reimbursement for cognitive interactions, with a decrease in payment for procedures.[139,140] Surprising changes are occurring in the area of physician performance assessment. Influential in this area is the Joint Commission on Accreditation of Health Care Organizations (JCAHCO); hospital accreditation will depend on the assessment of physician diagnostic and treatment performance. The JCAHCO plans a change of agenda from quality assurance (that is, quality by inspection) to quality assessment.[141] The latter is aimed at developing a cycle of continuous improvement. Institutions must establish acceptable thresholds or standards and develop total quality management by measuring patient outcomes. This feedback will then be used to improve care. Markers of performance must be utilized to evaluate quality of care. Examples of this for cardiac rehabilitation have been nicely provided by the American Association of Cardiopulmonary Rehabilitation.

In addition, certain procedures may be reimbursed only by Medicare at approved institutions that perform high volumes (hopefully still with a personal touch). The ultimate outcome of all this is difficult to predict. Although the public would like to chat with Dr. Welby, they want a diagnosis and treatment by Dr. McCoy without leaving the neighborhood to go to Cleveland. Moreover, when the latest medical test is announced to the public directly from the *New England Journal of Medicine,* they often demand it from their doctor. As a health care professional, one must read this journal just to appear "up to date."

In regard to research, molecular biochemistry

and genetics are the prime areas for funding. The only areas left for clinical research are in technological efficacy and outcome assessment, one would hope, as part of the quality assessment process. However, the results from such research will greatly influence medical practice.

In an effort to shape these changes, medical associations (such as the AHA, ACP, ACC, AACVPR, ACSM) are defining and refining guidelines for treatment and the use of technology and are becoming more involved in the accreditation of practioners. However, these guidelines have not led to adequate changes in practice, and thus governmental actions to effect these needed changes will no doubt be initiated.[142,143]

Health care planners have finally come to the realization that continued increases in health care costs are not resulting in improvements in the general health of our population. Since DRGs and RAM (disease-related groupings and the VA resource allocation model) have been dismal failures in controlling costs, more drastic measures will be enacted. Despite a rising proportion of the Gross National Product going to health care, 37 million Americans are denied access to health care for financial reasons. In addition, markers of public health (that is, infant mortality and life expectancy) are worsening relative to other modern countries.

Although some would blame the current expensive health care system on greed and lack of principles, that in general is not the case. The evolution of our costly system is not simply explained by Ogden Nash who said "every profession is a conspiracy against the public." Some of the overexpenditure has been caused by public expectations. Technology has replaced the "magic" the doctor dispensed in the past.[144] Modern technology fulfills our need to believe illness can be cured and death avoided or at least delayed.

Although practioners can accuse those in academia of being protected in our ivory tower, academics bear partial responsibility and are suffering the same pains as practioners as our world collapses in size and resources. For instance, we have taught and promoted intellectually satisfying concepts and technologies that have led to research support (silent ischemia, radionuclide testing, PET scanners) rather than teaching established facts. This has led to an implementation of ideas and hypotheses in clinical practice rather than scientific truths. Much of the medical literature has not had sufficient scientific rigor applied to it in order to achieve results that can be assimilated into practice. For example, ECG monitoring for cardiac rehabilitation was recommended unselectively, resulting in unjustifiable costs for exercise training. Electrophysiology studies are now recommended for nearly everyone with syncope, resulting in a threefold increase in billing through Medicare for this diagnosis. Because these excesses and competition with AIDS research, cardiovascular research support has dwindled, and we are hard pressed to defend continued financing of poor research. Academia is in crisis as expensive growth has been replaced by "damage control" in face of continuing losses.

But this is not a time to accuse one another but rather to participate in this process of change in order to ensure that our patients receive optimal health care. One advantage of these changes will be a lessening of the litigious nature of medical practice. With guidelines for the use of procedures and limitations of payments clearly defined, physicians will not have to practice defensive medicine or compete with the aggressive angiographer. However, the use of percutaneous transluminal coronary angioplasty continues to grow despite a 30% redo rate and the fact that many patients remain "disabled" and have to take antianginal agents after this intervention.

The changes that are coming in regard to exercise testing and cardiac rehabilitation are the following:

1. Exercise testing will be performed more by family practioners and internists than by cardiologists. In a recent American College of Physicians survey, 50% of internists were performing exercise tests.[145] The test will be used to decide which patients need to be referred to the cardiologist. It will serve as the "gatekeeper" to more expensive and invasive tests. A key need will be to educate these practioners to do testing properly.

2. Cardiac rehabilitation is being accepted as a standard of practice in the United States. "Inhospital" programs must be implemented for hospitals to be accredited. Physical and occupational therapists are critical in this process. "Outpatient" programs are being greatly curtailed by declining reimbursement. No longer can they generate revenue by charging for ECG monitoring of patients who really do not need it. Guidelines have greatly limited the percentage of patients who are to receive the ECG-monitored component. Each hospital has had its own outpatient program in order to compete with nearby hospitals, but eventually centralized programs responsible for a region will be the best approach. The practioners are changing as well. It is much more practical and realistic to teach cardiology and exercise physiology to physical medicine rehabilitation physicians and to family practioners than to expect cardiologists to

perform cardiac rehabilitation. In addition, research has demonstrated that exercise programs can be safely carried out in selected low-risk patients in the home setting.[146] The Multi-Fit program tested in the HMO settting by DeBusk and colleagues demonstrates that trained nurses can save health care costs using computer algorithms and telephone surveillance methods.

Some of the problems of modern medicine can be explained by the imposition of technology between practitioners and patients. Cardiac rehabilitation can ensure that humanistic concerns reverse these problems. It may well be that the guise of our implementation of these goals is changing and we should become part of the "outcome assessment" plan proposed by the JCAHCO. The agenda for change proposed by the JCAHCO is most exciting. The change involves replacement of the traditional quality assurance methods (inspection to find outliers) by quality assessment. This will develop a cycle of continual improvements. Rather than establishing acceptable thresholds or standards, quality assessment consists in measuring outcomes and utilizing this feedback to improve care. Indicators or markers of performance must be used to evaluate quality of care.

Scientifically, there is a sound basis for these changes and support for cardiac rehabilitation. In the United States, we will now have an opportunity to blend the best parts of current practice with a system that will reach all of our people with an appropriate mix of technology and humanistic concerns.

REFERENCES

1. ACC/AHA Task Force Report: Guidelines for the early management of patients with acute myocardial infarction. A report of the American College of Cardiology/American Heart Association Task Force on assessment of diagnostic and therapeutic cardiovascular procedures (subcommittee, *J Am Coll Cardiol* 16(2):249-292, 1990.
2. Maisel AS, Ahnve S, Gilpin E, et al: Prognosis after extension of myocardial infarct: the role of Q wave or non–Q wave infarction, *Circulation* 71:211-217, 1985.
3. Maisel AS, Gilpin E, Hoit B, et al: Survival after hospital discharge in matched populations with inferior or anterior myocardial infarction, *J Am Coll Cardiol* 6:731-736, 1985.
4. Lee TH, Weisberg MC, Brand DA, et al: Candidates for thrombolysis among emergency room patients with acute chest pain: potential true and false positives rates, *Ann Intern Med* 110:957-962, 1989.
5. Connolly DC, Elveback LR: Coronary heart disease in residents of Rochester, Minnesota. VI. Hospital and posthospital course of patients with transmural and subendocardial myocardial infarction, *Mayo Clin Proc* 60:375-381, 1985.
6. Ross, J, Gilpin EA, Madsen EB, et al: A decision scheme for coronary angiography after acute myocardial infarction, *Circulation* 79:292-303, 1989.
7. Ahnve S, Gilpin E, Ditrich H, et al: First myocardial in-

farction: age and ejection fraction identify a low-risk group, *Am Heart J* 116:925-932, 1988.
8. DeBusk RF: Specialized testing after recent acute myocardial infarction, *Ann Intern Med* 110:470-481, 1989.
9. Krone RJ: The role of risk stratification in the early management of a myocardial infarction, *Ann Intern Med* 116(3):223, 1992.
10. Miranda C, Froelicher V: An update on cardiac rehabilitation, *Eurorehab* 1:5-23, 1991.
11. Nicod P, Gilpin E, Dittrich H, et al: Short- and long-term clinical outcome after Q wave and non–Q wave myocardial infarction in a large patient population, *Circulation* 79:528-536, 1989.
12. Klein J, Froelicher VF, Detrano R, et al: Does the rest electrocardiogram after myocardial infarction determine the predictive value of exercise-induced ST depression? A 2 year follow-up study in a veteran population, *J Am Coll Cardiol* 14:305-311, 1989.
13. Krone RJ, Dwyer EM, Greenberg H, et al: The Multicenter Post-Infarction Research Group: Risk stratification in patients with first non–Q wave infarction: limited value of the early low level exercise test after uncomplicated infarct, *J Am Coll Cardiol* 14:31-37, 1989.
14. The TIMI Study Group: Comparison of invasive and conservative strategies after treatment with intravenous tissue plasminogen activator in acute myocardial infarction: results of the thrombolysis in myocardial infarction (TIMI) Phase II Trial, *N Engl J Med* 320:618-627, 1989.
15. Simoons ML, Arnold AER, et al: Thrombolysis with tissue plasminogen activator in acute myocardial infarction: no additional benefit from immediate percutaneous coronary angioplasty, *Lancet* 1:197-203, 1988.
16. DeBono DP, for the SWIFT Investigators Group: Should we intervene following thrombolysis? The SWIFT study of intervention versus conservative management after anistreplase thrombolysis, *Eur Heart J* 10(suppl):253, 1989.
17. Topol EJ, Burek K, O'Neill WW, et al: A randomized controlled trial of hospital discharge three days after myocardial infarction in the era of reperfusion, *N Engl J Med* 318:1083-1088, 1988.
18. Hammerman H, Schoen FJ, Kloner RA: Short-term exercise has a prolonged effect on scar formation after experimental acute myocardial infarction, *J Am Coll Cardiol* 2:979-982, 1983.
19. Kloner RA, Kloner JA: The effect of early exercise on myocardial infarct scar formation, *Am Heart J* 106:1009-1014, 1983.
20. Hochman JS, Healy B: Effect of exercise on acute myocardial infarction in rats, *J Am Coll Cardiol* 7:126-132, 1986.
21. Levine SA, Lown B: The "chair" treatment of acute coronary thrombosis, *Trans Assoc Am Physicians* 64:316-319, 1951.
22. Saltin B, Blomquist G, Mitchell JH, et al: Response to exercise after bed rest and after training, *Circulation* 37-38(suppl VII):1, 1968.
23. Convertino VA: Effect of orthostatic stress on exercise performance after bed rest: relation to inhospital rehabilitation, *J Cardiac Rehabil* 3:660-663, 1983.
24. Cain HD, Frasher WG, Stivelman R: Graded activity program for safe return to self-care after myocardial infarction, *JAMA* 177:111-120, 1961.
25. Torkelson LO: Rehabilitation of the patient with acute myocardial infarction, *J Chronic Disability* 17:685-704, 1964.
26. Sivarajan ES, Snydsman A, Smith B, et al: Low-level treadmill testing of 41 patients with acute myocardial infarction prior to discharge from the hospital, *Heart Lung* 6:975-980, 1977.

27. Hayes MJ, Morris GK, Hampton JR: Comparison of mobilization after two and nine days in uncomplicated myocardial infarction, *Br Med J* 3:10-13, 1974.
28. Bloch A, Maeder J, Haissly J, et al: Early mobilization after myocardial infarction: a controlled study, *Am J Cardiol* 34:152-157, 1974.
29. Sivarajan E, Bruce RA, Almes MJ, et al: A randomized study of cardiac rehabilitation, *N Engl J Med* 305:357-362, 1981.
30. World Health Organization (WHO), Report of Expert Committee: *Rehabilitation of patients with cardiovascular diseases,* Tech Rep no. 270, Geneva, 1964, World Health Organization.
31. American College of Sports Medicine: Guidelines for exercise testing and prescription, ed 4, Philadelphia, 1991, Lea & Febiger.
32. American Association of Cardiovascular and Pulmonary Rehabilitation: *Guidelines for cardiac rehabilitation programs,* Champaign, Ill, 1991, Human Kinetics.
33. Kelemen MH, Stewart KJ, Gillilan RE, et al: Circuit weight training in cardiac patients, *J Am Coll Cardiol* 7:38-42, 1986.
34. Sparling PB, Cantwell JD, Dolan CM, Niederman RK: Strength training in a cardiac rehabilitation program: a six-month follow-up, *Arch Phys Med Rehabil* 71:148, 1990.
35. Kallio V, Hämäläinen H, Hakkila J, Luurila OJ. Reduction in sudden deaths by a multifactorial intervention programme after acute myocardial infarction, *Lancet* 2:1091-1094, 1979.
36. Kentala E: Physical fitness and feasibility of physical rehabilitation after myocardial infarction in men of working age, *Ann Clin Res* 4:1-25, 1972.
37. Palatsi I: Feasibility of physical training after myocardial infarction and its effect on return to work, morbidity, and mortality, *Acta Med Scand* 599(suppl):1-100, 1976.
38. Wilhelmsen L, Sanne H, Elmfeldt D, et al: A controlled trial of physical training after myocardial infarction, *Prev Med* 4:491-508, 1975.
39. Shaw LW: Effects of a prescribed supervised exercise program on mortality and cardiovascular mortality in patients after a myocardial infarction, *Am J Cardiol* 48:39-46, 1981.
40. Shepard, RJ: Exercise regimens after myocardial infarction: rationale and results, *Cardiovasc Clin* 14:145-157, 1985.
41. Bengtsson K: Rehabilitation after myocardial infarction, *Scand J Rehabil Med* 15:1-9, 1983.
42. Carson P, Phillips R, Lloyd M, et al: Exercise after myocardial infarction: a controlled trial, *J R Coll Physicians London* 16:147-151, 1982.
43. Vermeulen A, Lie KI, Durrer D: Effects of cardiac rehabilitation after myocardial infarction: changes in coronary risk factors and long-term prognosis, *Am Heart J* 105:798-801, 1983.
44. Roman O: Do randomized trials support the use of cardiac rehabilitation? *J Cardiac Rehabil* 5:93-96, 1985.
45. Mayou RA: A controlled trial of early rehabilitation after myocardial infarction, *J Cardiac Rehabil* 3:397-402, 1983.
46. Hedback B, Perk J, Perski A: Effect of a post–myocardial infarction rehabilitation program on mortality, morbidity, and risk factors, *J Cardiopulmonary Rehabil* 5:576-583, 1985.
47. Goble AJ, Hare DL, Macdonald PS, et al: Effect of early programmes of high and low intensity exercise on physical performance after transmural acute myocardial infarction, *Br Heart J* 65:126-131, 1991.
48. Mary DA: Exercise training and its effect on the heart, *Rev Physiol Biochem Pharmacol* 109:62-144, 1987.
49. May GS, Eberlein KA, Furberg CD, et al: Secondary prevention after myocardial infarction: a review of long-term trials, *Prog Cardiovasc Dis* 24:331-352, 1982.
50. O'Connor GT, Buring JE, Yusuf S, et al: An overview of randomized trials of rehabilitation with exercise after myocardial infarction, *Circulation* 80:234-244, 1989.
51. Oldridge NB, Guyatt GH, Fischer ME, Rimm AA: Cardiac rehabilitation after myocardial infarction: combined experience of randomized clinical trials, *JAMA* 260:945-950, 1988.
52. Rochmis P, Blackburn H: Exercise tests: a survey of procedures, safety and litigation experience in approximately 170,000 tests, *JAMA* 217:1061, 1971.
53. Irving JB, Bruce RA: Exertional hypotension and postexertional ventricular fibrillation in stress testing, *Am J Cardiol* 39:849, 1977.
54. Yang JC, Wesley RC Jr, Froelicher VF: Ventricular tachycardia during routine treadmill testing, *Arch Intern Med* 151:349-353, 1991.
55. Gibbons L, Blair SN, Kohl HW, Cooper K: The safety of maximal exercise testing, *Circulation* 80(4):846-852, 1980.
56. Haskell WL: Cardiovascular complications during exercise training of cardiac patients, *Circulation* 57(5):920-924, 1978.
57. Hossack KF, Hartwig R: Cardiac arrest associated with supervised cardiac rehabilitation, *J Cardiac Rehabil* 2:404-408, 1982.
58. Cantwell JD, Murray PM, Thomas RJ: Exercise and the heart: current management of service exercise-related cardiac events, *Chest* 93(6):1264-1269, 1988.
59. Van Camp SP, Peterson RA: Cardiovascular complications of outpatient cardiac rehabilitation programs, *JAMA* 256:1160-1163, 1986.
60. Thompson PD, Funk EJ, Carleton RA, Sturner WQ: Incidence of death during jogging in Rhode Island from 1975 through 1980, *JAMA* 247:2535-2538, 1982.
61. Thompson PD: The benefits and risks of exercise training in patients with chronic coronary artery disease, *JAMA* 259:1537-1540, 1988.
62. Cobb LA, Weaver DW: Exercise: a risk for sudden death in patients with coronary heart disease, *J Am Coll Cardiol* 7:215, 1986.
63. Hlatky MA, Cotugno HE, Mark DB, et al: Trends in physician management of uncomplicated acute myocardial infarction, 1970 to 1987, *Am J Cardiol* 61:515-518, 1988.
64. Miller NH, Haskell WL, Berra K, DeBusk RF: Home versus group exercise training for increasing functional capacity after myocardial infarction, *Circulation* 70:645-649, 1984.
65. Kelbaek H, Eskildsen P, Hansen PF, Godtfredsen J: Spontaneous and/or training-induced hemodynamic changes after myocardial infarction, *Int J Cardiol* 1:205-213, 1981.
66. Dressendorfer RH, Smith JL, Amsterdam EA, Mason DT: Reduction of submaximal exercise myocardial oxygen demand post-walk training program in coronary patients due to improved physical work efficiency, *Am Heart J* 103:358-362, 1982.
67. Greenland P, Chu JS: Efficacy of cardiac rehabilitation services, with emphasis on patients after myocardial infarction, *Ann Intern Med* 109:650-666, 1988.
68. Scheuer J: Effects of physical training on myocardial vascularity and perfusion, *Circulation* 66:491-495, 1982.
69. Bloor CM, White F, Sanders T: Effects of exercise on collateral development in myocardial ischemia in pigs, *J Appl Physiol* 56:656-665, 1984.
70. Ferguson RJ, Petitclerc R, Choquette G, et al: Effect of physical training on treadmill exercise capacity, collateral

circulation and progression of coronary disease, *Am J Cardiol* 34:764-772, 1974.

71. Nolewajka AJ, Kostuk WJ, Rechnitzer PA, et al: Exercise and human collateralization: an angiographic and scintigraphic assessment, *Circulation* 60:114-122, 1979.

72. Sim DN, Neill WA: Investigation of the physiological basis for increased exercise threshold for angina pectoris after physical conditioning, *J Clin Invest* 54:763-770, 1974.

73. Verani MS, Hartung GH, Harris-Hoepfel J, et al: Effects of exercise training on left ventricular performance and myocardial perfusion in patients with coronary artery disease, *Am J Cardiol* 47:797-803, 1981.

74. Cobb FR, Williams RS, McEwan P, et al: Effects of exercise training on ventricular function in patients with recent myocardial infarction, *Circulation* 66:100-108, 1982.

75. DeBusk RF, Hung J: Exercise conditioning soon after myocardial infarction: effects on myocardial perfusion and ventricular function, *Ann NY Acad Sci* 382:343-351, 1982.

76. Todd IC, Bradnam MS, Cooke MBD, Ballantyne D: Effects of daily high-intensity exercise on myocardial perfusion in angina pectoris, *Am J Cardiol* 68:1593-1600, 1991.

77. Froelicher VF, Jensen D, Genter F, et al: A randomized trial of exercise training in patients with coronary heart disease, *JAMA* 252:1291-1297, 1984.

78. Atwood JE, Jensen D, Froelicher VF, et al: Agreement in human interpretation of analog thalium myocardial perfusion images, *Circulation* 64:601-609, 1981.

79. Sebrechts CP, Klein JL, Ahnve S, et al: Myocardial perfusion changes following 1 year of exercise training assessed by thallium-201 circumferential count profiles, *Am Heart J* 112:1217-1226, 1986.

80. Ehsani AA, Martin WH, Health GW, Coyle EF: Cardiac effects of prolonged and intense exercise training in patients with coronary artery disease, *Am J Cardiol* 50:246-254, 1982.

81. Sullivan M, Ahnve S, Froelicher VF, Myers J: The influence of exercise training on the ventilatory threshold of patients with coronary heart disease, *Am Heart J* 109:458-463, 1985.

82. Myers J, Ahnve S, Froelicher V, et al: A randomized trial of the effects of 1 year of exercise training on computer-measured ST segment displacement in patients with coronary artery disease, *J Am Coll Card* 4:1094-1102, 1984.

83. Malmborg R, Isacsson S, Kallivroussis G: The effect of beta-blockade and/or physical training in patients with angina pectoris, *Curr Therap Res* 16:171, 1974.

84. Obma RT, Wilson PK, Goebel ME, Campbell DE: Effect of a conditioning program in patients taking propranolol for angina pectoris, *Cardiology* 64:365-371, 1979.

85. Pratt CM, Welton DE, Squires WG Jr, et al: Demontration of training effect during chronic beta-adrenergic blockade in patients with coronary artery disease, *Circulation* 64:1125-1129, 1981.

86. Vanhees L, Fagard R, Amery A: Influence of beta-adrenergic blockade on the hemodynamic effects of physical training in patients with ischemic heart disease, *Am Heart J* 108:270, 1984.

87. Ewy GA, Wilmore JH, Morton AR, et al: The effect of beta-adrenergic blockade on obtaining a trained exercise state, *J Cardiac Rehabil*, 3(1):25-29, 1983.

88. Tesch PA, Kaiser P: Effects of beta-adrenergic blockade on O_2 uptake during submaximal and maximal exercise, *J Appl Physiol: Respirat Environ Exercise Physiol* 54:901-905, 1983.

89. Sable DL, Brammell HL, Shahan MV, et al: Attenuation of exercise conditioning by beta-adrenergic blockade, *Circulation* 65:679-684, 1982.

90. Gordon EP, Savin WM, Bristow MR, Haskell WL: Catecholamines and cardiac hypertrophy in exercise training, *Circulation* 68:III-376, 1983.

91. Froelicher VF, Sullivan M, Myers J, Jensen D: Can patients with coronary artery disease receiving beta blockers obtain a training effect? *Am J Cardiol* 55:155D-161D, 1985.

92. Rechnitzer PA, Cunningham DA, Andrew CM, et al: Relation of exercise to recurrence rate of myocardial infarction in men, Ontario Exercise-Heart Collaborative Study, *Am J Cardiol* 51:65-69, 1983.

93. Squires RW, Lavie CJ, Brandt TR, et al: Cardiac rehabilitation in patients with severe ischemic left ventricular dysfunction, *Mayo Clin Proc* 62:997-1002, 1987.

94. Conn EH, Williams RS, Wallace RG: Exercise responses before and after physical conditioning in patients with severely depressed left ventricular function, *Am J Cardiol* 49:296-300, 1982.

95. Judgutt BI, Michorowski BL, Kappagoda CT: Exercise training after anterior Q-wave myocardial infarction: importance of regional left ventricular function and topography, *J Am Coll Cardiol* 12:363-372, 1988.

96. Sullivan MJ, Higginbotham MB, Cobb FR: Clinical investigation: exercise training in patients with severe left ventricular dysfunction: hemodynamic and metabolic effects, *Circulation* 78(3):506-515, 1988.

97. Haines DE, Beller GA, Watson DD, et al: A prospective clinical, scintigraphic, angiographic, and functional evaluation of patients after inferior myocardial infarction with and without right ventricular dysfunction, *J Am Coll Cardiol* 6:995-1003, 1985.

98. Crosby L, Paternostro-Bayles M, Cottington E, Pifalo WB: Outpatient rehabilitation after right ventricular infarction, *J Cardiopulmonary Rehabil* 7:286-291, 1989.

99. Williams MA, Maresh CM, Esterbrooks DJ, et al: Early exercise training in patients older than age 65 years compared with that in younger patients after acute myocardial infarction or coronary artery bypass grafting, *Am J Cardiol* 55:263-266, 1985.

100. Adams WC, McHenry MM, Bernauer EM: Long term physiologic adaptations to exercise with special reference to performance and cardiorespiratory function in health and disease, *Am J Cardiol* 33:765-775, 1974.

101. Oldridge NB, Nagle FJ, Balke B, et al: Aortocoronary bypass surgery: effects of surgery and 32 months of physical conditioning on treadmill performance, *Arch Phys Med Rehabil* 59(6):268-275, 1978.

102. Soloff PH: Medically and surgically treated coronary patients in cardiovascular rehabilitation: a comparative study, *Int J Psychiatry Med* 9:93-106, 1980.

103. Horgan JH, Teo KK, Murren KM, et al: The response to exercise training and vocational counselling in post–myocardial infarction and coronary artery bypass surgery patients, *Irish Med J* 74:463-469, 1980.

104. Hartung GH, Rangel R: Exercise training in post–myocardial infarction patients: comparison of results with high risk coronary and post-bypass patients, *Arch Phys Med Rehabil* 62:147-153, 1981.

105. Dornan J, Rolko AF, Greenfield C: Factors affecting rehabilitation following aortocoronary bypass procedures, *Can J Surg* 25:677-680, 1982.

106. Fletcher BJ, Lloyd A, Fletcher GF: Outpatient rehabilitative training in patients with cardiovascular disease: emphasis on training method, *Heart Lung* 17:199-205, 1988.

107. Nakai Y, Kataoka Y, Bando M, et al: Effects of physical exercise training on cardiac function and graft patency after coronary artery bypass grafting, *J Thorac Cardiovasc Surg* 93:65-72, 1987.

108. Perk B, Hedback E, Engvall G: Effects of cardiac rehabilitation after CABS on readmissions, return to work, and physical fitness, *Scand J Soc Med* 18:45-53, 1990.

109. Robinson G, Froelicher VF, Utley JR: Continuing medical education rehabilitation of the coronary artery bypass graft surgery patient, *J Cardiac Rehabil* 4:74-86, 1984.

110. Foster C: Exercise training following cardiovascular surgery, *Exerc Sport Sci Rev* 14:303-323, 1986.

111. Holmes DR, Vliestra RE, Smith HC, et al: Restenosis after percutaneous transluminal coronary angioplasty (PTCA): a report from the PTCA registry of the National Heart, Lung, and Blood Institute, *Am J Cardiol* 53:77C-81A, 1989.

112. Fitzgerald ST, Becker DM, Celentano DP, et al: Return to work after percutaneous transluminal coronary angioplasty, *Am J Cardiol* 64:1108-1112, 1989.

113. Meier B, Gruentzig AR: Return to work after coronary artery bypass surgery in comparison to coronary angioplasty. In Walter PJ, editor: Return to work after coronary bypass surgery: psychosocial and economic aspects, New York, 1985, Springer-Verlag NY Inc, pp 171-176.

114. Ben-Ari E, Rothbaum DA, Linnemeier TJ, et al: Benefits of a monitored rehabilitation program versus physician care after percutaneous transluminal coronary angioplasty: follow-up of risk factors and rate of restenosis, *J Cardiopulmonary Rehabil* 7:281-285, 1989.

115. Ben-Ari E, Rothbaum DA, Linnemeier TA, et al: Return to work after successful coronary angioplasty: comparison between a comprehensive rehabilitation program and patients receiving usual care, *J Cardiac Rehabil* 12.20-24, 1992.

116. Haskel WL: Restoration and maintenance of physical and psychosocial function in patients with ischemic heart disease, *J Am Coll Cardiol* 12:1090-1121, 1988.

117. Dennis C, Houston-Miller N, Schwartz RG, et al: Early return to work after uncomplicated myocardial infarction: results of a randomized trial, *JAMA* 260:214-220, 1988.

118. Picard MH, Dennis C, Schwartz RG, et al: Cost-benefit analysis of early return to work after uncomplicated acute myocardial infarction, *Am J Cardiol* 63:1308-1014, 1989.

119. Ades P, Huang D, Weaver SO: Cardiac rehabilitation participation predicts lower rehospitalization costs, *Am Heart J* 123(4):916-920, 1992.

120. Siegel D, Grady P, Browner WS, Hulley SB: Risk factor modification after myocardial infarction, *Ann Intern Med* 109:213-218, 1988.

121. LaRosa JC, Cleary P, Muesing RA, et al: Effect of long-term moderate physical exercise on plasma lipoproteins: the National Exercise and Heart Disease Project, *Arch Intern Med* 142:2269-2274, 1982.

122. Pekkanen J, Linn S, Meiss G, et al: Ten year mortality from cardiovascular disease in relation to cholesterol level among men with and without preexisting cardiovascular disease, *N Engl J Med* 332:1700-1707, 1990.

123. Hämäläinen H, Luurila OJ, Kallio V, et al: Long-term reduction in sudden deaths after a multifactorial intervention programme in patients with myocardial infarction: 10-year results of a controlled investigation, *Eur Heart J* 10:55-62, 1989.

124. Levy RI, Breniske JF, Epstein SE, et al: The influence of changes in lipid values induced by cholestyramine and diet on progression of coronary artery disease, *Circulation* 69:325-337, 1984.

125. Blankenhorn DH, Nessim SA, Johnson RL, et al: Beneficial effect of combined colestipol-niacin therapy on coronary atherosclerosis and coronary venous bypass grafts, *JAMA* 257:3233-3240, 1987.

126. Hammond KH, Kelly TL, Froelicher VF, Pewen W: Use of clinical data in predicting improvement in exercise capacity after cardiac rehabilitation, *J Am Coll Cardiol* 6:19-26, 1985.

127. Van Dixhoorn E, Duivenvoorden H, Pool G: Success and failure of exercise training after myocardial infarction: Is the outcome predictable? *J Am Coll Cardiol* 15:974-980, 1990.

128. Myers J, Froelicher VF: Predicting outcome in cardiac rehabilitation, *J Am Coll Cardiol* 15:983-985, 1990.

129. Gattiker H, Goins P, Dennis C: Cardiac rehabilitation: current status and future directions, *West J Med* 156(2):183-188, 1992.

130. Mann C: Meta-analysis in the breech, *Science* 249:476-480, 1990.

131. Froelicher VF, Perdue S, Pewen W, Risch M: Application of meta-analysis using an electronic spread sheet to exercise testing in patients after myocardial infarction, *Am J Med* 83:1045-1054, 1987.

132. Brown G, Albers JJ, Fisher LD, et al: Regression of coronary artery disease as a result of intensive lipid-lowering therapy in men with high levels of apolipoprotein B, *N Engl J Med* 323:1289-1298, 1990.

133. Schuler G, Hambrect R, Schlierf G, et al: Progression of coronary stenoses in patients on intensive physical exercise and low fat diet, *Circulation* 4:III-238, 1990.

134. Ornish D, Brown SE, Scherwitz LW, et al: Can lifestyle changes reverse coronary heart disease? *Lancet* 336:129-133, 1990.

135. Schuler G, Shlierf G, Wirth A, et al: Low-fat diet and regular, supervised physical exercise in patients with symptomatic coronary artery disease: reduction of stress-induced myocardial ischemia, *Circulation* 77:172, 1988.

136. Ross J, Gilpin EA, Madsen EB, et al: A decision scheme for coronary angiography after acute myocardial infarction, *Circulation* 79:292, 1989.

137. DeBusk RF: Specialized testing after recent acute myocardial infarction, *Ann Intern Med* 110.470, 1989.

138. McHenry PL, Ellestad MH, Fletcher GF, et al: A position statement for health professionals by the committee on exercise and cardiac rehabilitation of the Council on Clinical Cardiology, American Heart Association, *Circulation* 81:396-398, 1990.

139. Detsky AS, Naglie IG: A clinician's guide to cost-effectiveness analysis, *Ann Intern Med* 113:147-154, 1990.

140. Hadorn DC: The future of the American health care system, *N Engl J Med* 10:752, 1990.

141. Clinical outcomes: managing patients and the total cost of care, *Clin Outcomes* 1:1-8, 1990.

142. McGuire LB: A long run for a short jump: understanding clinical guidelines, *Ann Intern Med* 113:705-708, 1990.

143. Audet AM, Greenfield S, Field M: Medical practice guidelines: current activities and future directions, *Ann Intern Med* 113:709-714, 1990.

144. Fuchs VF, Garber AM: The new technology assessment, *N Engl J Med* 10:673-677, 1990.

145. Wigton RS et al: Procedural skills of the general internist: a survey of 2500 physicians, *Ann Intern Med* 111:1023, 1990.

146. DeBusk FR, Haskell WL, Miller NH, et al: Medically directed at-home rehabilitation soon after clinically uncomplicated acute myocardial infarction: a new model for patient care, *Am J Cardiol* 55:251, 1985.

Index